# Digestive Disease Pathology

☐ VOLUME I

# Digestive Disease Pathology

☐ VOLUME I

---

Editors

Shaw Watanabe, M.D.

Chief for Epidemiology Division
National Cancer Center Research Institute
and Professor of Pathology
Keio University School of Medicine
Tokyo, Japan

Marianne Wolff, M.D.

Professor of Clinical Surgical Pathology
Columbia University
College of Physicians & Surgeons
New York, New York, and
Pathology Department
Morristown Memorial Hospital
Morristown, New Jersey

Sheldon C. Sommers, M.D.

Clinical Professor of Pathology
Columbia University
College of Physicians & Surgeons
New York, New York, and
University of Southern California
School of Medicine
Los Angeles, California

MACMILLAN PUBLISHING COMPANY
New York

Distributed by:
Macmillan Publishing Company
866 Third Avenue
New York, N.Y. 10022

ISBN: 0-02-424570-4

# Contents

# Contributors to Digestive Disease Pathology, Volume I

**Hitoshi Asakura, M.D.**
Assistant Professor, Internal Medicine
Keio University School of Medicine
Tokyo, Japan

**Yasuyoshi Enomoto, Ph.D.**
Chief Technician, Department of Pathology
Keio University School of Medicine
Tokyo, Japan

**Hidemasa Ishikawa, M.D.**
Department of Internal Medicine
Postgraduate School of Fukushima
Medical College
Fukushima, Japan

**Kotaro Kaneko, M.D.**
Department of Internal Medicine
Keio University School of Medicine
Tokyo, Japan

**J. Lindeman, M.D., Ph.D.**
Chairman, Department of Pathology
Stichting Samenwerking Delftse Siekenhuizen
Delft,
The Netherlands

**C.J.L.M. Meijer, M.D., Ph.D.**
Chairman & Director, Pathological Institute
Free University Hospital
Amsterdam,
The Netherlands

**Soichiro Miura, M.D.**
Internal Medicine
Keio University Hospital
Tokyo, Japan

**Akira Morita, M.D.**
Department of Internal Medicine
Tokyo Metropolitan Hiroo
Tokyo, Japan

**Hiroshi Nagura, M.D., Ph.D.**
Professor
Laboratory of Germfree Life
Research Institute for Disease
Mechanism and Control
Nagoya University School of Medicine
Nagoya, Japan

**Masahiko Nakamura, M.D.**
Department of Internal Medicine
Tokyo Electric Power Co. Hospital
Tokyo, Japan

**Masaya Oda, M.D.**
Assistant Professor, Internal Medicine
Keio University School of Medicine
Tokyo, Japan

**Manuel Moutinho-Ribeiro, M.D.**
Assistant Professor of Surgery
Department of Cirurgia 4
The Medical Faculty; Attending Surgeon
Hospital S. Joao
Porto, Portugal

**Ricardo V. Lloyd, M.D., Ph.D.**
Associate Professor of Pathology
University of Michigan Hospitals
Ann Arbor, Michigan

**Mário Seixas, M.Sc., Ph.D.**
Assistant Professor of Biophysics
Department of Biophysics
The Medical Faculty
Porto, Portugal

**Manuel Sobrinho-Simões, M.D., Ph.D.**
Professor of Pathology
Department of Pathology
The Medical Faculty and Hospital S. Joao
Porto, Portugal

**Yukiko Sumi, M.D.**
Assistant Professor
Laboratory of Germfree Life
Research Institute for Disease
Mechanism and Control
Nagoya University School of Medicine
Nagoya, Japan

**Eiichi Tahara, M.D.**
Professor
Department of Pathology
Hiroshima University School of Medicine
Hiroshima, Japan

**Masaharu Tsuchiya, M.D.**
Professor
Internal Medicine
Keio University School of Medicine
Tokyo, Japan

**Yutaka Tsutsumi, M.D.**
Assistant Professor
Department of Pathology
Tokai University School of Medicine
Bonseidai, Isehara-city
Kanagawa, Japan

**J.P. van Spreeuwel, M.D.**
Department of Internal Medicine
Division of Gastroenterology
University Hospital
Maastricht,
The Netherlands

**P. van der Valk, M.D., Ph.D.**
Pathological Institute
Free University Hospital
Amsterdam,
The Netherlands

**Haruki Wakasa, M.D.**
Professor
Department of Pathology
Fukushima Medical College
Fukushima, Japan

**Hikaru Watanabe, M.D.**
Chief
Division of Gastroenterology
National Sendai Hospital
Sendai, Japan

# 1

# Differentiation of Gastric Cancer Cells: Analysis Using Immunohistochemistry and Mucin Histochemistry

Yutaka Tsutsumi

Most, even all neoplasms are known to show variable degrees of cellular differentiation, not only biologically, but also morphologically.[1] Thus, we pathologists can recognize the histological type of each tumor on the basis of morphological similarities to its normal or nonneoplastic counterparts. Carcinoma of the stomach, the most common cancer in Japan,[2,3] shows a variety of histological appearances, although it has been roughly grouped into two types, diffuse carcinoma vs. adenoplastic carcinoma.[4,5] The diffuse cancer is characterized by its scirrhous growth pattern and the occurrence of signet ring cells, a peculiar cancer morphology in the stomach. The histological heterogeneities of gastric cancer possibly reflect the fact that the gastric mucosa shows a bidirectional cell renewal pattern, (i.e., the generative (stem) cells differentiate upward to the foveolar epithelium and downward to the gastric gland).[6–9] The frequent occurrence of intestinal metaplasia in the aged gastric mucosa[2,10] makes the situation more complicated.

Studies of cell kinetics of normal gastric mucosa have proved that fundic gland cells (and endocrine cells) move in a stochastic flow system, while pyloric gland cells and foveolar cells move in a pipe line system.[6–9] Chief cells, parietal cells, and endocrine cells ultrastructurally show poorly developed junctional complexes, interdigitations, and necessarily connect to each other with a weak binding ability.[9] Thus, they can change their position with a random velocity as dissociative cells.[6,8,9] On the contrary, pyloric gland cells and surface epithelial cells ultrastructurally show well-developed junctional complexes and interdigitations, and necessarily connect to each other with a strong binding ability.[9] Thus, they change their position with a constant rate as associative cells.[7–9] Signet ring (diffuse type) cancer cells are typical of dissociative cells, whereas adenoplastic cancer cells belong to associative cells.[8,9]

Speaking of the histogenesis of gastric cancer, it has been pointed out that signet ring cell carcinomas often arise from the intact oxyntic mucosa, while adenoplastic carcinomas are intimately related to intestinal metaplasia of the gastric mucosa.[2,5,10] Nakamura et al specified the former as gastric-proper (or undifferentiated) type and the latter as intestinal (or differentiated) type.[5,11] Through the histological and mucin histochemical studies of minute mucosal cancer, Matsukura et al postulated that the incomplete type of intestinal metaplasia (devoid of Paneth cells) is more likely precancerous than the complete type (with Paneth cells).[12]

Functional and phenotypic expressions of human gastric cancer have been investigated concerning lysozyme,[13–15] secretory component (SC)[13] and IgA[13,16], pepsinogen II,[17,18] carcinoembryonic antigen (CEA),[16,19–21] α-fetoprotein (AFP),[21–23] human chorionic gonadotropin (HCG),[21,23,24] placental alkaline phosphatase (PALP),[21,25,26] mucins,[27–30] hormones,[31–34] and so on. We have also studied the expression of various histochemical markers of gastric epithelium in gastric cancer tissues.[35–40] These include mucin histochemistry for pyloric gland cells and goblet cells and immunoperoxidase staining for lysozyme, lactoferrin, SC, pepsinogen II, CEA, AFP, HCG, PALP, chromogranin, and five gastrointestinal hormones. Such a series of histochemical studies greatly contributes to investigating not only the histogenesis, but also the functional differentiations of gastric cancer or gastric cancer cells. In the present review, attempts were thus centered on clarifying the functional differentiations of gastric cancer cells by analyzing the expression of those markers.

## MATERIALS AND METHODS

Surgically removed gastric tissues were routinely fixed in 10% formalin for 2–7 days and embedded in paraffin wax. Sections of 4 μm thickness from a representative site of cancer (mainly at the cancer–noncancer junction) were prepared for hematoxylin and eosin (H&E) staining, mucin histochemistry, silver methods for endocrine cells with light green counterstaining after Grimelius,[41] and Masson,[42] and immunoperoxidase method. The diagnosis of the histological type of cancer was applied corresponding to "the general rules of the gastric cancer study in surgery and pathology" of the Japanese Research Society for Gastric Cancer.[3,43] The typing was made on the basis of the predominance of histological varieties. An exception was as follows: scirrhous carcinoma mainly consisting of isolated small and immature-looking cancer cells with a small amount of intracytoplasmic mucin was included in signet ring cell carcinoma (sig), so that poorly differentiated carcinoma (por) means a solid carcinoma with a medullary growth pattern.

*Mucin histochemistry:* Alcian blue-periodic acid Schiff (AB-PAS), PAS with or without diastase digestion, and high iron diamine-alcian blue (HID-AB)[44] were employed. To detect mucins of pyloric glands and mucous neck cells specifically, Concanavalin A paradoxical staining (CPS) class III after Katsuyama and Spicer[45] was used. Briefly, diastase digested deparaffinized sections were oxidized in 0.5% periodic acid (PA) for 60 minutes, followed by the reduction in 0.3% sodium borohydride (SB)-1%$NA_2HPO_4$ solution for 3 minutes. The sections were then incubated with 0.1% Concanavalin A-phosphate buffered-saline (PBS) solution, pH 7.4 for 15 minutes, and, after rinsing in PBS, were dipped in 0.0005% horseradish peroxidase (HRP, Sigma type VI)-PBS solution. Finally, HRP was visualized by incubation in 30mg% 3,3′-diaminobenzidine tetrahydrochloride (DAB)-0.05M Tris-HCl solution, pH 7.6. Nuclei were counterstained with 1% methyl green buffered by veronal acetate at pH 4.0 or lightly with hematoxylin.

To identify N-acetyl neuraminic acid (NANA), mild periodate oxidation-Schiff (MOS) reaction by Katsuyama et al[30] was employed. The C8-9 vicinal hydroxyls of NANA are extremely susceptible to periodate oxidation. Thus, the periodate oxidation at an extremely low concentration (1 mM) and low temperature (0–2°C) and for a short time (5 minutes) in 0.05M acetate buffer, pH 5.5, provides a method for the selective demonstration of NANA. The MOS reaction after neuraminidase digestion was carried out as a control procedure.

To demonstrate O-acylated NANA (or O-acylated sialic acid), which is specific for gut goblet cell mucin especially of the large intestine, the sequence of PA-SB-PH-PAS after Culling et al[46] was employed. PH means potassium hydroxide. Oxidation by 0.5% PA was performed for 90 minutes, reduction by

**TABLE 1-1**
Primary Antibodies Used in this Chapter

| Antigen | Animal Immunized | Final Dilution | Source |
|---|---|---|---|
| SC | rabbit | ×200 | Behringerwerke, AG, Marburg |
| lysozyme | rabbit | ×200 | DAKO Immunoglobulins, Copenhagen |
| lactoferrin | rabbit | ×200 | DAKO |
| pepsinogen II | rabbit | ×500 | Dr. K. Miki* |
| CEA | rabbit | ×400 | DAKO |
| AFP | rabbit | ×200 | DAKO |
| HCG | rabbit | ×200 | DAKO |
| PALP | rabbit | ×200 | Green Cross Co., Osaka |
| chromogranin (bovine) | rabbit | ×200 | Immuno Nuclear Co., Stillwater, MN |
| glicentin 49–69 (porcine) | rabbit | ×500 | Prof. N. Yanaihara** |
| glucagon 19–29 | rabbit | ×1500 | Japan Immunoresearch Laboratores, Takasaki |
| PP (bovine)† | rabbit | ×20000 | Dr. R.E. Chance*** |
| somatostatin | rabbit | ×2000 | DAKO Co., Santa Barbara, CA |
| gastrin (human) | guinea pig | ×500 | Prof. N. Yanaihara |

* Department of Internal Medicine, University of Tokyo Faculty of Medicine, Tokyo

** Laboratory of Bioorganic Chemistry, Shizuoka College of Pharmacy, Shizuoka

*** Lilly Research Laboratories, Indianapolis

† pancreatic polypeptide

Concerning the specificity of antiglicentin 49–69 and antiglucagon 19–29 antibodies, see references 38 and 57.

0.3% SB in 1%$Na_2HPO_4$ was for 5 minutes, alkaline hydrolysis by 1% PH in 70% ethanol was for 10 minutes and the PAS reaction was performed in a conventional condition. Nuclei were lightly counterstained with hematoxylin. Negative control procedure was done, in which the step of PH was omitted.

*Immunoperoxidase method:* Immunohistochemistry was performed either with the indirect HRP-labeled antibody method after Nakane[47] or, for the study mainly in Parts 2 and 3, with the peroxidase-antiperoxidase (PAP) method after Sternberger et al.[48] Primary antibodies used are listed in Table 1-1 together with the animal immunized, final dilution and their source. A minor contaminating activity against alpha-chain of immunoglobulin in antiSC antibody was absorbed by mixing it with 1% normal human serum. The commercial antiCEA antibody contains a high antibody activity against nonspecific cross-reacting antigen (NCA).[49] The antiCEA was used with or without previous absorption by a perchloric acid (PCA) extract of human spleen, as described previously.[49,50]. HRP-labeled Fab against rabbit IgG was prepared in our laboratory, and HRP-labeled antiguinea pig IgG was purchased from Miles Laboratories, Naperville, IL. Unlabeled secondary antibody and PAP complexes were obtained from DAKO Immunoglobulins, Copenhagen. Time of antibody incubation and rinsing in each step was 30 minutes. Endogenous peroxidase was inactivated by dipping sections in 0.5% PA for 10 minutes. For the purpose of coloration, the sections were incubated in the DAB solution for 5–10 minutes. Nuclear counterstaining was done with 1% methyl green or, in the case of the PAP method, with hematoxylin. For control immunostaining, the primary antibody was replaced by nonimmune rabbit or guinea pig serum at a 1:200 dilution. Staining results obtained by the indirect immunoperoxidase and PAP method were fundamentally identical.

**TABLE 1-2**
Expression of Various Histochemical Markers in Nonneoplastic Gastrointestinal Tissues

| | Stomach | | | | | | Intestine | |
|---|---|---|---|---|---|---|---|---|
| | | | | | Intestinal Metaplasia | | | |
| | Surface Epithelium | Generative Cell | Fundic Gland | (Pseudo) Pyloric Gland | Incomplete | Complete | Small | Large |
| SC | – | N – G(+) | – | N – G(+)/– | + (L≥U) | + (L≥U) | + (L>U) | + (L>U) |
| Lysozyme | – | + | – | N+/– G + | PG+ | P+ | BG,P+ | – |
| Lactoferrin | – | – | +/– | +/– | – | – | – | – |
| Pepsinogen II | – | + | + | + | PG+ | – | BG+ | – |
| CEA | + (L<U) | – | – | – | + (L<U) | + (L<U) | + (L<U) | + (L<U) |
| Neutral mucin | + | +/– | MNC+ | + | +/– | – | BG+ | – |
| Sialomucin | N – G(+)/– | – | – | – | + | + | + | + |
| Sulfomucin | – | – | – | N- G+/– | +/– | – | – | + |
| CPS class III | – | – | MNC+ | + | PG+ | – | BG+ | – |
| MOS | – | – | – | – | + | + | + | +/– |
| PA-SB-PH-PAS | – | – | – | – | +/– | +/– | +/– | + |

–: negative
(+): weakly positive
+: positive
(+)/– or +/–: occasionally positive
BG: Brunner's gland
MNC: mucous neck cell
N: normal
G: gastritis, nonmetaplastic
L: lower layer
U: upper layer
P: Paneth cell
PG: pyloric gland

## RESULTS

### 1. Histochemical Markers of Noncancerous Gastric Epithelial Cells

Table 1-2 shows the expression of various immunohistochemical and mucin histochemical markers in nonneoplastic gastric and intestinal tissues. Figures 1-1 and 1-2 illustrate representative features of the marker localization in nonneoplastic gastric mucosa with or without intestinalization.

Secretory component (SC), a key substance for secretory immunity, is a good epithelial marker for various exocrine tissues including intestinal, respiratory, pancreatobiliary, and genitourinary tracts as well as mammary, salivary, nasal, lacrimal, and sweat glands.[51] SC is produced by the epithelial cells and acts as a receptor for dimeric IgA on their basolateral plasma membranes.[52,53] Gastric mucosal epithelium under normal conditions, which means gastric mucosa with negligible inflammatory changes, is devoid of SC, probably owing to high acidity in the gastric lumen.[13,37,54] The high acid condition must be a "natural defense" of the gastric mucosa instead of secretory immunity.[13,54] However, cells in the generative zone, the junctional area between foveolar cells and gastric glands, turn weakly positive for SC when chronic inflammatory changes occur.[13,37,54] Infrequently, atrophic pyloric glands in the mucosa with chronic gastritis are faintly positive for SC. Intestinal metaplasia is immunohistochemically characterized by the prominent expression of SC, especially in Golgi areas of intes-

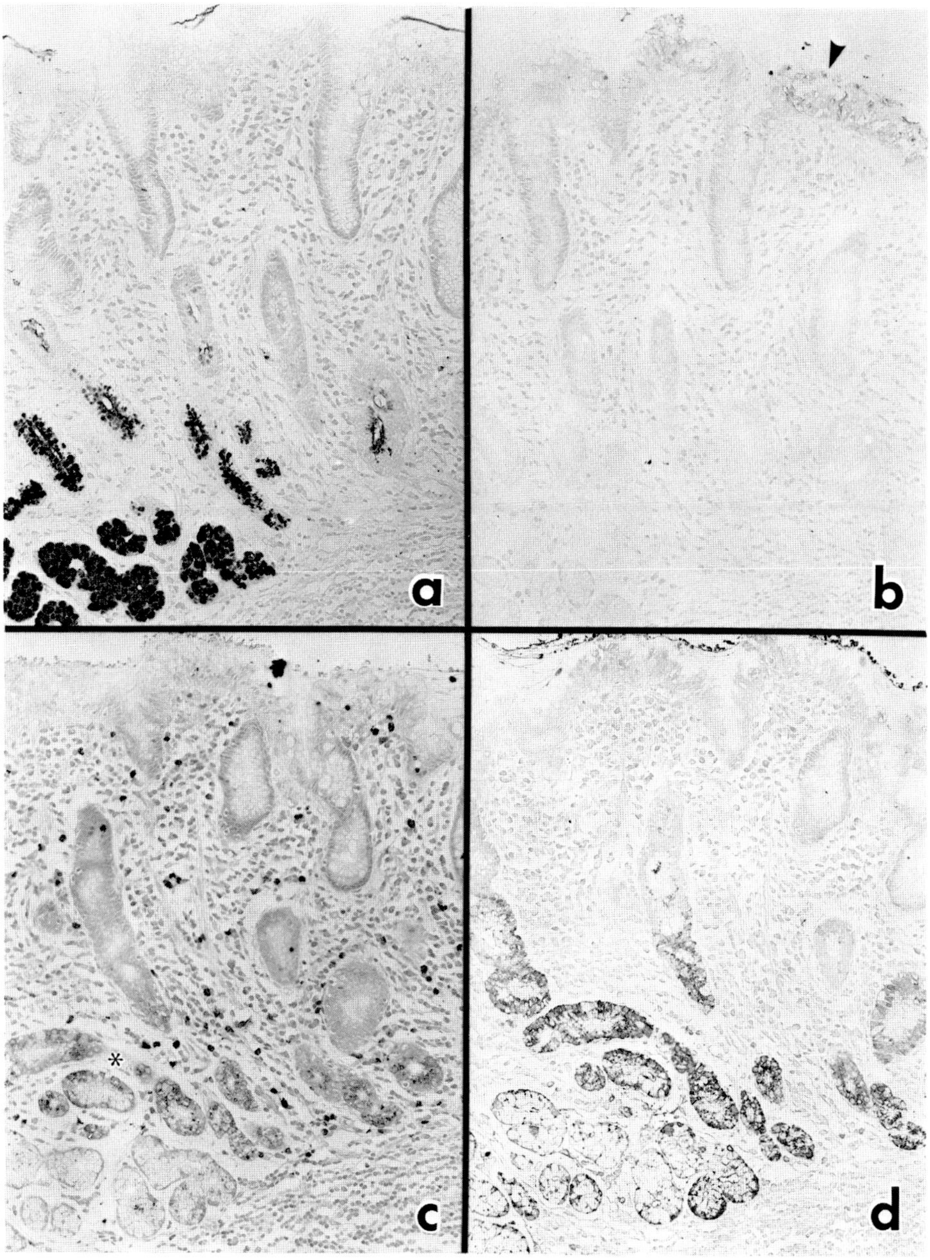


**Fig. 1-1.** Marker expression in nonintestinalized gastric mucosa. CPS class III (a) and indirect immunoperoxidase method for CEA (b), lysozyme (c) and pepsinogen II (d). Methyl green counterstain, ×120

CPS class III specifically stains pyloric gland cells where pepsinogen II is localized. Atrophic pyloric glands at the right side of each picture and cells of the glandular neck region (generative zone, asterisk) are positive for lysozyme. Mature pyloric glands at the left side are devoid here of lysozyme, which is also positive for granulocytes and histiocytes in the stroma. CEA, detected by antiCEA antibody after absorption with the PCA extract of spleen, is focally positive in the uppermost part of foveolar cells (arrowhead). Granulocytes and histiocytes are not stained with the absorbed antiCEA antibody.

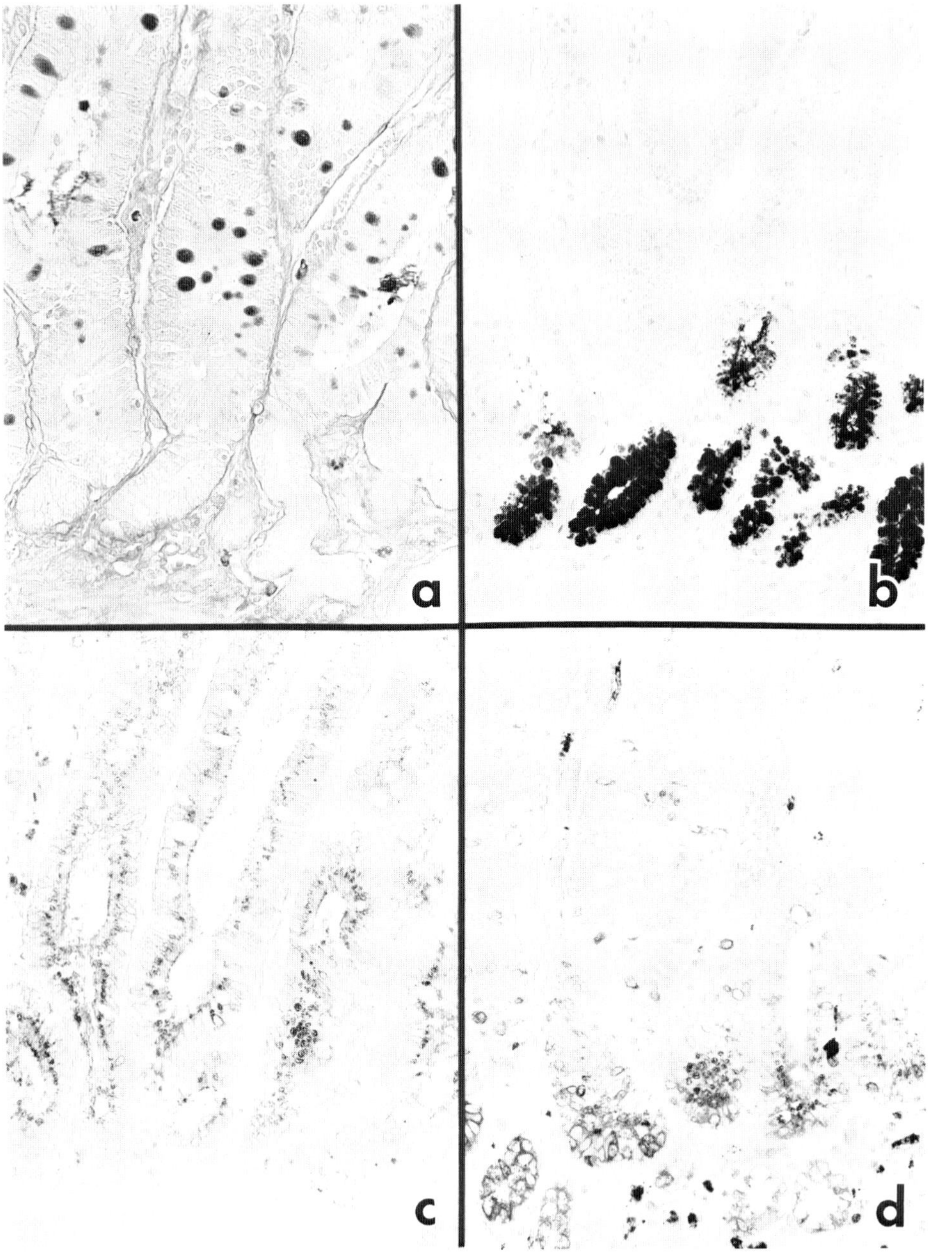



**Fig. 1-2.** Marker expression in intestinal metaplasia (incomplete type[12] or type B[57]). HID-AB (a), CPS class III (b) and indirect immunoperoxidase method for SC (c) and lysozyme (d). Methyl green counterstain, ×200.

Both sialomucin (blue) and sulfomucin (black) are seen in goblet cells. CPS class III and lysozyme are positive in atrophic pyloric glands remaining at the bottom of the mucosa. SC positivity is evident in intestinalized cells.

tinalized cells (Fig. 1-2c),[13,37,54] as seen in normal intestinal epithelium. A minority of intestinalized mucosal cells shows a polarity of the SC expression, as seen in normal intestinal epithelium,[53] i.e., SC immunoreactivity is stronger in cells in the lower half layer of the mucosa than in cells in the upper layer. But the majority shows strong immunoreactivity of SC throughout the intestinalized epithelium without the polarity.[54]

Lysozyme is a bacteriolytic enzyme, muramidase,[55] and is known to cooperate with secretory immunoglobulins.[56] In the small intestine and intestinal metaplasia of the complete type, Paneth cells are strongly positive for lysozyme, in addition to such inflammatory cells as neutrophils, eosinophils, and histiocytes.[13,35,55] Lysozyme is further localized in glandular neck cells at the generative zone of the gastric mucosa with minimal inflammation and pyloric gland cells, especially those showing atrophic changes (Fig. 1-1c).[13,35] Lysozyme immunoreactivity is also observed in the atrophic pyloric glands located at the bottom of intestinal metaplasia, (A and B of Tsutsumi et al[57]) (Fig. 1-2d) and in metaplastic pseudopyloric glands in the fundus.

Lactoferrin is an iron-containing bacteriostatic glycoprotein substance,[58] and is one of the major components of neutrophil granules.[59] Being similar to lysozyme,[55] lactoferrin is widely distributed in various exocrine glands such as salivary, nasal, bronchial, prostatic and lactating mammary glands and renal tubules.[51,58] In the stomach, pyloric gland cells and fundic gland cells except for parietal cells inconsistently show lactoferrin immunoreactivity.[35,60]

Pepsinogen II, an isozyme of gastric digestive enzyme, is consistently positive in pyloric glands including the glandular neck region (Fig. 1-1d), pseudopyloric glands, mucous neck cells, chief cells, and Brunner's glands.[17,61] Foveolar cells and intestinalized epithelia are negative for pepsinogen II.[17,61]

Carcinoembryonic antigen (CEA), an excellent tumor marker, was first described by Gold and Freedman in 1965.[62] Conventional antiserum against CEA including ours used in this study is known to contain antibody activities against several CEA-related substances and blood group substances.[49] The antigenicity of the latter, having antigenic determinants on sugar moieties, is destroyed mostly by the periodate treatment of sections, which was used for endogenous peroxidase inactivation in the present study. The most important CEA-related substance is a nonspecific cross-reacting antigen (NCA), which is present in neutrophils. Thus, the PCA extract of human spleen[50] was used for the elimination of antiNCA activity in the commercial antiCEA antibody. In this chapter the antigenicity recognized by the absorbed antiCEA antibody that does not stain neutrophils is regarded as "CEA" in a broad sense. Strictly speaking, however, "CEA" by this definition includes such CEA-related substances as NCA-2 and normal fecal cross-reacting antigen (NFCA).[49] Normal or metaplastic gastric mucosa has been shown to be positive with the antibody even after the absorption procedure, as reported previously.[37,49] CEA-related substances ("CEA" and NCA) are mainly present in the superficial mucosal part of the foveolar epithelium (Fig. 1-1b).[35,37,49] The antigenicity turns weaker after the absorption of the antibody. Goblet cells and cells in the generative zone are always negative for the antigens. The expression of the CEA-related substances is stronger in intestinalized gastric epithelium than in nonintestinalized epithelium.[35,37]

The AB-PAS procedure differentiates neutral mucin (stained red) from acidic mucin (stained blue or purple). The HID-AB procedure is useful to differentiate sialomucin (stained blue) from sulfomucin (stained black).[44] It is well known that normal human gastric epithelium such as foveolar cells, pyloric glands, mucous neck cells and Brunner's gland in the duodenum exclusively contain neutral mucin. When the foveolar epithelium shows a hyperplastic or regenerative change, however, it sometimes turns faintly alcianophilic. HID-AB staining further confirms the presence of a small amount of sialomucin in such altered foveolar cells. Atrophic pyloric

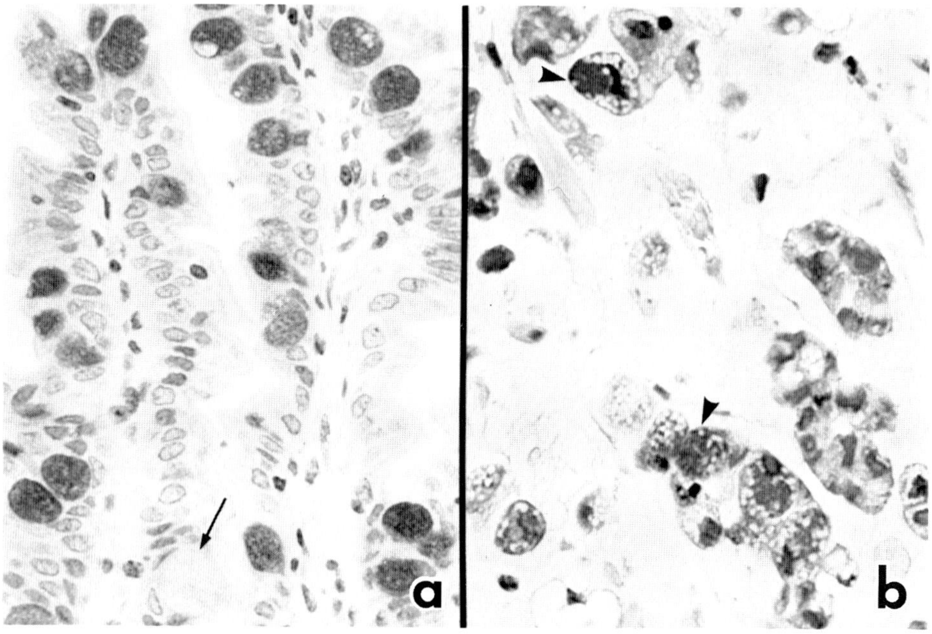


**Fig. 1-3.** PA-SB-PH-PAS reaction in goblet cells of intestinal metaplasia (a) and mucinous adenocarcinoma (b). ×480.
Goblet cells in some, but not all, intestinalized mucosa stain positive for O-acylated sialic acids. Arrow indicates a negative goblet cell. Mucin of signet ring cells in mucinous adenocarcinoma (arrowheads) mostly belong to the goblet cell type.

glands in inflamed antral mucosa or pseudopyloric glands in inflamed fundic mucosa are occasionally positive for sulfomucin.[35] The situation is the same in atrophic pyloric glands remaining at the bottom in intestinal metaplasia. Goblet cells in intestinalized glands are commonly positive for sialomucin, but sulfomucin-containing goblet cells are often noted in intestinal metaplasia of the incomplete type[12] (or types A and B of Tsutsumi et al (Fig. 1-2a).

CPS class III has been confirmed to be highly specific for mucins of pyloric glands (Fig. 1-1a) including those remaining at the bottom of intestinalized epithelium (Fig. 1-2b), pseudopyloric glands, mucous neck cells and Brunner's glands.[30,45,54,57]

Most of the goblet cells in the small intestine and intestinalized mucosa and some in the large intestine stain positive with the MOS sequence.[30,35] The PA-SB-PH-PAS sequence specifically detects mucins of all colonic goblet cells, some goblet cells in the small intestine and intestinal metaplasia of the stomach (Fig. 1-3a).[35]

Nonmetaplastic mucosal cells including hyperplastic or regenerative foveolar cells and sulfomucin-positive atrophic pyloric glands are equally negative for the goblet cell type mucins.

Negative staining results are to be obtained in all of the control specimens including those for immunoperoxidase staining incubated with nonimmune sera, for the MOS sequence followed by the neuraminidase treatment, and for the PA-SB-PH-PAS sequence with omission of the PH step. The same is true in the following Parts.

## 2. EXPRESSION OF HISTOCHEMICAL MARKERS IN GASTRIC CANCER CELLS

A total of 51 surgical specimens of gastric carcinoma of various histological types in-

**TABLE 1-3**
Gastric Carcinomas Histochemically Analyzed

| | m | sm | pm~ | Total |
|---|---|---|---|---|
| sig | 1 | 2 | 8 | 11 |
| muc | 0 | 0 | 5 | 5 |
| pap | 0 | 2 | 4 | 6 |
| $tub_1$ | 3 | 3 | 3 | 9 |
| $tub_2$ | 4 | 2 | 9 | 15 |
| por | 0 | 0 | 5 | 5 |
| total | 8 | 9 | 34 | 51 |

sig: signet ring cell carcinoma
muc: mucinous adenocarcinoma
pap: papillary adenocarcinoma
$tub_1$: well-differentiated tubular adenocarcinoma
$tub_2$: moderately differentiated tubular adenocarcinoma
por: poorly differentiated adenocarcinoma (with medullary growth pattern)
m: intramucosally localized early cancer
sm: early cancer invading into the submucosal layer
pm~: advanced cancer invading into the proper muscle layer or into the serosa

cluding 17 early carcinomas (Table 1-3) were histochemically examined for SC, lysozyme, lactoferrin, CEA/NCA, CPS class III, MOS, and PA/SB/PH/PAS reactivities.[35] Three adenocarcinomas with lymphoid stroma were included in "$tub_2$" (moderately differentiated tubular adenocarcinoma). CEA/NCA means the immunoreactivity detected by an antiCEA polyclonal antibody without absorption with the PCA extract of the spleen. Results are summarized in Table 1-4.

SC and lysozyme were at least focally positive in more than 80% of cancer tissues. The frequency of positivity was principally independent of the histological typing, excepting for less SC immunoreactivity in mucinous adenocarcinoma (muc). Lysozyme can be regarded as a marker relatively specific for gastric epithelium, because intestinal epithelial cells other than Paneth cells and Brunner's glands are commonly negative for lysozyme. In H&E preparations of the gastric cancer tissues examined, no typical Paneth cell granules were seen. It is noteworthy that the expression of lysozyme was quite common even in adenoplastic or "intestinal-type" carcinomas (pap, $tub_1$ and $tub_2$). In a separate study, however, some crypt epithelium of either the small or large intestine was infrequently and inconsistently immunostained for lysozyme, and a very small number of lysozyme-positive cancer cells were identified in 11 of 28 adenocarcinomas (39%) of the colon and rectum (unpublished observation). Klockars et al[63] reported lysozyme-positive crypt epithelial cells in the lesion of ulcerative colitis.[60] Therefore, the significance of lysozyme as a gastric marker should be considered relative.

The demonstration of lactoferrin immunoreactivity in gastric carcinomas was quite inconstant. Only a few lactoferrin-positive cancer cells were detected in 18 of 51 carcinomas (35%) irrespective of histological typing. On the contrary, CEA/NCA or CEA-related substance(s) were positive in all carcinoma tissues, and the positive cells were generally plentiful. Poorly differentiated adenocarcinomas with a medullary growth pattern (por) were apt to show a lesser number of CEA/NCA-positive cancer cells. The positivity of CEA/NCA was noted on the plasma membranes in principle, whereas cancer cells showing a strongly positive cytoplasmic staining were not rarely encountered.

Intracytoplasmic mucins specifically demonstrated by CPS class III (for pyloric gland type) and MOS and/or PA/SB/PH/PAS (for goblet cell type) were positive in many cancer cells, again irrespective of histological typing. Mucins of the pyloric gland-type and goblet cell-type were fairly frequently detected in both diffuse and adenoplastic carcinomas. For the evaluation of MOS reaction, only intracytoplasmic staining was regarded as positive and positive staining of the surface coat of some neoplastic glands was neglected.

Mucinous adenocarcinomas were characterized by the constant occurrence of goblet cell type mucin. In other words, most signet ring cells in mucinous adenocarcinomas could be categorized as the goblet cell type, while a few small-sized cells containing neutral mucin and/or CPS class III mucin were also found in four of five tumors. The detection of PA/SB/PH/PAS reactivity in gastric

**TABLE 1-4**
Expression of Glycoprotein Markers and Mucins in 51 Gastric Carcinomas

| | | SC | | | | Lysozyme | | | | Lactoferrin | | | | CEA/NCA | | | |
|---|---|---|---|---|---|---|---|---|---|---|---|---|---|---|---|---|---|
| | | − | (+) | + | ++ | − | (+) | + | ++ | − | (+) | + | ++ | − | (+) | + | ++ |
| sig | 11 | 1 | 3 | 7 | 0 | 1 | 2 | 6 | 2 | 6 | 5 | 0 | 0 | 0 | 0 | 3 | 8 |
| muc | 5 | 2 | 3 | 0 | 0 | 1 | 2 | 1 | 1 | 4 | 1 | 0 | 0 | 0 | 0 | 0 | 5 |
| pap | 6 | 1 | 2 | 2 | 1 | 2 | 2 | 1 | 1 | 3 | 3 | 0 | 0 | 0 | 0 | 1 | 5 |
| $tub_1$ | 9 | 1 | 0 | 4 | 4 | 1 | 1 | 7 | 0 | 6 | 3 | 0 | 0 | 0 | 0 | 1 | 8 |
| $tub_2$ | 15 | 2 | 4 | 7 | 2 | 1 | 2 | 6 | 6 | 10 | 5 | 0 | 0 | 0 | 0 | 4 | 11 |
| por | 5 | 0 | 2 | 1 | 2 | 2 | 1 | 0 | 2 | 4 | 1 | 0 | 0 | 0 | 1 | 3 | 1 |
| total | 51 | 7 | 14 | 21 | 9 | 8 | 10 | 21 | 12 | 33 | 18 | 0 | 0 | 0 | 1 | 12 | 38 |

| | | CPS Class III | | | | PA/SB/PH/PAS | | | | MOS | | | |
|---|---|---|---|---|---|---|---|---|---|---|---|---|---|
| | | − | (+) | + | ++ | − | (+) | + | ++ | − | (+) | + | ++ |
| sig | 11 | 2 | 4 | 4 | 1 | 10 | 1 | 0 | 0 | 4 | 4 | 3 | 0 |
| muc | 5 | 4 | 1 | 0 | 0 | 2 | 1 | 2 | 0 | 0 | 3 | 1 | 1 |
| pap | 6 | 3 | 2 | 1 | 0 | 5 | 0 | 1 | 0 | 3 | 1 | 2 | 0 |
| $tub_1$ | 9 | 3 | 2 | 3 | 1 | 8 | 1 | 0 | 0 | 4 | 5 | 0 | 0 |
| $tub_2$ | 15 | 3 | 6 | 3 | 3 | 14 | 1 | 0 | 0 | 7 | 6 | 2 | 0 |
| por | 5 | 4 | 0 | 0 | 1 | 5 | 0 | 0 | 0 | 3 | 1 | 0 | 1 |
| total | 51 | 19 | 15 | 11 | 6 | 44 | 4 | 3 | 0 | 21 | 20 | 8 | 2 |

−: negative
(+): positive in only a few cells
+: positive in a modest number of cells
++: positive in many cells

cancer was infrequent except for mucinous adenocarcinomas (Fig. 1-3b).

The present series included three adenocarcinomas with marked infiltration of small lymphocytes and plasma cells in the stroma. The cancer cells revealed constant morphological features showing a microalveolus, trabecular, or irregular small tubule-like arrangement with the formation of small lumina (categorized as $tub_2$ in this study).[64] The nuclear pleomorphism was not so marked. The formation of lymphoid follicles in the stroma and the infiltration of small lymphocytes inside cancerous nests were common, while necrosis of cancer cells was hardly seen (Fig. 1-4). The margin of invasion was well-demarcated, and the biological behavior was reported to be relatively less malignant.[64] Histochemical properties of the cancer cells corresponded to those of the pyloric glands. Most tumor cells possessed intracytoplasmic neutral mucin with weak CPS class III reactivity. Lysozyme was positive in addition to SC and CEA/NCA. Surface coat-type mucin was occasionally seen along the lumen of cancerous tubules, but goblet cell-type mucin was hardly noted especially in the invading site.

A separate study has disclosed that IgG is predominantly shown in the plasma cells, and plasma cells containing IgM or IgA are minor components. With monoclonal antibodies, MB-1 and MT-1, from Bio-Science Products AG, Emmenbrücke, Switzerland, which are applicable to formalin-fixed and paraffin-embedded tissue, lymphocytes forming lymphoid follicles are mostly composed of B cells, while small lymphocytes scattered in the stroma and in cancer nests are largely T cells. It seems important to note that the morphology and histochemical features of cancer cells

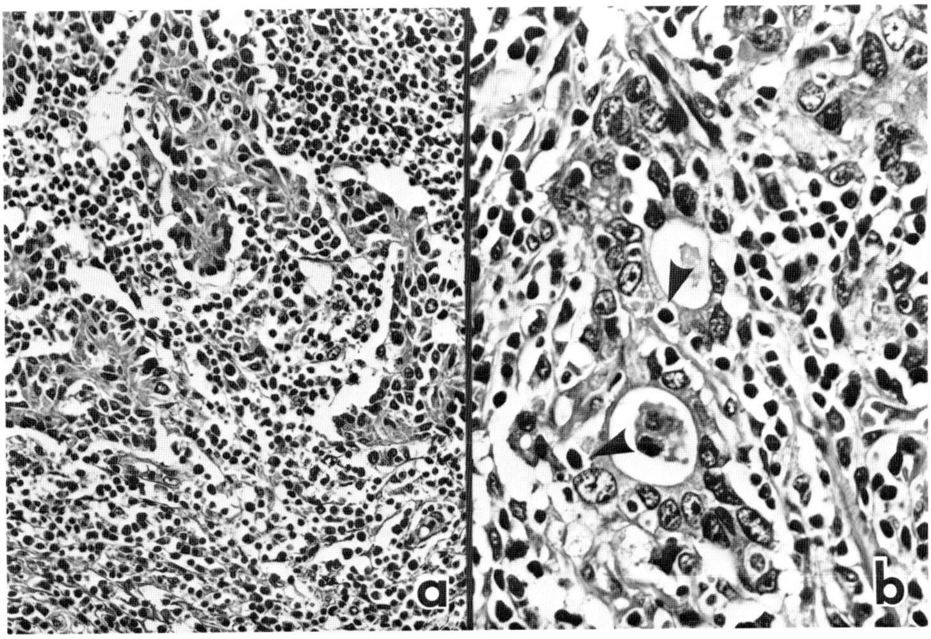


**Fig. 1-4.** Adenocarcinoma with lymphoid stroma. H&E, ×200 (a) and ×400 (b).
Cancer cells form a trabecular or abortive tubular arrangement. Marked stromal infiltration of lymphocytes and plasma cells is characteristic. The presence of intraepithelial lymphocytes (arrowheads) is a common finding.

of this special type are quite uniform, as seen in medullary carcinoma with lymphocytic infiltration of the breast.[65] In addition to the possibility of tumor immunity, the production of some factors chemotactic to lymphocytes and plasma cells (lymphoegresin)[66] by the specifically differentiated cancer cells should also be taken into consideration when we discuss the pathological significance of the lymphoid stroma.

In fact, the presence of "intraepithelial lymphocytes" (small T lymphocytes among epithelial cells) reflects an important function of nonneoplastic gastrointestinal mucosa.[54,67] We have reported the universal occurrence of "intraepithelial lymphocytes" in every colonic adenocarcinoma without evidence of tumor cell damage.[68] Additionally, the production of colony-stimulating and neutrophil chemotactic factor(s) has been clarified in poorly differentiated cancers with marked neutrophilic infiltration from a variety of primary sites.[69,70]

Table 1-5 summarizes the mode of mucin expression (the predominance of surface coat mucin, intracytoplasmic mucin or both) in the above 51 carcinomas. Nearly half (13/30) of the adenoplastic carcinomas showed the

**TABLE 1-5**
Predominant Type of Mucin in 51 Gastric Carcinomas: Surface Coat Type, Intracytoplasmic Type or Both

| | | Mainly SCM | SCM + ICM | Mainly ICM | Paucity of Mucin |
|---|---|---|---|---|---|
| sig | 11 | 0 | 3 | 8 | 0 |
| muc | 5 | 0 | 0 | 5 | 0 |
| pap | 6 | 4 | 2 | 0 | 0 |
| $tub_1$ | 9 | 6 | 3 | 0 | 0 |
| $tub_2$ | 15 | 3 | 7 | 5 | 0 |
| por | 5 | 1 | 0 | 2 | 2 |
| total | 51 | 14 | 15 | 20 | 2 |

SCM: surface coat-type mucin
ICM: intracytoplasmic mucin

**TABLE 1-6**
Expression of Intracytoplasmic Mucins of Gastric and Intestinal Type in 35 Gastric Carcinomas

| | | Intramucosal Lesion (m) | | | | Invasive Lesion (sm⁻) | | | | |
|---|---|---|---|---|---|---|---|---|---|---|
| | | G | G+I | I | NS | G | G+I | I | NS | NL |
| sig | 11 | 5 | 5 | 1 | 0 | 5 | 2 | 3 | 0 | 1 |
| muc | 5 | 0 | 4 | 1 | 0 | 0 | 4 | 1 | 0 | 0 |
| pap | 2 | 1 | 1 | 0 | 0 | 1 | 1 | 0 | 0 | 0 |
| $tub_1$ | 3 | 1 | 2 | 0 | 0 | 0 | 0 | 0 | 0 | 3 |
| $tub_2$ | 12 | 5 | 6 | 0 | 1 | 5 | 1 | 0 | 2 | 4 |
| por | 2 | 0 | 1 | 1 | 0 | 1 | 0 | 1 | 0 | 0 |
| total | 35 | 12 | 19 | 3 | 1 | 12 | 8 | 5 | 2 | 8 |

G: gastric type [neutral mucin and/or CPS class III mucin]
I: intestinal (or goblet cell) type [MOS and/or PA-SB-PH-PAS]
NS: not specified
NL: no lesion seen

predominance of surface coat-type mucin, while all diffuse carcinomas showed intracytoplasmic mucin. Five $tub_2$ adenocarcinomas predominantly with intracytoplasmic mucin included three adenocarcinomas with lymphoid stroma and two adenocarcinomas simulating an acinus-like arrangement.

Thirty-five carcinomas with intracytoplasmic mucin worth evaluating (ICM and SCMICM in Table 1-5) were further analyzed for the occurrence of mucins of the gastric or intestinal type. Neutral mucin (stained red both by the AB-PAS sequence and PAS after diastase digestion) and CPS class III mucin were regarded as gastric type, while PA/SB/PH/PAS and MOS reactions were regarded as intestinal (goblet cell) type. Results are summarized in Table 1-6 in which the reaction for the mucin in question was judged as positive even when only a few cells stained. About half of carcinomas of any histological type revealed an admixture of gastric and intestinal mucins. The dual expression of gastric and intestinal mucins was clearer in the mucosal lesion than in the submucosal or deeper lesion.

*Comment:* The division of gastric cancer into diffuse and adenoplastic types has been widely accepted so far because it allegedly reflects both biological behaviors and the histogenesis of the cancer.[4,5,11] The adenoplastic type is closely related to intestinal metaplasia, especially of the incomplete type,[12] while the diffuse type is believed to arise from nonintestinalized mucosa proper to the stomach.[5,11]

In the present study, however, the dual expression of gastric- and intestinal-type mucins was confirmed in gastric cancer cells irrespective of histological typing. Signet ring cell carcinoma occasionally contains cancer cells of the goblet cell type, while the demonstration of pyloric gland mucin in adenoplastic carcinoma is fairly common. Mucinous adenocarcinoma is predominantly composed of signet ring cells of the goblet cell type, and cancer cells of adenocarcinoma with lymphoid stroma, classified as $tub_2$, mainly show the properties of pyloric gland cells. Therefore, it is concluded that any type of gastric cancer possesses similar properties with regard to the bidirectional differentiation into gastric and intestinal type epithelial cells.[28,35,36]

As commented in the introduction, the most apparent cell biological difference between the two types is whether the cancer cell acts as a dissociative cell in a stochastic flow system or if it acts as an associative cell in a

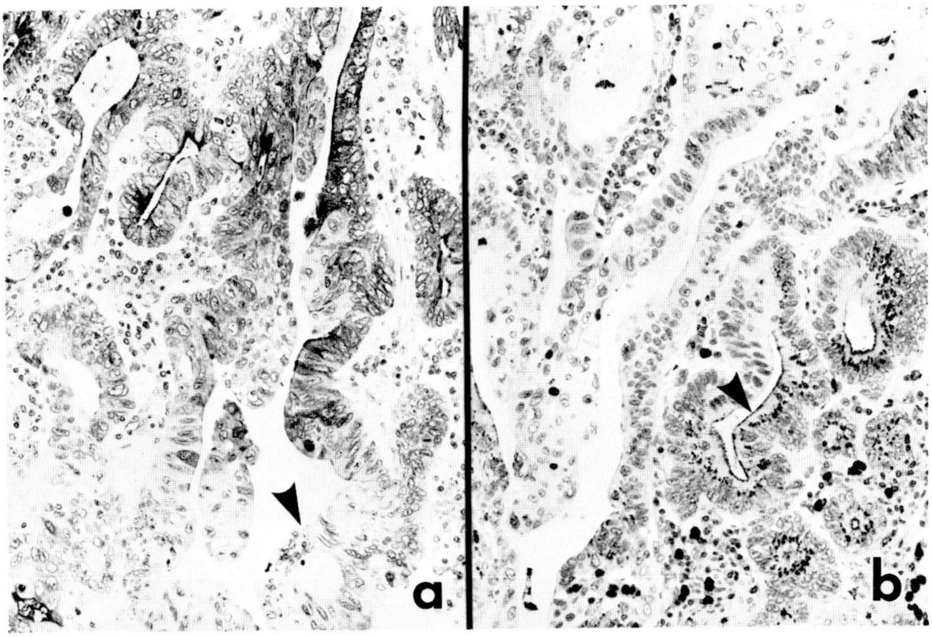


**Fig. 1-5.** Organoid marker expression in invasive tubular adenocarcinoma. PAP method for SC (a) and lysozyme (b). Hematoxylin counterstain, ×150.

Longitudinally arranged tubular area is positive for SC and negative for lysozyme, whereas the localization pattern is reversed in an associated gland-like area (arrowheads). The latter area is also reactive to CPS class III.

pipe line system.[8,9] In noncancerous gastric mucosa, the generative cells of intestinal metaplasia with remaining atrophic pyloric glands at the bottom (types A and B of Tsutsumi et al,[57] corresponding to the incomplete type),[12] differentiate bidirectionally upward to intestinal-type cells including goblet cells and downward to pyloric gland cells.[57] Accordingly, the similarity of the mode of differentiation among proliferative cells in gastric cancer of any histological type and generative cells in "incompletely" intestinalized mucosa is quite meaningful.

## 3. ORGANOID DIFFERENTIATION IN ADVANCED GASTRIC CANCER

The expression of the various histochemical markers in advanced gastric cancer is not necessarily discordant. Some degrees of organoid or polarized differentiation have been demonstrated in certain tumors. Several representative pictures of the organoid differentiation are shown below.

Figure 1-5 displays immunostaining for SC and lysozyme in a tubular adenocarcinoma. Cancerous epithelium is arranged in elongated and irregularly branching tubules associated with small glandular structures. SC immunoreactivity is mainly seen in the elongated tubular areas, while lysozyme is localized predominantly in the associated gland-like areas. The latter part is also focally positive for CPS class III reactivity. Although neoplastic goblet-like cells are absent, the morphological and histochemical features strongly suggest that the adenoplastic cancer cells imitate the "incompletely" intestinalized epithelium, which consists of strongly SC-reactive absorptive-type cells and lysozyme-positive atrophic pyloric glands at the bottom. A similar organoid differentiation has sometimes been observed at the invading site of other adenoplastic carcinomas, in which tumor cells protruding papillarily into cancerous lumina exhibit the properties of neutral mucin-containing surface epithelium or MOS-positive goblet-like cells, while tumor cells forming an associated gland-like structure and facing toward the interstitium reveal CPS class III reactivity, as described by Katsuyama et al.[30]

Regarding the differentiation toward Paneth cells in adenoplastic carcinomas, see below.

Figure 1-6 shows consecutive sections of adenocarcinoma (classified as $tub_2$) stained for HID-AB, lysozyme, SC, and CEA/NCA. The upper half is composed of both scattered goblet-like cells predominantly containing sialomucin (MOS reaction being also positive) and lysozyme immunoreactive cells with an abortive trabecular or tubular arrangement. In this area, CPS class III mucin is further identified (see Fig. 1-7d), but CEA/NCA is only focally and weakly positive in goblet-like cells. On the contrary, most cancer cells in the lower half show strong CEA/NCA immunoreactivity, but almost no mucin or lysozyme. SC is localized in both areas with stronger staining in the lower half. H&E stain does not discriminate morphologic differences between these two areas except for the presence of goblet-like cells in the former. The number of mitoses and the degree of nuclear atypia are nearly the same. Cancer cells in the former area may have characteristics of glandular neck cells differentiating toward the pyloric gland and goblet cells, while the latter area is solely composed of cancer cells differentiating toward surface-lining cells probably of intestinal absorptive type.

Figure 1-7 illustrates a high power view of the upper area of Figure 1-6. The cancer cells consist of both goblet-like large cells and small immature-looking cells. The goblet-like cells contain predominantly sialomucin and partially sulfomucin; they show a positive MOS reaction and weak CEA/NCA immunoreactivity. The small cells reveal neutral mucin with a positive CPS class III reaction. Lysozyme and SC are further localized predominantly in the small cells. The small cells are likely to have the properties of generative cells partially expressing pyloric gland nature. These histochemical findings indicate that cancer cells are capable of retaining their cellular characteristics, which they are destined to express even after the structural organization is completely lost. A similar phenomenon has been commonly encountered in mucinous adenocarcinomas or signet ring cell carcinomas with histochemical characteristics of goblet cell mucin. Namely, cancer cells reactive to lysozyme, SC, and CPS class III are often small in size and haphazardly intermingled with goblet-like mature signet ring cells.

Figure 1-8 illustrates a remarkable regional distribution of CEA/NCA and lysozyme in signet ring cell carcinoma.[35] The expression pattern of both markers forms a good contrast; CEA/NCA immunoreactive cancer cells are small in size, look immature and show numerous mitotic figures (Fig. 1-8c), whereas cells in the lysozyme-positive area reveal a fairly typical appearance of signet ring cells and scarcely show mitoses (Fig. 1-8d). The latter cells further focally display SC immunoreactivity, sulfomucin, and CPS class III reactivity, representing rather mature cells differentiating toward the pyloric gland. Almost no mucin is identified in the CEA/NCA positive immature cancer cells, which probably represents an actively proliferating component in the signet ring cell carcinoma. Infiltrating diffuse carcinomas with a scirrhous growth pattern are commonly composed of small-sized and immature-looking cancer cells with striking immunoreactivity for CEA/NCA. The concurrent occurrence of CEA/NCA and lysozyme, SC or CPS class III mucin in these scirrhous cancer cells is not infrequently seen.

Figure 1-9 shows a rather exceptional expression of lysozyme in goblet-like mature signet ring cells, which are also positive for CEA/NCA. The expression of CEA/NCA in goblet-like cancer cells is a very common phenomenon. Many of the signet ring cells in mucinous adenocarcinoma react positively to

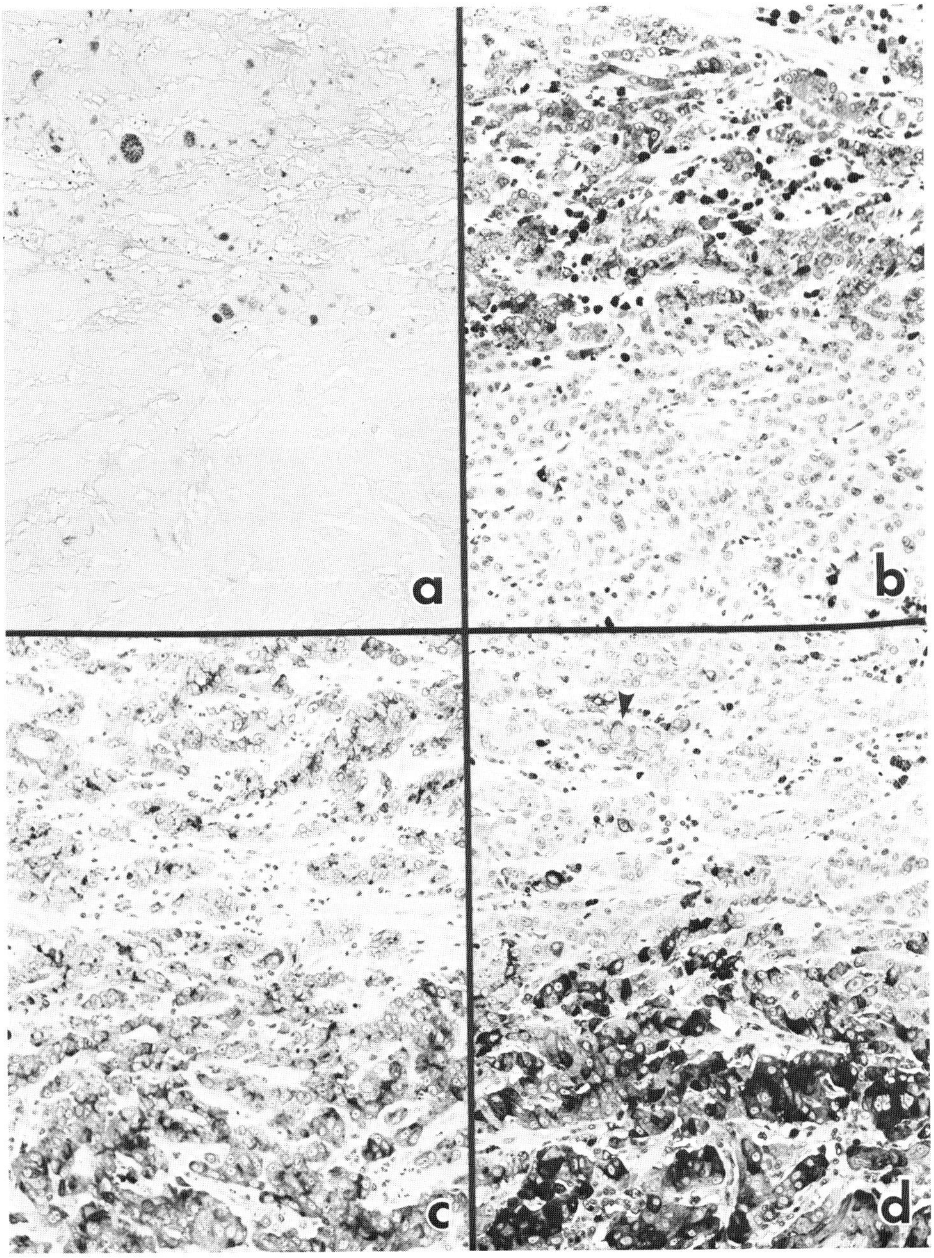


**Fig. 1-6.** Contrasted marker localization in rather poorly differentiated area of $tub_2$ adenocarcinoma. HID-AB (a) and PAP method for lysozyme (b), SC (c) and CEA/NCA (d). Hematoxylin counterstain (b–d), ×150.

Cancer cells in the upper half area are positive for lysozyme but negative for CEA/NCA except for a few goblet-like cells (arrowhead), in which acidic mucin (predominantly sialomucin) is demonstrated. The lower half is composed of cells strongly positive for CEA/NCA but unreactive to lysozyme and mucin. SC is detected in both halves with stronger staining of the latter.

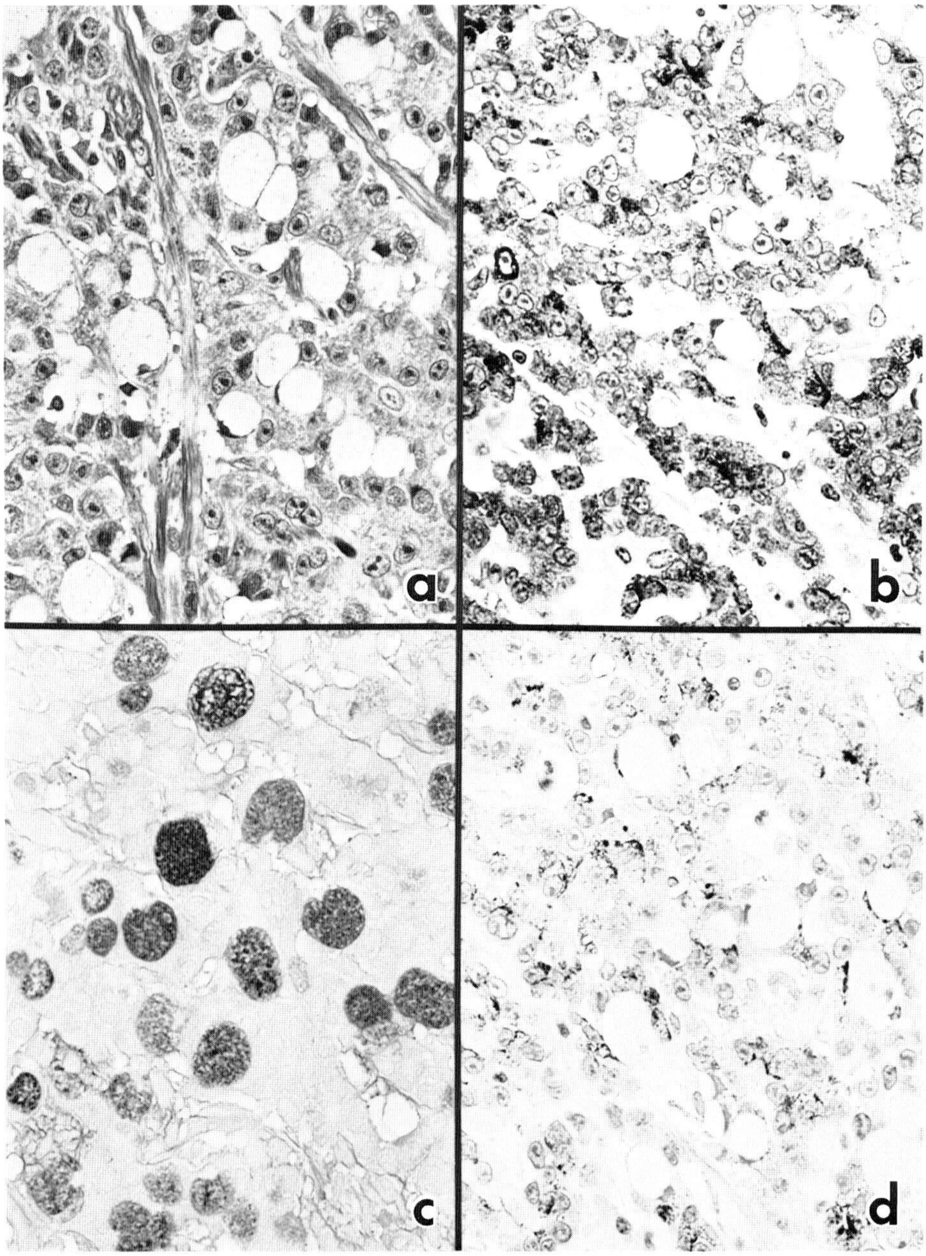


**Fig. 1-7.** Mixed differentiation toward goblet cells and pyloric gland cells in the upper half area of Figure 1-6. H&E (a), PAP method for SC (b), HID-AB (c) and CPS class III (d). Hematoxylin counterstain, ×400.
The tumor consists of both goblet-like large cells containing acidic mucin and immature-looking small cells with positive reactions to SC, lysozyme, and CPS class III. The former cells are also reactive to MOS. Even after the loss of structural organization, haphazardly differentiated tumor cells retain the nature of marker expression in their nonneoplastic counterparts.

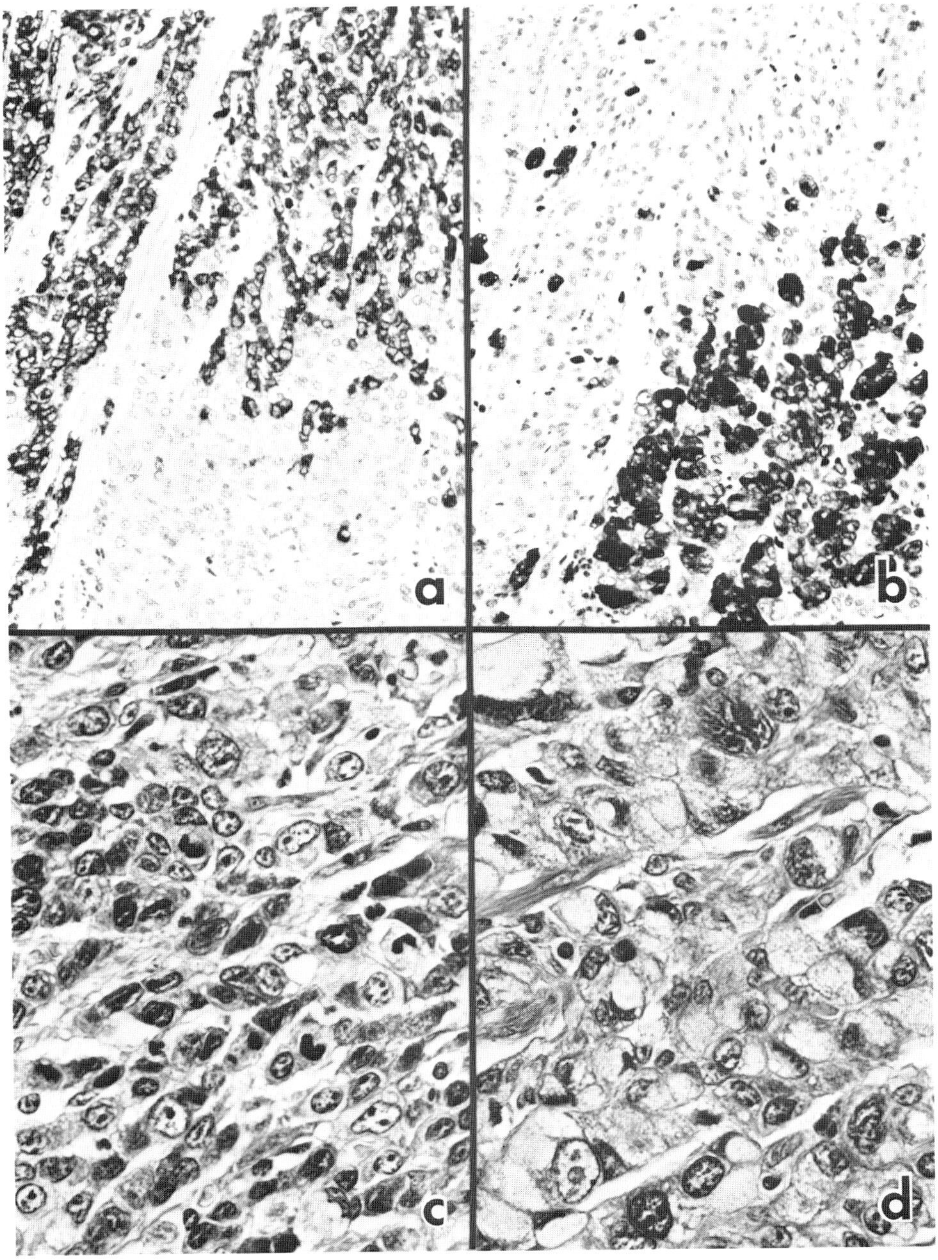


**Fig. 1-8.** Reciprocal distribution pattern of CEA/NCA (a) and lysozyme (b) and high power view of CEA/NCA-positive area (c) and lysozyme-positive area (d). a & b: PAP method with hematoxylin counterstain, ×150; c & d: H&E, ×480.

Cancer cells in the CEA/NCA-positive area are small in size and look immature, while the lysozyme-positive area is solely composed of fairly large signet ring cells with CPS class III reactivity. Mitotic figures are frequently noted in the former area.

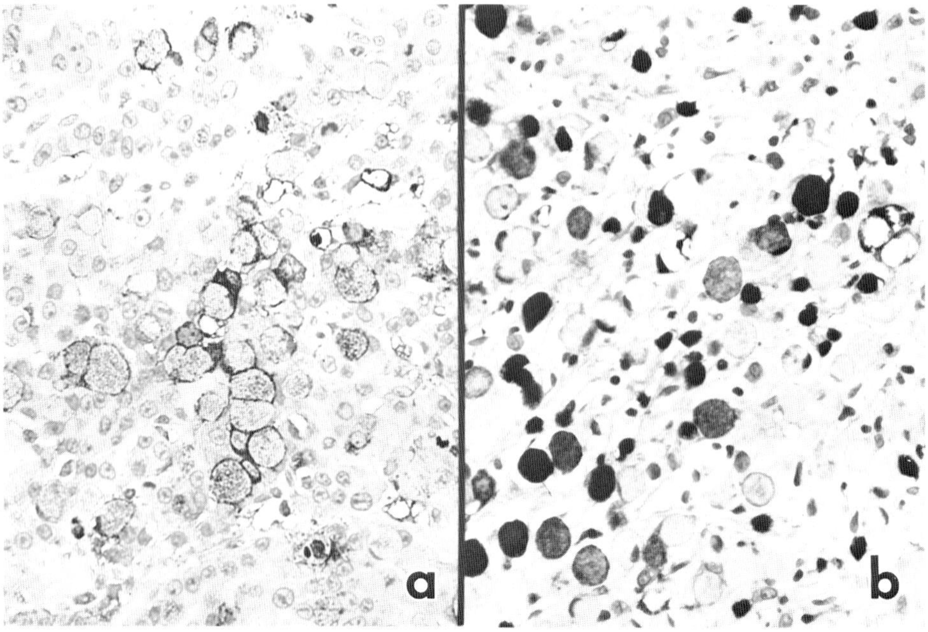


**Fig. 1-9.** Disorganized expression of CEA and lysozyme in mature signet ring cells of the goblet cell type. PAP method for CEA/NCA (a) and lysozyme (b). Hematoxylin counterstain, ×300.
Mature signet ring cells, which are strongly reactive to alcian blue and MOS, are occasionally positive for lysozyme deep in their cytoplasm. CEA/NCA shows cell membrane staining. These marker expressions are unexpected, since nonneoplastic goblet cells lack both markers.

antiCEA antibody. However, this is also regarded as a deviation occurring during the neoplastic progression, since nonneoplastic goblet cells lack the antigen. Although such unexpected and disorganized expressions of the marker substances are one of the characteristic features of advanced cancer cells, the above-mentioned rather organized or polarized differentiations of cancer cells should be emphasized again.

## 4. ZONAL DIFFERENTIATION OF SIGNET RING CANCER CELLS IN THE MUCOSA

Here, peculiar zonal (lamellar or layered) differentiations shown by intramucosally located gastric cancer cells are described.[35,36] Careful observation of 40 intramucosal lesions from the above series disclosed a characteristic zonal (lamellar or layered) distribution pattern of the markers in some cancers. No mucosal lesions worth evaluating were left in 11 advanced carcinomas, especially of pap and por types. As shown in Table 1-7, lysozyme and CPS class III reactivities tended to localize in cancer cells occupying the bottom or lower half layer of the mucosa, whereas CEA/NCA and MOS reactivities had a tendency to be localized in cancer cells occupying the upper layer of the mucosa. Immunoreactive SC was found to be localized in cancer cells occupying either the lower or upper layer of the mucosa. It is apparent that the zonation pattern of the markers reflects well those seen in noncancerous gastric mucosa. The localization of SC in the lower layer of cancerous mucosa is likely to be a reflection of that attribute of nonmetaplastic gastric mucosa with chronic inflammation, while SC seen in the upper layer of the cancerous mucosa probably mimics the pattern in intestinalized epithelia with SC-negative pyloric glands at their bot-

**TABLE 1-7**
Zonal Differentiation of Gastric Carcinomas in the Mucosa

| | Marker | SC | | Lysozyme | CEA/NCA | CPS,III | MOS |
|---|---|---|---|---|---|---|---|
| | Zonation | Lower | Upper | Lower | Upper | Lower | Upper |
| sig | 11(3) | 4(3) | 1 | 5(2) | 5(3) | 6(2) | 2(2) |
| muc | 5(0) | 0 | 0 | 0 | 0 | 1 | 0 |
| pap | 2(1) | 0 | 0 | 1(1) | 0 | 1(1) | 0 |
| $tub_1$ | 8(6) | 2(2) | 2(2) | 4(4) | 3(2) | 6(5) | 4(3) |
| $tub_2$ | 13(6) | 3(2) | 3(2) | 6(4) | 7(3) | 6(3) | 4(3) |
| por | 1(0) | 0 | 0 | 0 | 0 | 0 | 0 |
| total | 40(16) | 9(7) | 6(4) | 16(11) | 15(8) | 20(11) | 10(8) |

( ): indicates the number of early carcinomas

toms. Early carcinomas more frequently showed the organized differentiation pattern than advanced carcinomas (Table 1-7). This fact suggests that less severely destroyed mucosal structures are required for the formation of the above-mentioned zonation pattern. The intramucosal zonation pattern, however, was seen only focally in most tumors judged positive. The exception included two of three early signet ring cell carcinomas, which clearly revealed the organized zonation pattern of the markers including SC, lysozyme, CEA/NCA and CPS class III mucin in any area of the mucosal lesion (Fig. 1-10). In addition, two of 22 adenoplastic carcinomas ($tub_1$ and $tub_2$ confined to the mucosa) also displayed the zonal distribution of lysozyme and CEA/NCA widely but not in every area of the cancerous mucosa, whereas the zonation of SC and CPS class III mucin was focal and abortive. Generally, the zonal differentiation shown by adenoplastic carcinomas was often partial (Fig. 1-11a). The expression of CEA/NCA in adenoplastic carcinomas was frequently so marked and exaggerated that all of the cancer cells stained strongly for the antigen (Fig. 1-11b). In a similar sense, we clarified the abnormal ultrastructural localization of CEA on the plasma membranes of individual adenoplastic cancer cells.[37]

To confirm the universality of the above-mentioned phenomenon seen in early signet ring cell carcinomas, an additional 50 tumors (38 mucosal cancers and 12 submucosally invading cancers) were analyzed both with the indirect immunoperoxidase method for SC, lysozyme, pepsinogen II, and CEA and with mucin histochemistry by AB-PAS, HID-AB, and CPS class III. CEA was visualized by a conventional antiCEA antibody previously absorbed with the PCA extract of human spleen. Results are summarized in Table 1-8. Representative pictures are shown in Figure 1-12, in which a rather well developed pyloric gland-like zone is observed in the lower half of the mucosa. Compare the width of CPS class III-positive zone of Figure 1-12b with that of Figure 1-10a.

Many signet ring cell carcinomas revealed a fairly constant zonation pattern of the marker expression as expected. The frequency and degree of the organized differentiation were not related to the degree of intestinalization in the surrounding mucosa, the site of cancer in the stomach, or to the age and sex of patients. The perfection of the organized differentiation was apparently dependent on the degree of persistence of noncancerous epithelial cells. Namely, in the lamina propria mucosae with well-preserved noncancerous epithelium, signet ring cancer cells differentiate quite well in a like manner to noncancerous cells. The zonal expression for CEA was most stable, then reactivities to lysozyme, CPS class III

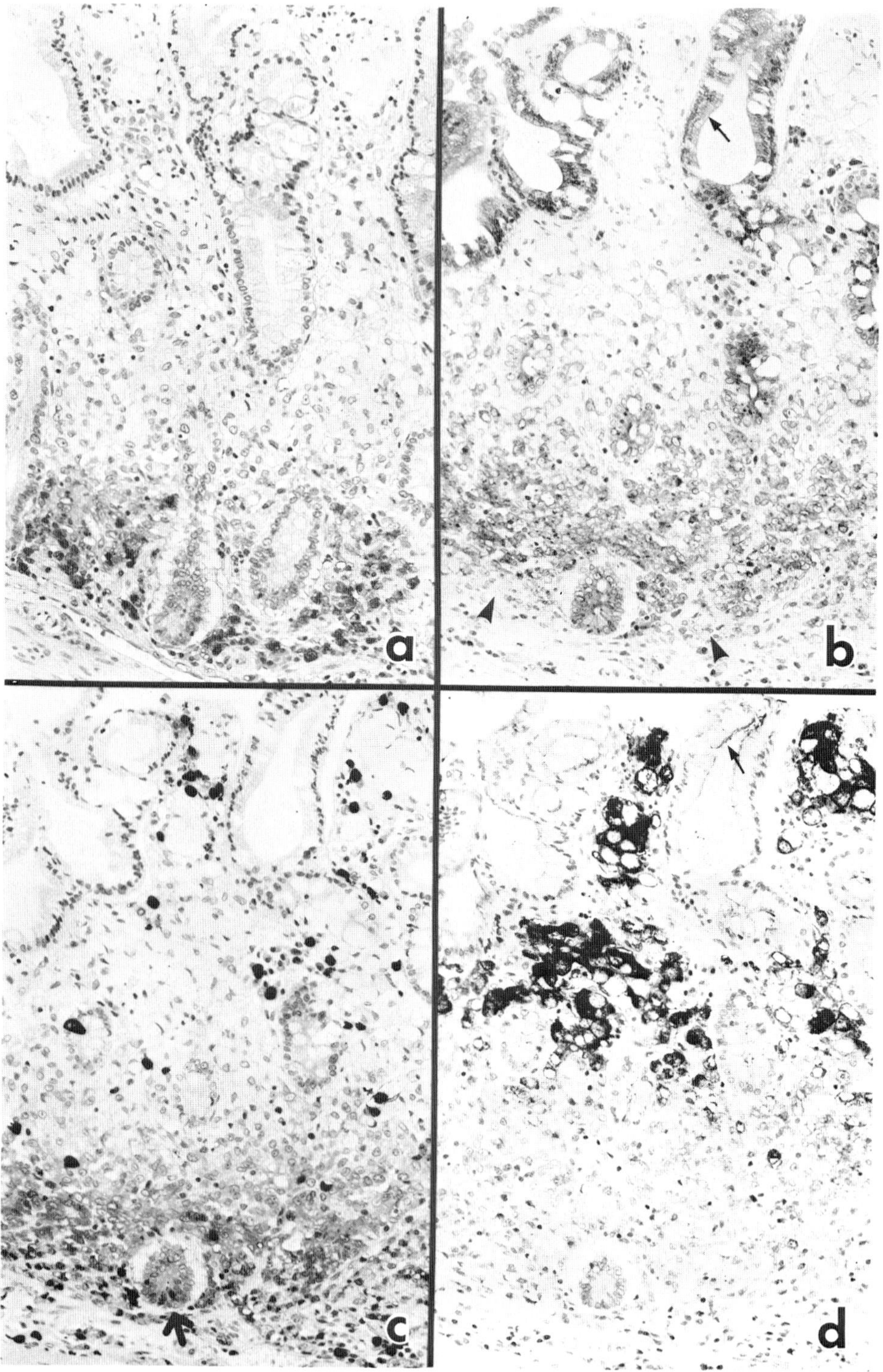
a
b
c
d

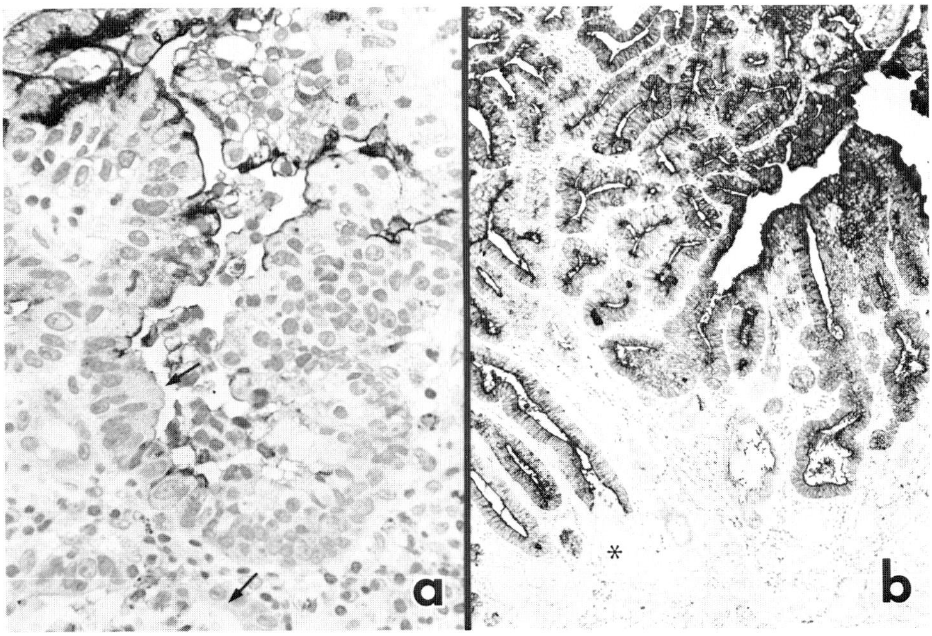


**Fig. 1-11.** CEA/NCA in adenoplastic carcinoma. PAP method with hematoxylin counterstain, ×300 (a) and ×60 (b).

Polarized expression of CEA/NCA is focally visualized in (a) where the antigen is localized on the apical plasma membranes of cells in the upper part of the cancerous tubule but cells in the lower part are negative (arrows). CEA/NCA is occasionally expressed so excessively in every adenoplastic cancer cell as to lose the polarized pattern (b). Asterisk indicates noncancerous pyloric glands remaining at the bottom of cancerous epithelium.

and SC followed it. Among the latter three markers, the width of the positive zone was broadest for SC and narrowest for CPS class III mucin, representing well the expression pattern in noncancerous epithelium. When carefully observed, cancer cells at the lowermost narrow zone of the mucosa were only weakly positive or even negative for SC (see Fig. 1-10), especially in the tumors with a wide CPS class III reactive zone. This certainly reflects the negative SC staining of mature pyloric gland cells in noncancerous mucosa.

CEA immunoreactivity in mature signet ring cells and submucosally invading immature-looking cells shown by the absorbed antibody was fundamentally identical to CEA/NCA immunoreactivity as detected by the

←

**Fig. 1-10.** Typical zonal differentiation of signet ring cell carcinoma in the mucosa. CPS class III (a) and PAP method for SC (b), lysozyme (c) and CEA/NCA (d). Hematoxylin counterstain, ×150.

Layered distribution of markers is evident in any mucosal area of this signet ring cell carcinoma. Small-sized cells in the bottom layer are positive for CPS class III, SC and lysozyme, while CEA/NCA is strongly expressed in mature signet ring cells in the upper layer. SC is almost negative in the lowermost narrow zone (arrowheads) where CPS class III-reactive slightly larger-sized cells are distributed. SC-positive cancer cells may represent mitogenic cancer cells (see text). Intestinalized epithelia are positive for SC and CEA/NCA (thin arrows). Scattered cells strongly positive for lysozyme are granulocytes and macrophages in the stroma, and Paneth cells (thick arrow).

**TABLE 1-8**
Zonal Differentiation of Signet Ring Cancer Cells in the Mucosa: Analysis Using 50 Early Carcinomas

| Marker | Zonation* | +++ | ++ | + | − | Reversed** |
|---|---|---|---|---|---|---|
| SC | lower | 10(3) | 9(2) | 13(2) | 13(5) | 5(0) |
| lysozyme | lower | 17(4) | 18(4) | 10(1) | 5(3) | 0(0) |
| pepsinogen II*** | lower | 2(0) | 9(3) | 9(1) | 27(6) | 0(0) |
| CEA | upper | 32(7) | 13(4) | 5(1) | 0(0) | 0(0) |
| CPS class III | lower | 17(4) | 13(1) | 13(3) | 7(4) | 0(0) |
| sulfomucin | lower | 5(4) | 7(2) | 8(1) | 30(5) | 0(0) |

( ): indicates the number of "sm" cancer (total 12 cases)

* The zonal distribution of marker is seen in most (+ + +), less than two thirds (+ +), less than one third (+), or none (-) of areas of the mucosal lesion.

** The reversed pattern of SC is seen in five tumors, in which SC immunoreactivity is demonstrated in the upper layer of the mucosa.

*** Immunostaining of pepsinogen II was not done for three specimens.

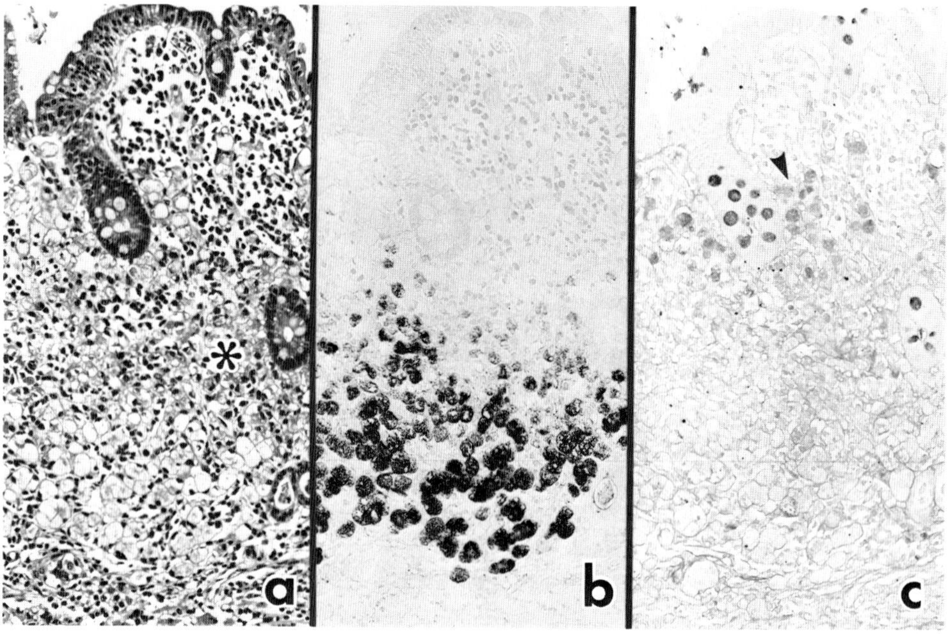


**Fig. 1-12.** Zonal differentiation of signet ring cell carcinoma in the mucosa. H&E (a), CPS class III with methyl green counterstain (b) and HID-AB (c), ×120.

Bidirectional differentiation of intramucosally occupying signet ring cells is evident. The lower half layer contains well matured signet ring cells of the pyloric gland type, while signet ring cells distributed in the upper layer are faintly alcianophilic (arrowhead) without CPS class III reactivity. The middle zone marked by asterisk is composed of small-sized immature-looking cells intermingled with CPS class III-reactive cells.

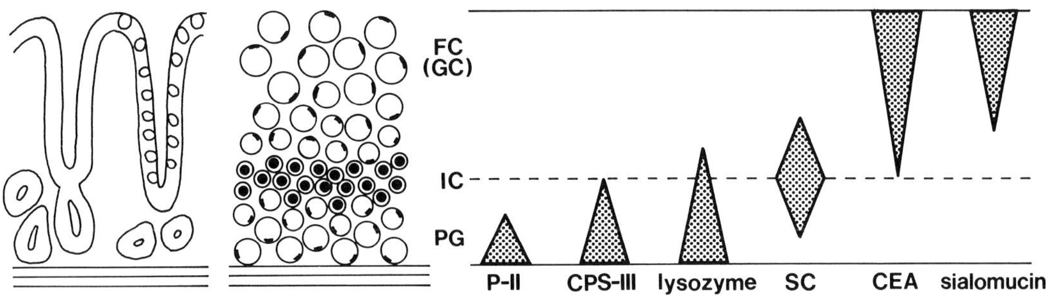


**Fig. 1-13.** Schematic representation of the zonal expression of markers in signet ring cell carcinoma in the mucosa.

**FC(GC):** signet ring cells of the surface epithelial cell type (occasionally goblet cell type)
**IC:** immature-looking cancer cells
**PG:** signet ring cells of the pyloric gland type
**P-II:** pepsinogen II

unabsorbed antibody, although some decrease of the number and staining intensity of positive cells was noted. The width of the CEA-positive zone in the "upper" layer varied from tumor to tumor: In some tumors, CEA was positive in most cells except for the lowermost narrow zone of the mucosa, while other tumors contained CEA-positive signet ring cells only in the uppermost zone. Less pronouncedly, the variation of the width of the positive zone was noted for SC, lysozyme, and CPS class III mucin. Thus, double positivity for CEA and SC, lysozyme or CPS class III mucin in cells in the same layer was occasionally noted. The zonation pattern of the markers is schematically illustrated in Figure 1-13.

Pepsinogen II, a marker of both pyloric and fundic glands, was less frequently expressed in signet ring cancer cells, but if positive, it showed a distinct zonation pattern at the lower layer of the mucosa. Sulfomucin in cancer cells occupying the bottom layer of the mucosa certainly reflects the fact that atrophic pyloric glands are occasionally positive for sulfomucin. Furthermore, by AB-PAS staining 39 of 50 tumors showed a predominance of neutral mucin in signet ring cancer cells. Acid mucin predominance was seen only in four tumors. Sialomucin-positive mature signet ring cells were fairly consistently scattered in the upper layer of the mucosa in all but three tumors, although the staining intensity with alcian blue was mostly weak (Fig. 1-12c). The sialomucin-positive signet ring cancer cells are not necessarily a counterpart of goblet cells, since hyperplastic or regenerative foveolar cells without intestinal metaplasia often stain weakly positive for sialomucin.

When we observe intramucosal lesions of signet ring cell carcinoma, taking into account the above information, the multilamellar pattern formed by signet ring cancer cells is easily recognized even in H&E preparations (Figs. 1-12a and 1-14a). Typical signet ring cells occur in the upper and bottom layers of the mucosa, whereas immature-looking small cancer cells with scanty or finely vacuolated cytoplasm are distributed at the junctional zone between the above two layers, which correspond to the level of the generative zone of normal or inflamed antral mucosa. The immature-looking cancer cells in the junctional zone occasionally show mitoses. Signet ring cells in the upper layer are generally larger than those in the bottom layer. In many specimens with tumors arising from the fundic mucosa, the oxyntic glands especially adjacent to the tumors showed antralization, resulting in the formation of pseudopyloric glands with or without remaining parietal cells. Chief cells were absent from the antralized mucosa.

In a few cancers arising from the fundic mucosa with fairly intact oxyntic glands, the immature cancer cell layer occupied the level

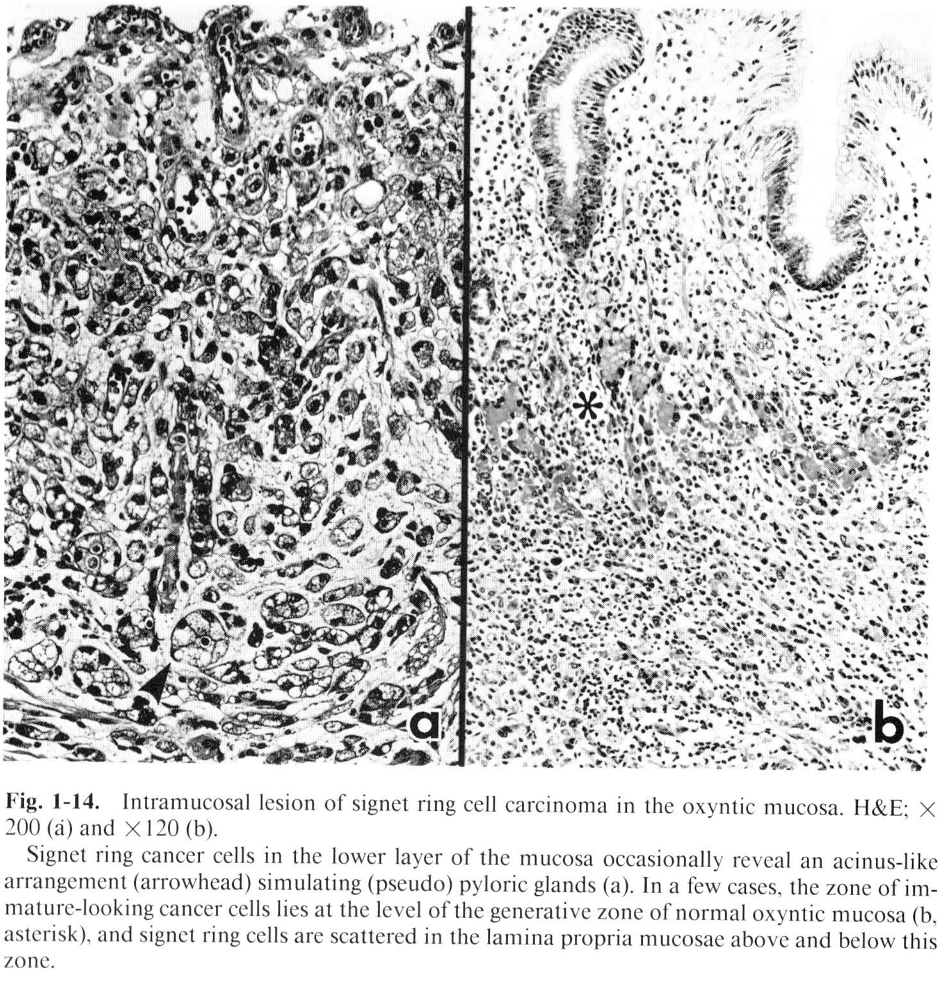


**Fig. 1-14.** Intramucosal lesion of signet ring cell carcinoma in the oxyntic mucosa. H&E; × 200 (a) and ×120 (b).

Signet ring cancer cells in the lower layer of the mucosa occasionally reveal an acinus-like arrangement (arrowhead) simulating (pseudo) pyloric glands (a). In a few cases, the zone of immature-looking cancer cells lies at the level of the generative zone of normal oxyntic mucosa (b, asterisk), and signet ring cells are scattered in the lamina propria mucosae above and below this zone.

of the generative zone of normal fundic mucosa, but the differentiation toward parietal cells or chief cells by cancer cells occupying the lower half layer was hardly evident (Fig. 1-14b).[17,71] The cancer cells in the bottom layer with histochemical characteristics of pyloric gland cells (pyloric gland-type signet ring cells) varied in their morphological features from case to case. In some tumors, (e.g., the tumor in Figure 1-10), the pyloric gland-type cancer cells looked so immature and small-sized that we were unable to recognize the junctional zone. In many such tumors, not only lysozyme and CPS class III but also SC reactivities were seen with a bottom-layered pattern.

In other tumors, the pyloric gland-type cancer cells were so well developed as to form an acinus-like arrangement (Fig. 1-14a). In the latter case, pepsinogen II immunoreactive pyloric gland-type cancer cells were rather frequently encountered, while immunoreactivity for SC was scarcely seen. In one tumor, cancer cells in the lower half mucosal layer showed quite a well organized arrangement simulating normal pyloric glands, while cancer cells in the upper half layer were arranged in abortive tubules consisting of columnar atypical cells (Fig. 1-15). SC was exclusively detected in the latter cancer cells, resulting in a reversed distribution pattern of SC. The mature pyloric gland-like cancer cells were posi-

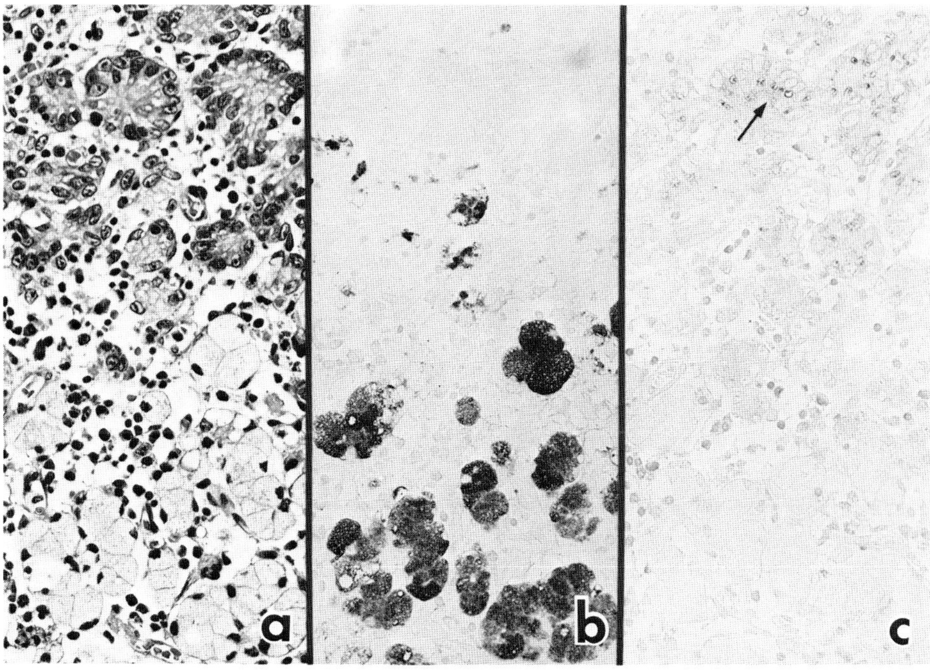


**Fig. 1-15.** Signet ring cell carcinoma with a reversed SC expression in the mucosa. H&E (a), CPS class III (b) and indirect immunoperoxidase method for SC (c). Methyl green counterstain (b & c), ×240.

This intramucosal cancer looks like mature pyloric glands (SC-negative) in the lower half of the mucosa, while cells in the upper layer display a tubular differentiation with SC immunoreactivity (arrow). The mode of marker expression corresponds to that in "incompletely" intestinalized mucosa.

tive for lysozyme, while the tubularly arranged part contained scattered goblet-like cells of small size and showed CEA immunoreactivity in cancer cells near the gastric lumen. Therefore, this cancer tissue resembled intestinalized mucosa with remaining pyloric glands at the bottom, not only morphologically, but also histochemically. The reversed pattern of SC staining was encountered in five tumors, three of which were focally associated with characteristics of adenoplastic carcinomas.

A varying number of signet ring cells with intracytoplasmic lumen (ICL) were seen in 29 of 50 early signet ring cell carcinomas examined. Four tumors showed many signet ring cells of the ICL type, 10 tumors showed a modest number, and 15 tumors contained a few. Ultrastructurally, the plasma membranes of ICL have been described as comparable to the absorptive surface of intestinal-type epithelial cells.[30] ICL has been reported as a specific structure of various adenocarcinoma cells, especially of breast carcinoma.[72] In fact, signet ring cells with ICL were easily detected in tumors with admixed adenoplastic components. However, with AB-PAS staining the mucin in ICL was often neutral, but not acidic. Signet ring cells of the pyloric gland type also occasionally formed ICLs, as Figure 1-16 illustrates. Therefore, the detection of signet ring cells of the ICL type does not necessarily indicate their intestinal differentiation.

*Discussion:* It is worthy of note that gastric cancer cells in the mucosa often simulate the polarity of differentiation of their noncancer-

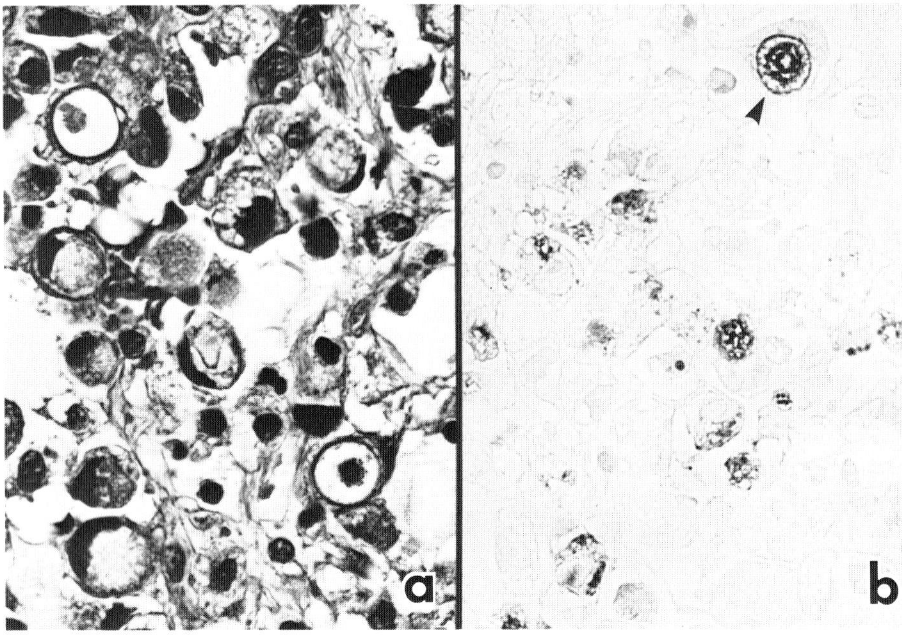


**Fig. 1-16.** Signet ring cells of the intracytoplasmic lumen (ICL) type. H&E (a) and CPS class III (b), ×600.

A varying number of signet ring cells with ICL are not infrequently intermingled with ordinary signet ring cells. They are often present in tumors focally showing a tubular component. Signet ring cells of the ICL type reactive to CPS class III are occasionally observed (b, arrowhead).

ous counterparts. The polarity is expressed as the zonal (lamellar or layered) distribution of the glycoprotein antigens and mucins of the pyloric gland and goblet cell types.[9,29,30,35,36] Such organized differentiation in the mucosa is more stable and more synchronized in signet ring cell carcinoma than in adenoplastic carcinoma.[35] Early cancer with rather intact noncancerous epithelial structures more clearly shows the zonation pattern than advanced cancer with severely distorted noncancerous epithelium. These findings suggest that the cancer cell differentiation is regulated by the microenvironment in the mucosa, as is shown in normal tissues.[73] In other words, stromal elements in the lamina propria mucosae are able to control the differentiation and growth of cancer cells, as has been described by Fujita.[8,9,74]

Tsuchihashi has clearly proved that mucosal microvascular networks in the stomach form a functional trilayered zonation corresponding to three such epithelial layers as glands, generative cells and surface lining cells.[75] Watanabe emphasized with experimental models of radiation pneumonia the importance of preceding changes of vascular and lymphatic microcirculation in pulmonary alveoli for the progression of interstitial inflammation and the formation of fibrosis.[76] Intact mucosal microcirculatory networks should, therefore, be greatly involved in establishing the cancer-regulating microenviroment. Meanwhile, certain degrees of the organoid differentiation were demonstrated at the site of invasion of some advanced carcinomas. This fact suggests a partial induction of cancer cell differentiation by the stromal elements even at extramucosal sites.

Quite interestingly, it has been clarified with [$^3$H]-thymidine autoradiography that cancer cells with proliferation ability in the mucosal lesion of early signet ring cell carcinoma are solely distributed in the zone of the generative cells found in noncancerous mucosa.[9,77] These mitogenic cells are equivalent to immature cancer cells located between mature signet ring cells in the upper layer and pyloric gland-type signet ring cells in the bottom layer. With rare exceptions, typical signet ring cells filled with cytoplasmic mucin have been shown to lack mitotic activity.[9,77] Thus, the initial site of carcinogenesis in signet ring cell carcinoma must be logically in the zone of generative cells, as has been pointed out by Fujita.[9] CEA-positive mature signet ring cells in the upper layer of the mucosa react strongly to PAS, and weakly and inconsistently to alcian blue in most cases. Such histochemical reactions probably reflect the properties of hyperplastic or regenerative gastric foveolar epithelium. Katsuyama et al demonstrated the properties of gastric surface epithelial cell-type mucin in these mature signet ring cells with the galactose oxidase-Schiff (GOS) sequence.[30]

From our limited experience, MOS-positive and strongly alcianophilic signet ring cells (goblet cell-type), which are frequently present in mucinous adenocarcinoma, are also found in some early signet ring cell carcinomas. The presence of PA-SB-PH-PAS reactive goblet cell mucin in such signet ring cells has been described by Katsuyama et al.[30] It is concluded that neoplastic cells in the mucosa with signet ring cell carcinoma proliferate in the generative immature cell layer and differentiate upward to the surface to become surface epithelial-type cells or goblet-type cells, and downward to the deeper layer to become pyloric gland-type cells, as has been reported independently by groups of Katsuyama,[29,30] Fujita[9,74] and ourselves.[35,36] It is quite reasonable that the mitogenic and immature-looking cancer cells in the mucosa are a neoplastic counterpart of totipotent stem cells in the nonneoplastic mucosa. They, which may be called "malignant stem cells,"[78-81] are capable of mitosis and of differentiation under the appropriate influence of the mucosal microenvironment.

On the other hand, it has been shown by Fujita that adenoplastic cancer cells in the mucosa are able to incorporate [$^3$H]-thymidine into DNA in any layer of the mucosa.[9] Namely, the proliferation site of adenoplastic carcinoma is not related to the generative zone of the noncancerous mucosa. This fact necessarily corresponds to our observation that the zonation pattern of histochemical markers is often focal and abortive in adenoplastic carcinomas.

Of great interest is the difference of CEA expression between lesions in the mucosa and lesions at the invading site of signet ring cell carcinoma. In noncancerous mucosa, CEA is localized in the uppermost surface lining cells with or without intestinalization, the cells without mitotic activity, as occurs in normal intestine.[49,82] Cells in the generative zone are negative for CEA. As discussed above, in the mucosal lesion of many signet ring cell carcinomas, CEA is expressed on mature signet ring cells without mitotic activity occupying the upper layer of the mucosa, while immature-looking proliferative cells are usually devoid of CEA immunoreactivity. On the other hand, the morphology of invading cancer cells in advanced signet ring cell carcinomas with scirrhous growth usually resembles that of immature-looking proliferative cells in the mucosa. It is quite different from the mucosal lesion, in that the immature-looking cancer cells at the invading site almost always display strong immunoreactivity for CEA or CEA/NCA in addition to occasional reactivities to lysozyme, SC and/or CPS class III.

Such a discrepancy of CEA expression between the mucosal and invading lesions is a genuine problem that must be solved. It is assumed that the expression of CEA in a given cell is time-dependent, but is not directly related to the cell cycle (i.e., CEA is a substance appearing on the cell membranes with a fixed time lag after the mitotic event, whether the cell has proliferative ability or not).

It has been described that both leukemia cells[83] and gastric cancer cells[9] show a decrease of the ratio of cells in the generative cycle and an elongation of cellular life span in comparison with their normal counterparts. It has further been disclosed that the [$^3$H]-thymidine-labeling index is lower in invading cancer cells of scirrhous carcinomas than in mucosally located cancer cells.[84] The presence of postmitotic and nonproliferating tumor stem cells in $G_0$ phase has been described in invasive mammary adenocarcinoma of mice.[85] The maturation or differentiation of immature cancer cells should be quite reasonably restricted by the presence of thick fibrous tissue at the invading site. Consequently, the cancer cells with an elongated life span come to express CEA excessively with maturation in the upper layer of the mucosa, and with restricted maturation at the invading site.

## 5. DIFFERENTIATION TO ENDOCRINE CELLS IN SCIRRHOUS CARCINOMA

A wide variety of carcinomas, especially adenocarcinomas, are known to contain neoplastic cells with endocrine nature, even when they are not categorized as so-called neuroendocrine tumors.[31,86] Scirrhous carcinoma of the stomach is one of the representatives of such tumors, since plentiful endocrine-like cells with a positive argyrophil reaction have been detected among scirrhously invading cancer cells.[32,34,40] Such cancers are called as argyrophilic carcinoma.[32,34]

In this part, the differentiation to endocrine cells in scirrhous carcinoma is analyzed and characterized with the indirect immunoperoxidase method. First, the properties of endocrine cells in nontumorous mucosa are presented.[38,57,87] The specificity of the immunostaining was confirmed by absorption experiments using synthetic or purified antigens, as reported previously.[38,57]

In both antral and oxyntic mucosa, there are scattered argyrophil cells and argentaffin (enterochromaffin, EC) cells identified by Grimelius silver and Masson's silver, respectively. Argentaffin cells are argyrophilic, but argyrophil cells are not necessarily argentaffin. Argentaffin cells in nonmetaplastic gastric mucosa (gastric EC cells) are marked by their closed position (without direct contact to the gland lumen). These cells are fairly evenly distributed in the generative zone through the pyloric or oxyntic glands.

Gastrin cells and somatostatin cells are present mainly in the generative zone of antral mucosa and occasionally among the pyloric glands. Somatostatin cells are also scattered in the oxyntic glands where gastrin cells are absent. The occurrence of gastrin cells in pseudopyloric glands in fundic mucosa is exceptional. Glicentin (enteroglucagon or proglucagon) cells, in which pancreatic glucagon immunoreactivity is frequently, but not consistently detected, are distributed in fetal fundic mucosa, while adult oxyntic glands are devoid of glicentin immunoreactive cells.[38] Drastic changes of endocrine cells occur in the mucosa with intestinal metaplasia, as reported previously.[38,57] Selective and often hyperplastic increase of glicentin cells, argyrophil cells, and intestinal EC cells is quite characteristic of intestinal metaplasia. Intestinal EC cells with an open position (showing direct contact to the gland lumen) are easily recognized as basal granulated cells in H&E preparations.[57] The occurrence of pancreatic glucagon and PP immunoreactivities in the glicentin cells is infrequent.[38] Gastrin cells, somatostatin cells, and gastric EC cells are rarely present after the metaplastic change.[57]

Chromogranin is a substance present in cored granules of various endocrine cells including adrenomedullary cells and parathyroid cells,[40,88] and is known to be cosecreted with a variety of peptide hormones and amines.[89,90] In the gastrointestinal tract, chromogranin-positive endocrine cells correspond fairly well to the argyrophil and argentaffin cells.[40] Some of the gastrin cells and glicentin cells are chromogranin-positive, whereas most of the peptide-containing cells are argyrophobic.[40]

The occurrence of endocrine-like cells in the mucosal lesion of early signet ring cell carcinoma[33] is now commented on. Immunoperoxidase staining for chromogranin and Grimelius silver are used to detect such a

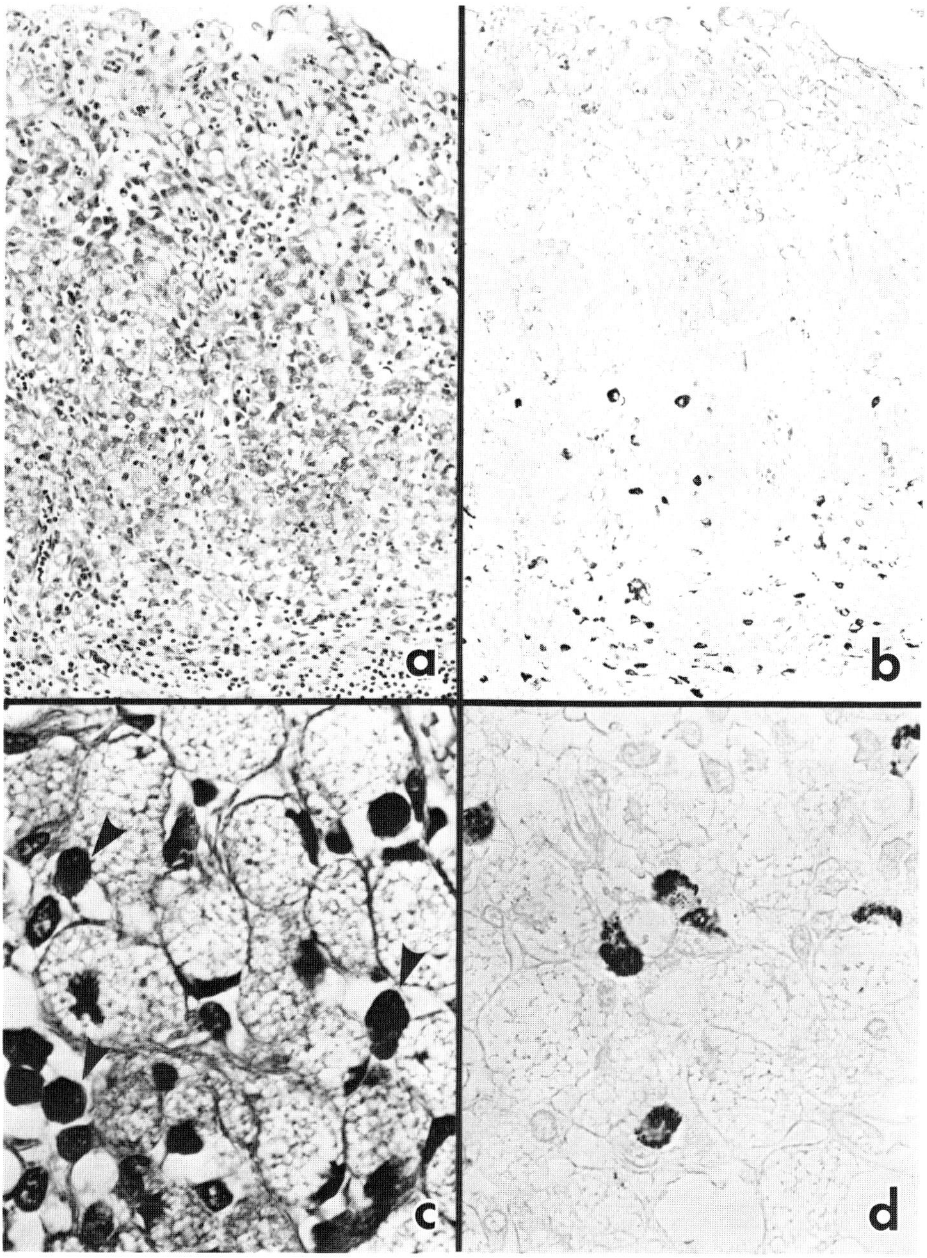


**Fig. 1-17.** Differentiation of intramucosal signet ring cell carcinoma to endocrine-like cells. H&E (a) and Grimelius silver (b), ×150. H&E (c) and indirect immunoperoxidase method for chromogranin (d), ×750.

Argyrophilic cancer cells are predominantly distributed in the bottom layer of the mucosa. High power view reveals that the endocrine-like cells with granular cytoplasmic reaction to chromogranin are small in size and correspond to small non-signet ring cells with eosinophilic granularity in the cytoplasm (arrowheads).

component. Both methods gave almost the same results for the detection of endocrine-like cells. Keen attention was paid to evaluation of whether the positive cells were neoplastic or not, since (1) atrophic pyloric glands commonly persist in the cancerous mucosa and (2) isolated micronodules of endocrine cells are frequently distributed in the lamina propria of the mucosa with atrophic gastritis.[33,57,87] Of 59 lesions examined, 14 showed many endocrine-like cancer cells, 20 showed scattered cells, nine showed only a few cells, and 16 were devoid of such cells. It is noteworthy that the endocrine-like cells were almost always distributed in the lower half layer or, more frequently, at the bottom of the mucosa, as are endocrine cells in noncancerous mucosa.

This distribution pattern of endocrine-like cells should be another example of the zonal differentiation shown by signet ring cancer cells in the mucosa. Figure 1-17(a,b) shows a representative picture of intramucosally located cancer differentiating to argyrophilic endocrine-like cells. Figure 1-17(c,d) illustrates a high power view of the bottom layer of the mucosa of another case, where numbers of chromogranin-positive cells are intermingled with signet ring cells of the pyloric gland-type. Characteristically, the endocrine-like cells have small amounts of granular cytoplasm without mucin in H&E preparations.

Table 1-9 summarizes results of histochemical analysis of endocrine-like cells in 26 scirrhous carcinomas of the stomach. Seven scirrhous carcinomas contained numbers of cells with a positive Grimelius reaction in the gastric wall, and could be categorized as argyrophilic carcinoma (Fig. 1-18). Varying numbers of argyrophilic neoplastic cells were seen at the invading site of 15 of 26 tumors. An additional five tumors exhibited argyrophilic cancer cells only in the mucosa. Thus, the occurrence of argyrophilic cancer cells in scirrhous carcinoma is quite frequent.[32,34,38]

On the contrary, Masson's silver-positive argentaffin tumor cells were infrequently noted in those specimens. Of five peptide hormones examined, glicentin immunoreactive cells were most frequently demonstrated (Fig. 1-18c). Cancers with two-plus or one-plus glicentin cells in Table 1-9 were all argyrophilic carcinomas, although most, if not all, glicentin cells have been shown to be argyrophobic.[38] Pancreatic glucagon immunoreactivity was detected in the glicentin-containing cells in two tumors, while no PP immunoreactive cells were noted. A small to modest number of somatostatin-containing cells were present in six of 16 tumors (Fig. 1-18d).[34] The infrequency of gastrin-positive scirrhous cancer cells possibly reflects the fact that most tumors originated from the oxyntic mucosa. However, Tahara et al described the rather frequent occurrence of gastrin-positive cells in scirrhous carcinomas.[34]

The occurrence of glicentin immunoreactive cells in scirrhous carcinoma is preferably interpreted to be an expression of fetalism in cancer cells, since glicentin is present in endocrine cells of fetal oxyntic mucosa, but it is absent from those of adult oxyntic mucosa.[38]

**TABLE 1-9**
Endocrine-like Cells at Invading Site of 26 Scirrhous Carcinomas of the Stomach

| | ++ | + | (+) | − | ND |
|---|---|---|---|---|---|
| Argyrophil | 7 | 4 | 4 | 11[5] | 0 |
| Argentaffin | 0 | 0 | 2 | 20 | 4 |
| Glicentin 49–69 | 2 | 2 | 4 | 18[1] | 0 |
| Glucagon 19–29 | 0 | 2 | 0 | 21 | 3 |
| PP | 0 | 0 | 0 | 13 | 13 |
| Somatostatin | 0 | 3 | 3 | 10 | 10 |
| Gastrin | 0 | 0 | 1 | 15 | 10 |

++: plentiful positive cells seen
+: positive cells scattered
(+): only a few cells positive
−: negative
ND: not done
Glicentin 49–69: enteroglucagon or proglucagon
Glucagon 19–29: pancreatic-type glucagon
PP: pancreatic polypeptide
[ ]: the number of tumors with positive cells only in the mucosa

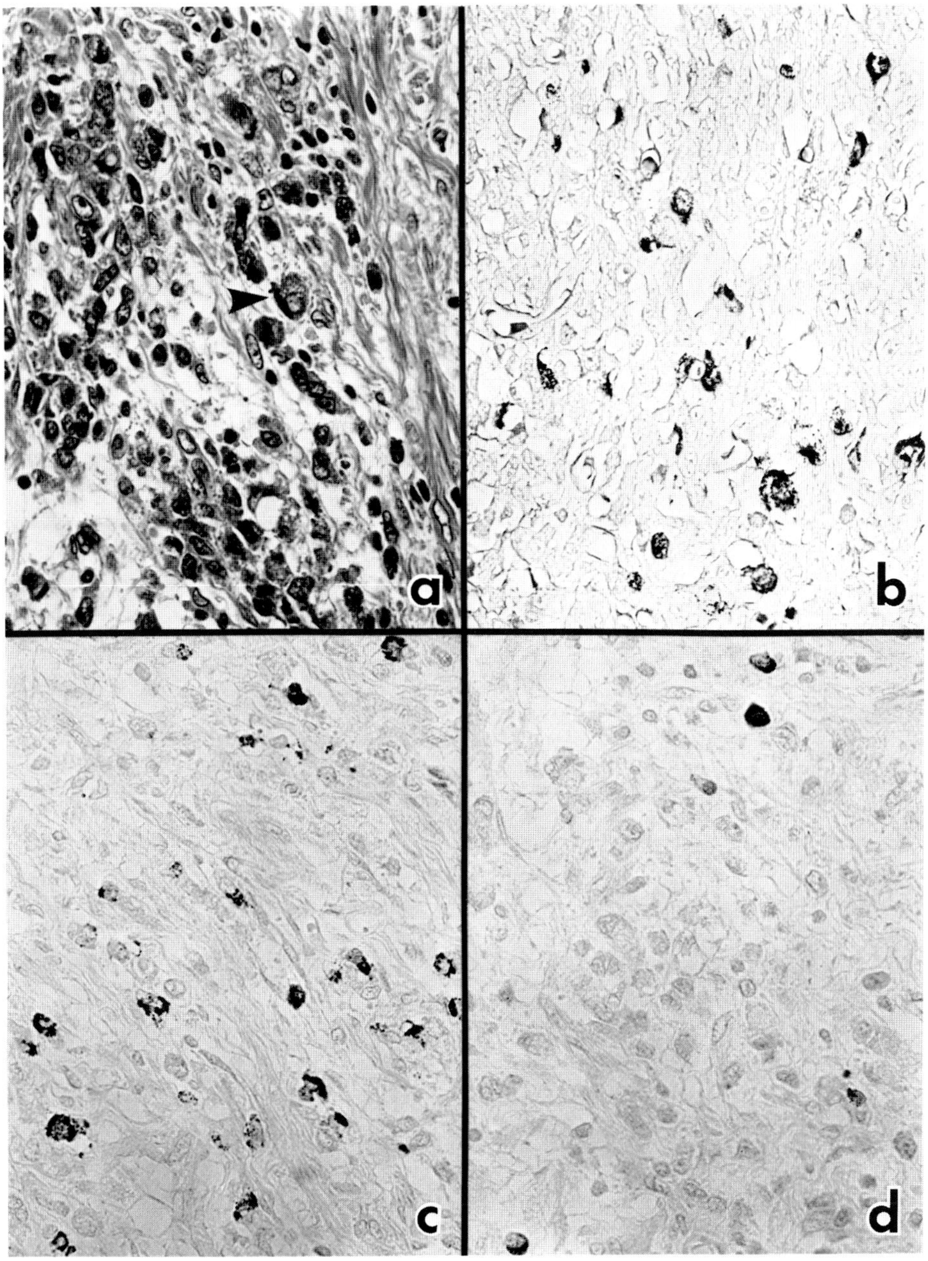


**Fig. 1-18.** Scirrhous argyrophil carcinoma of the stomach. H&E (a), Grimelius silver (b) and immunoperoxidase method for glicentin (c) and somatostatin (d). Methyl green counterstain (c & d), ×400.

Scirrhously infiltrating cancer cells usually look immature and occasionally show a cytoplasmic granularity (arrowhead). Argyrophil reaction and peptide hormone immunoreactivity (especially of glicentin) are often positive in such cancer cells.

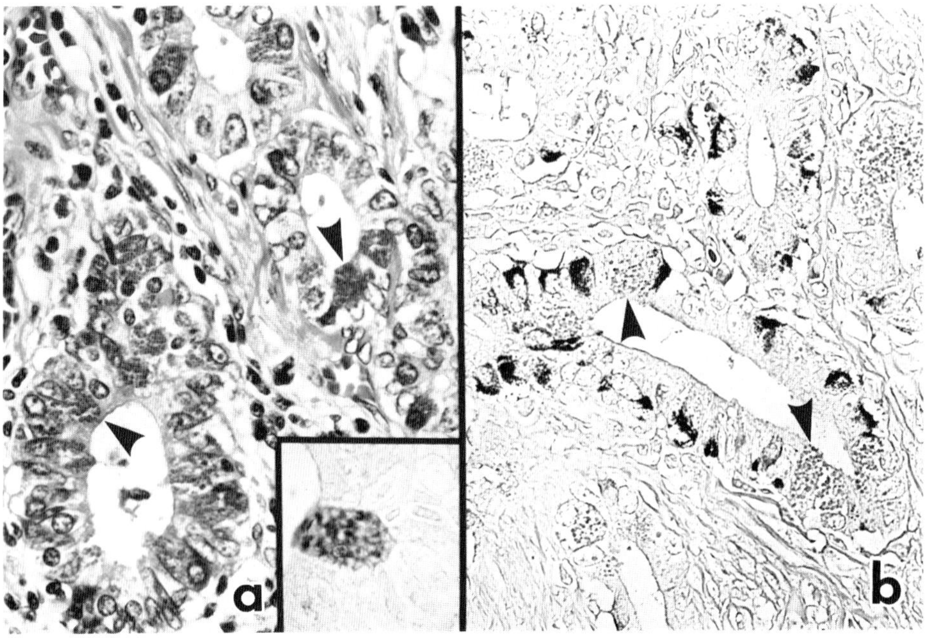

**Fig. 1-19.** Advanced adenoplastic carcinoma ($tub_1$) partially differentiating toward Paneth cells and endocrine-like cells. H&E (a) and Grimelius silver (b), ×400. Indirect immunoperoxidase method for lysozyme (inset), ×750.

Infiltrating tubular adenocarcinoma contains numbers of Paneth cells (arrowheads) with immunoreactive lysozyme. In addition, the existence of plentiful argyrophil cells is characteristic of this tumor.

Intestinalized mucosa has been proved to exhibit a number of glicentin-containing endocrine cells,[38,57] but the above phenomenon is unlikely to represent an intestinal phenotype, because most scirrhous carcinomas have their origin in nonintestinalized oxyntic mucosa. The frequent association of endocrine differentiation in diffuse carcinoma of the stomach is closely related to the facts that (1) from the standpoint of cell kinetics, the endocrine cell in the gastric mucosa belongs to a dissociative cell group,[91] and the tumor cell of diffuse carcinoma is literally an extreme expression of a dissociative cell;[8,9] and that (2) nontumorous endocrine cells under fibrotic conditions frequently show hyperplastic proliferations, including islet cells in chronic pancreatitis,[92] endocrine cell micronodules in chronic gastritis,[33,57,87] and pulmonary tumorlets with fibrotic derangement of peribronchial tissue.[93,94]

On the other hand, the detection of endocrine-like cells in adenoplastic carcinomas is a rare occasion. In fact, of 23 adenoplastic carcinomas invading into the submucosa or deeper areas, only three tumors exhibited a few or scattered Grimelius-positive cancer cells at the invading site, whereas four of seven intramucosally located adenoplastic carcinomas contained scattered endocrine-like cells in the cancerous glands. Adenoplastic carcinomas with plentiful endocrine-like cells as a neoplastic component are very limited in our experience so far. In a few adenoplastic carcinomas, such cells were easily recognized in H&E preparations as basal granulated cells, which clearly revealed both argyrophil and argentaffin reactions. Interestingly enough, many of such tumors also contained typical Paneth cells with strong immunoreactivity for lysozyme as shown in

Figure 1-19.[95] Immunohistochemically, most argyrophilic tumor cells stained positive for chromogranin, while a number of cells immunoreactive to glicentin were also commonly distributed in the cancerous glands.[40] Cells immunoreactive to pancreatic glucagon, PP, somatostatin, or gastrin were less or a few in number. The expression pattern is intimately related to that of intestinal metaplasia.

*Comment:* When we note the occurrence of endocrine-like cells in nonneuroendocrine carcinoma, it is quite fascinating to suppose there is a totipotent neoplastic stem cell, as has been vigorously investigated in hematopoietic malignancies.[96] The carcinogenesis occurs at the level of the tumor stem cell or differentiation-committed immature cell,[78–81] and it then differentiates, under the influence of mucosal microenvironment, into various epithelial cell types such as surface epithelial cell, absorptive cell, goblet cell, pyloric gland cell, Paneth cell, and endocrine cell. The same assumption has been proposed in teratocarcinoma[97] and in other nonhematopoietic malignancies[78,79] including lung cancer.[80,81]

In fact, the endodermal origin of dispersed endocrine cells in the alimentary and respiratory tracts has been clarified,[79,98] denying the original Pearse hypothesis of their neural crest (neuroectodermal) origin. He proposed the concept of the APUD (amine precursor uptake and decarboxylation) system.[99] With the assumption of the totipotent tumor stem cell,[78–81] we as pathologists can reasonably understand our frequent experiences of such mixed forms of endocrine and nonendocrine tumors as goblet cell carcinoid of the vermiform appendix,[100] an intermediate form of papillary and medullary carcinoma of the thyroid gland,[101] small cell lung carcinoma with glandular and squamous cells,[102] and a variety of adenocarcinomas with endocrine-like cells.[31,86] We have further disclosed that SC-immunoreactive nonneuroendocrine neoplastic cells are occasionally present in ordinary gastrointestinal carcinoid tumors and in pancreatic islet cell tumors.[94]

## 6. PRODUCTION OF ALPHA-FETOPROTEIN AND HUMAN CHORIONIC GONADOTROPIN BY GASTRIC CANCER: EXPRESSION OF "RETRODIFFERENTIATION"

Production of $\alpha$-fetoprotein (AFP) is characteristic of hepatocellular carcinoma, hepatoblastoma, and teratocarcinoma.[103] Increased levels of serum AFP have been described repeatedly, however, in patients with neoplasms of foregut origin.[21–23,104] Especially in Japan, many of these patients suffer from gastric cancer.[104] About 15% of patients with gastric cancer are known to show elevated serum AFP levels.[105] AFP has been directly demonstrated in gastric cancer tissue by both immunoassay[106] and immunohistochemistry.[21–23,39]

Our immunohistochemical analyses to characterize AFP-producing gastric cancer are presented below, in which 20 surgical specimens of gastric cancer with elevated serum AFP levels and 10 control surgical specimens of gastric cancer with negative serum AFP were studied.[39] Samples from metastatic sites (lymph nodes, livers or pancreas) including autopsy materials were also examined. Serum AFP was measured by the enzyme immunoassay, and 20 ng/ml or more were judged as positive.

Group A included 11 cases with preoperatively elevated levels of serum AFP. Group B included nine cases whose preoperative sera failed to show the elevation of AFP, but AFP levels were elevated after surgery. Group C included 10 unselected serial cases with negative serum AFP levels throughout the clinical course. The indirect immunoperoxidase staining was performed to detect CEA, human chorionic gonadotropin (HCG), placental alkaline phosphatase (PALP), SC and lysozyme as well as AFP. AntiCEA was prepared to be unreactive to NCA by previous absorption. AntiHCG is reactive to both alpha and beta subunits of HCG. AntiPALP partially cross-reacts to alkaline phosphatase of the intestinal type,[107] since the brush border of normal duodenal lining cells and of some, but not all, intestinalized epithelia stains positive in addition to plasma membranes of normal placental syncytiotrophoblasts and seminoma cells.[108] To demonstrate glycogen and mucin, PAS reactions with or without diastase treatment and the AB-PAS sequence were employed.

Clinical and histochemical data are summarized in Table 1-10. With regard to immunostaining of AFP, nine of 11 tumors in group A, five of nine tumors in group B, and none of 10 in group C were positive. Noncancerous gastric tissue was uniformly negative for AFP. Serum AFP levels of AFP stain-negative cases in groups A and B were relatively low (211 ng/ml maximum). In contrast with the observation by Kodama et al,[23] a rough correlation between serum AFP levels and staining tendency for AFP was noted. Namely, all four tumors accompanying extremely high levels of serum AFP (more than 10,000 ng/ml) immunohistochemically revealed a number of AFP-positive tumor cells (++ or +++). A case with relatively low serum AFP (141 ng/ml) but with two-plus AFP stain (case 4 in Table 1-10) suffered from early gastric cancer invading into the submucosa. Positive AFP staining was demonstrated in all nine cases with serum AFP levels of more than 1,000 ng/ml, in four of six cases with serum AFP levels between 100–1,000 ng/ml, and in only one of five cases with serum AFP levels between 20–100 ng/ml. In group B, there were two cases whose AFP staining was positive in the metastatic site but negative in the primary. This possibly reflects the postoperative elevation of serum AFP. All tumors with positive AFP staining in the primary site showed AFP-positive cells also in the metastatic site.

High incidence of liver metastasis in AFP producing gastric cancer has been pointed out.[26,104] Since mild to moderate elevation of serum AFP in patients with chronic hepatitis or liver cirrhosis has been described,[109] the production of AFP by nonneoplastic hepatocytes should also be considered,[104] especially in AFP stain-negative cases. In five liver tissues immunohistochemically examined, however, AFP was localized only in the metastatic tumors, and no hepatocytes were stained.

AFP immunoreactivity was mainly observed as vesicular or granular structures in the cytoplasm, which probably correspond to rough endoplasmic reticula and Golgi apparati as its localization sites. This intracytoplasmic pattern of positivity is totally identical to that in fetal hepatocytes and yolk sac tumor cells.[110]

It has been noted that histologically, AFP-producing gastric cancer tends to show a poorly differentiated medullary or well-differentiated papillary growth pattern.[23] In the present series, medullary carcinomas with paucity of mucin were often strongly positive for AFP (Fig. 1-20a,b). Four tumors were at least focally papillary adenocarcinomas, three of which were positive for AFP staining (Fig. 1-20c). Six tumors were signet ring cell (scirrhous) carcinomas including three with positive AFP staining (Fig. 1-20d). It is noteworthy that four neoplasms focally or diffusely showed histological features of embryonal carcinoma with positive AFP staining, as is shown and discussed later.

The common cytological feature of AFP-positive cancer cells was a clear and finely granular appearance of the cytoplasm, and the cells possessed abundant glycogen (Fig. 1-20a). The abundance of glycogen was also true for the AFP-positive tumor cells in signet ring cell carcinoma. On the basis of such a cytological feature, we can anticipate the occurrence of immunoreactive AFP in a given gastric cancer. Gitlin et al disclosed a small amount of AFP in gastrointestinal tissue extracts of human fetus.[111] Lee et al[22] and Miyayama and Miyayama[21] observed AFP immunoreactivity in fetal gastrointestinal epithelium of 9 to 16 or 21 gestational weeks. The gastrointestinal epithelium of the fetus is known to be rich in glycogen. Namely, fetal cells are shown to be relatively resistant to hypoxia and to have a well-developed anaerobic glycolysis system.[112] Accordingly, it is appro-

## TABLE 1-10

Immunohistochemical Analysis of AFP-Producing Gastric Cancer

| Case Age/ Sex | Site | Histology | Serum AFP Level (ng/ml) | | Mucin/ Glycogen | Immunohistochemistry | | | | | |
|---|---|---|---|---|---|---|---|---|---|---|---|
| | | | Pre-op. | Post-op. | | AFP | CEA | HCG | PALP | SC | Lysozyme |
| group A | | | | | | | | | | | |
| 1. 62M | St(sm) | por(med) | 1000< | 1000< | −** | +++ | + | − | − | (+) | − |
| | Liver | por(med) | | | −** | +++ | ++ | − | + | − | − |
| | Liver# | por(med) | | | −** | +++ | − | − | − | − | − |
| 2. 68M | St(se) | emb | 99.3 | 20.4–28200 | −** | ++ | + | (+) | (+) | − | − |
| | LN | emb | | | −** | ++ | + | (+) | (+) | − | − |
| | LN | $tub_2$ | | | ++(c) | − | +++ | − | − | +++ | ++ |
| | Liver# | emb | | | −** | ++ | + | − | | − | − |
| 3. 52M | St(se) | por(med) | 3500 | 54–15100 | +(s)* | ++ | +++ | + | + | (+) | − |
| | LN | por(med) | | | +(s)** | + | ++ | (+) | − | (+) | (+) |
| | Liver# | por(med) | | | +(s)** | (+) | +++ | − | | − | − |
| 4. 67M@ | St(sm) | por(med) | 141 | 67–3.2 | (+)(s/c)** | ++ | + | (+) | − | + | + |
| | | emb | | | −** | ++ | + | − | − | − | − |
| 5. 54F | St(se) | por(med) | 430 | 4300 | +(s/c)** | + | ++ | − | + | + | (+) |
| | LN | por(med) | | | −** | (+) | (+) | − | − | − | (+) |
| 6. 72F@ | St(se) | pap | 160 | 13.5–49 | +++(s) | (+) | +++ | − | − | + | − |
| | | por(med) | | | +(s) | − | (+) | − | − | − | − |
| | LN | por(med) | | | +(s)** | + | + | − | − | (+) | (+) |
| 7. 72M | St(se) | $tub_1$ | 36.4 | 168–1800 | +(s/c) | − | +++ | − | ++ | +++ | (+) |
| | | emb | | | −** | (+) | ++ | (+) | + | − | − |
| 8. 73M | St(pm) | $tub_1$/pap | 161 | 51.5–2.8 | (+)(s/c)** | + | +++ | (+) | +++ | + | − |
| | LN | pap | | | −** | ++ | +++ | − | +++ | + | − |
| | LN | por(med) | | | ++(c)** | ++ | ++ | − | − | − | +++ |
| 9. 69F | St(se) | pap | 38.0 | 21.1–1.0 | +++(s)* | − | ++ | (+) | (+) | ++ | + |
| | LN | pap | | | +++(s)* | − | +++ | (+) | (+) | + | (+) |
| | Liver | pap | | | +++(s)* | − | ++ | (+) | (+) | (+) | +++ |
| 10. 42F | St(se) | sig(sci) | 46.0 | 3.3–2300 | ++(s/c)** | + | +++ | (+) | +++ | ++ | (+) |
| | LN | sig | | | ++(s/c)** | (+) | +++ | − | +++ | +++ | (+) |
| 11. 29F | St(se) | sig(sci) | 211 | 27.7 | +++(s/c)* | − | +++ | + | ++ | +++ | + |
| | LN | sig | | | +++(s/c) | − | ++ | + | +++ | +++ | ++ |

| Case Age/ Sex | Site | Histology | Serum AFP Level (ng/ml) Pre-op. | Post-op. | Mucin/ Glycogen*,** | Immunohistochemistry AFP | CEA | HCG | PALP | SC | Lysozyme |
|---|---|---|---|---|---|---|---|---|---|---|---|
| group B | | | | | | | | | | | |
| 12. 78M | St(ss) | emb | negative | 10000< | –** | ++ | + | – | – | (+) | – |
| | LN | emb | | | –** | +++ | + | – | + | (+) | – |
| | Panc# | emb | | | –** | + | – | – | | – | – |
| 13. 58F | St(se) | por(med) | 13.0 | 108 | (+)(s) | – | (+) | – | – | (+) | (+) |
| | LN | por(med) | | | (+)(s)* | (+) | – | – | – | – | – |
| 14. 60F@ | St(sm) | $tub_1$ | 1.0 | 91–14.0 | +++(s) | – | +++ | – | (+) | +++ | – |
| | | por(med) | | | (+)(s) | – | +++ | – | (+) | + | – |
| | LN | por(med) | | | ++(s) | – | +++ | – | + | ++ | (+) |
| 15. 68F | St(se) | $tub_1$/pap | 6.0 | 1600–3550 | +(s/c)** | + | +++ | (+) | (+) | + | – |
| | LN | pap | | | +++(s/c)** | + | +++ | – | – | + | – |
| | Liver# | $tub_1$/pap | | | +(s/c)** | (+) | +++ | – | | – | – |
| 16. 39F | St(se) | sig(sci) | 3.8 | 168–1200 | ++(s/c)** | (+) | +++ | (+) | +++ | + | (+) |
| | LN | sig | | | +++(s/c)** | + | +++ | – | +++ | + | ++ |
| 17. 32F | St(se) | sig(sci) | 9.0 | 78 | +++(c) | – | +++ | – | ++ | ++ | – |
| | LN | sig | | | ++(c)** | + | +++ | + | +++ | (+) | (+) |
| 18. 32F | St(se) | sig(sci) | 2.0 | 2.8–48 | ++(c)** | – | +++ | – | +++ | ++ | (+) |
| | LN | sig | | | ++(c) | – | +++ | – | | + | – |
| 19. 62F | St(ss) | sig(sci) | negative | 22–2.0 | +++(c) | – | ++ | – | – | ++ | ++ |
| | Panc# | sig | | | +++(c) | – | +++ | – | | ++ | (+) |
| 20. 48M | St(ss) | sig(sci) | negative | 41–122 | ++(s/c) | – | ++ | (+) | + | ++ | + |
| | LN | sig | | | ++(c) | – | +++ | – | – | +++ | + |
| | LN# | $tub_1$ | | | ++(s) | – | +++ | – | | ++ | – |

| | | | | | | | | | | | | |
|---|---|---|---|---|---|---|---|---|---|---|---|---|
| group C | | | | | | | | | | | | |
| 21. | 68M | St(se) | pap | 3.4 | 15.5 | + +(c)* | − | + + + | − | + | + + + | (+) |
| 22. | 59M@ | St(m) | $tub_1$ | 2.1 | 2.3 | + + +(s) | − | + + | − | − | + + + | (+) |
| 23. | 42M | St(se) | $tub_1$ | 2.8 | 1.9 | + + +(s) | − | + + | (+) | − | + + + | + |
| 24. | 64M@ | St(ss) | $tub_2$ | 1.1 | 5.9 | + + +(s) | − | + | (+) | (+) | + | (+) |
| | | LN | $tub_1$ | | | + + +(s) | − | + + + | − | + | + + | (+) |
| 25. | 61F | St(se) | $tub_2$ | 1.1 | 2.0 | + +(s) | − | + + + | − | + + + | (+) | + + + |
| | | LN | $tub_2$ | | | + +(s) | − | + + | − | + + | − | + + |
| 26. | 62M@ | St(m) | sig | 1.0 | 1.5 | + + +(c) | − | + + + | (+) | (+) | + | + |
| 27. | 48M@ | St(sm) | sig | negative | 1.4 | + + +(c) | − | + + | (+) | − | + + + | + + |
| 28. | 47M | St(se) | por(med) | 1.0 | 1.8 | +(s/c)* | − | + + + | + | + + + | + | − |
| | | LN | sig | | | + + +(c) | − | + + + | − | + | (+) | (+) |
| 29. | 48M@ | St(se) | sig | negative | 1.0 | + +(s/c)* | − | + + + | − | (+) | − | (+) |
| 30. | 56F | St(se) | sig(sci) | 2.2 | 7.6 | + + +(s/c) | − | + + + | − | + | + | (+) |

+ + +: Many cancer cell are positive (>2/3).

+ +: A moderate number of cancer cells are positive (1/3 ~ 2/3).

+: A small number of cancer cells are positive (<1/3).

(+): Only a few cancer cells are positive.

−: No cancer cells are positive.

@: Patient alive

#: Autopsy material

med: medullary; sci: scirrhous; emb; embryonal carcinoma

(s): surface coat-type mucin

(c): intracytoplasmic mucin

** Many cancer cells are glycogen-rich.

* Glycogen-rich cancer cells are focally seen.

St: stomach; LN: lymph node; Panc: pancreas; m, sm, pm, ss, se: indicate the depth of invasion: m: mucosa, sm: submucosa, pm: proper muscle layer, ss: subserosa, and se: exposure onto the serosa

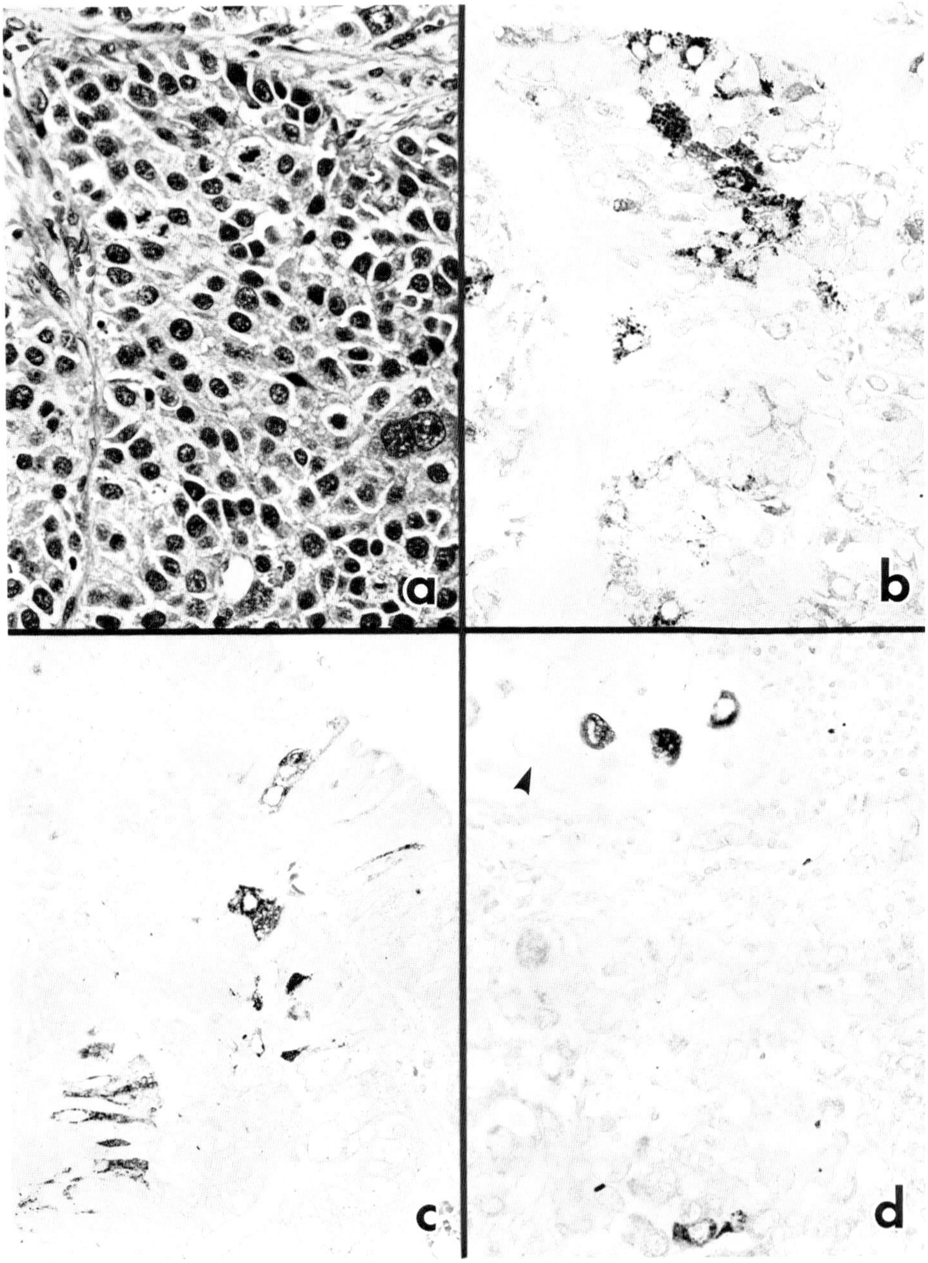


**Fig. 1-20.** Morphological variation of AFP-producing gastric carcinoma. Medullary carcinoma (case 1), a: H&E, b: AFP, ×300; papillary adenocarcinoma (case 15), c: AFP, ×240; and signet ring cell carcinoma (case 17, lymph node metastasis), d: AFP, ×300. Indirect immunoperoxidase method with methyl green counterstain.

Poorly differentiated medullary carcinoma consisting of cells with clear and finely granular cytoplasm frequently is accompanied by high serum AFP levels and numbers of AFP-positive cancer cells. Well-differentiated papillary adenocarcinoma and signet ring cell carcinoma occasionally show scattered AFP-positive cells. Mature signet ring cells (arrowhead) are usually devoid of AFP.

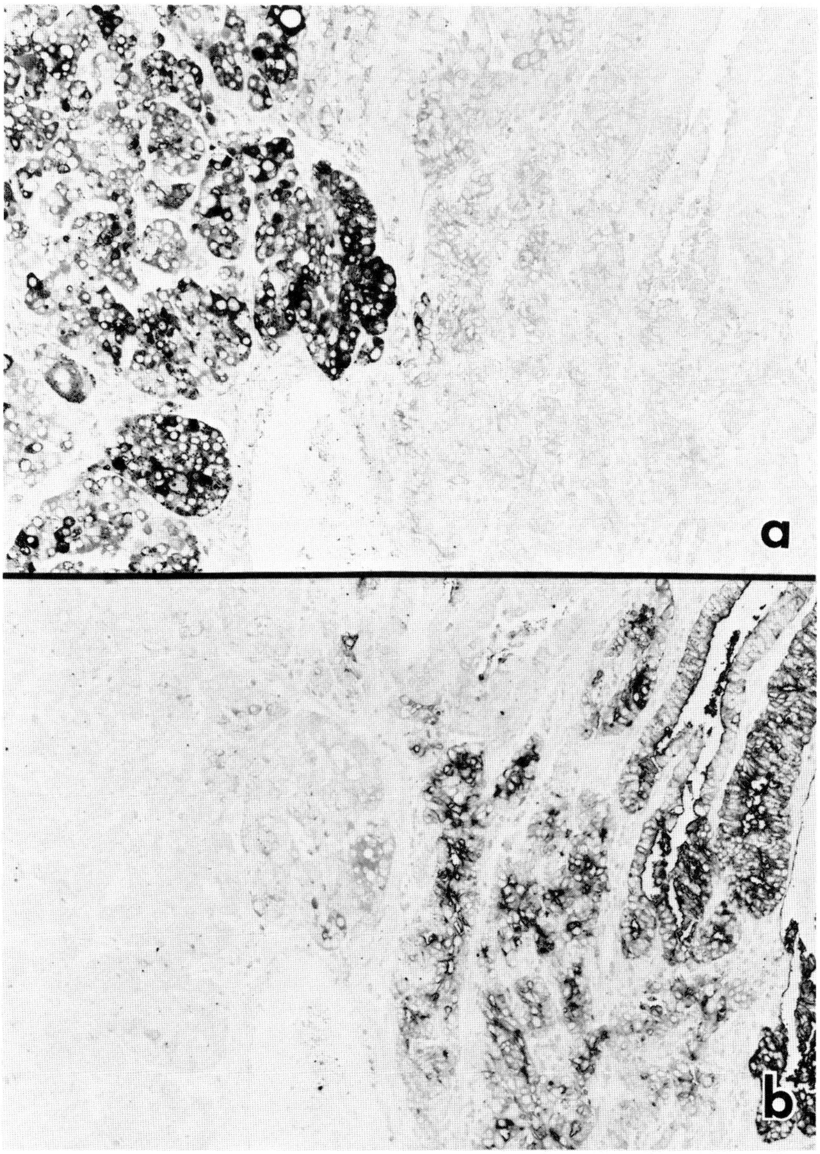


**Fig. 1-21.** Reciprocal localization of AFP (a) and CEA (b) in the mucosal lesion of case 4. Indirect immunoperoxidase method with methyl green counterstain, × 120.

AFP-positive area shows a medullary growth pattern whereas CEA-positive cancer cells proliferate in a papillotubular fashion.

priate to assume that AFP-producing gastric cancer has regained the properties of fetal gastrointestinal epithelium.

The intriguing contrast of the staining pattern between AFP and CEA[39] is presented next. CEA was again positive in all tumors examined. In tumors with a number of AFP-positive cells, however, CEA showed a tendency to be only focally positive (Table 1-10). Figure 1-21 demonstrates a reciprocal localization pattern of AFP and CEA in a poorly differentiated carcinoma (case 4 in Table 10). Namely, AFP-positive cells proliferate in a medullary growth pattern and are CEA-negative, whereas the CEA-positive area shows a papillotubular growth pattern and is AFP-negative. The latter area seems to represent an ordinary type of adenocarcinoma. The specialities of AFP-positive gastric cancer cells as cells retrodifferentiating toward fetal gastrointestinal cells become herein evident. SC and lysozyme are also regarded as strict markers of the ordinary type of gastric carcinoma, although their expression was less consistent than CEA. AFP-positive cells hardly revealed any immunoreactivities with SC and lysozyme.

Immunoreactive PALP was detected in a varying number of gastric cancer cells in 23 of 30 tumors (Fig. 1-22a, b), as has already been pointed out.[21,25,26] The plasma membranes were the main site of staining for PALP, but some signet ring cancer cells showed positivity in Golgi areas. Cancers with plentiful PALP-positive cells were often diffuse carcinomas strongly positive for CEA. A reciprocal staining pattern was noted between PALP and lysozyme (Table 1-10). PALP staining in cancer with a pronounced AFP reactivity was often focal.

Regarding immunoreactive HCG, a few cancer cells were positive in 17 of 30 cases without evidence of a correlation with the staining for AFP, CEA, and PALP. HCG-positive cancer cells in the series of Table 1-10 never showed syncytiotrophoblastic morphology, as seen in Figure 1-22(c,d). Similar results have been reported by other investigators.[21,23,24,34] In a separate study, we have observed that the HCG-like substance in some gastric carcinomas is predominantly an alpha-subunit of HCG. The Alpha-subunit of HCG is further demonstrated in some endocrine-like cells of noncancerous antral mucosa. Unbalanced synthesis and secretion of HCG subunits are well known characteristics of cultured tumor cell lines[113,114] and various endocrine neoplasms.[40,115] Therefore, the detection of HCG immunoreactivity with antiHCG conventional antibody by itself does not necessarily indicate the retrodifferentiation toward trophoblastic cells.

In the next condition, embryonal carcinoma arising from the stomach as a AFP-producing tumor is shown and discussed.[39] As Figure 1-23 illustrates, the tumor cells (case 2 in Table 1-10) possess clear and finely granular cytoplasm. They proliferate with a sheet-like solid arrangement, and the formation of glandular structures with papillary projections is characteristic. Other areas reveal those glomeruloid structures with a few hyaline globules that are typical of yolk sac tumor. Glycogen is abundant in the tumor cells, and mucin is completely negative. AFP is positive in many tumor cells, while CEA is focally detected along the surface of the papillary projections. This peculiar tumor further shows foci of tubular adenocarcinoma both in the mucosa of the primary tumor and in lymph node metastasis. As shown in Figure 1-24, these foci are positive for mucin and immunoreactive for CEA, SC, and lysozyme, but negative for AFP. In the present series, another three tumors focally (two cases) or almost totally (one case) showed features resembling embryonal carcinoma, an admixture of solid and papillary areas without the glomeruloid structures. The cells were uniformly glycogen-rich, mucin-negative, and AFP-positive.

These phenomena can be regarded as the retrodifferentiation of gastric cancer cells toward yolk sac or very immature embryonal cells. A similar hypothesis has been proposed for the histogenesis of choriocarcinoma of the stomach,[116] which is presented below. Endo et al found with the Concanavalin A binding analysis that the sugar moiety of serum AFP in patients with gastrointestinal cancer is very similar to that of yolk sac tumor, but is different from that of fetal liver and hepatocellular carcinoma.[117] Therefore, it may be relevant that while the degree of retrodifferentiation in AFP-producing nonembryonal carcinoma of the stomach comes toward fetal gastrointestinal cells (fetalism), the degree of retrodifferentiation in AFP-producing embryonal carci-

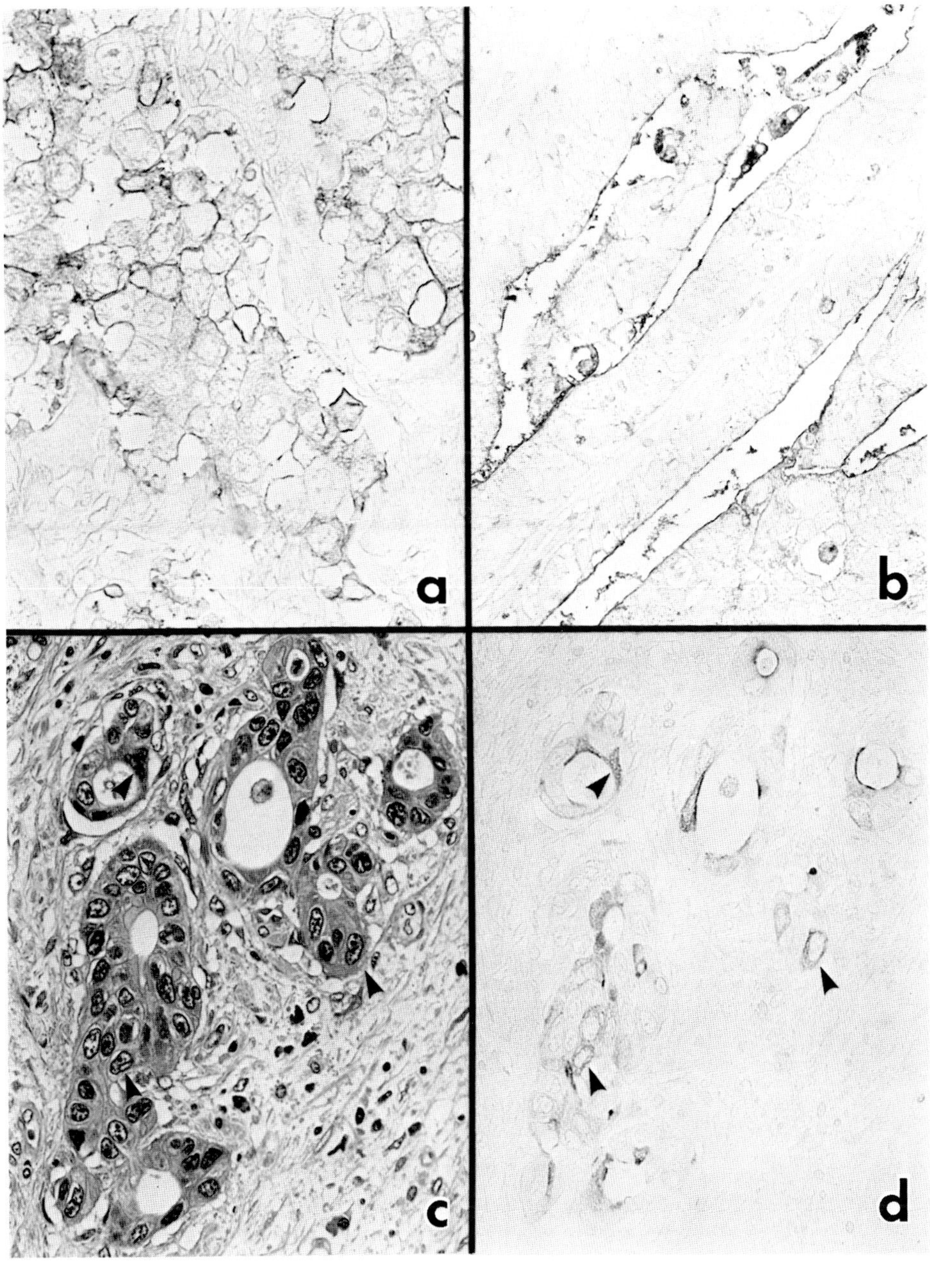


**Fig. 1-22.** Immunohistochemical localization of PALP and HCG in gastric cancer. Signet ring cell carcinoma (case 11, a: PALP), ×400; papillary adenocarcinoma (case 8, b: PALP), ×300; papillary adenocarcinoma (case 9, c: H&E, d: HCG), ×300. Indirect immunoperoxidase method with methyl green counterstain.

PALP is often strongly positive on the plasma membranes of scirrhous cancer cells. PALP is also demonstrated on the apical surface of some adenoplastic carcinoma cells. HCG-positive gastric cancer cells are not necessarily syncytiotrophoblastic (arrowheads).

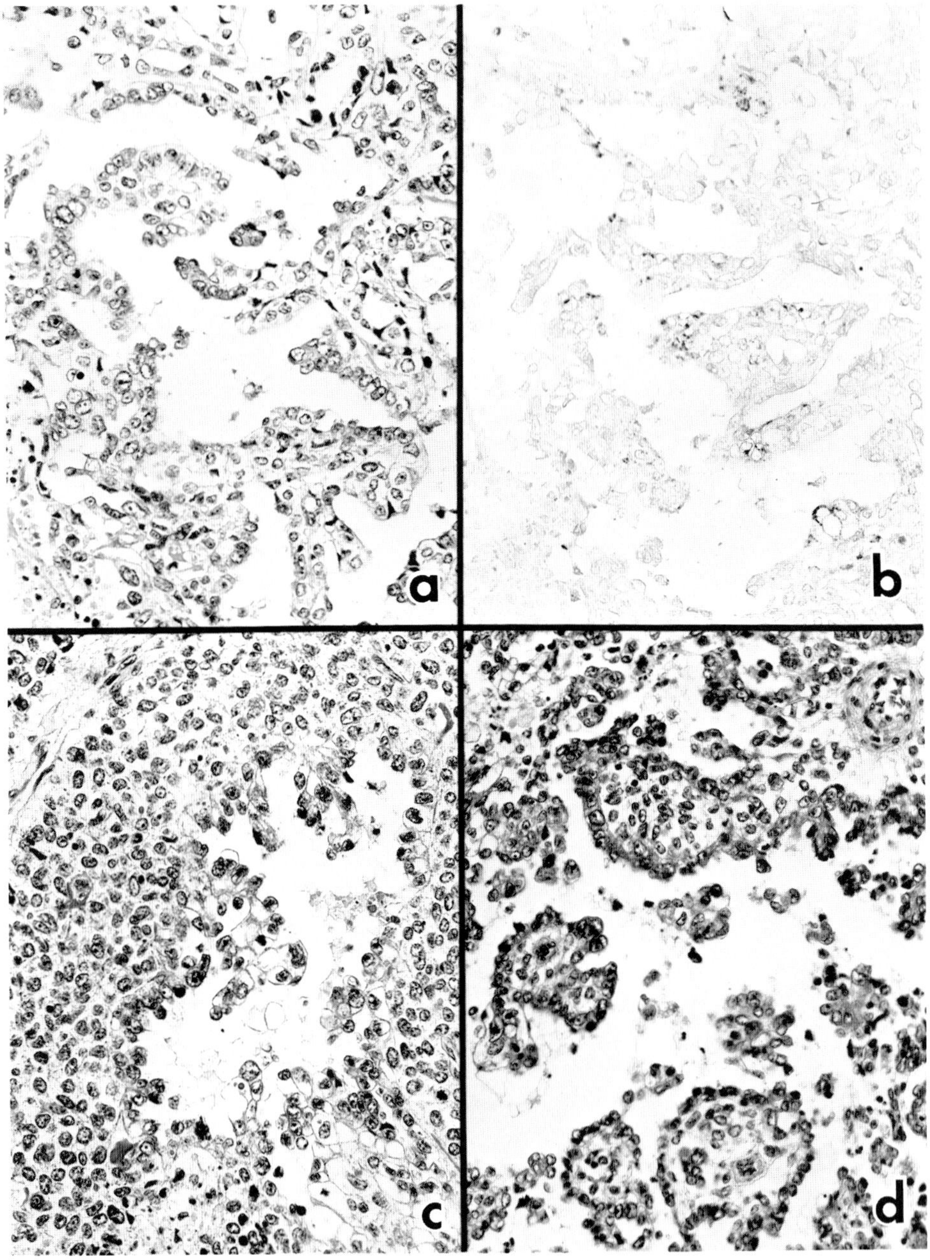


**Fig. 1-23.** Primary embryonal carcinoma of the stomach (case 2). H&E (a, c and d) and indirect immunoperoxidase method for AFP (b), ×200.

The tumor is composed of an admixture of solid and papillary areas. Glomeruloid structure is focally noted (d). Granular or vesicular positivity of AFP is easily seen in the papillary area (a and b). CEA is focally positive along the apical surface of a lumen in (c). Mucin, SC and lysozyme are negative in these areas.

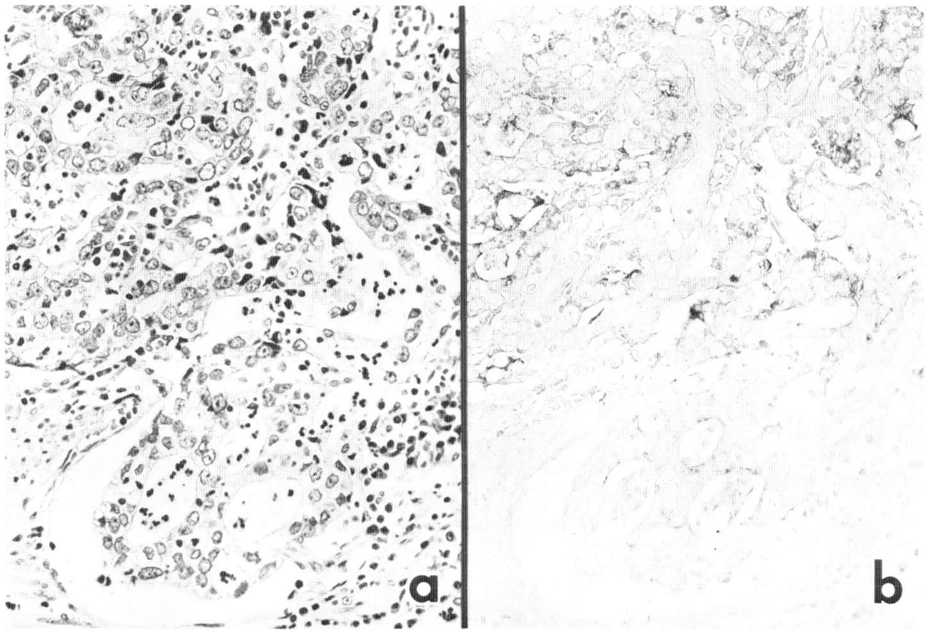


**Fig. 1-24.** Component of adenoplastic carcinoma in a case of primary gastric embryonal carcinoma. Intramucosal lesion of case 2. H&E (a) and indirect immunoperoxidase method for SC (b), ×200.

Not only in the mucosa but also in lymph node metastasis, foci of adenoplastic carcinoma with SC immunoreactivity are found, although the predominant histology is embryonal carcinoma. Note lymphatic invasion.

noma of the stomach comes back to yolk sac cells or very immature embryonal cells (embryonism).

Meanwhile, primary gastric choriocarcinoma has been described, whose histological pictures are identical to those of ordinary choriocarcinoma.[116,118] So far, we have experienced one surgical and two autopsy specimens of primary gastric choriocarcinoma with clinical and laboratory manifestations of HCG overproduction. All patients died within a short clinical period of generalized metastases including to the liver. Large volumes of the tumors showed massive hemorrhagic necrosis intermingled with syncytiotrophoblastic and cytotrophoblastic tumor cells. Immunohistochemically, the syncytiotrophoblastic cells were strongly positive for HCG (and its alpha and beta subunits), but were negative for CEA, AFP, PALP, SC, and lysozyme (Fig. 1-25). The cytotrophoblastic cells were devoid of such markers (keratin is clearly positive). In metastatic lesions, two cases further showed a component of yolk sac tumor with typical histological and immunohistochemical features (AFP and CEA positive but PALP, HCG, SC, and lysozyme negative).

A similar case has recently been presented by Yonemura et al.[119] The components of choriocarcinoma and yolk sac tumor were detected as separate metastatic nodules in the lymph node and/or liver. The co-occurrence of choriocarcinoma and yolk sac tumor from a single primary is very common phenomenon in gonadal and extragonadal malignant germ cell tumors.[120] Quite distinct from the ordinary malignant germ cell tumors is the consistent existence of a component of adenocarcinoma in the gastric tumor,[116,118,119] as was mentioned above for embryonal carcinoma of the stomach. All three cases of gastric choriocarcinoma disclosed foci of adenoplastic (tubular or papillary) carcinoma with pos-

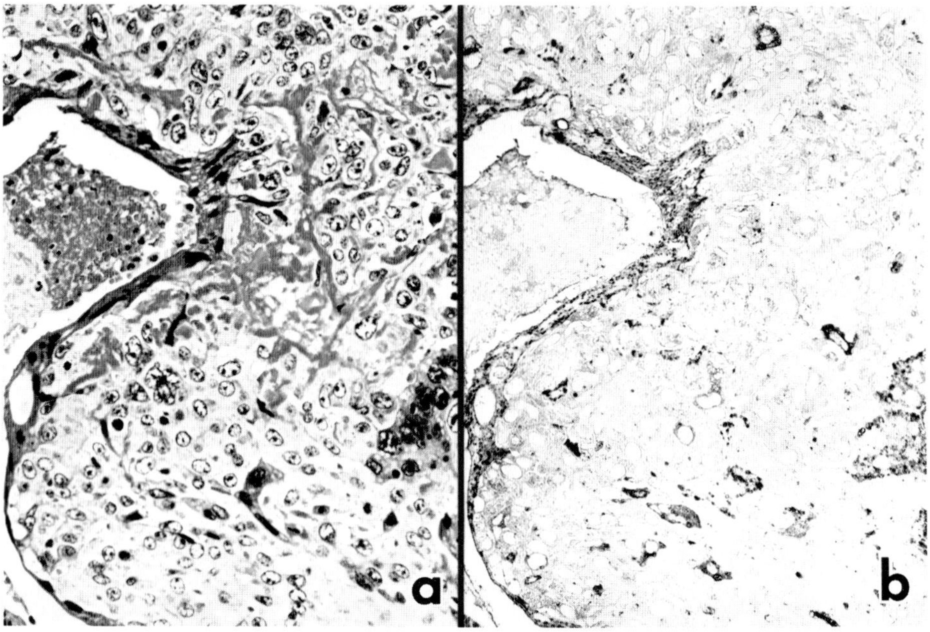

**Fig. 1-25.** Primary gastric choriocarcinoma. H&E (a) and indirect immunoperoxidase method for HCG (b), ×200.

Syncytiotrophoblastic tumor cells are clearly positive for HCG. Foci of yolk sac tumor and adenoplastic carcinoma are also seen in both the primary and metastatic sites.

itive reactions to mucin, CEA, SC, and/or lysozyme within the gastric wall, including the mucosa. Lymph node metastasis of adenoplastic carcinoma was also noted in one case.

The clinical and morphological transformation of papillary thyroid cancer into anaplastic cancer is regarded as "malignant transformation of less malignant cancer cells."[121] Similarly, the occurrence of malignant germ cell tumors from the stomach may be understood when such a concept is extended to the gastric cancer (i.e., the transformation occurs at the stem cell level of ordinary adenoplastic cancer), resulting in retrodifferentiation into highly malignant cancer of embryonal, yolk sac, or trophoblastic nature.

## OVERALL SUMMARY AND CONCLUSIONS

In this chapter, highly variegated but harmonized differentiations of gastric cancer cells were presented and analyzed with the aid of immunohistochemistry and mucin histochemistry. The demonstration of dual differentiation toward gastric and intestinal epithelial cells in both diffuse and adenoplastic carcinomas supports questioning the view of histogenesis that diffuse carcinoma arises from almost intact gastric mucosa, while adenoplastic carcinoma arises from intestinalized mucosa. In fact, not only carcinomas predominantly composed of signet ring cells with an intestinal phenotype, but also tubular adenocarcinomas predominantly with a gastric phenotype (e.g., adenocarcinoma with lymphoid stroma) were identified.

It is very surprising that many signet ring cell carcinomas in the mucosa reveal well organized zonal (lamellar or layered) differentiations, especially when the destruction of preexisting mucosal structures is minimal. The marker substances are expressed in the intramucosal cancer cells with a consistent localization pattern similar to that of nonneoplastic epithelial cells.

These observations are very important in a

sense that the differentiation of cancer cells is possibly controlled by the appropriate mucosal microenvironment that contains well developed microcirculatory networks. Such a notion becomes most understandable when we take the cell kinetics in the lesion carefully into account. The proliferative cells of intramucosal signet ring cell carcinoma occupy solely the layer that corresponds to the generative zone of noncancerous mucosa, and mature signet ring cells, which occupy the upper and bottom layers of the mucosa are no longer mitogenic. Consequently, immature-looking proliferative cancer cells, "neoplastic stem cells," in the mucosa differentiate upward to signet ring cells of the surface epithelial cell-type or goblet cell-type and downward to those of the pyloric gland-type. The incompletion of the zonal differentiation in adenoplastic carcinoma in the mucosa may reflect the random distribution of mitogenic cancer cells.

The differentiation toward endocrine-like cells is another characteristic of diffuse (scirrhous) carcinoma, in which argyrophilic and chromogranin-immunoreactive cells are frequently encountered. Some argyrophilic carcinomas exhibited a number of glicentin-immunoreactive cells. This probably represents a fetal-type expression (fetalism), since most scirrhous carcinomas occur in scarcely intestinalized oxyntic mucosa, and the demonstration of glicentin cells in the oxyntic mucosa is peculiar to fetal stomach. The presence of multipotent tumor stem cells that differentiate into various cell components including endocrine cells should be speculated upon again.

Finally, the notion of "retrodifferentiation" of gastric cancer cells was insistently favored. Tumors with extremely high levels of serum AFP or a number of AFP stain-positive cells mostly belonged to poorly differentiated medullary carcinoma or embryonal carcinoma arising from the stomach, while papillary adenocarcinoma or signet ring cell carcinoma was also occasionally AFP-positive. A component of yolk sac tumor was seen in two of three primary gastric choriocarcinomas. Clear cytoplasm with abundance of glycogen was a common cytological feature of AFP-positive cancer cells. For these tumors, the acquisition of the properties of fetal gastrointestinal epithelium, which has been reported to be AFP-positive, or of more immature retrodifferentiated embryonal cells would be a relevant explanation. The common existence of a component of ordinary adenoplastic carcinoma in tumor tissues of embryonal carcinoma and choriocarcinoma of the stomach may lead to the concept of "malignant transformation" of ordinary gastric cancer cells into highly retrodifferentiated embryonal, yolk sac or trophoblastic tumor cells.

## ACKNOWLEDGEMENTS

The author expresses gratitude to Professor Keiichi Watanabe, Department of Pathology, Tokai University School of Medicine, Isehara, for his efforts in reviewing and criticizing the manuscript. The author is also deeply indebted to Professor Hiroshi Nagura, Laboratory of Germfree Life Research, Institute for Disease Mechanism and Control, Nagoya University School of Medicine, Nagoya, and to Associate Professor Tsutomu Katsuyama, Pathology Division of Central Clinical Laboratories, Shinshu University Hospital, Matsumoto, for their valuable advice and suggestions. The skillful technical assistance of Mr. Johbu Ito, Cell Biology Research Laboratory, Tokai University School of Medicine, Isehara, for taking photographs is also gratefully acknowledged. This work was in part supported by the Grant-in-Aid from the Ministry of Education, Japan #61010035.

## REFERENCES

1. Markert C.L.: Cell differentiation in neoplasia, in: Tumor Cell Heterogeneity. Origins and Implications (eds. Owens A.H. Jr, Coffey D.S., Baylin S.B.), New York, London, Academic Press, 1982, pp 237–247
2. Sugano H., Nakamura K., Kato Y.: Pathological studies of human gastric cancer. Acta Pathol Jpn 32 (Suppl **2**):329–347, 1982
3. Osamura R.Y.: Review: gastric carcinoma in Japan. Tokai J. Exp Clin Med **8**:405–410, 1983
4. Lauren P.: The two histologic main types of gastric carcinoma; diffuse and so-called intestinal-type car-

cinoma. An attempt at a histoclinical classification. Acta Pathol Microbiol Scand **64**:31–49, 1965
5. Nakamura K.: Structure of the gastric cancer. Igaku-Shoin, Tokyo, 1982 (in Japanese)
6. Hattori T., Fujita S.: Tritiated thymidine autoradiographic study on cellular migration in the gastric gland of the golden hamster. Cell Tiss Res **172**:171–184, 1976
7. Hattori T., Fujita S.: Tritiated thymidine autoradiographic study of cellular migration and renewal in the pyloric mucosa of golden hamsters. Cell Tiss Res **175**:49–57, 1976
8. Fujita S., Hattori T.: Cell proliferation, differentiation, and migration in the gastric mucosa: a study on the background of carcinogenesis, in: Pathophysiology of Carcinogenesis in Digestive Organs (eds. Farber F., Kawachi T., Nagayo T., Sugano H., Sugimura T., Weisburger J.H.), Tokyo University/Park Press, 1977, pp 21–36
9. Fujita S.: Histogenesis and progression of gastric cancer from a viewpoint of cell kinetics. Tr Soc Pathol Jpn **70**:23–54, 1981 (in Japanese)
10. Imai T., Kubo T., Watanabe H.: Chronic gastritis in Japanese with reference to high incidence of gastric carcinoma. J Natl Cancer Inst **47**:179–195, 1971
11. Nakamura K., Sugano H., Takagi K.: Carcinoma of the stomach in incipient phase. Its histogenesis and histological appearances. Gann **59**:251–258, 1968
12. Matsukura N., Suzuki K., Kawachi T., Aoyagi M., Sugimura T., Kitaoka H., Numajiri H., Shirota A., Itabashi M., Hirota T.: Distribution of marker enzymes and mucin in intestinal metaplasia in human stomach and relation of complete and incomplete types of intestinal metaplasia to minute gastric carcinomas. J Natl Cancer Inst **65**:231–240, 1980
13. Isaacson P.: Immunoperoxidase study of the secretory immunoglobulin system and lysozyme in normal and diseased gastric mucosa. Gut **23**:578–588, 1982
14. Kittas C., Aroni K., Kotsis L., Papadimitriou C.S.: Distribution of lysozyme, $\alpha_1$-antichymotrypsin and $\alpha_1$-antitrypsin in adenocarcinomas of the stomach and large intestine. An immunohistochemical study. Virchows Arch [Pathol Anat] **398**:139–147, 1982
15. Tahara E., Ito H., Shimamoto F., Iwamoto T., Nakagami K., Niimoto H.: Lysozyme in human gastric carcinoma: a retrospective immunohistochemical study. Histopathology **6**:409–421, 1982
16. Ejeckam G.C., Huang S.N., McCaughey W.T.E., Gold P.: Immunohistopathologic study on carcinoembryonic antigen (CEA)-like material and immunoglobulin A in gastric malignancies. Cancer **44**:1606–1614, 1979
17. Tome Y., Hirohashi S., Sekine T., Itabashi M., Hirota T., Shimosato Y.: Production of pepsinogen by gastric carcinoma. Igaku-no-ayumi **123**:999–1000, 1982 (in Japanese)
18. Reis W.A., Thompson W.D., Kay J.: Pepsinogen in gastric carcinoma cells. J Clin Pathol **36**:137–139, 1983
19. Denk H., Tappeiner G., Davidovits A., Eckerstorfer R., Holzner J.H.: Carcinoembryonic antigen and blood group substances in carcinomas of the stomach and colon. J Natl Cancer Inst **53**:933–942, 1974
20. Mori T., Lee P.-K., Nakajo Y., Awata K., Kosaki G.: Biological features of CEA-positive cells in gastric cancer and fetal tissues, in: Carcino-Embryonic Proteins: Chemistry, Biology, Clinical Applications, vol II (ed. Lehmann F.G.), Elsevier/North Holland Biomedical Press, New York, 1979, pp 23–28
21. Miyayama H., Miyayama Y.: Immunohistochemical study of $\alpha$FP, CEA, hCG, and placental A1-P expressed in human gastrointestinal cancers in comparison to embryo-fetal gastrointestinal mucosa. Pathol Clin Med **3**:905–915, 1985 (in Japanese with English abstr)
22. Lee P.-K., Mori T., Fujimoto N., Nakamura T., Kosaki G.: Relationships of AFP-producing cells in gastric cancer, hepatocellular cancer and fetal tissues, in: Carcino-Embryonic Proteins: Chemistry, Biology, and Clinical Applications (ed. Lehmann FG), vol II, Elsevier/North Holland Biomedical Press, New York, 1979, pp 373–378
23. Kodama T., Kameya T., Hirota T., Shomosato Y., Ohkura H., Mukojima T., Kitaoka H.: Production of alpha-fetoprotein, normal serum protein, and human chorionic gonadotropin in stomach cancer: histologic and immunohistochemical analyses of 35 cases. Cancer **48**:1647–1655, 1981
24. Ito H., Tahara E.: Human chorionic gonadotropin in human gastric carcinoma. A retrospective immunohistochemical study. Acta Pathol Jpn **33**:287–296, 1983
25. Kawasaki H., Takeuchi M., Kimoto E.: Immunofluorescent staining of placental alkaline phosphatase in gastric and rectal carcinoma. Gann **65**:473–479, 1974
26. Kojima J., Kanatani M., Yamamoto T., Tateishi R., Nakamura N.: Carcinoembryonic proteins in gastric carcinoma metastatic to the liver. Gastroenterol Jpn **14**:596–603, 1979
27. Rapp W., Windisch M., Peschke P., Wurster K.: Purification of human intestinal goblet cell antigen (GOA): its immunohistological demonstration in the intestine and in mucus producing gastrointestinal adenocarcinomas. Virchows Arch [Pathol Anat] **382**:163–177, 1979
28. Furihata C., Tatematsu M., Miki K., Katsuyama T., Sudo K., Miyagi N., Kubota T., Jin S.-S., Kodama K., Ito N., Konishi Y., Suzuki K., Matsushima T.: Gastric-and intestinal-type properties of human gastric cancers transplanted into nude mice. Cancer Res **44**:727–733, 1984
29. Katsuyama T., Tsukahara M., Nasu T.: Application of paradoxical Concanavalin A staining to gastrointestinal pathology. II. Mucosubstance histochemistry of human gastric carcinoma. Igaku-no-ayumi **111**:156–158, 1979 (in Japanese)
30. Katsuyama T., Ono K., Nakayama J., Kanai M.: Recent advances in mucosubstance histochemistry, in: Gastric Mucus and Mucus Secreting Cells (ed. Kawai K), Excerpta Medica, Tokyo, 1985, pp 3–18
31. Azzopardi J.G., Pollock D.J.: Argentaffin cells and argyrophil cells in gastric carcinoma. J Pathol Bacteriol **86**:443–452, 1963
32. Kubo T., Watanabe H.: Neoplastic argentaffin cells in gastric and intestinal carcinomas. Cancer **27**:447–454, 1971
33. Tahara E., Ito H., Shimamoto F., Taniyama K., Iwamoto T., Sumiyoshi H., Kajihara H., Yamamoto M.: Argyrophil cells in early gastric carcinoma: an immunohistochemical and ultrastructural study. J Cancer Res Clin Oncol **103**:187–202, 1982
34. Tahara E., Ito H., Nakagami K., Shimamoto F., Yamamoto M., Sumii K.: Scirrhous argyrophil cell carcinoma of the stomach with multiple production of polypeptide hormone, amine, CEA, lysozyme and HCG. Cancer **49**:1904–1915, 1982
35. Tsutsumi Y., Nagura H., Kamoshida E., Ishii M., Mikata A.: Immunohistochemical studies on secre-

tory glycoproteins produced by gastric cancer. Digest Org Immunol **7**:168–174, 1981 (in Japanese)
36. Tsutsumi Y., Mikata A., Nagura H.: Histochemical studies on mucins and secretory glycoproteins in early gastric carcinoma. Acta Histochem Cytochem **14**:82, 1981 (Abstract)
37. Nagura H., Tsutsumi Y., Shioda Y., Watanabe K.: Immunohistochemistry of gastric carcinomas and associated diseases: novel distribution of carcinoembryonic antigen and secretory component on the surface of gastric cancer cells. J Histochem Cytochem **31**:193–198, 1983
38. Tsutsumi Y.: Immunohistochemical studies on glucagon, glicentin and pancreatic polypeptide in human stomach: normal and pathological conditions. Histochem J **16**:869–883, 1984
39. Tsutsumi Y., Sato T., Kondo Y., Ogoshi K.: Immunohistochemical analysis of alpha-fetoprotein producing gastric carcinomas. Digest Org Immunol **13**:31–39, 1984 (in Japanese)
40. Tsutsumi Y.: Immunohistochemistry of hormone (4). Neuroendocrine-related substances. Pathol Clin Med **2**:1610–1623, 1984 (in Japanese)
41. Grimelius L.: A silver nitrate stain for $\alpha_2$ cells in human pancreatic islets. Acta Soc Med Upsal **73**:243–270, 1968
42. Masson P.: Carcinoids (argentaffin cell tumors) and nerve hyperplasia of the appendicular mucosa. Am J Pathol **4**:181–212, 1928
43. Japanese Research Society of Gastric Cancer: The general rules for the gastric cancer study in surgery and pathology (11th ed), Kanehara-Shuppan, Tokyo, 1985 (in Japanese)
44. Spicer S.S.: Diamine methods for differentiating mucosubstances histochemically. J Histochem Cytochem **13**:211–234, 1965
45. Katsuyama T., Spicer S.S.: Histochemical differentiation of complex carbohydrates with variants of the Concanavalin A-horseradish peroxidase method. J Histochem Cytochem **26**:233–250, 1978
46. Culling C.F.A., Reis P.E., Dunn W.L.: A new histochemical method for the identification and visualization of both side chain acylated and nonacylated sialic acids. J Histochem Cytochem **24**:1225–1230, 1976
47. Nakane P.K.: Recent progress in peroxidase-labeled antibody method. Ann NY Acad Sci **254**:203–211, 1975
48. Sternberger L.A. Hardy P.H. Jr, Cuculis J.J., Meyer H.G.: The unlabeled antibody enzyme method of immunohistochemistry. Preparation and properties of soluble antigen-antibody complex (horseradish peroxidase-antihorseradish peroxidase) and its use in identification of spirochetes. J Histochem Cytochem **18**:315–333, 1970
49. Tsutsumi Y., Nagura H., Watanabe K.: Immunohistochemical observations of carcinoembryonic antigen (CEA) and CEA-related substances in normal and neoplastic pancreas. Pitfalls and caveats in CEA immunohistochemistry. Am J Clin Pathol **82**:535–542, 1984
50. Wagener C., Csaszar H., Totović V., Breuer H.: A highly sensitive method for the demonstration of carcinoembryonic antigen in normal and neoplastic colonic tissue. Histochemistry **58**:1–11, 1978
51. Tourville D.R., Adler R.H., Bienenstock J., Tomasi T.B. Jr: The human secretory immunoglobulin of $\gamma$A, secretory "piece", and lactoferrin in normal human tissue. J Exp Med **129**:411–429, 1969
52. Brandzaeg P., Bahlien K.: Immunohistochemical studies of the formation and epithelial transport of immunoglobulins in normal and diseased human intestinal mucosa. Scand J Gastroenterol 11 (Suppl **36**):1–45, 1976
53. Brown W.R., Isobe Y., Nakane P.K.: Studies on translocation of immunoglobulins across intestinal epithelium. II. Immunoelectronmicroscopic localization of immunoglobulins and secretory component in human intestinal mucosa. Gastroenterology **71**:985–995, 1976
54. Tsutsumi Y., Nagura H., Watanabe K.: Immune aspects of intestinal metaplasia of the stomach: an immunohistochemical study. Virchows Arch [Pathol Anat] **403**:345–359, 1984
55. Mason D.Y., Taylor C.R.: The distribution of muramidase (lysozyme) in human tissues. J Clin Pathol **28**:124–132, 1975
56. Adinolfi M., Glynn A.A., Lindsay M., Milne C.M.: Serological properties of $\gamma$-A antibodies to *Escherichia coli* present in human colostrum. Immunology **10**:517–526, 1966
57. Tsutsumi Y., Nagura H., Watanabe K., Yanaihara N.: A novel subtyping of intestinal metaplasia of the stomach, with special reference to the histochemical characterizations of endocrine cells. Virchows Arch [Pathol Anat] **401**:73–88, 1983
58. Mason D.Y., Taylor C.R.: Distribution of transferrin, ferritin, and lactoferrin in human tissues. J Clin Pathol **31**:316–327, 1978
59. Parmley R.T., Takagi M., Barton J.C., Boxer L.A., Austin R.L.: Ultrastructural localization of lactoferrin and iron-binding protein in human neutrophils and rabbit heterophils. Am J Pathol **109**:343–358, 1982
60. Nishida O., Kano T., Tsukada H., Yasuda N., Kobayashi Y., Sakai M., Uchino H., Miyake T.: Localization of lactoferrin in gastric mucosa. Jap J Gastroenterol **82**:1–8, 1985 (in Japanese with English abstr)
61. Samloff I.M., Liebman W.M.: Cellular localization of the group II pepsinogens in human stomach and duodenum by immunofluorescence. Gastroenterology **65**:36–42, 1973
62. Gold P., Freedman S.O.: Specific carcinoembryonic antigens in human digestive system. J Exp Med **122**:467–481, 1965
63. Klockars M., Reitamo S., Reitamo J.J., Möller C.: Immunohistochemical identification of lysozyme in intestinal lesions in ulcerative colitis and Crohn's disease. Gut:**18**:377–381, 1977
64. Watanabe H., Enjoji M., Imai T.: Gastric carcinoma with lymphoid stroma. Cancer **38**:232–243, 1976
65. Ridolfi R.L., Rosen P.P., Port A., Kinne D., Miké V.: Medullary carcinoma of the breast. A clinicopathologic study with 10 years follow-up. Cancer **40**:1365–1385, 1977
66. Higuchi Y., Ishida M., Hayashi H.: A lymphocyte chemotactic peptide released from immunoglobulin G by neutrophil neutral thiol protease. Cell Immunol **46**:297–308, 1979
67. Selby W.S., Janossy G., Jewell D.P.: Immunohistochemical characterization of intraepithelial lymphocytes of human gastrointestinal tract. Gut **22**:169–176, 1981
68. Sato T., Yamazaki H., Tsutsumi Y., Mori I., Hata J., Tamaoki N., Noto T., Nagura H.: Quantitative analysis of subsets of intraepithelial T lymphocytes in carcinoma of the colon. Digest Org Immunol **13**:61–65, 1984 (in Japanese)
69. Asano S., Sato N., Mori M., Ohsawa N., Kosaka K.,

Ueyama Y.: Detection and assessment of human tumors producing granulocyte-macrophage colony-stimulating factor (GM-CSF) by heterotransplantation into nude mice. Br J Cancer **41**:689–694, 1980
70. Tamaoki N.: Pathology of human cancer transplanted into nude mice. Experimental approach to the pathology of tumor-bearing individuals. Tr Soc Pathol Jpn **93**:93–125, 1985 (in Japanese)
71. Tsutsumi Y.: Application of parietal cell autoantibody to histopathological studies. Acta Pathol Jpn **35**:823–829, 1985
72. Fisher E.R.: Ultrastructure of the human breast and its disorders. Am J Clin Pathol **66**:291–305, 1976
73. Ruoslahti E.: Cell-matrix interactions as determinants of differentiation and tumor invasion, in: Oncodevelopmental Markers. Biologic, Diagnostic, and Monitoring Aspects (ed. Fishman W.H.), Academic Press, New York, London, 1983, pp 21–35
74. Fujita S.: Stroma as a rate limiting factor for growth of tumors *in vivo*. Gann Monogr Cancer Res **25**:57–66, 1980
75. Tsuchihashi Y.: Studies on structure and function of the mucosal microvascular system of the gastrointestinal tract with special references to their relations to epithelial functions. J Kyoto Pref Univ Med **92**:59–81, 1983 (in Japanese with English abstr)
76. Watanabe K.: Microcirculation in lung, in: Microcirculation (eds. Azuma T., Tsuchiya M., Mishima Y.), Lifetime Education Series 6, Nakayama Books, Tokyo, 1979, pp 186–196 (in Japanese)
77. Sugihara H.: Proliferation and differentiation of human signet ring cell carcinoma in gastric mucosa. Fine structural basis of the morphogenesis of "layered structure." J Kyoto Pref Univ Med **93**:591–605, 1984 (in Japanese with English abstr)
78. Pierce G.B., Nakane P.K., Mazurkiewicz J.E.: Natural history of malignant stem cells, in: Differentiation and Control of Malignancy of Tumor Cells. Proceedings of the 4th International Symposium of the Prince Takamatsu Cancer Research Fund, Tokyo, 1973, University of Tokyo Press, Tokyo, 1974, pp 453–469
79. Pierce G.B., Nakane P.K. Martinez-Hernandez A., Ward J.M.: Ultrastructural comparison of differentiation of stem cells of murine adenocarcinomas of colon and breast with their normal counterparts. J Natl Cancer Inst **58**:1329–1345, 1977
80. Yesner R.: Spectrum of lung cancer and ectopic hormones. Pathol Annu **13**:(Part 1)217–240, 1978
81. Gazdar A.F., Carney D.N., Guccioni J.G., Baylin S.B.: Small cell carcinoma of the lung: cellular origin and relationship to other pulmonary tumors, in: Small Cell Lung Cancer (eds. Greco F.A., Oldham R.K., Bunn P.A. Jr), Grune & Stratton, New York, 1981, pp 145–175
82. Ahnen D.J., Nakane P.K., Brown W.R.: Ultrastructural localization of carcinoembryonic antigen in normal intestine and colon cancer. Abnormal distribution of CEA on the surface of colon cancer cells. Cancer **49**:2077–2090, 1982
83. Schumacher H.R., McFeely A.E., Davis K.D., Maugel T.K.: The acute leukemia cell. IV. DNA synthesis in peripheral blood and bone. Am J Clin Pathol **56**:508-514, 1971
84. Nakamura S., Kino I., Baba S.: *Ex vivo* autoradiographic study on the labeling index of gastric cancers. Proc Jap Cancer Assoc, the 44th Annual Meeting, 1985, p 379 (Abstr)
85. Wylie C.V., Nakane P.K., Pierce G.B.: Degree of differentiation in nonproliferating cells in mammary carcinoma. Differentiation **1**:11–20, 1973
86. Hamperl H.: Über die "gelben" (chromaffinen) Zellen in gesunden und kranken Magendarmschlauch. Virchows Arch [Pathol Anat] **266**:509–548, 1927
87. Solcia E., Cappela C., Buffa R., Usellini L., Frigerio B., Fontana P.: Endocrine cells of the gastrointestinal tract and related tumors. Pathobiol Annu **9**:163–204, 1979
88. O'Connor D.T., Burton D., Deftos L.J.: Immunoreactive human chromogranin A in diverse polypeptide hormone producing human tumors and normal endocrine tissues. J Clin Endocrinol Metab **57**:1084–1086, 1983
89. Cohen D.V., Elting J.: Biosynthesis, processing, and secretion of parathormone and secretory protein-I. Recent Prog Horm Res **39**:181–209, 1983
90. O'Connor D.T., Frigon R.P., Sokoloff R.L.: Human chromogranin A. Purification and characterization from catecholamine storage vesicles of human pheochromocytoma. Hypertension **6**:2–12, 1984
91. Fujimoto S., Hattori T., Kimoto K., Yamashita S., Fujita S., Kawai K.: Tritiated thymidine autoradiographic study on origin and renewal of gastrin cells in antral area of hamsters. Gastroenterology **79**:785–791, 1980
92. Bartow S.A., Mukai K., Rosai J.: Pseudoneoplastic proliferation of endocrine cells in pancreatic fibrosis. Cancer **47**:2627–2633, 1981
93. Torikata C., Kawai T., Yakumaru K., Kageyama K.: Histopathological studies on the tumorlet of the lung with special reference to the cytogenesis of proliferating cells. Acta Pathol Jpn **25**:539–553, 1975
94. Tsutsumi Y., Osamura R.Y., Watanabe K., Yanaihara N.: Cytogenesis and pathological alterations of human bronchial neuroendocrine cells: an immunohistochemical study. Pathol Clin Med **1**:298–319, 1983 (in Japanese with English abstr)
95. Heitz P.U., Wegmann W.: Identification of neoplastic Paneth cells in an adenocarcinoma of the stomach using lysozyme as a marker, and electron microscopy. Virchows Arch [Pathol Anat] **386**:107–116, 1980
96. Clarkson B., Marks P.A., Till J.E. (eds): Differentiation of Normal and Neoplastic Hematopoietic Cells. Cold Spring Harbor Laboratory, 1978
97. Pierce G.B., Wills R.S.: Embryonic microenvironment in the regulation of cancer cells, in: Tumor Cell Heterogeneity. Origins and Implications (eds. Owens A.H. Jr, Coffey D.S., Baylin S.B.), Academic Press, New York, London, 1982, pp 249–258
98. Sidhu G.S.: The endodermal origin of digestive and respiratory tract APUD cells. Histopathologic evidence and a review of the literature. Am J Pathol **96**:5–20, 1979
99. Pearse A.G.E.: the cytochemistry and ultrastructure of polypeptide hormone-producing cells of the APUD series and the embryologic, physiologic, and pathologic implications of the concept. J Histochem Cytochem **17**:303–313, 1969
100. Subuswamy S.G., Gibbs N.M., Ross C.F., Morson B.C.: Goblet cell carcinoid of the appendix. Cancer **34**:338–344, 1974
101. Ljungberg O., Bondeson L., Bondeson A-G: Differentiated thyroid carcinoma, intermediate type: a new tumor entity with features of follicular and parafollicular cell carcinoma. Hum Pathol **15**:218–228, 1984
102. Matthews M.J., Hirsch F.R.: Problems in the diag-

nosis of small cell carcinoma of the lung. In: Small Cell Lung Cancer (eds. Greco F.A., Oldham R.K., Bunn P.A. Jr), Grune & Stratton, New York, 1981, pp 35–50

103. Masopust J., Kithier K., Rádl J., Koutecký J., Kotal L.: Occurrence of fetoprotein in patients with neoplasms and non-neoplastic diseases. Int J Cancer **3**:364–373, 1968
104. Mori H., Onji M., Yoshida A., Fukunishi R.: Serum alpha-fetoprotein-positive gastric carcinoid with liver metastasis. Virchows Arch [Pathol Anat] **387**:107–116, 1980
105. McIntire K.R., Walsmann T.A., Moertel C.G., Co V.L.W.: Serum $\alpha$-fetoprotein in patients with neoplasms of the gastrointestinal tract. Cancer Res **35**:991–996, 1975
106. Kitaoka Y., Hattori N., Mukojima T., Ohkura H., Nakayama N., Okada H.: Alpha-fetoprotein content in tissues from patients with gastric cancer. Tumor Res **8**:171–177, 1973
107. Lehmann F.G.: Immunological relationship between human placental and intestinal alkaline phosphatase. Clin Chim Acta **65**:257–269, 1975
108. Uchida T., Shjimoda T., Miyata H., Shikata T., Iino S., Suzuki H., Oda T., Hirano K., Sugiura M.: Immunoperoxidase study of alkaline phosphatase in testicular tumor. Cancer **48**:1455–1462, 1981
109. Ishii M.: Radioimmunoassay of $\alpha$-fetoprotein. Gann Monogr Cancer Res **14**:89–98, 1973
110. Hata J., Ueyama Y., Tamaoki N., Akatsuka A., Yoshimura S., Shimizu K., Morikawa Y., Furukawa T.: Human yolk sac tumor serially transplanted in nude mice: its morphologic and functional properties. Cancer **46**:2446–2455, 1980
111. Gitlin D., Perricelli A., Gitlin G.M.: Synthesis of $\alpha$-fetoprotein by liver, yolk sac, and gastrointestinal tract of the human conceptus. Cancer Res **32**:979–982, 1972
112. Villee C.A., Hagerman D.D., Holmberg N., Lind J., Villee D.B.: The effects of anoxia on the metabolism of human fetal tissues. Pediatrics **22**:953–971, 1958
113. Tashjian A.H. Jr, Weintraub B.D., Barowsky N.J., Rabson A.S, Rosen S.W.: Subunits of human chorionic gonadotropin: unbalanced synthesis and secretion by clonal cell strains derived from a bronchogenic carcinoma. Proc Natl Acad Sci USA **70**:1419–1422, 1973
114. Stanbridge E.J., Rosen S.W., Sussman H.H.: Expression of the $\alpha$-subunit of human chorionic gonadotropin is specifically correlated with tumorigenic expression in human cell hybrids. Proc Natl Acad Sci USA **79**:6242–6245, 1982
115. Heitz P.V., Kasper M., Klöppel G., Polak J.M., Vaitukaitis J.L.: Glycoprotein-hormone alpha-chain production by pancreatic endocrine tumors: a specific marker for malignancy. Immunocytochemical analysis of tumors of 155 patients, Cancer **51**:277–282, 1983
116. Kameya T., Shimosato Y., Tsumuraya M., Ohsawa N., Nomura T.: Human gastric choriocarcinoma serially transplanted in nude mice. J Natl Cancer Inst **56**:325–332, 1976
117. Endo Y., Tsuchida Y., Miyazaki J., Kaneko M.: Analysis of lectin affinity of alpha-fetoprotein. Application to diagnosis. Jap J Cancer Chemother **10**:636–641, 1983 (in Japanese)
118. Mori H., Soeda O., Kamano T., Tsunekawa K., Ueda N., Yoshida A., Fukunishi R.: Choriocarcinomatous change with immunohistochemically HCG-positive cells in the gastric carcinoma of the males. Virchows Arch [Pathol Anat] **396**:141–153, 1982
119. Yonemura Y., Hashimoto T., Sawa T., Shimizu K., Miyazaki I.: A case of gastric carcinoma producing chorionic gonadotropin and alpha fetoprotein. Pathol Clin Med **3**:541–545, 1985 (in Japanese with English abstr).
120. Teilum G.: Special Tumors of Ovary and Testis. Comparative Pathology and Histologic Identification (2nd ed), Philadelphia, J.B., Lippincott, 1976
121. Hutter R.V.P., Tollefsen H.R., De Cosse J.J., Foote F.W., Frazell E.L.: Spindle and giant cell metaplasia in papillary carcinoma of the thyroid. Am J Surg **110**:660–668, 1965

# 2

# Prognosis in Gastric Carcinoma
## The preeminence of staging and futility of histological classification.

Manuel Moutinho Ribeiro
Mário Seoxas
Manuel Sobrinho-Simões

Numerous studies dealing with the predictive value of epidemiological and morphological factors in gastric carcinoma are on record.[1-53] Excluding a few of the earliest published papers,[2,11,25,35] all of the aforementioned studies stress the major prognostic significance of the extent of the neoplastic disease. From this agreement on, however, controversy is the rule.

Some authors claim that the finding of lymphatic and/or venous invasion carries a worse prognosis[18,27,32,38,56] while others stress the lack of influence of this finding,[3] and most do not mention it at all.

Sex and age of patients have been considered either as meaningful[6,8,14] or as meaningless prognostic factors.[4,11,23,38]

Most authors stress that patients with tumors located in the cardia and/or fundus do worse than those with tumors located elsewhere.[7,10,12,13,17,23,31,33] Discrepant results are reported, however, in the comparison of the relative survival of patients with tumors located in the antrum and in body of the stomach.[11-13,23,33,51]

Size and/or shape of tumors are regarded as major prognostic factors in some papers,[2,13,15,18,23,25,31,38] as minor in others,[27,35] and as nonsignificant in a few.[17,19]

The prognostic significance of some quite specific features such as the "breach of the capsule of metastatic lymph nodes" and "tumor necrosis" has been emphasized by a few authors[3,30,53] and ignored by the majority.

The predictive value of the analysis of the so-called host immunologic response (lymphoid infiltration of the primary tumor, predominant pattern of regional lymph nodes and degree of nodal histiocytosis) has been found either as (very) rewarding[3,4,17,30,35,36,47,49] or as relatively useless.[5,12]

The controversy attains its maximum in the discussion of the prognostic significance of several microscopical features of the tumors.

Some authors claim that the histological grading provides valuable prognostic information,[11,17,22,25] while others deny it.[8]

The prognostic significance of nuclear grading has only been reported once[4] and the influence on survival of the morphological pattern of tumoral growth is not equally estimated in different studies.[35,37,41,49]

The predictive value of most (if not all) the

histological classifications still is an open question, [8,12,15,19,31,41,42,46] despite the general agreement on the dreadful prognosis carried by the so-called scirrhous carcinoma.[15,18,21,30,36,44]

Several reasons contribute to these discrepancies. First, there is too large a variation of factors, as well as of the criteria employed in their definition, from series to series. Second, the evaluation of the prognostic significance of the different factors is frequently performed without controlling the influence of the interrelated variables. Third, many authors concentrate on a single surgical, pathological, or clinico-pathologic entity and are, therefore, prone to overemphasize the significance of their findings. Finally, the misuse of statistics, namely in what concerns the utilization of linear multivariable regression analysis without checking the adequacy of the models, has frequently contributed to increase the confusion.

We undertook the present study of prognostic factors in gastric carcinoma using several methods of analysis in an attempt to settle the aforementioned controversies. In addition, we intended to see if the accuracy of the TNM method might be improved and if histology kept any predictive value when survival was adjusted for the extent of neoplastic disease. Finally, we also intended to find which of the available histological classifications should be considered the best for prognostic purposes.

## MATERIAL AND METHODS

From 1960 to 1983, 610 patients were operated on for gastric carcinoma in the Serviço de Cirurgia—4 of Hospital S. João in Portugal. Two-hundred and fifty eight patients were submitted to "curative" resection, 29 to "palliative" resection, 174 to bypass procedures and 149 patients to laparotomy. The diagnosis of gastric carcinoma was histologically confirmed in every case. The procedure was considered as "palliative" whenever there were distant metastases to lymph nodes, peritoneal surface or liver, and/or neoplastic invasion of neighboring structures that made radical tumor resection impossible. The gastrectomy was also regarded as "palliative" whenever there was histological demonstration of neoplastic invasion of the surgical border.

This study is based on the detailed analysis of the cases submitted to "curative" resection. Twelve post-operative deaths and 10 cases of severe dysplasia/*in situ* carcinoma were excluded from the series. Any death occurring within the first month after surgery was considered as "post-operative." Follow-up information was obtained in 227 of the 236 patients (96.1%). Patients were followed until death, loss to follow-up, or end of study (October 1985). Treatment was strictly surgical; no chemotheraphy was used. Operative procedures were recorded as distal, subtotal gastrectomy (n = 176), total gastrectomy (n = 47), and proximal, subtotal gastrectomy (n = 13).

Sex and age of patients were always recorded. The mean age of patients was 55.1 ± 11.7 (mean ± SD) with a range from 22 to 79 years. The mean age of women (52.2 ± 14.2 years) was significantly lower than that of men (56.3 ± 10.5 years).

The macroscopical appearance of the tumors was classified according to the surgical and pathological descriptions as polypoid and/or fungating (n = 17), ulcerating (n = 62), ulcero-fungating (n = 64), ulcero-infiltrative (n = 54) and infiltrative (n = 26). In 13 cases there was not enough information about the shape of the tumors.

Tumor site was recorded as follows: antrum, including the pyloric region (n = 146), body (n = 50), fundus (n = 23) and cardia (n = 12). Four cases occurred in previously operated stomachs. In one case the bulk of tumor could not be located precisely. Size of the tumors as measured in the surgical specimens was classified in "less than 3 cm" (n = 30), "from 3 to 6 cm" (n = 65) and "6 cm or larger than 6 cm" (n = 96). There was no information on size in 45 cases.

The original descriptions and the microscopic slides from all cases were reviewed for staging purposes. The extent of penetration of gastric wall was evaluated according to the criteria of the A.J.C.[1] Ten cases were classified as T1m (mucosa), 18 as T1sm (submucosa), 84 as T2 (muscularis propria), 94 as T3 (serosa), and 30 as T4a (direct extension of immediately adjacent tissues). An attempt to subdivide T3 tumors according to the extent of penetration of the outer layer of the gastric wall ("invasion of the subserosa," "suspected invasion of the serosa", and "invasion of the serosa") as defined by the WHO International Reference Center[50] was abandoned due to its lack of reproducibility. Cases classified as T4b were excluded from the present series since they were considered as having been submitted to "palliative" resection.

The extent of lymph node involvement was evaluated according to the criteria of the A.J.C.[1] The NO group was further divided according to the absence or presence of definite signs of lymphatic permeation within the primary tumor (NO and NO1p, respectively), and the N1 group was subdivided in N1(1) (only one lymph node with metastasis) and N1(>1) (two or more than two lymph nodes with metastases). After these criteria, 66 cases were classified as NO, 22 as NO1p, 30 as N1(1), 54 as N1(>1), and 54 cases as N2. In 10 cases, lymph node involvement could not be evaluated at all (NX). Cases with metastases to distant, intraabdominal lymph nodes—so-called N3 group—were not included in the present series, since they were regarded as having been submitted to "palliative" resection.

No attempt was made to evaluate the "breach of the capsule of metastatic nodes," which was only found in highly advanced cases (N2-3).

The presence of blood vessel invasion was scrutinized in 206 cases by an experienced histopathologist not aware of the staging and follow-up data. Sections from all these cases were stained with orcein for elastic fibers. A case was regarded as positive for venous invasion (n = 76) only if there were unequivocal clusters of neoplastic cells within the lumina of elastic walled vessels. In some cases the presence of an adjacent artery was useful confirmatory evidence.

Sections stained with hematoxylin-eosin, PAS, and Alcian-blue at pH 2.5 were used for the histological classification of the tumors according to the criteria advanced by Laurén[54] Oota and Sobin (WHO booklet)[55] and Ming.[37]

One hundred and thirty eight carcinomas were classified as intestinal, 59 as diffuse, and 39 as unclassified according to Laurén.[54] In 10 cases there coexisted intestinal and diffuse patterns; in 9 of these cases the intestinal pattern was found on the surface and the diffuse pattern in the deeper portion of the tumors, whereas in the remaining case, both patterns were found "side by side." For statistical purposes these cases were included in the group of diffuse carcinomas.

According to the WHO classification,[55] 88 cases were labeled as well/moderately differentiated (tubular and/or papillary) adenocarcinomas, 64 as poorly differentiated carcinomas, 12 as mucinous carcinomas, and 72 as signet ring-cell carcinomas. Whenever there was more than one pattern, tumors were classified according to the less differentiated pattern.

One hundred and twenty seven carcinomas were classified as expanding and 109 as infiltrative according to Ming criteria.[37]

The reproducibility of Laurén and Ming classifications was evaluated through the comparison of the diagnosis made in 1981 and in the present study by the same observers (MMR and MSS) in a consecutive series of 244 gastric carcinomas. The percentage of disagreement was greater with Laurén classification than with Ming's (15.2% and 9.0%, respectively) (Sobrinho-Simões and Ribeiro, unpublished results).

The degree of desmoplastic reaction was subjectively scored as follows: 157 cases were regarded as having absent/minimal desmoplasia and the remaining 79 cases as having moderate/abundant desmoplasia. The lymphoid infiltration of the primary tumors was semiquantitively evaluated as abundant (n = 42), moderate (n = 68), and minimal or absent (n = 126).

The histological pattern of regional lymph nodes was evaluated according to the degree of sinusal histiocytosis (absent/minimal, 72

**TABLE 2-1**
Factors Evaluated for their Influence on Survival with Cox Model

| Factors | Definition |
|---|---|
| Stage | 1 = T1m NO; 2 = T1sm NO<br>3 = T2 NO; 4 = T3 NO<br>5 = T1-2 NOLp N1(1); 6 = T3 NOLp N1(1)<br>7 = T1-3 N1(>1); 8 = T1-3 N2<br>9 = T4a N1-2 |
| Venous invasion | 1 = absent; 2 = present |
| Sex | 1 = male; 2 = female |
| Age | 1 = < 40 yr; 2 = 40–59 yr; 3 = ≥ 60 yr |
| Type of resection | 1 = distal; 2 = total; 3 = proximal |
| Site | 1 = antrum; 2 = body; 3 = fundus; 4 = cardia |
| Histology/Laurén | 1 = intestinal; 2 = diffuse; 3 = unclassified |
| Histology/WHO | 1 = mucinous; 2 = well/moderately dif.; 3 = poorly dif.; 4 = signet ring cell |
| Histology/Ming | 1 = expanding; 2 = infiltrative |
| Desmoplasia | 1 = abundant/moderate; 2 = minimal/absent |
| Lymphoid infiltration | 1 = abundant/moderate; 2 = minimal/absent |
| Follicular hyperplasia | 1 = abundant/moderate; 2 = minimal/absent |
| Sinusal histiocytosis | 1 = abundant/moderate; 2 = minimal/absent |

cases; and moderate/abundant, 129) and to the number of germinal centers. Cases having the cortex of any regional lymph node occupied by numerous germinal centers were classified as "follicular hyperplasia" (n = 120) according to the criteria advanced by Black et al.[4] This group corresponds grossly to the "germinal center predominance" group of Tsakraklides et al,[56] whereas most of the cases with less numerous germinal centers (n = 81) fit in the groups of "lymphocyte predominance" and "unstimulated nodes" of Tsakraklides et al.[56] In 35 cases there was not enough evidence to label the pattern of nodal response.

The initial prognostic screening of the individual factors was performed using both the death rates and the crude survival curves. Death rates were calculated dividing the number of deaths by the total number of patient months of follow-up (×100). Survival rates were calculated according to Berkson's actuarial method.[57]

The evaluation of the prognostic significance of several factors acting simultaneously was performed using two different methods: comparison of the survival curves of stratified groups and multivariable regression techniques. The Cox proportional hazards model[58] was employed to evaluate the influence on survival of 13 factors (Table 2-1). The MPLR (maximum partial likelihood ratio) method was employed to perform a linear stepwise multivariate regression of the factors, which are significantly or suggestively related to survival. The assumed limit for significance to enter a term was 0.10 and the limit to remove a term 0.15.

A stepwise procedure was also used to evaluate the prognostic significance of each histological classification alone and in combination with the other ones after adjusting survival for stage and venous invasion.

Results were expressed in percentage or in mean ± standard error. Chi-square method after Yates correction and Student's two sided *t* test were used to perform statistical analysis. Significance tests relating to the hypothesis that a specific regression coefficient was zero were based on the assumption that the regression coefficient divided by its estimated standard error is distributed according to the Student's *t* distribution.

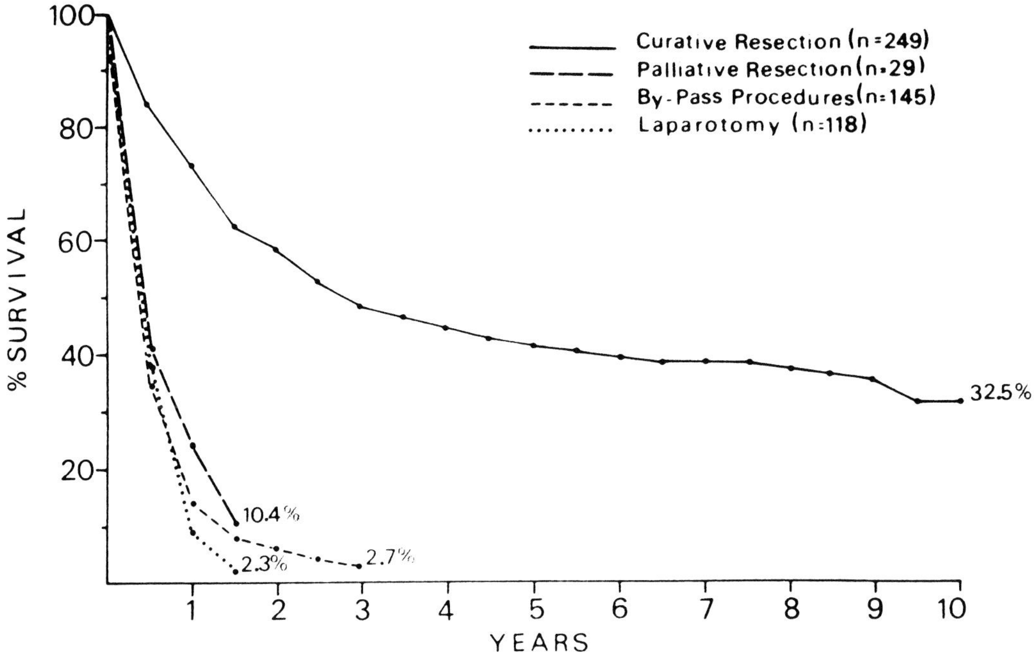


**Fig. 2-1.** Survival curves of the 541 patients submitted to surgery for gastric carcinoma.

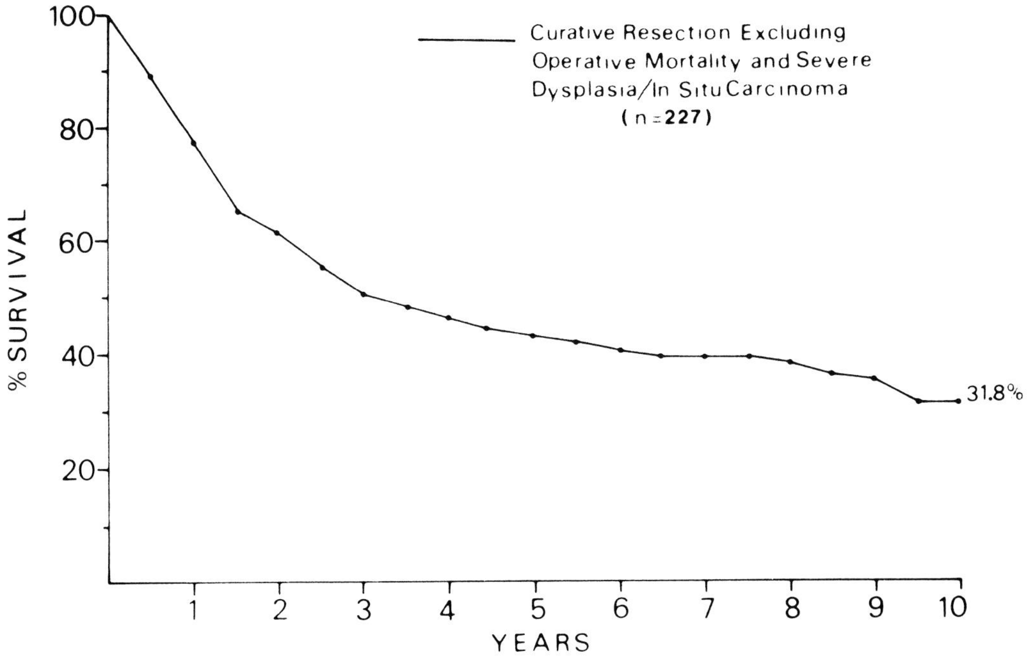


**Fig. 2-2.** Survival curve of the 227 patients used as basis for the evaluation of the prognostic factors.

**TABLE 2-2**
Summary of the Results Obtained with the Multivariate Analysis of Prognostic Factors with Cox Model

| Factors | Regression Coefficient | Coeff/st. error | p value |
|---|---|---|---|
| Stage | 0.3647 | 5.85 | $p < 0.001$ |
| Venous invasion | 0.6714 | 3.18 | $p < 0.001$ |
| Sex | −0.1924 | −0.85 | NS |
| Age | 0.1431 | 0.81 | NS |
| Type of resection | −0.1863 | −0.55 | NS |
| Site | 0.4018 | 1.97 | $p < 0.05$ |
| Histology/Laurén | 0.1930 | 0.94 | NS |
| Histology/WHO | 0.0159 | −0.09 | NS |
| Histology/Ming | 0.1007 | 0.32 | NS |
| Desmoplasia | −0.6013 | −2.38 | $p < 0.02$ |
| Lymphoid infiltration | −0.0812 | 0.39 | NS |
| Follicular hyperplasia | 0.3807 | 1.63 | $p \simeq 0.10$ |
| Sinusal histiocytosis | −0.2137 | −0.92 | NS |

**TABLE 2-3**
Summary of the Results Obtained with the Stepwise Multivariate Regression of Prognostic Factors with MPLR Method

| | Improvement | | |
|---|---|---|---|
| Factors | Log Likelihood | Chi-Square | p Value |
| 0 | −472.0 | | |
| Stage | −441.8 | −60.38 | 0.001 |
| Venous invasion | −434.8 | −14.02 | 0.001 |
| Desmoplasia | −431.7 | −6.24 | 0.013 |
| Site | −428.5 | −6.48 | 0.011 |
| Follicular hyperplasia | −426.9 | −3.14 | 0.076 |

## RESULTS

As is to be expected, the survival curve of patients submitted to "curative" resection is clearly better than those of patients submitted to other types of surgery (Fig. 2-1). Excluding post-operative deaths, the 5 and 10-year survival rates of the 227 patients with invasive carcinomas submitted to curative resection are 42.3% and 31.8%, respectively (Fig. 2-2).

## STAGE AND VENOUS INVASION

The multivariate analysis of prognostic factors shows that stage (extent of neoplastic disease as measured according to the TNM criteria) and venous invasion are, by far, the most important factors (Tables 2-2 and 2-3).

The prognostic value of both the depth of tumor invasion (T) and the status of nodal metastases (N) is shown in Figures 2-3 and 2-4 and Table 2-4.

The survival experience of patients with carcinomas lacking nodal metastases and showing definite signs of lymphatic permeation (NO1p) is much worse than that of patients with NO carcinomas and no signs of lymphatic permeation (Fig. 2-4) (Table 2-4). Patients with NO1p carcinomas were, therefore, grouped together with those having metastasized to a single lymph node (N1(1)). This grouping was used in the evaluation of the prognostic meaning of the combination of T and N factors, as well as in the study of the prognostic value of the other factors (Fig. 2-5) (Tables 2-1–4).

Most of the patients with carcinomas showing signs of venous invasion have advanced stages of the neoplastic disease (Table 2-5). These patients do much worse than those having similarly advanced carcinomas and lacking venous invasion (Fig. 2-6) (Table 2-5). The presence of blood vessel invasion worsens also the survival of patients with less advanced carcinomas, but the difference is, in these cases, lesser than in the group of advanced carcinomas (Fig. 2-6) (Table 2-5).

## SITE, DESMOPLASIA AND PATTERN OF LYMPH NODE RESPONSE

The multivariate analysis shows that site of tumors and degree of desmoplasia are significantly ($p<0.05$) correlated with survival (Tables 2-2 and 2-3). The pattern of regional nodes is also correlated with survival, though

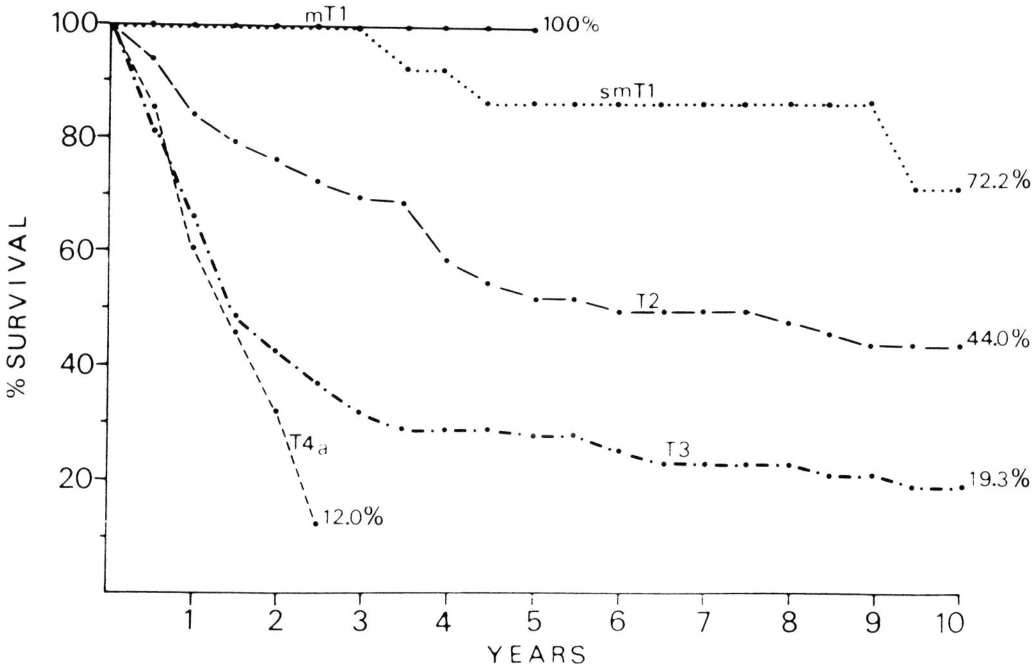


**Fig. 2-3.** Survival curves of the 227 patients according to the depth of penetration of gastric wall. (Abbrev: m = mucosa, sm = submucosa).

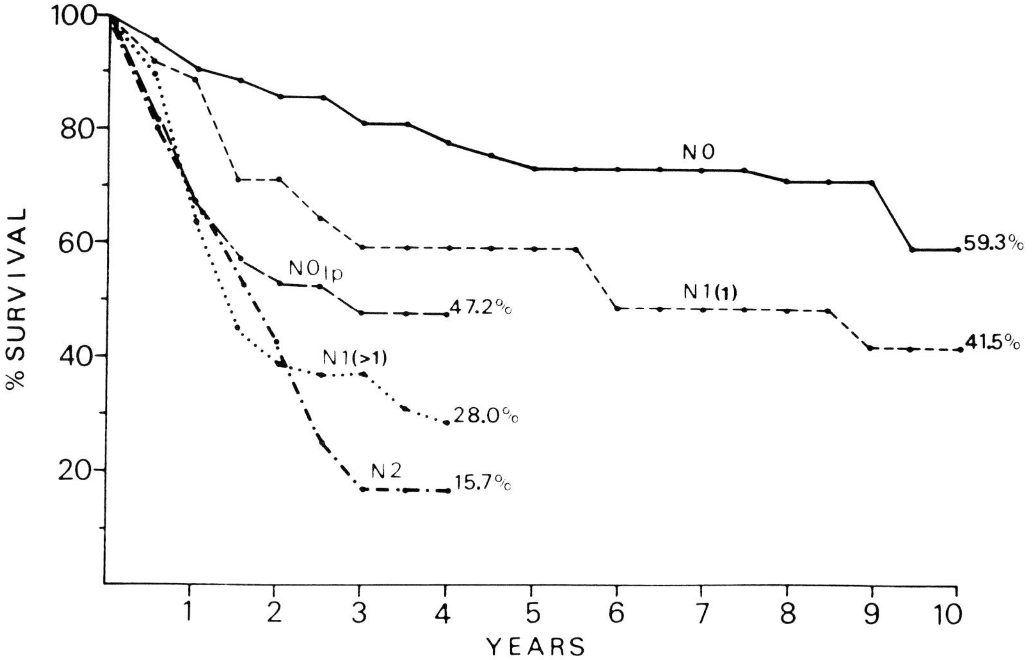


**Fig. 2-4.** Survival curves of 218 patients according to the status of nodal metastases. (Abbrev: lp = lymphatic permeation). No information was available in 9 patients.

## TABLE 2-4

Death Rates According to Depth of Invasion, Nodal Metastases and Stage

| Depth of Invasion | Death Rate | Nodal Metastases | Death Rate | Stage | Death Rate |
|---|---|---|---|---|---|
| T1m (10) | 0.0 | NO (64) | 0.43 | T1m NO (8) | 0.0 |
| T1sm (18) | 0.33 | NOLp (21) | 1.59 | T1sm NO (7) | 0.37 |
| T2 (80) | 0.83 | N1 (1) (29) | 0.86 | T2 NO (30) | 0.30 |
| T3 (91) | 2.02 | N1 (>1) (52) | 2.48 | T3 NO (18) | 0.79 |
| T4a (28) | 4.13 | N2 (52) | 3.82 | T4a NO (2) | 6.45 |
| | | Nx (9) | 0.69 | T1-2 NOLp N1(1) (24) | 0.68 |
| | | | | T3 NOLp N1 (1) (18) | 1.60 |
| | | | | T1-3 N1 (>1) (44) | 2.34 |
| | | | | T1-3 N2 (41) | 3.78 |
| | | | | T4a NOLpN1-2 (26) | 4.0 |

The number of patients is recorded in parentheses.

only at a suggestive ($p<0.10$) level (Tables 2-2 and 2-3).

### Site

Patients with tumors located in the antrum have better prognosis (5 and 10-year survival rates of 48.3% and 36.3%, respectively) than those with tumors originating in the body of the stomach (39.2% and 28.2%, respectively). The prognosis worsens clearly when the bulk of the tumor is located in the fundus or in the cardia (2-year survival rates of 36.1% and

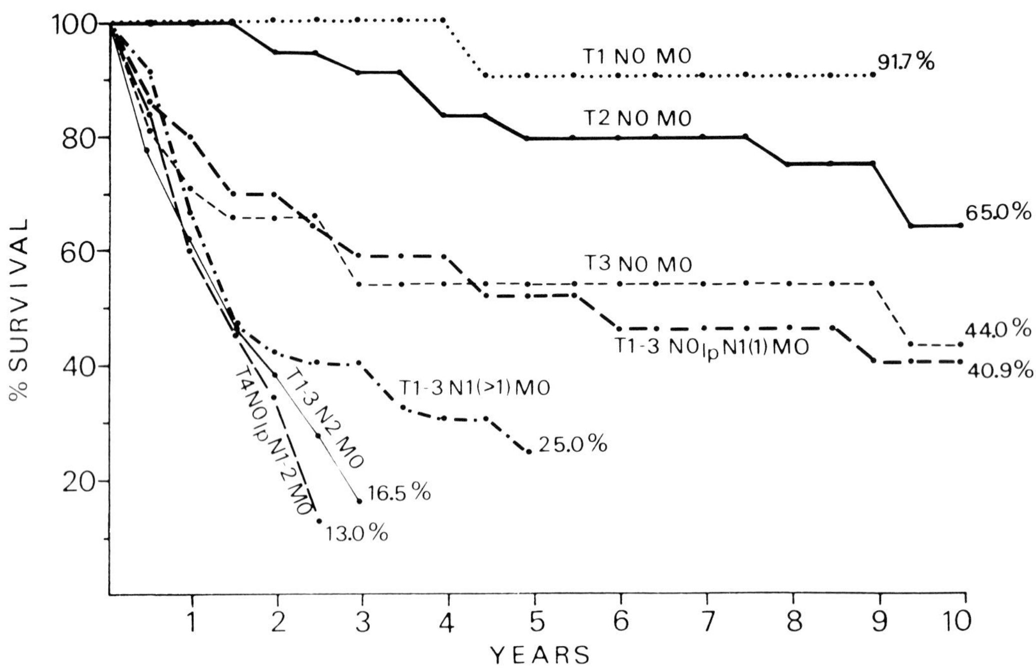


**Fig. 2-5.** Survival curves of 216 patients according to the TNM stage. (Abbrev: lp = lymphatic permeation). Two T4NOMO cases and 9 NX cases were excluded.

**TABLE 2-5**
Death Rates According to Stage and Venous Invasion

| T1-3 NO | | T1-3 NOLp N1 (1) | | T1-4a N1 (> 1)N2 | |
|---|---|---|---|---|---|
| Venous Invasion | Death Rate | Venous Invasion | Death Rate | Venous Invasion | Death Rate |
| Absent (46) | 0.29 | Absent (20) | 0.88 | Absent (54) | 2.33 |
| Present (8) | 1.04 | Present (13) | 1.21 | Present (46) | 5.40 |

The number of patients is recorded in parentheses.

45.5%, respectively). This worse prognosis is confirmed by the evaluation of death rate (Table 2-6).

The prognostic significance of the site of tumors depends upon the type of resection. The putative influence of other factors (technical problems related to the operative procedures, topography of the upper part of the abdomen, and "special" routes of lymphatic drainage in the proximal stomach) will be discussed in detail elsewhere (Ribeiro et al in preparation).

Desmoplasia

Patients with carcinomas showing moderate to abundant desmoplastic reaction do worse (5 and 10-year survival rates of 21.7% and 17.4%, respectively) than those with tumors lacking this histologic feature (51.8% and 38.6%, respectively). The analysis of death rate provides similar results (Table 2-6). The presence of moderate to abundant desmoplasia is significantly correlated with the size and shape of tumors, being particularly frequent in large tumors displaying an infiltrative or ulcero-infiltrative macroscopical appearance.

Pattern of Lymph Node Response

The 5 and 10-year survival rates of patients with "follicular hyperplasia" of regional

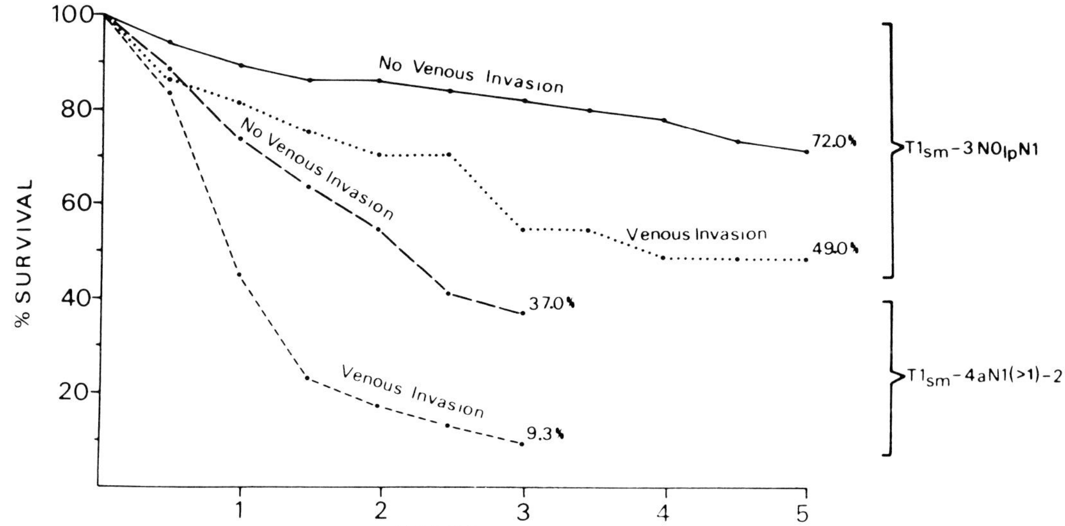


**Fig. 2-6.** Survival curves of 184 patients according to TNM stage and venous invasion (Abbrev: sm = submucosa, lp = lymphatic permeation). Ten intramucosal (T1m) carcinomas, 2 T4NOMO carcinomas, 9 NX carcinomas, and 22 cases without information on venous invasion were excluded.

**TABLE 2-6**
Death Rates According to Site, Desmoplasia and Pattern of Regional Lymph Nodes (Follicular Hyperplasia)

| Factors | | No of Patients | Death Rate |
|---|---|---|---|
| Site | Antrum | 142 | 1.02 |
| | Body | 47 | 1.36 |
| | Fundus | 22 | 2.66 |
| | Cardia | 11 | 2.80 |
| Follicular Hyperplasia | Abund./Moderate | 119 | 0.97 |
| | Min./Absent | 77 | 1.80 |

nodes (53.8% and 38.1%, respectively) are higher than those of patients lacking this feature (25.8% and 21.7%, respectively). These results were confirmed by death rate analysis (Table 2-6). Follicular hyperplasia is significantly correlated with the presence of moderate to abundant sinusal histiocytosis and independent from the degree of lymphoid infiltration of the tumors and extent of neoplastic disease.

## Histology

The multivariate analysis reveals that none of the histological classifications is significantly correlated with survival (Tables 2-2 and 2-3). This lack of prognostic significance does not depend upon the presence of desmoplasia as a covariate, since similar results were obtained when desmoplasia was removed from the regression equation.

The evaluation of the prognostic value of each histological classification shows that, *per se*, Ming[37] classification appears to be the most discriminating (Figs. 2-7–2-9) (Table 2-7). The combined use of WHO[55] and Ming classifications reveal that patients with poorly differentiated carcinomas of expanding pattern do better than those with well/moderately differentiated carcinomas of infiltrative pattern (Fig. 2-10).

Ming classification also provides better prognostic information than Laurén[54] and

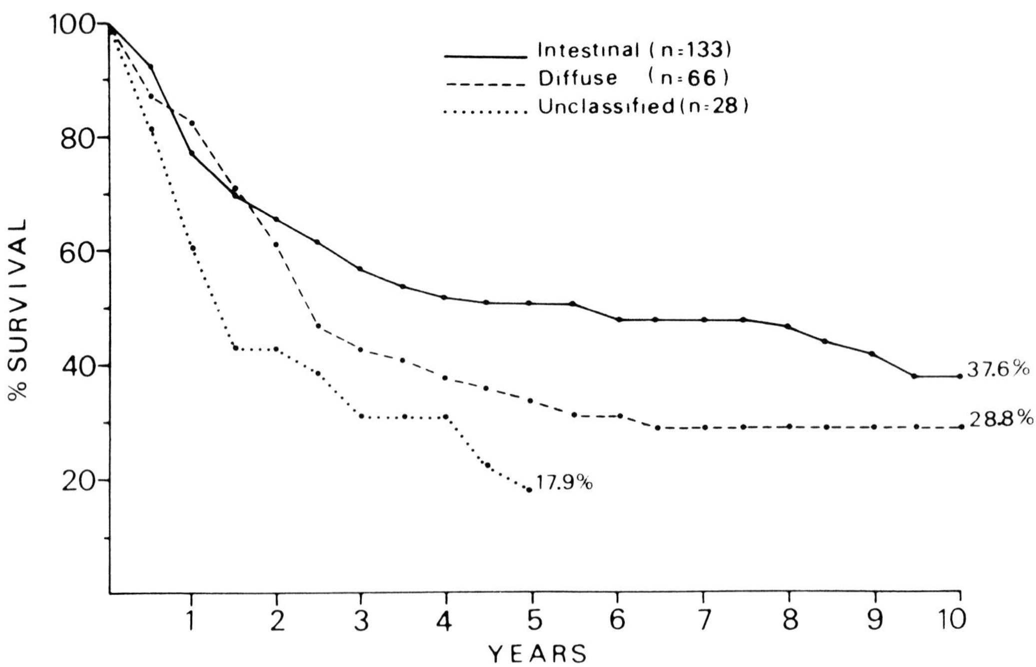


**Fig. 2-7.** Survival curves of the 227 patients according to Laurén classification.

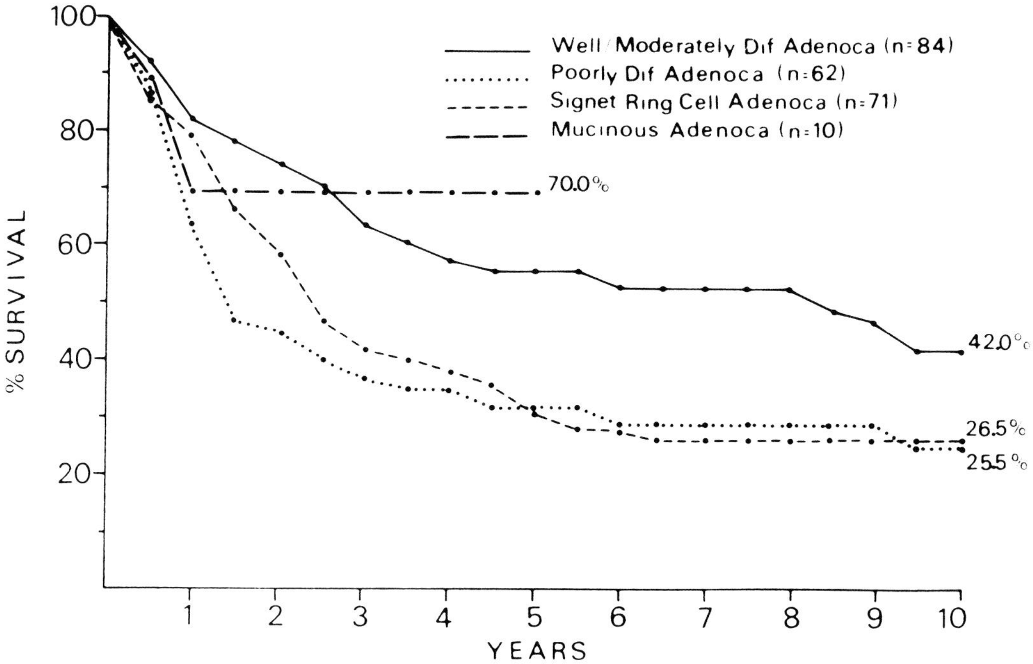


**Fig. 2-8.** Survival curves of the 227 patients according to WHO classification.

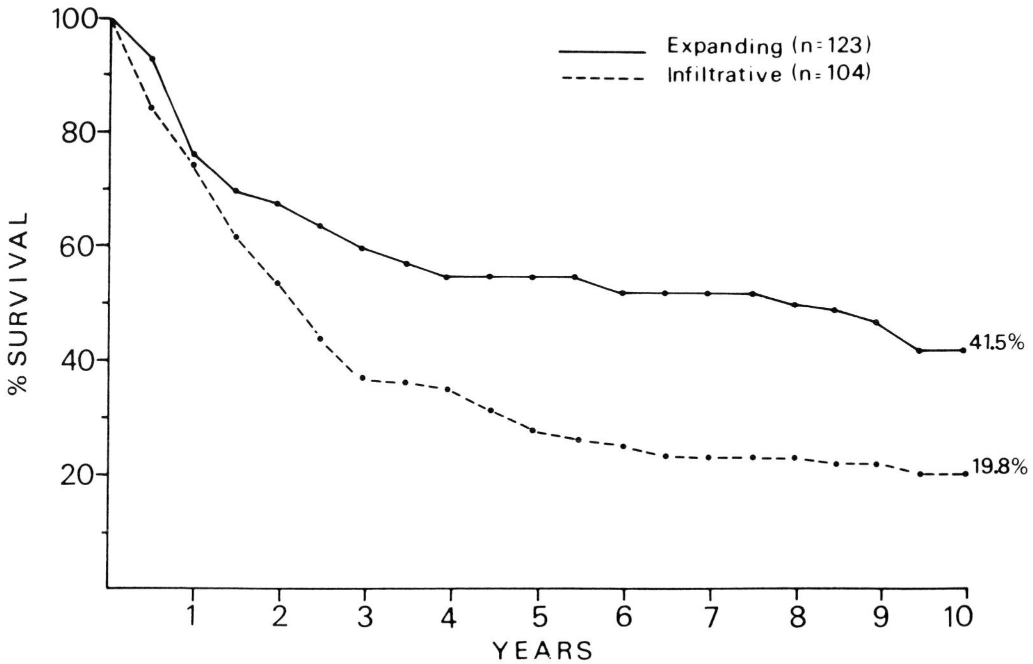


**Fig. 2-9.** Survival curves of the 227 patients according to Ming classification.

**TABLE 2-7**
Death Rates According to Histological Classification

| | Factors | No of Patients | Death Rate |
|---|---|---|---|
| Laurén | Intestinal | 133 | 0.97 |
| | Diffuse | 66 | 1.53 |
| | Unclassified | 28 | 2.74 |
| WHO | Mucinous | 10 | 1.07 |
| | Well/Moderately dif. | 84 | 0.79 |
| | Signet ring cell | 70 | 1.66 |
| | Poorly dif. | 63 | 1.77 |
| Ming | Expanding | 122 | 0.87 |
| | Infiltrative | 105 | 1.88 |

WHO classifications when stage and venous invasion are kept as the sole covariates of the regression equation (Table 2-8). Using this model, no further improvement is obtained when two classifications are used instead of one (Table 2-8).

## Other Factors

### Sex and Age of Patients

The 5 and 10-year survival rates of women (44.9% and 34.9%) are slightly better than those of men (40.0% and 29.7%, respectively). Death rate is also slightly lower in women than in men (Table 2-9).

The 5-year survival rate of patients less than 40 years (38.2%) is slightly lower than those of patients from 40 to 60 years (42.3%) and older than 60 years (43.4%). The analysis of death rate shows the worse prognosis of the youngest patients (Table 2-9). The multivariate analysis demonstrates that neither sex nor age are significantly correlated with survival (Tables 2-2 and 2-3).

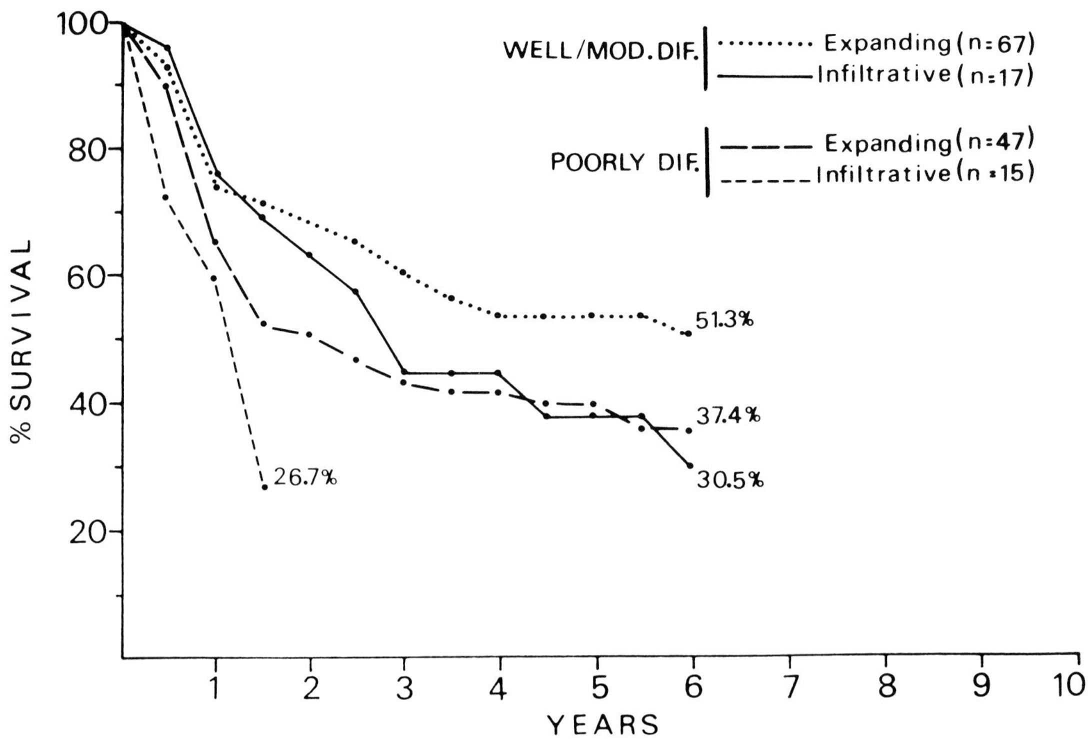


**Fig. 2-10.** Survival curves of 146 patients according to Ming and WHO classifications. Ten mucinous carcinomas and 71 signet ring cell carcinomas were excluded.

## TABLE 2-8

Summary of the Results Obtained with the Multivariate Analysis of the Prognostic Significance of Histological Classifications

| Factors | Improvement: Log Likelihood | Improvement: p Value |
|---|---|---|
| Stage + Ven. Inv. | −515.8 | |
| Stage + Ven. Inv. + Laurén | −515.3 | NS |
| + WHO | −515.6 | NS |
| + Ming | −514.2 | $p < 0.10$ |
| Stage + Ven. Inv. + Laurén + WHO | −515.3 | NS |
| + Laurén + Ming | −514.1 | NS |
| + WHO + Ming | −514.1 | NS |

## TABLE 2-9

Death Rates According to Sex, Age, Type of Resection, Shape, Size, Lymphoid Infiltration, and Sinusal Histiocytosis

| Factors | | No of Patients | Death Rate |
|---|---|---|---|
| Sex | Women | 85 | 1.18 |
| | Men | 142 | 1.28 |
| Age | < 30 | 7 | 2.10 |
| | 30–39 | 16 | 1.13 |
| | 40–49 | 42 | 0.96 |
| | 50–59 | 68 | 1.29 |
| | 60–69 | 71 | 1.42 |
| | 70–79 | 23 | 1.19 |
| Type of Resection | Distal | 170 | 1.10 |
| | Total | 45 | 1.70 |
| | Proximal | 12 | 3.66 |
| Shape | Polyp./Fungating | 17 | 0.82 |
| | Ulcerative | 57 | 0.86 |
| | Ulc./Fungating | 61 | 0.91 |
| | Ulc./Infiltrative | 53 | 2.19 |
| | Infiltrative | 26 | 2.76 |
| Size | < 3 cm | 29 | 0.70 |
| | ≥ 3 < 6 cm | 64 | 0.94 |
| | ≥ 6 cm | 92 | 1.74 |
| Lymphoid Infiltration | Abundant | 40 | 0.97 |
| | Moderate | 67 | 1.22 |
| | Min./Absent | 120 | 1.36 |
| Sinusal Histiocytosis | Abundant/Moderate | 125 | 0.87 |
| | Min./Absent | 70 | 1.51 |

### Type of Resection

Patients submitted to distal gastrectomy do better (5-year survival of 46.0%) than those submitted to total gastrectomy (5-year survival of 32.8%) and proximal gastrectomy (2-year survival of 41.7%). The 10-year survival rate of patients submitted to distal gastrectomy (33.0%) is, however, similar to that of patients submitted to total gastrectomy (32.8%). The analysis of death rate also demonstrates the worse prognosis of patients submitted to proximal gastrectomy (Table 2-9). The prognostic value of this factor is closely related to that of "tumor site" as mentioned previously and does not stand when the multivariate analysis is performed (Tables 2-2 and 2-3).

### Shape and Size of Tumors

The 5 and 10-year survival rates of patients with polypoid/fungating tumors (59.3% and 48.5%, respectively) are similar to those of patients with ulcerating (68.5% and 52.4%) and ulcero-fungating tumors (63.6% and 48.9%). The prognosis is clearly worse in patients with ulcero-infiltrative tumors (5 and 10-year survival rates of 23.4% and 14.9%, respectively) and even much worse in those bearing infiltrative carcinomas (3-year survival rate of 27.0%). These results are confirmed by death rate analysis (Table 2-9).

Patients with tumors 6 cm, or larger than 6 cm, do worse (5 and 10-year survival rates of 35.0% and 21.9%, respectively) than those with smaller tumors (3 to 6 cm, 49.0% and 38.4%; less than 3 cm, 58.6% and 51.7%, respectively). Death rate analysis provides similar results (Table 2-9).

The prognostic value of both the macroscopical appearance and the size of tumors almost disappears when the influence of stage, venous invasion, and desmoplasia is controlled.

### Lymphoid Infiltration of the Tumors and Histiocytosis of Regional Nodes

The 5 and 10-year survival rates of patients with carcinomas showing abundant lymphoid infiltration (55.6% and 38.9%, respectively) do better than those with carcinomas displaying moderate (44.2% and 33.9%, respectively) and minimal/absent lymphoid infiltration (38.6% and 29.9%, respectively). These results are confirmed by death rate analysis (Table 2-9). Lymphoid infiltration is independent of the stage of tumors and correlates negatively with mucin producing carcinomas (so-called mucinous and signet ring cell carcinomas).

Patients with abundant/moderate nodal histiocytosis do better (5 and 10-year survival rates of 46.5% and 32.7%, respectively) than those with minimal/absent histiocytosis (34.0% and 27.0%, respectively). Death rate analysis provides similar results (Table 2-9).

The multivariate analysis demonstrates that neither lymphoid infiltration nor nodal histiocytosis are significantly correlated with survival (Tables 2-2 and 2-3).

## DISCUSSION

As it usually happens with papers dealing with statistical analysis of interrelated clinicopathological variables, our study offers a number of conclusions that will be tentatively discussed in a stepwise fashion.

The first of such conclusions concerns the major prognostic significance of the evaluation of the extent of neoplastic disease as measured according to the TNM criteria defined by the American Joint Committee.[1] This finding might be anticipated from most of the results obtained elsewhere[1,9,12,16,17,20,22,26,28,29,38,40,41,45,51] and does not justify, therefore, any special comment.

Our second conclusion regards the advantage of adding the evaluation of lymphatic permeation and status of nodal metastases to the traditional TNM criteria. In fact, the survival experience of patients with "N0 carcinomas plus lymphatic permeation" is sufficiently bad to advise the inclusion of these cases, for staging purposes, in the group of N1 carcinomas. The subdivision of N1 carcinomas according to the number of positive nodes was also found to provide additional and valuable prognostic information.

These results reinforce the concept of neoplastic development, which forms the rational basis for the TNM method and demonstrate that the predictive value of this method can still be improved. It is likely that further improvement would have been achieved if more detailed information on the number and localization of metastatic lymph nodes had been available. However, the possibility of testing this hypothesis, which has already been confirmed in several other models (e.g., breast carcinoma), rests beyond the limits of a retrospective study like this.

The exceedingly important prognostic role played in our series by the presence of unequivocal signs of venous invasion within the primary tumors also deserves a special mention. The search for venous invasion is easily performed in slides stained with orcein and does not require the study of extramural veins unlike what happens in colorectal carcinoma.[59] It seems, therefore, quite surprising that most authors apparently ignore the study of this factor.

The major predictive value of venous invasion had been previously reported.[18,32,38,44] Kodama et al[27] obtained similar results in a study of early gastric carcinoma, thus supporting our assumption that venous invasion worsens the outcome of patients regardless of the extent of neoplastic disease. The negative findings of Bedikian et al[3] may reflect different criteria in judging blood vessel invasion which, in our experience, should only be affirmed if clusters of neoplastic cells are seen within the lumina (often distending the walls) of elastic walled vessels.

Desmoplasia was the third most important prognostic factor disclosed in our series. This finding is in keeping with the dreadful prognosis that is generally linked to the well-known "linitis plastica" and to its histological counterpart, the so-called scirrhous carcinoma.[4,8,11,18,21,30,36,44] The predictive value of the desmoplastic reaction goes far beyond those of signet ring cell carcinomas and diffuse carcinomas. Desmoplasia correlates with size and macroscopical appearance of tumors. One can therefore assume that the predictive value of the presence of desmoplastic reaction may be due, partly at least, to the large size and the infiltrative (or ulcero-infiltrative) growth of the tumors displaying such reaction.

The site of carcinomas was also found to carry significant prognostic information. This is particularly obvious in what concerns the poor outcome of patients with high-seated tumors and has been repeatedly reported in the literature.[7,10,12,13,17,23,31,33] This worse prognosis cannot be merely ascribed to a more advanced extent of the neoplastic disease. It expresses probably the concurrence of several "negative" factors related to the anatomy and topography of the cardioeosophageal junction and to some specific problems of the surgical approach to such tumors (Ribeiro et al, in preparation).

The pattern of regional lymph nodes as measured through the evaluation of the degree of follicular hyperplasia was the last factor carrying some prognostic value, though at a suggestive level only. Our findings support therefore those of Black et al[4] who claim the superiority of follicular hyperplasia over nodal histiocytosis for prognostic purposes. They clearly contradict, on the other hand, those authors that stress the prognostic significance of nodal histiocytosis.[3]

The absence of any predictive value of the lymphoid infiltration of the tumors also contradicts many previous reports.[4,15,17,30,35,49] This does not mean, however, that we question the existence of a special type of tumor successively coined as "blue cell carcinoma," "medullary carcinoma with lymphoid infiltration," and "gastric carcinoma with lymphoid stroma" (for a thorough review see Watanabe et al[49]). This type of carcinoma, which is slightly more prevalent in our series (5.4%) than in Watanabe et al[49] series (4%), indeed carries an excellent prognosis.[15,35,49]

Such benign behavior should not be ascribed in our opinion to the abundance of lymphoid infiltrate, since our cases, like those of Watanabe et al,[49] have such limited extent of the neoplastic disease that this fact might, per se, explain their good prognosis (as it does in similarly well circumscribed carcinomas lacking moderate to abundant lymphoid infiltration). Most of these carcinomas are well circumscribed tumors with pushing margins that do not infiltrate deeply the gastric wall and do not have nodal metastases. It is of course impossible to decide whether or not the lymphoid infiltration plays any decisive role in the limitation of the neoplastic extension in these tumors.

It is also difficult to draw any definite conclusions from the contradictory prognostic results obtained in the study of the factors admittedly linked to the so called host-immunologic "response" that suggest positive findings with follicular hyperplasia and negative findings with nodal histiocytosis and lymphoid infiltration. The study of this "response" with other methods did not provide conclusive results either,[5] and the problem rests, therefore, unsolved, namely in what concerns advanced carcinomas.[5] Our attitude in this area remains pragmatic: the use of follicular hyperplasia as a prognostic factor is justified by its suggestive influence on the outcome of the patients without necessarily implying any specific relationship with the host-immunologic response.

Our last conclusions will concentrate on the most impressive negative finding of the study—the lack of prognostic significance of any of the most well-known histological classifications. In fact, our results demonstrate that none of them provides valuable prognostic information. They demonstrate also that no additional information is obtained when two histological classifications are used in combination. This lack of predictive value cannot be ascribed to the presence of desmoplasia as a covariable, since the results were almost the same when desmoplasia was removed from the regression equation. Our results confirm, therefore, those[8,31] who stressed the lack of prognostic significance of histology when the influence of staging was controlled. They contradict, on the other hand, most of the papers published so far on the subject in which the prognostic value of histology in general, or of some histological types of carcinoma in particular (e.g. signet ring cell carcinoma), is stressed.[3,8,12,15,19,41,42,46]

We feel somewhat embarrassed with these results since one of the main goals of the study was actually to decide the best classification for prognostic purposes. This lack of prognostic significance does not mean, however, that histological classifications of gastric carcinoma are useless and should be abandoned. Several reasons support this opinion. First, the three classifications provide valuable information for the study of the neoplastic transformation of gastric epithelium. In this field Laurén classification appears to be, in spite of its relatively low reproducibility,[37,60] Sobrinho-Simões and Ribeiro, (unpublished results), the most rewarding as it has been repeatedly proven in epidemiological studies.[41,54] Second, all of them provide the indispensable morphologic basis for further histochemical and immunocytochemical characterization of gastric carcinoma cells. Finally, and this is probably the most interesting conclusion of our study within this area, all of them are closely related with the extent of neoplastic disease. That is the reason why they lose their prognostic significance when survival is adjusted for stage and venous invasion.

The existence of a significant correlation between histology and extent of disease means that these classifications do indeed "measure" some biological properties of the neoplastic cells. In our hands, as well as in others, Ming classification was found to be, *per se,* the most discriminating. It is also noteworthy that the combination of Ming and WHO classifications were found the best "pair" under these circumstances (read: no adjustment for stage and venous invasion). One might anticipate this result from the fact that Ming and WHO "measure" two quite different morphological variables (pattern of growth and differentiation, respectively), whereas both of them more or less overlap Laurén classification.[15,37,55,41]

## CONCLUSIONS

Staging together with the assessment of lymphatic permeation and venous invasion is, by far, the most valuable prognostic factor in gastric carcinoma. The evaluation of the tumoral desmoplasia and pattern of regional lymph node response also provides significant prognostic information.

None of the available histological classifications seems to add any meaningful information regarding prognosis.

High seated tumors carry a worse prognosis, whereas the remaining factors (age and sex of patients, type of resection, tumor shape, tumors size and lymphoid infiltration of the tumors, and histiocytosis of the regional nodes) do not influence significantly the outcome of the patients.

## ACKNOWLEDGMENT

This work was supported by Instituto Nacional de Investigačão Científica (Centro MbP3). The authors thank Dr. Carlos Menezes for his help in the statistical analysis of the results, and Mrs. Olga Ferreira, Miss Fátima Magalhães and Mrs. Odete Ferreira da Costa for technical assistance.

## REFERENCES


1. American Joint Committee for Cancer Staging and End-Results Reporting, In: Manual for Staging of Cancer, Chicago, American Joint Committee, 1978, pp 71–76
2. Barber Jr K.W., Gage R.P., Priestley J.T.: Significance of duration of symptoms and size of lesion in the prognosis of gastric carcinoma. Surg Gynecol Obstet **113**:673–676, 1961
3. Bedikian A.Y., Chen T.T., Khankhanian N., Heilbrun L.K., McBride C.M., McMurtrey M.J., Bodey G.P.: The natural history of gastric cancer and prognostic factors influencing survival. J Clin Oncol **2**:305–310, 1984
4. Black M.M., Freeman C., Mork T., Harvei S., Cutler S.: Prognostic significance of microscopic structure of gastric carcinomas and their regional lymph nodes. Cancer **27**:703–711, 1971
5. Blanca I., Grases P.J., Matos M.V., Contreras C.E., Ochoa M., Wright H., Bianco N.C.: Immunology of human gastric cancer: a preliminary report. Cancer **49**:1810–1816, 1982
6. Bloss R.S., Miller T.A., Copeland III EM: Carcinoma of the stomach in the young adult. Surg Gynecol Obstet **150**:883–886, 1980
7. Brookes V.S., Waterhouse J.A.H., Powell D.J.: Carcinoma of the stomach: a 10-year survey of results and of factors affecting prognosis. Br Med J **1**:1577–1583, 1965
8. Curtis R.E., Kennedy B.J., Myers M.H., Hankey B.F.: Evaluation of AJC stomach cancer staging using the Seer Population. Semin Oncol **12**:21–31, 1985
9. Douglass H.O., Nava H.R.: Gastric adenocarcinoma: management of primary disease. Semin Oncol **12**:32–45, 1985
10. Dupont J.B., Lee J.R., Burton G.R., Cohn I.: Adenocarcinoma of the stomach: review of 1,497 cases. Cancer **41**:941–947, 1978
11. Eker R., Efskind J.: The pathology and prognosis of gastric carcinoma. Acta Chir Scand, suppl 264, 1960
12. Gennari L., Bonfanti G., Salvadori B.: Prognostic factors in gastric cancer. In: International Congress on Diagnosis and Treatment of Upper Gastrointestinal Tumors, International Congress Series 542, Mainz, Excerpta Medica, 1980, pp 173–184
13. Goldenberg I.S., Cohen J.M., Skinner D.G.: A study of survival patterns in patients with gastric carcinoma. Surg Gynecol Obstet **124**:241–250,, 1967
14. Grabiec J., Owen D.A.: Carcinoma of the stomach in young persons. Cancer **56**:388–396, 1985
15. Hoat J., Degels M.A.: Cancer gastrique. Classification anatomopathologique des tumeurs épithéliales malignes de l'estomac. Acta Gastro-Enterol Belg **42**:433–449, 1979.
16. Hautefeuille P., Valleur P., Castaing D., Piel J.-L., Gérum A., Houdart R., Villet R., Galian A.: Influence de l'extension ganglionnaire sur la survie après resection de cancers gastriques infiltrants. Gastroenterol Clin Biol **6**:849–856, 1982
17. Hawley P.R., Westerholm P., Morson B.C.: Pathology and prognosis of carcinoma of the stomach. Br J Surg **57**:877–883, 1970
18 Higgins Jr G.A., Serlin O., Amadeo J.H., McElhinney J., Keehn J: Gastric cancer: factors in survival. Chir Gastroenterol **10**:393–398, 1976
19. Hillon P., Faivre J., Milan C., Justrabo E., Piard F., Michiels R., Klepping C.: Traitement et pronostic des carcinomes gastriques. Étude de la population du département de la Côte-d'Or. Gastroenterol Clin Biol **7**:585–590, 1983
20. Hoerr S.O.: Prognosis for carcinoma of the stomach. Surg Gynecol Obstet **137**:205–209, 1973
21. Hoerr S.O., Hazard J.B., Bailey D.: Prognosis in carcinoma of the stomach in relation to the microscopic type. Surg Gynecol Obstet **122**:485–494, 1966
22. Huguier M., Lacaine F.: Cancer de l'estomac. Facteurs de survie. La Nouv Presse Méd **9**:231–234, 1980
23. Inberg M., Laurén P., Viikari S.J.: Factors influencing survival after radical operation for gastric carcinoma. Acta Chir Scand **132**:195–199, 1966
24. Inberg M.V., Vuori J., Viikari S.J.: Carcinoma of the stomach. A follow-up study of 1963 patients. Acta Chir Scand **138**:195–201, 1972
25. Inlow R.P., Dockerty M.B., Priestley J.T.: Large gastric cancers. Surg Gynecol Obstet **120**:725–730, 1965
26. Kennedy B.J.: TNM classification for stomach cancer. Cancer **26**:971–983, 1970
27. Kodama Y., Inokuchi K., Soejima K., Matsusaka T., Okamura T.: Growth patterns and prognosis in early gastric carcinoma. Superficially spreading and penetrating growth types. Cancer **51**:320–326, 1983
28. Kodama Y., Sugimachi K., Soejima K., Matsusaka T., Inokuchi K.: Evaluation of extensive lymph node dissection for carcinoma of the stomach. World J Surg **5**:241–248, 1981
29. Lambert R.: Les bases rationnelles du pronostic du cancer gastrique opéré. Arch Fr Mal App Dig **64**:679–696, 1975
30. Larmi T.K.I., Saxén L.: "Host Reactions" in gastric cancer. A preliminary study of 119 cases of gastrectomy. Acta Chir Scand **125**:144–146, 1963
31. Lawrence W.T., Lawrence Jr W.: Gastric cancer: The surgeon's viewpoint. Semin Oncol **7**:400–414, 1980
32. Lewin E.: Gastric cancer. Acta Clin Scand Suppl 262, 1960
33. Lumpkin W.M., Crow R.L., Hernandez C.M., Cohn I.: Carcinoma of the stomach: Review of 1,035 cases. Ann Surg **159**:919–932, 1964
34. MacDonald W.C.: Clinical and pathologic features of adenocarcinoma of the gastric cardia. Cancer **29**:724–732, 1972
35. Martin C., Kay S.: The prognosis of gastric carcinoma as related to its morphologic characteristics. Surg Gynecol Obstet **119**:319–322, 1964
36. Mehrotra M.L., Gupta I.M., Khanna S., Vaidya M.P.: Host response and tumor biological behaviour in the two histological types of gastric carcinoma. Histopathology **2**:373–382, 1978
37. Ming S.-C.: Gastric carcinoma: a pathobiological classification. Cancer **39**:2475–2485, 1977
38. Öhman U., Wetterfors J., Moberg A.: Primary gastric cancer and its prognosis. Acta Chir Scand **138**:378–383, 1972
39. Papachristou D.N., Agnanti N., D'Agostino H., Fortner J.G.: Histologically positive esophageal margin in the surgical treatment of gastric cancer. Amer J Surg **139**:711–713, 1980
40. Remine W.H., Gomes M.M.R., Dockerty M.B.: Long-term survival (10 to 56 years) after surgery for carcinoma of the stomach. Amer J Surg **117**:177–184, 1969
41. Ribeiro M.N., Sarmento J.A., Sobrinho-Simões M.A.,

Bastos J.: Prognostic significance of Laurén and Ming classifications and other pathologic parameters in gastric carcinoma. Cancer **47**:780–784, 1981
42. Ribeiro M.M., Sobrinho-Simões M.A., Bastos J.: Analysis of 242 cases of gastric carcinoma. World J Surg **5**:97–102, 1981
43. Roux M., Vayrè P., Lassau J.-P., Chevallard A.: Une série de 100 cancers de l'estomac opérés avec un recul de 5 ans. Commentaires et réflexions. J Chir (Paris) **101**:377–388, 1971
44. Serlin O., Keehn R.J., Higgins G.A. Jr, Harrower H.W., Mendeloff G.L.: Factors related to survival following resection for gastric carcinoma: analysis of 903 cases. Cancer **40**:1318–1329, 1977
45. Soga J., Kobayashi K., Saito J., Fujimaki M., Muto T.: The role of lymphadenectomy in curative surgery for gastric cancer. World J Surg **3**:701–708, 1979
46. Stemmermann G.N., Brown C.: A survival study of intestinal and diffuse types of gastric carcinoma. Cancer **33**:1190–1195, 1974
47. Teglbjaerg P.S., Vetner M.: Gastric carcinoma: an analysis of morphological and prognostic parameters correlated to the classification proposed by Masson, Rember & Mulligan. Acta Path Microbiol Scand (A) **85**:528–534, 1977
48. Wanke M., Schwan H.: Pathology of gastric cancer. World J Surg **3**:675–684, 1979
49. Watanabe H., Enjoji M., Imai T.: Gastric carcinoma with lymphoid stroma. Its morphologic characteristics and prognostic correlations. Cancer **38**:232–243, 1976
50 WHO International Reference Center to evaluate methods of diagnosis and treatment of stomach cancer. Report of the Meeting National Cancer Center Publ., Tokyo, 1972
51. Yamada E., Miyaishi S., Nakazato H., Kato K., Kito T., Takagi H., Yasue M., Kato T., Morimoto T., Yamauchi M.: The surgical treatment of cancer of the stomach. Internat Surg **65**:387–399, 1980
52. Zacho A., Cederovist C., Fishermann K.: Surgical treatment of gastric malignancies: a twenty-year series comprising mainly far advanced and high-seated tumors. Ann Surg **1**:94:101, 1974
53. Zacho A., Fischermann K., Sorensen B.L.: Prognostic role of breach of lymph node capsule in nodal metastases from gastric carcinoma. Acta Chir Scand **125**:365–369, 1963
54. Laurén P.: The two histological main types of gastric carcinoma: diffuse and so-called intestinal-type carcinoma. An attempt at a histo-clinical classification. Acta Path Microbiol Scand **64**:31–49, 1965
55. Oota K., Sobin L.H.: Histological Typing of Gastric and Oesophageal Tumours. International Histological Classification of Tumours no 18, World Health Organization, Geneva, 1977
56. Tsakraklides V., Anastassiados O.T., Kersey J.H.: Prognostic significance of regional lymph nodes histology in uterine cervical cancer. Cancer **31**:860–868, 1973
57. Berkson J., Gage R.P.: Calculation of survival rates for cancer. Mayo Clin Proc **25**:270, 1950
58. Cox D.R.: Regression models and life tables. J Roy Soc Stat, Series B, **34**:187–220, 1972
59. Talbot I.C., Ritchie S., Leighton M., Hughes A.O., Bussey H.J.R., Morson B.C.: Invasion of veins by carcinoma of rectum: method of detection, histological features and significance. Histopathology **5**:141–163, 1981
60. Pagnini C.A., Rugge M.: Gastric cancer: problems in histological diagnosis. Histopathology **6**:391–398, 1982

# 3

# Varioliform Gastritis Revisited

J.P. van Spreeuwel M.D., Ph.D.
C.J.L.M. Meijer M.D., Ph.D.
J. Lindeman M.D., Ph.D.

Gastritis is very commonly encountered in both asymptomatic individuals and in patients with upper abdominal discomfort; its frequency increases with age. It is the result of various endogenous and exogenous and often poorly defined noxes to the gastric mucosa. It represents a diagnostic and therapeutic problem for the clinician, since correlation between symptoms and histologically proven gastritis is poor, correlation between endoscopic and histological findings is poor, and there is no effective therapy.

Several classifications of gastritis have been proposed and attempts have been made to discriminate certain more or less specific forms of gastritis. One of these is the so called varioliform gastritis, alternatively known as chronic erosive gastritis, dellen gastritis, superficial hypertrophic gastritis, aphthous ulcers, or complete erosions, which has been claimed to be an entity characterized by an increased number of IgE containing cells in the gastric mucosa and requiring specific treatment.[1] Varioliform gastritis, especially whether or not it represents a specific entity, will be the subject of this paper.

## CLINICAL FEATURES

Varioliform gastritis is characterized by usually multiple, round, or oval lesions of the gastric mucosa, 5–10 mm in diameter, consisting of a central erosion surrounded by an elevated border (Fig. 3-1). Varioliform or chronic erosions as opposed to acute erosions have elevated margins and are predominantly located in the gastric antrum along the greater curvature.[2,3] They may, on the other hand, occur diffusely throughout the stomach and be accompanied by congested swollen rugae. The name gastritis has been argued because the surrounding gastric mucosa may be entirely normal. Although they have already been described in autopsy studies in the 18th century,[4] the first demonstration by gastroscopy and radiology dates back to 1933.[5]

The diagnosis varioliform gastritis has become relatively common since the 70s when endoscopy became widely available in the workup of patients with upper abdominal complaints. The prevalence in patients subjected for some reason to diagnostic gastroduodenoscopy varies from 0.3 to 12.7% with an average of 3%.[3,6–13] It is three-fold more common in males than in females, and its frequency reaches a maximum in the 5th and 6th decades, thereby resembling very much the age profile of gastric and duodenal ulcer disease.[14] Although varioliform gastritis has been diagnosed in asymptomatic persons during cancer screening procedures the majority of patients reported have periodic symptoms reminiscent of peptic ulcer disease such as epigastric pain, pyrosis, nausea, and food intolerance often of many years standing. Atypical complaints and considerable weight loss

**Fig. 3-1.** Endoscopic view of a varioliform erosion.

have also been reported especially in patients with the diffuse type.

In a considerable number, 30–40% of the patients, peptic ulceration of the duodenum or the stomach is diagnosed simultaneously[3] or during follow-up.[3,6,15] Gastrointestinal bleeding, common in acute erosions, is rare. Occasionally, varioliform gastritis is complicated by protein losing enteropathy.[9,12,17] Association with recurrent oral aphthous ulcers has been described.[19] Long-term observations in 64 patients with varioliform gastritis[3] showed that the condition remained stable in 26, deteriorated in 12, improved in 13; whereas in 13 other patients the lesions healed completely. In 16 patients a gastric or duodenal ulcer developed during follow-up but this was not shown to arise from a varioliform erosion. In some patients erosions fuse together to form hypertrophic folds in the gastric antrum (Fig. 3-2). Evolution to gastric polyps has been suggested, but this was not confirmed.[3] Although varioliform erosions have been shown to heal in several days, most authors have confirmed the persistent or recurrent nature of the lesions.[1,12,16,20]

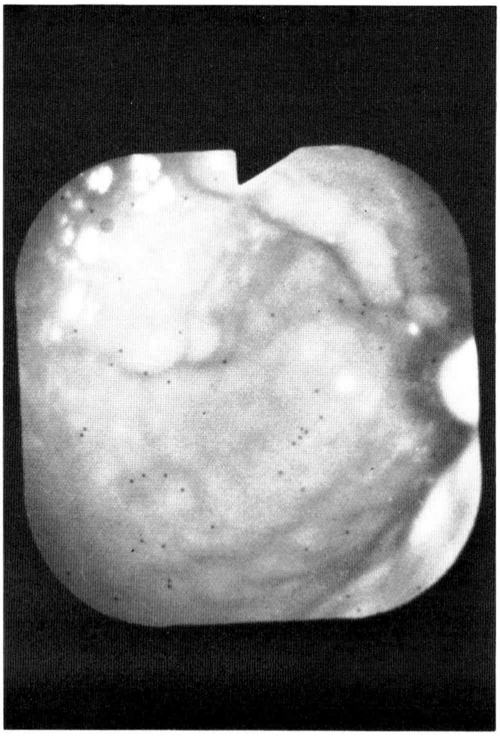

**Fig. 3-2.** Endoscopic view of the gastric antrum showing a swollen mucosal fold as a result of fusion of varioliform erosions.

## HISTOPATHOLOGICAL FEATURES

Histologically varioliform gastritis is characterized by a central epithelial defect not penetrating the muscularis mucosae (Fig. 3-3). The lamina propria is infiltrated by mononuclear cells: plasma cells, lymphocytes, macrophages, and eosinophilic and neutrophilic granulocytes. The latter often infiltrate both surface and glandular epithelium. Marked foveolar hyperplasia and sometimes cystic dilatation of glands in the margins of the lesion explain the macroscopical appearance. Metaplasia of the intestinal type may be found, as well as atrophy of the glandular layer of the epithelium. Specific histological features such as a marked preponderance of eosinophils or granulomas are absent. The surrounding gastric epithelium, may likewise show features of chronic nonspecific gastritis (Fig. 3-4) or be completely normal.

Immunohistochemically Rösh and colleagues[21] found a decrease of IgM and an increase of IgG containing cells, whereas André and colleagues demonstrated a marked increase of IgE containing cells (Fig. 3-5), both plasma cells and activated mast cells, in gastric biopsies of patients with varioliform gastritis.[22] Other studies, however, failed to confirm this.[23-25] Ultrastructural examination failed to reveal specific abnormalities, especially no virus particles could be detected.[14,26] Sometimes microorganisms can be observed in the mucus overlying the gastric mucosa. Recently the presence of campylobacter-like microorganisms in upper gastrointestinal biopsies from patients with gastritis and peptic ulcer disease was given much attention in the literature. These organisms could also be found in 4 of 10 patients with varioliform gastritis.[25] In one histological study of chronic gastric erosions, completely removed by diathermy, a greatly thickened muscularis mucosae, dissociated by fibrous bundles, was observed as well as thickening of vessel walls in the submucosa and occasional cystic gastric glands penetrating the submucosa.[15]

## DIFFERENTIAL DIAGNOSIS

The differential diagnosis of varioliform gastritis should not pose too big a problem. It can reliably be diagnosed by radiological examination,[26,28] preferably by the double contrast method, and by endoscopical examination, the latter probably being more sensitive.[16,25] Varioliform erosions can be differentiated from acute erosions by their elevated margins. Otherwise they differ from true ulcers, since they do not penetrate the muscularis mucosae and, therefore, do not interfere with the peristalsis of the gastric wall.

Crohn's disease may produce varioliform or aphthous erosions in the stomach as well.[29] Differentiation relies both on the demonstration of granulomas in the gastric mucosa, which can be found in two-thirds of patients, as well as the demonstration of Crohn's disease elsewhere in the gastrointestinal tract, as this is invariably present. This, however, applies only to those patients in whom on clinical grounds more extensive disease of the intestine is suspected, and in our experience this is a rare occasion.

Varioliform erosions sometimes fuse to form enlarged folds of the gastric mucosa, and in such cases multiple forceps biopsies should be obtained to exclude other disorders such as infiltrating gastric carcinoma or lymphoma. Other hypertrophic gastropathies such as Menetrier's disease or the Zollinger-Ellison syndrome present with more diffuse abnormalities, but they can be confused with diffuse varioliform gastritis. Large sized biopsies, as well as serum gastrin determination (normal levels are found in varioliform gastritis)[1] should allow differentiation from the Zollinger-Ellison syndrome. A differentiation from Menetrier's disease that relies on histological examination showing hyperplasia of the foveolar layer of the gastric mucosa in the presence of inflammation may be more difficult.

## IS VARIOLIFORM GASTRITIS A SPECIFIC ENTITY?

Arguments to consider varioliform gastritis as a specific entity have been put forward by André and coworkers.[22] They found increased

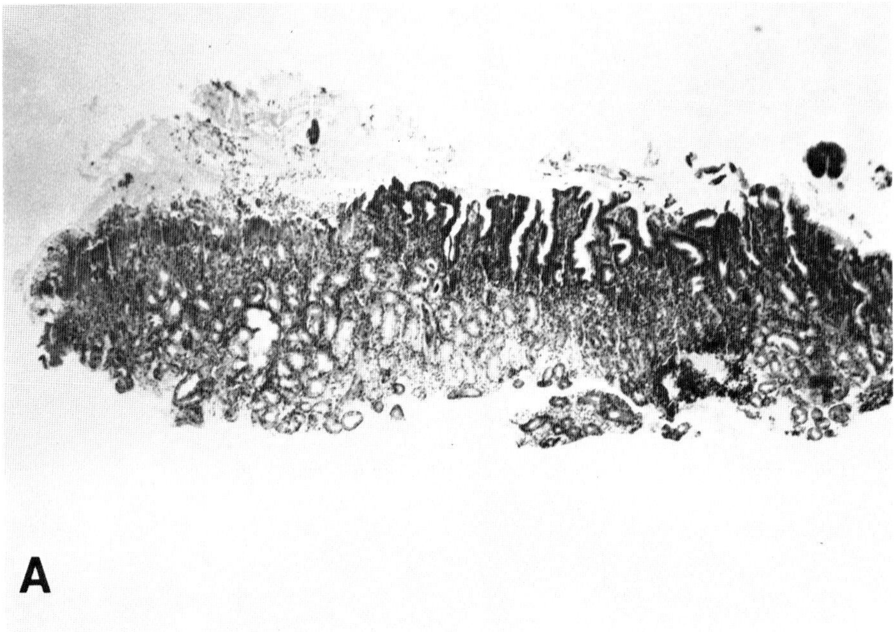


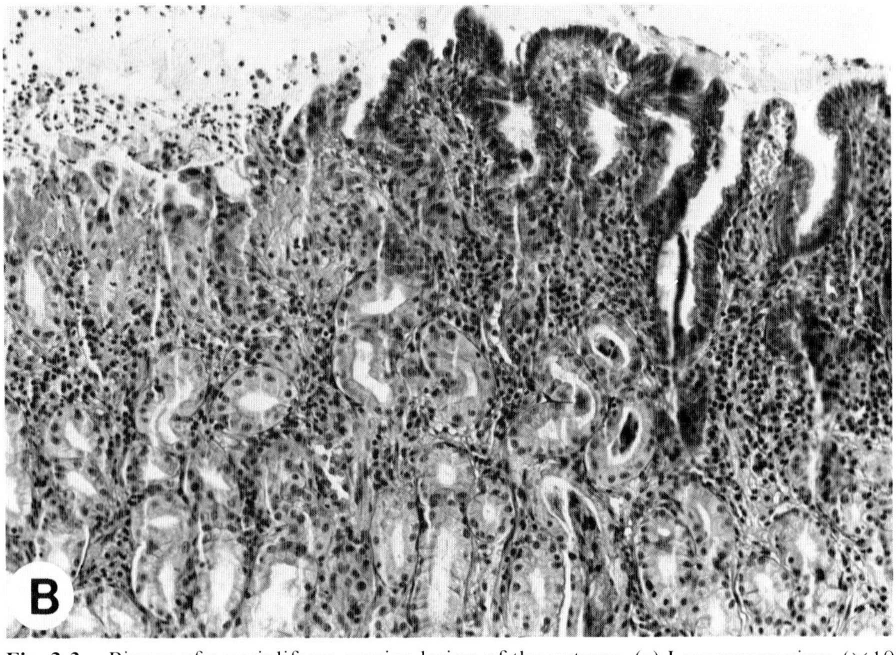


**Fig. 3-3.** Biopsy of a varioliform erosive lesion of the antrum. (a) Low power view. (×10) Note the fibrinoid necrosis of the surface epithelium on the left part of this biopsy. (b) Detail of the transitional area of the erosion (left) and the inflamed adjacent foveolar layer. (×100) (c) Detail of the fibrinoid necrosis of the surface epithelium. (×250)

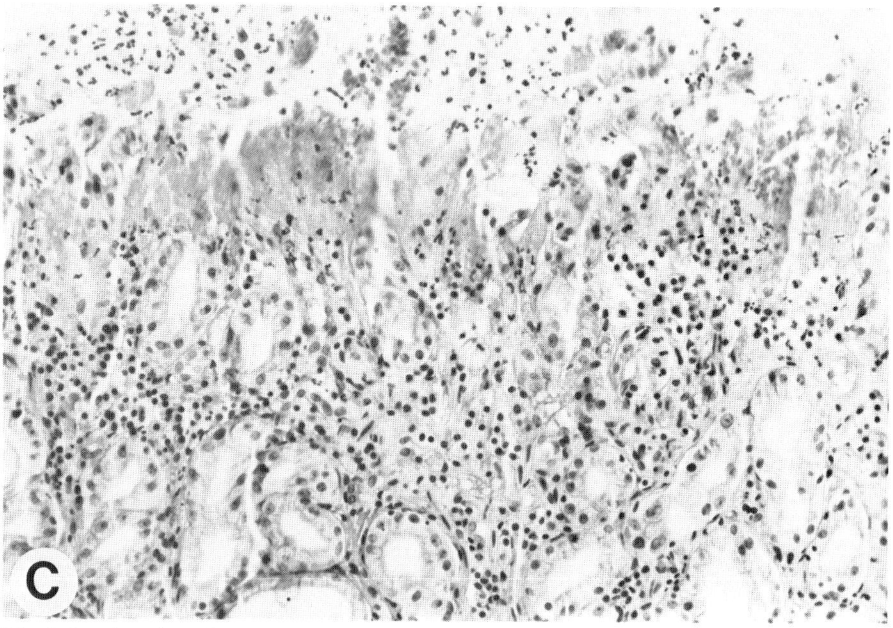


**Fig. 3-3.** *(continued)*

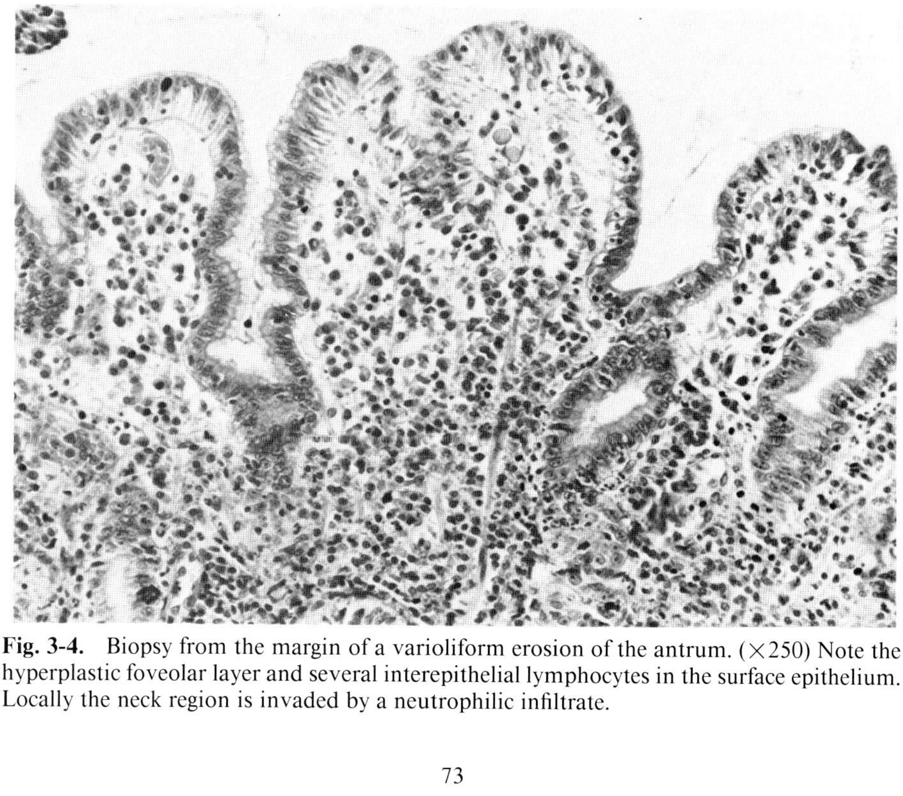

**Fig. 3-4.** Biopsy from the margin of a varioliform erosion of the antrum. (×250) Note the hyperplastic foveolar layer and several interepithelial lymphocytes in the surface epithelium. Locally the neck region is invaded by a neutrophilic infiltrate.

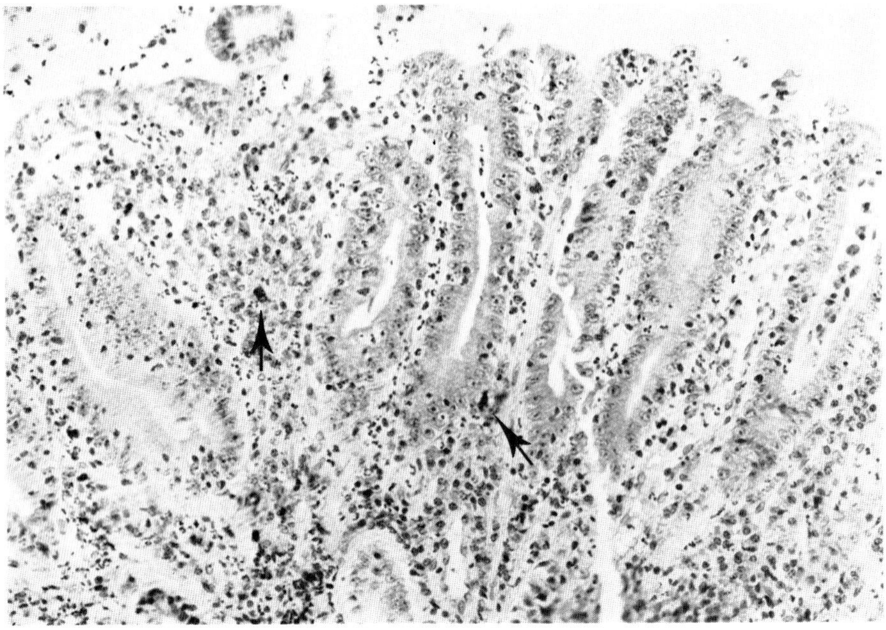

**Fig. 3-5.** Biopsy from a varioliform erosion of the antrum. Note two IgE-containing plasma cells (arrows). (×250)

numbers of IgE-containing cells in gastric biopsies of patients with varioliform gastritis, as compared to patients with chronic nonspecific gastritis. Moreover, some patients had raised serum IgE levels and those who were treated with disodium cromoglycate showed a favorable response.[1,22] Therefore, they proposed an allergic (type I, IgE-mediated hypersensitivity) immune reaction as the pathophysiological mechanism. This hypothesis was further substantiated by the demonstration of anaphylaxis producing gastric ulceration,[30,31] and the successful treatment of varioliform gastritis with disodium cromoglycate[1] and prednisolone.[32]

Increased numbers of IgE-containing cells have been shown in the jejunal mucosa of patients with food allergy[33,34] and in the tonsils of patients with atopy[36] and are, therefore, associated with type I IgE-mediated hypersensitivity. As far as the stomach is concerned, however, an increased number of IgE-containing cells in the mucosal biopsies specimens has, besides in varioliform gastritis, also been demonstrated at the base of gastric and duodenal ulcers[37] and in gastritis[38] especially gastritis due to biliary reflux.[39]

Moreover, in a survey of gastric biopsies of 2543 patients IgE-containing cells were increased in 2.6% of the patients who suffered from a variety of chronic inflammatory disorders of the stomach of various etiology.[24] This finding was fairly reproducible in time within the same patient. Since an increase of IgE-containing cells in mucosal biopsies was observed in various disorders it was considered unlikely that type I IgE-mediated hypersensitivity played a primary role and suggested that it could be an epiphenomenon, reflecting allergy probably towards food constituents, secondary to chronic non-specific inflammation as a result of increased antigen exposure to the intestinal mucosa. Therefore, increased numbers of IgE containing cells in mucosal biopsies cannot be considered to be definite proof of an allergic type I IgE-mediated immune reaction as the primary mechanism. Moreover, an increase of IgE-containing cells in gastric biopsies of patients with varioliform gastritis has not been confirmed in other studies.[23,24]

It should be stated, however, that André et al[22] initially made their observations in patients with diffuse varioliform gastritis. In the other studies the type of varioliform gastritis was not further specified in one[23] and concerned antral varioliform gastritis in the other.[24] Therefore, varioliform gastritis of the diffuse type may be different from antral varioliform gastritis.

André and coworkers, however, have subsequently extended their observation of an increase of IgE-containing cells to antral varioliform gastritis. Uncontrolled therapeutic trials with either disodium cromoglycate or prednisolone[22,32] that showed a favorable response of the gastritis have their obvious drawbacks in a disorder, which may have spontaneous remissions. The one placebo-controlled trial in varioliform gastritis, however, exploring the effect of disodium cromoglycate and cimetidine, showed a favorable response to disodium cromoglycate.[1] Again it concerned patients with diffuse varioliform gastritis. Studies of gastric acid production failed to show a distinct pattern.[6,7,9,26] Gastric acid production ranged from hyper- to normo-acidity, whereas in one study even some patients with anacidity were described. The age distribution of patients with varioliform gastritis is very similar to that of patients with peptic ulcer disease.[3,14] Moreover, benign gastric and duodenal ulcers are frequently associated with varioliform erosions, suggesting that the two disorders are related. Therapy with cimetidine, ranitidine, or pirenzipine, however, has been shown to produce healing of the peptic ulcers, whereas the coexisting varioliform erosions persisted.[15] Furthermore, it has never been documented that peptic ulcers arose from varioliform erosions and indeed both lesions have a different topographical distribution in the stomach.

Other associated and possibly etiological factors observed in varioliform gastritis are the use of coffee and tea, smoking as well as corticosteroids.[14] The same author failed to show an association with acetylsalicylic acid that by interfering with local prostaglandin synthesis may damage the mucosal barrier.

Finally, based upon histological similarities with solitary rectal ulcers and colitis cystica profunda an ischemic origin of varioliform erosions has been suggested.[15]

Summarizing the available data on varioliform gastritis, it appears the clinical and histological features are nonspecific, whereas various etiological mechanisms have been incriminated. Therefore, since evidence is lacking to support the statement that varioliform gastritis is a specific entity, varioliform gastritis should be considered as a heterogeneous disorder. Probably it merely represents a morphological variant of chronic nonspecific gastritis.

## SUMMARY

Varioliform gastritis has been claimed to represent a specific entity, characterized by an increased number of IgE-containing cells in the gastric mucosa, which requires specific therapy. The clinical and histological features of varioliform gastritis are reviewed and considered nonspecific. It is argued that the increase of IgE-containing cells in mucosal biopsies cannot be considered as definite proof for a type I IgE-mediated immune mechanism and may represent an epiphenomenon. Moreover, other etiological factors have been incriminated. It is, therefore, concluded that varioliform gastritis is a heterogeneous disorder that probably merely represents a morphological variant of chronic nonspecific gastritis.

## ACKNOWLEDGMENT

The authors express their gratitude to Mrs. W. van Golde who prepared the manuscript.

# REFERENCES


1. André G., Gillon J., Moulinier B., Martin A., Fargier M.C.: Randomised placebo-controlled doubleblind trial of two dosages of sodium cromoglycate in the treatment of varioliform gastritis: comparison with cimetidine. Gut **23**:348–352, 1982
2. Roesch W.: Erosions of the upper gastrointestinal tract. Clinics in Gastroenterology Vol 7, nr. **3**:623–634, 1978
3. Freise J., Hofmann R., Gebel H., Huchzermeyer M.: Follow-up study of chronic gastric erosions. Endoscopy **1**:13–17, 1979
4. Morgagni G.B.: De sedibus et causis morborum per anatomem indagatis. Tomus II. Vet EP Anat Med **30**:20, 1756
5. Henning N., Schatzki R.: Gastrophotographisched und roentgenologisches Bild der Gastritis erosiva. Fortschr Roentgenstrahle **48**:177–182, 1933
6. Kawai K., Shimamoto K., Misaki F., Hurakami K., Masuda M.: Erosions of gastric mucosa: Pathogenesis, incidence and classification of the erosive gastritis. Endoscopy **3**:168–174, 1970
7. Roesch W., Ottenjahn R.: Gastric erosions. Endoscopy **2**:93–98, 1970
8. Seifert E., Paul F., Schmidt W.C.: Akute und chronischen Magenerosionen. Med Klin **3**:83–87, 1971
9. Filippini L., Isliker K. Gastritis varioliformis mit Proteinverlust. Dtsch Med Wrschr **98**:1892–1894, 1973
10. Bosseckert H., Koppe P., Heid R. Die endoskopische Diagnostik von Magenerosionen und ihre klinische Bedeutung. Z inn Med **29**:888–891, 1974
11. Hauzeur F., Arendt R., Leithauser W.: Die kompletten Magenerosionen—ein relativ haufiger gastroskopischer Befund. Z inn Med **30**:353–355, 1975
12. Krentz K., Gohrband G. Klinik und Verlauf gastraler Erosionen. Med Klin **71**:156–162, 1976
13. Green P.H.R., Feure D.I., Barrett P.J., Hunt J.H., Gillespie P.E., Nagy G.S.. Chronic erosive (verrucous) gastritis. A study of 108 patients. Endoscopy **9**:74–78, 1977
14. Walinga H. Varioliforme erosies. Thesis, Amsterdam, 1985
15. Franzin G., Manfrini C., Musola R., Rodella S., Fratton A. Chronic erosions of the stomach. A clinical, endoscopic and histological evaluation. Endoscopy **16**:1–5, 1984
16. Roesch W. Erosions of the upper gastrointestinal tract. Clinics in Gastroenterology **7**:623–634, 1978
17. Clarke A.C., Lee S.P., Nicholson G.I. Gastritis varioliformis. Chronic erosive gastritis with protein-losing gastropathy Am J Gastroenterol **68**:599–602, 1977
18. Walk L. Polyps caused by gastric erosions. Radiologe **15**:354–355, 1975
19. O'Brian T.K., Saunders D.R., Templeton F.E. Chronic gastric erosions and oral aphthae. Am J Dig Dis **17**:447–454, 1972
20. Walk L. Long-term prognosis of idiopathic gastric erosions. Radiologe **15**:356–359, 1975
21. Rösch W., Warnatz H. Immunofluorescenzmikroskopische Untersuchungen bei Magenerosionen, in: Lindener H. Fortschritte in der gastroenterologische Endoskopie, 1974 Baden-Baden, Witztrock, 194–251.
22. André C., Moulinier B., Lambert R., Bugnon B.: Gastritis varioliformis, allergy and disodium cromoglycate. Lancet **I**:964–965, 1976
23. Dekker W., Walinga H., Balk T., Tytgat G.N.J.: Chronische varioliforme laesies van de maag: een onderzoek naar de aethiologie, Ned Tijdschr v Geneeskd **127**:240–244, 1983
24. Spreeuwel van J.P., Lindeman J., Maanen van J., Meijer C.J.L.M.: Increased numbers of IgE containing cells in gastric and duodenal biopsies, 1984 J Clin Pathol **37**:601–606.
25. Price A.B., Levi J., Dolby J.N., Dunscombe P.L., Smith A., Clark J., Stephenson M.J.: Campylobacter pyloridis in peptic ulcer disease: Microbiology, pathology and scanning electron microscopy. Gut **26**:1183–1188, 1985
26. Morgan A.G., Mc Adam W.A.F., Pypah R.D., Tinsley E.G.F.: Multiple recurring gastric erosions (aphthous ulcers). Gut **17**:633–637, 1976
27. Laufer I., Hamilton J., Mullens J.E.: Demonstration of superficial gastric erosions by double contrast radiography. Gastroenterology **68**:387–391, 1975.
28. Op den Orth J.O., Dekker W.: Gastric erosions: radiological and endoscopical aspects. Radiol Clin **45**:88–99, 1976
29. Rutgeerts P., Ponette E., Vantrappen G., Geboes K., Broeckaert L., Taleven L.: Crohn's disease of the stomach and duodenum: a clinical study with emphasis on the value of endoscopy and endoscopic biopsies. Endoscopy **12**:288–294, 1980
30. André F., André C.: Gastric ulcer induced by mucosal anaphylaxis in ovalbumin-sensitized Proamys (Mastomys) natalensis. Am J Pathol **102**:133–135, 1981
31. André F., André C., Vialard J.L.: Role of homocytotrophic antibodies in the pathogenesis of gastric ulcer. Digestion **19**:175–179, 1979
32. Farthing M.J.G., Fairclough P.D., Hegarthy J.E., Swarbrick E.T., Dawson A.M.: Treatment of chronic erosive gastritis with prednisolone. Gut **22**:759–762, 1981
33. Shiner M., Ballard, J., Smith M.E.: The small intestinal mucosa in cows with intolerance. Lancet I; 136–140, 1975
34. Rosekrans P.C.M., Meijer C.J.L.M., Cornelisse C.J., Wal van der A.M., Lindeman J.: Use of morphometry and immunohistochemistry of small intestinal biopsy specimens in the diagnosis of food allergy. J Clin Pathol **33**:155–130, 1980
35. Spreeuwel van J.P., Meijer C.J.L.M., Rosekrans P.C.M., Lindeman J.: Immunoglobulin containing cells in gastrointestinal pathology. Diagnostic applications. Pathol Ann 1986, **21**:(Part 2)295–310, 1985
36. Feltkamp Vroom T.M., Stallman P.J., Aalbers R.C., Reerink Brongers E.E.: Immunofluorescence studies on renal tissue, tonsils, adenoids, nasal polyps and skin of atopic and non-atopic patients with special reference to IgE. Clin Immunol Immunopathol **4**:392–404, 1975
37. Brown W.R., Borthistle V.K., Chen S.T.: Immunoglobulin E (IgE) and IgE-containing cells in human gastrointestinal fluids and tissues Clin Exp Immunol **20**:227–237, 1975.
38. Niedobitek F., Volkheimer G., Dumke K., Schlecht

Martine: Zur Haufigkeit and Verteilung IgE-haltiger Zellen in der Magenschleimhaut. Pathologe **5**:212–215, 1984

39. André C., Vilart J.L., Fargier M.C.: IgE mediated reactions in inflammation of the stomach, in: Pepys J., Edward A.M., The Mast Cell, its Role in Health and Disease. Kent, Pitman Medical Publishing Comp Ltd 642–646, 1980
40. André C., Moulinier B., André F., Daniere S.: Evidence for anaphylactic reactions in peptic ulcer and varioliform gastritis. Ann Allergy **51**:325–328, 1983

# 4

# Aminergic and Peptidergic Innervation of the Gastric Mucosa—Its Possible Relevance to Ulcerogenesis

Masaya Oda M.D.
Masahiko Nakamura M.D.
Kotaro Kaneko M.D.
Masaharu Tsuchiya M.D.

A number of studies on the relationship between autonomic nervous abnormalities and gastric ulcer formation were performed since the pioneering reports of Cushing[1] and Bergamann.[2] However, further investigation of this pathognomonic relationship from a different angle or using a newly developed technique is still warranted in order to clarify the mechanism of gastric ulceration.

Recently, a balance theory was proposed,[3] whereby peptic ulcer formation is dependent upon an equilibrium between aggressive and defensive factors. The former comprise acid and pepsin, the latter mucus, $HCO_3^-$ and the gastric mucosal microcirculatory system.[4]

It is proposed that ulcer formation occurs mainly due to the hypersecretion of gastric acid as an aggressive factor, possibly triggered by stress-induced overactivity of the sympathetic and/or parasympathetic (vagal) nerves.[5] On the other hand, disruption of the gastric mucosal barrier,[6] which is caused or aggravated by disturbances of the mucosal microcirculation[4,7] and $H^+$ back-diffusion[8] are considered to be crucial in gastric ulcerogenesis.

It is established that the mucosal microcirculation supporting the defensive mechanism of the stomach is regulated by sympathetic and parasympathetic nerves.[9,10] Thus both aggressive and defensive factors in the stomach are directly or indirectly influenced by the functional state of the autonomic nerves.

The gastrointestinal tract is richly innervated by the enteric or peptidergic nervous system,[11,12,13] which is partly independent of the central autonomic nervous system and is supposed to act as "gut brain." These enteric autonomic nerves possess a variety of neurotransmitters. It is well known that the classical neurotransmitters, acetylcholine[14] and noradrenaline,[15] are widely distributed in the nervous system throughout the gastrointestinal wall. However, since a pioneering immunohistochemical study demonstrating the existence of substance P in the intramural plexuses in mammalian intestine,[16] a variety of the gastrointestinal peptides such as vasoactive intestinal polypeptide (VIP)[17,18] and gastrin releasing peptide (GRP)[19,27a] are also found to exist in the enteric nervous system, and they are considered to play an important

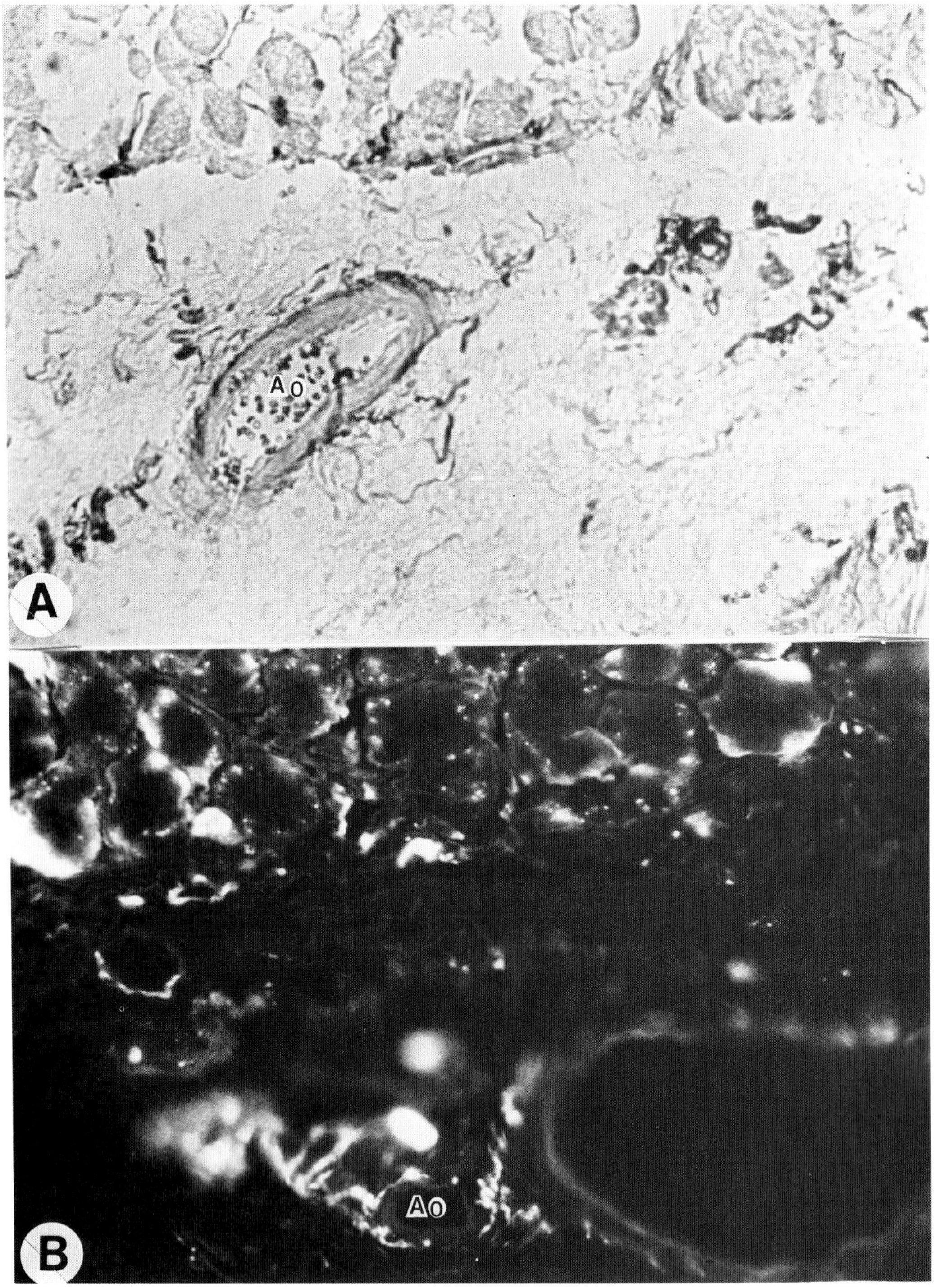


**Fig. 4-1.** The autonomic nerve plexuses in the submucosal layer of the rat fundic mucosa. (a) Karnovsky-Roots stain. The AChE-positive nerve fibers are noted in the submucous plexuses near the arterioles (Ao). ×800. (b) A modification of Falck-Hillarp method. The noradrenaline-specific fluorescence is seen in the perivascular plexuses of the arterioles (Ao). ×800.

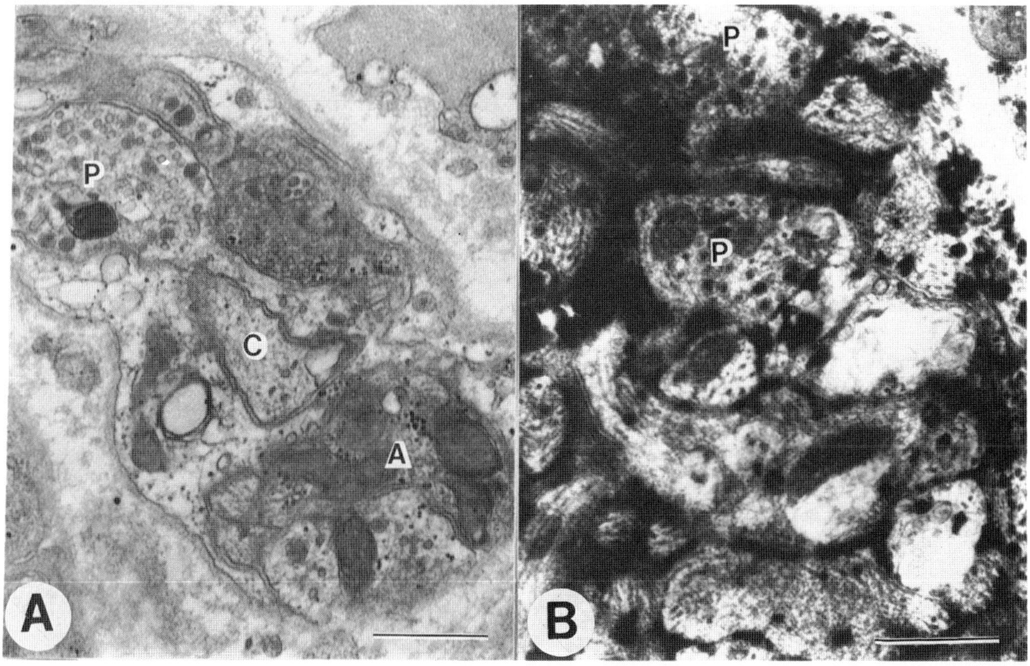


**Fig. 4-2.** Electron micrographs of the unmyelinated nerve endings in the submucosal layer of the rat stomach. (a) A typical plexus composed of adrenergic (A), cholinergic (C) and peptidergic (P) nerve endings. Routine fixation. Most of the nerve fibers in these plexuses include agranular small synaptic vesicles, corresponding to the cholinergic nerves. Some of these nerves contain small granular vesicles characteristic to adrenergic nerves and large granular vesicles probably corresponding to peptidergic nerves. ×18,000. (b) On the axonal membranes of the peptidergic nerve endings (P), AChE reaction products are also recognized. × 20,000.

role in the regulation of gastrointestinal functions.[20] The existence of histaminergic,[21] serotonergic,[22] dopaminergic[23] and purinergic nerves[24] are also postulated. There is little known about the detailed innervation of epithelial cells and microvessels in the mucosal layer of the stomach. It is essential for better understanding of pathophysiology of the stomach, particularly ulcerogenesis, to clarify the morphological and functional properties of these aminergic and peptidergic nerves in the stomach.

In this chapter, the distribution of cholinergic, adrenergic, VIP-ergic and histaminergic nerves, and the localization of their receptors in the gastric mucosa in the rat are described according to our recent studies. Functions of these nerves are also discussed.

## DISTRIBUTION OF THE CHOLINERGIC NERVES AND THEIR RECEPTORS

The parasympathetic nerve supply to the stomach is via the vagal nerves. The histochemical localization of the cholinergic nerves was identified by acetylcholinesterase (AChE) activity[25,26] and choline acetyltransferase (ChA) immunoreactivity.[27]

In the submucosal layer, the AChE-positive nerves are recognized in the submucous plexuses (Meissner plexuses) near the arterioles (Fig. 4-1A). Most of the nerve fibers in these plexuses include agranular small synaptic vesicles specific for cholinergic nerves. Some of these nerves also contain small granular vesicles characteristic of adrenergic nerves and

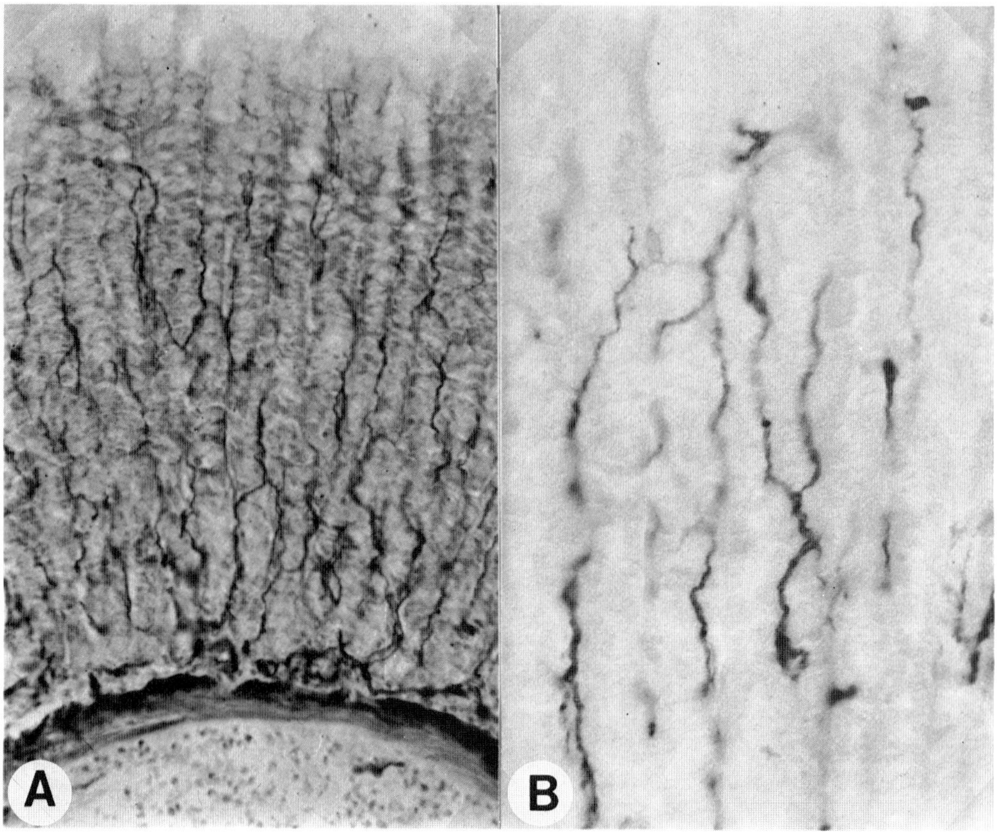


**Fig. 4-3.**. Histochemical distributions of the AChE-positive nerve fibers in the rat fundic mucosa. (a) In the vertical section of the gastric mucosa, cholinergic nerves are noted in the lamina propria mucosae between the gastric epithelial cells. ×400. (b) At high magnification, the AChE-positive nerve fibers are observed up to the top portion of the gastric mucosa. ×800. (c) In the cross section, cholinergic nerves are noted in dot form between the epithelial cell columns. ×400. (d) Fluorescence micrographs obtained by the indirect immunofluorescence antibody method using the anti-ChA serum. ChA-positive nerve fibers and cell bodies are seen between the gastric epithelial cells. ×400.

large granular vesicles probably corresponding to peptidergic nerves (Fig. 4-2A&B).

The nerve fibers arising from the submucosa extend to the basal part of the gastric mucosa and then form plexuses near the terminal arterioles. They are noted in linear form in the longitudinal section (Fig. 4-3A&B) and some in dot form in the cross-sections (Fig. 4-3C) between the gastric epithelial cell columns.[28] According to the AChE histochemical findings, only linear nerve fibers are recognized in the adult rat stomach. By the histofluorescence study using anti-ChA antiserum, however, these cholinergic nerves are found to consist of the nerve cell body and nerve fibers (Fig. 4-3D).

Recent embryological studies using isolated cultured cells show that autonomic nerve cells and their effectors affect each others' differentiation.[29] In an attempt to clarify a relationship between the activity of autonomic nerves and the differentiation of parietal cells, histochemical studies were performed in the rat in the embryonic and postnatal periods.

The AChE-positive nerve cells appeared in the rat glandular stomach by the 14th day of the embryonic period (Fig. 4-4A), and ganglia formed on the 18th to 20th day. The ganglia,

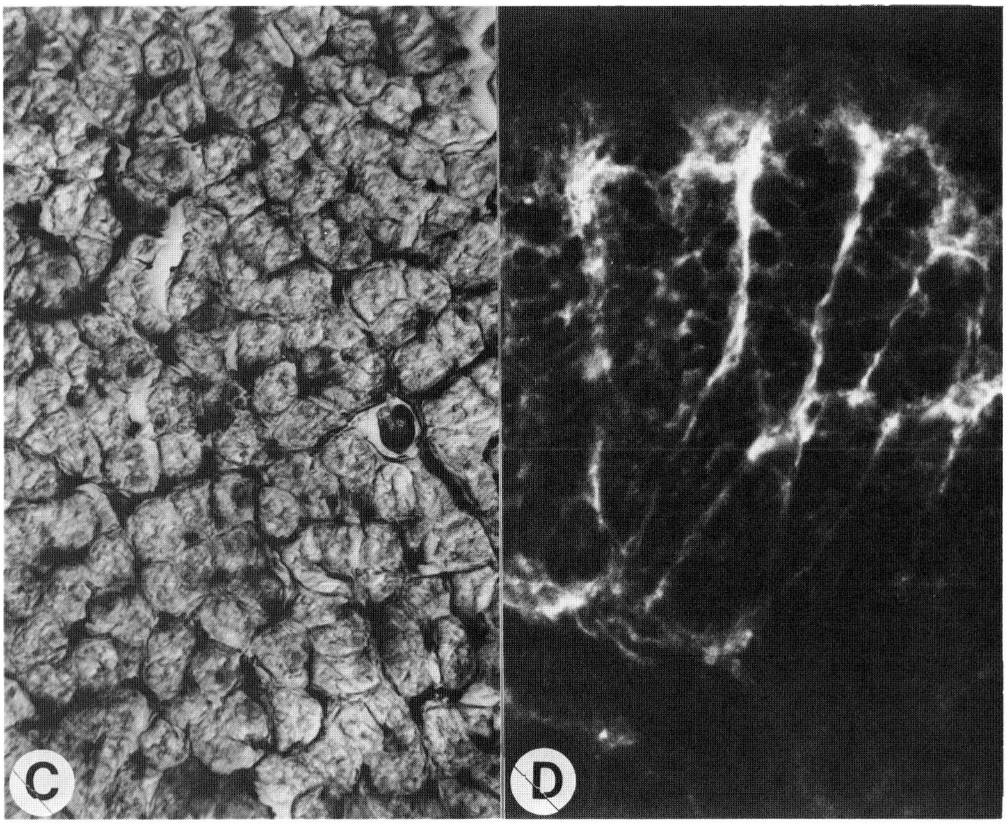


which were very large on the fourth day after birth, became reduced in size during the third postnatal week, largely corresponding to those found in adult rat stomach. AChE-positive nerve cells and their neural processes are clearly demonstrated between the gastric epithelial cells (Fig. 4-4B), and electron microscopically, the huge AChE-positive nerves are seen just under the epithelial cells (Fig. 4-4C&D).[30]

Regarding the regulation of differentiation of effectors by peripheral nerves, there is a report that differentiation of striated muscle cells is enhanced by noradrenaline released from adrenergic nerves, while it is suppressed by acetylcholine from cholinergic nerves.[31] Hence the chronological observations described above suggest that differentiation of parietal cells may be induced by cholinergic nervous activity. Further studies on neural degeneration or using appropriate inhibitors are needed to establish this possibility.

These observations suggest that cholinergic nerves may induce both the proliferation of the epithelial cells such as parietal and chief cells and the development of microcirculatory system comprising arterioles, true capillaries and collecting venules, leading to the hypothesis of dual action of cholinergic nerves in the gastric mucosa, (i.e., direct regulation of gastric mucosal microcirculation as well as acid and pepsinogen secretion).[32,33] By histochemical studies, the distribution pattern of the autonomic nerves is found to be largely similar to that in human stomach and in rat stomach.[32,34]

In an attempt to determine the effectors of the cholinergic nerves morphologically in the stomach wall, it is useful to clarify the localization of the AChE reaction products, since AChE is released from the nerve terminals to the effector cell plasma membrane. It is also essential for the determination of the cholinergic effector cells to identify the localization

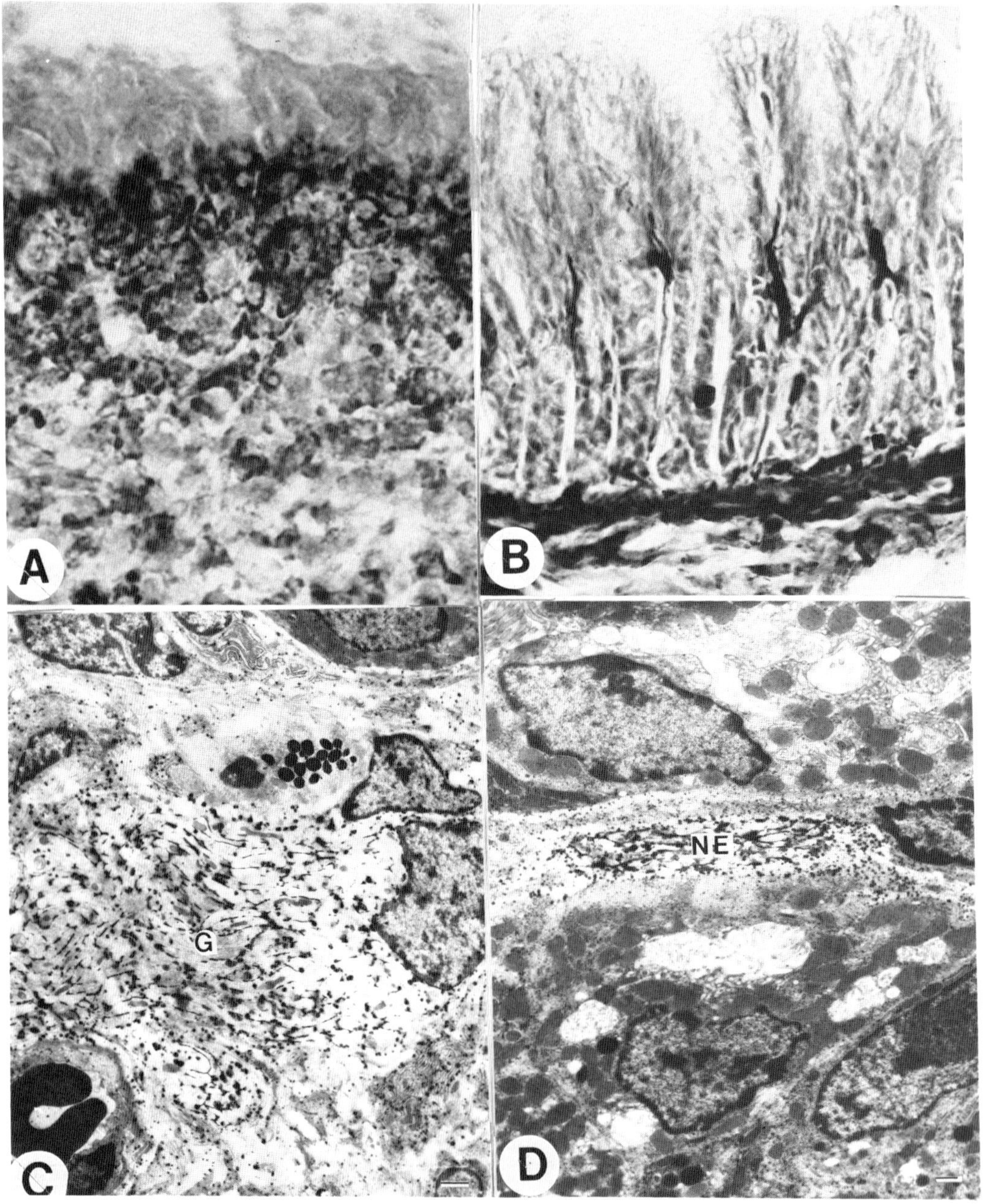


**Fig. 4-4.** Embryological observations of the AChE-positive nerves in the rat fundic mucosa. (a) In the 14-day-old rat embryo, the AChE-positive cells are clustered under the epithelial cells. ×160. (b) In the 4-day-old rat, the AChE-positive nerve cells and their neural processes are clearly observed between the gastric epithelial cells. ×400. (c) Electron microscopically, the huge AChE-positive ganglion (G) is seen just under the epithelial cells in the 4-day-old rat. ×5,000. (d) Unmyelinated nerve endings between the parietal cells in the 18-day-old rat. AChE reaction products are located on the axonal membrane of the unmyelinated nerve endings (NE). ×5,000.

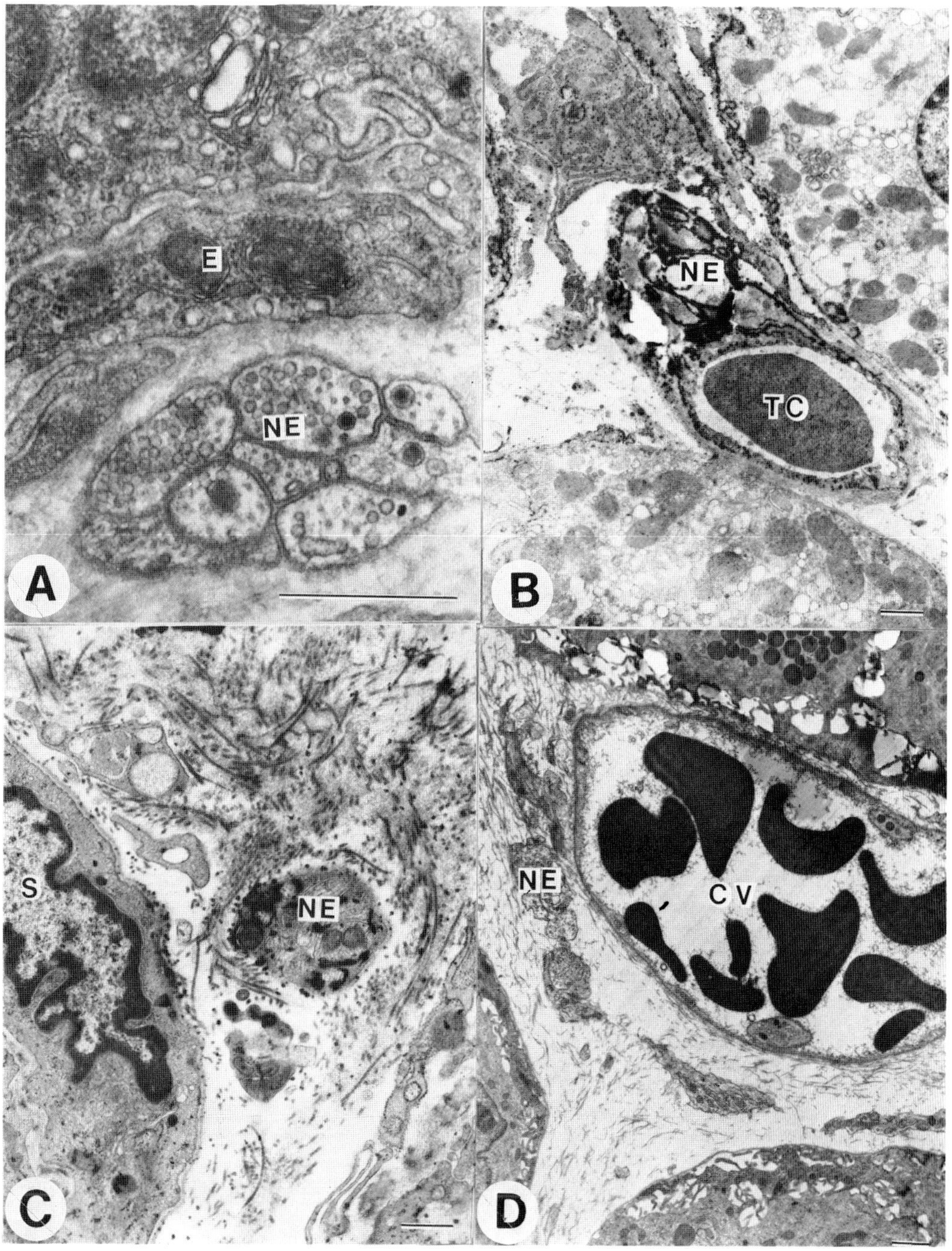


**Fig. 4-5.** Electron micrographs of the unmyelinated nerve endings near the microvessels. (a) Unmyelinated nerve endings (NE) near the true capillary endothelium (E). Synaptic vesicles in this nerve are small agranular, corresponding to the cholinergic nerves. ×30,000. (b) AChE reaction products are seen on the axonal membranes of the unmyelinated nerve endings (NE) as well as on the abluminal surface of the endothelial plasma membrane. TC: true capillary ×8,000. (c) Unmyelinated nerve endings (NE) near the smooth muscle cell (S) of the arteriole. The AChE reaction products are present on the smooth muscle cell. × 10,000. (d) Unmyelinated nerve endings near the collecting venule (CV). ×7,000.

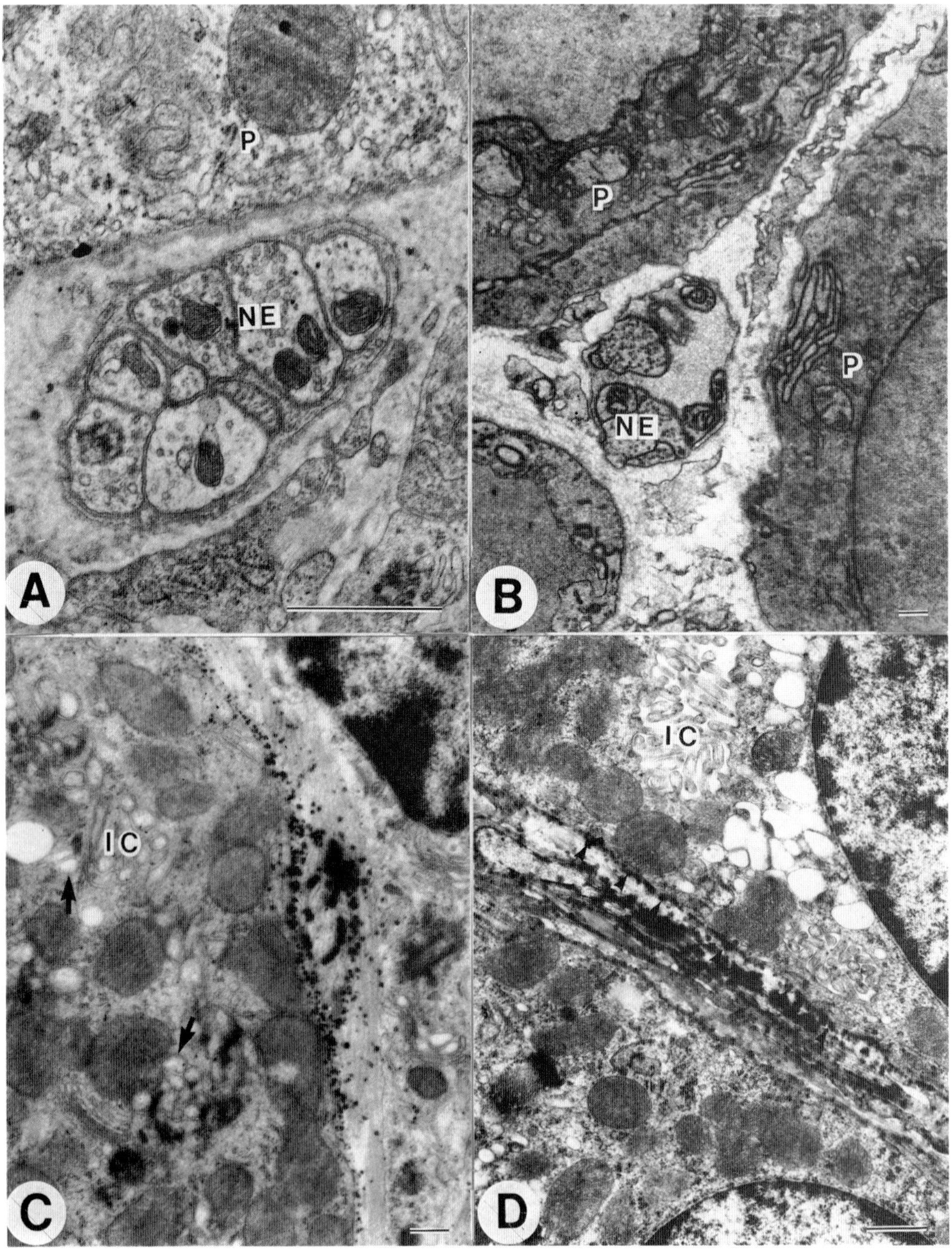


**Fig. 4-6.** Electron micrographs of the nerve endings near the parietal cells. (a) Unmyelinated nerve endings (NE) near the parietal cell (P). Routine fixation. ×26,000. (b) The synaptic vesicles of these nerve endings are agranular, corresponding to the cholinergic nerves. $KMnO_4$ fixation. ×5,000. (c) The AChE reaction products surrounding the nerve endings are decreased by truncal vagotomy. The tubulovesicles are clearly increased (arrows). IC: intracellular canaliculi. ×7,000. (d) In the control, the AChE reaction products are normally present on the axonal membrane of unmyelinated nerve endings. IC:intracellular canaliculi. ×7,000.

of muscarinic acetylcholine receptors (m-AChRs) on the cell plasma membrane in the close vicinity of the nerve terminals.

The AChE reaction products are demonstrated both on the axonal membranes of the unmyelinated nerve endings containing small agranular synaptic vesicles and on the plasma membrane of the true capillary endotherium (Fig. 4-5A–D). Also the AChE reaction products are noted on the basal plasma membrane of the parietal cell and on the smooth muscle cell plasma membrane (Fig. 4-6A–D). These distributions of the AChE reaction products suggest the direct cholinergic innervation of the mucosal capillaries, parietal cells, and arterioles.

The radioautographic study using the tritium-labelled muscarinic antagonist, $^3$H-quinuclidinyl benzilate (QNB), and $^3$H-pirenzepine (PZ) is very useful for proving the localization of m-AChRs in the gastric mucosa.[37] Under light anesthesia with intraperitoneal injection of sodium pentobarbital, aqueous solutions of $^3$H-QNB were infused for 30 min through an aortic catheter by an infusion pump at a constant rate, followed by an infusion of saline to wash out the unbound ligand. Immediately after the infusion, the small tissue blocks of the stomach were quickly frozen in isopentane cooled with liquid nitrogen, and were freeze-dried at $-50°C$ and evacuated at $9 \times 10^{-3}$ Torr. The freeze-dried tissue blocks were then exposed to osmium vapor, followed by infiltration of Epon in a dripping unit. Thereafter, the tissue blocks were embedded in Epon.

Semithin or ultrathin sections were cut with LKB ultramicrotome using ethylene glycol instead of water.[35] The emulsion film (Sakura NR-H2 or M2) was then applied to the glass plates or meshes on which sections were mounted. They were exposed in a refrigerator in the dark for 4 to 8 weeks. After development, they were examined with light or electron microscopy. As shown in Figs. 4-7 and 4-8, the silver grains indicating the $^3$H-QNB-binding sites (i.e., the localization of m-AChRs) are mainly located in the basal two-thirds of the gastric mucosa, coinciding with the localization of the cholinergic nerves in the gastric mucosa. Electron microscopically the silver grains indicating the presence of m-AChRs are recognized on the parietal cells as well as on the endothelial cell plasma membranes of the true capillaries.[36] (Figs. 4-9A-C, 4-10A-C). The cellular ulstrastructures in these radiographs are not well maintained, since the radioautographic method for soluble compounds[35] applied in this study avoids fixation to prevent the migration of radiolabelled receptor antagonists defining the receptor sites. These silver grains were significantly increased in number after truncal vagotomy, while they were diminished by atropine pretreatment, supporting the specificity of these radioautographic reactions. Moreover, these grains were not noticed in the rat stomach infused with unlabelled QNB. The localization of the silver grains is therefore thought to be specific for the m-AchRs. The radioautography using $^3$H-PZ reveals that the localization sites of a high dose of $^3$H-PZ showing the distribution of m-AchRs are almost the same as those of $^3$H-QNB (Fig. 4-11A-C).[37]

## GASTRIC MUCOSAL MICROCIRCULATION AND CHOLINERGIC CONTROL

In vivo microscopy revealed the hemodynamics in the microvasculature of the gastric mucosal surface in the control rat.[34,38] Blood is seen flowing rapidly and uniformly in the anastomosing capillary network surrounding the gastric pits, and ultimately draining into the collecting venules, forming a functional unit in the mucosal microvasculature. In the rat restrained by the plaster bandage method,[34] the blood flow is not uniform in the mucosal capillaries, and a variety of vasomotor disturbances such as sludge, regurgitation, and stasis are observed concomitant with hemorrhagic changes, particularly in the area surrounding the hemorrhagic erosive lesions induced by the restraint stress.[33,34,39]

In an experimental model of stress ulcer induced by restraint using a plaster bandage,[34]

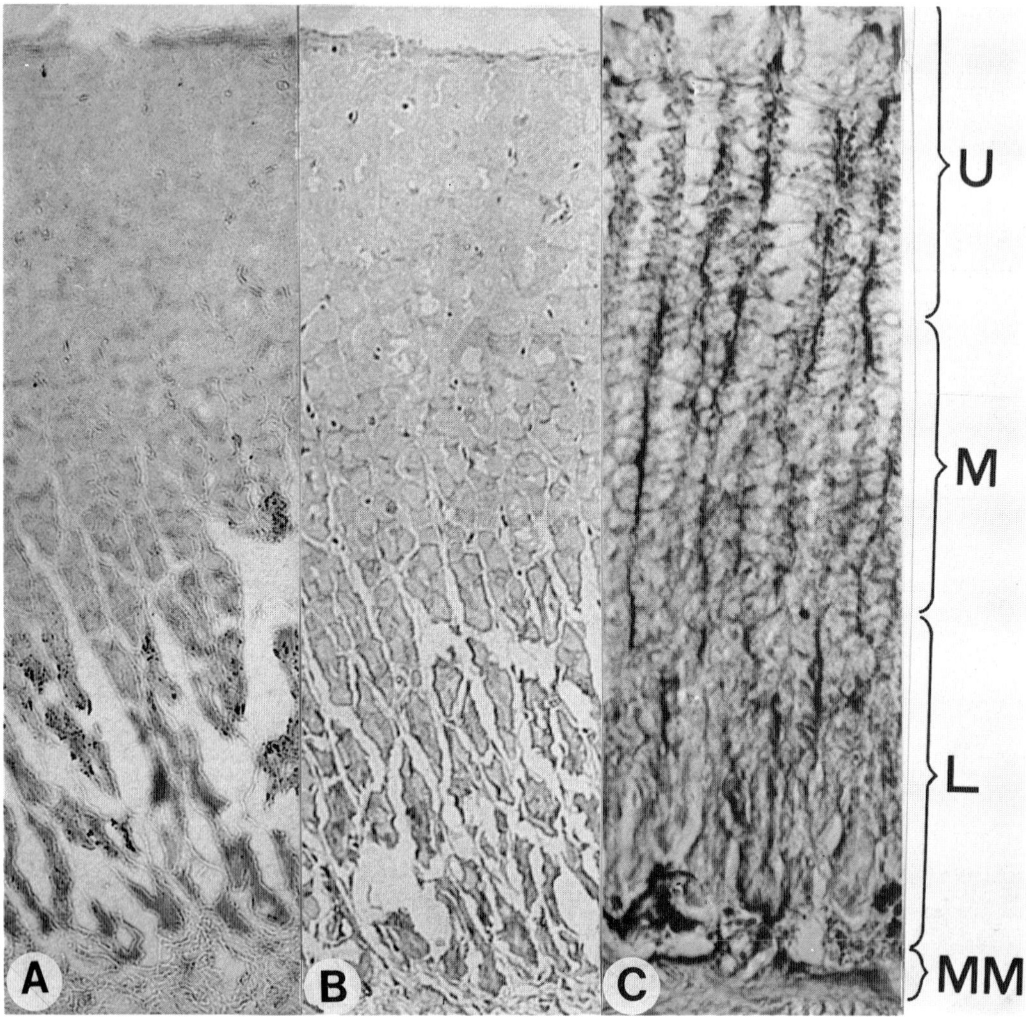


**Fig. 4-7.** Light microscopic radioautographs of the $^{3}$H-QNB-binding sites in the fundic mucosa. The silver grains are mainly found in the basal two-thirds of the gastric mucosa. U: upper, M: middle, L: lower gastric mucosa; MM: muscularis mucosae. (a) control group. ×400. (b) In the atropine-treated group, few grains are seen compared with control group. ×400. (c) AChE stain. ×400.

hemorrhagic erosions were formed in the glandular stomach of the rat eight hours after starting the restraint. The AChE reaction products were increased, both on the axonal membranes of the unmyelinated nerve endings and on the basal site of the plasma membrane of the parietal cell, implying an enhanced transmission of ACh from the former to the latter via m-AChRs demonstrated on the parietal cell plasma membrane under restraint stress.[36] On the other hand, the noradrenaline fluorescence, indicating sympathetic nervous activity, was decreased in the mucosal layer.[34] The dye-4% pontamine sky blue, or horseradish peroxidase (HRP), administered via an aortic catheter, had permeated remarkably from the collecting venules and capillaries in the mucosal layer, particularly around the hemorrhagic erosions where AChE activity was greatly activated. Electron microscopic observation revealed a widening of the gaps between the capillary en-

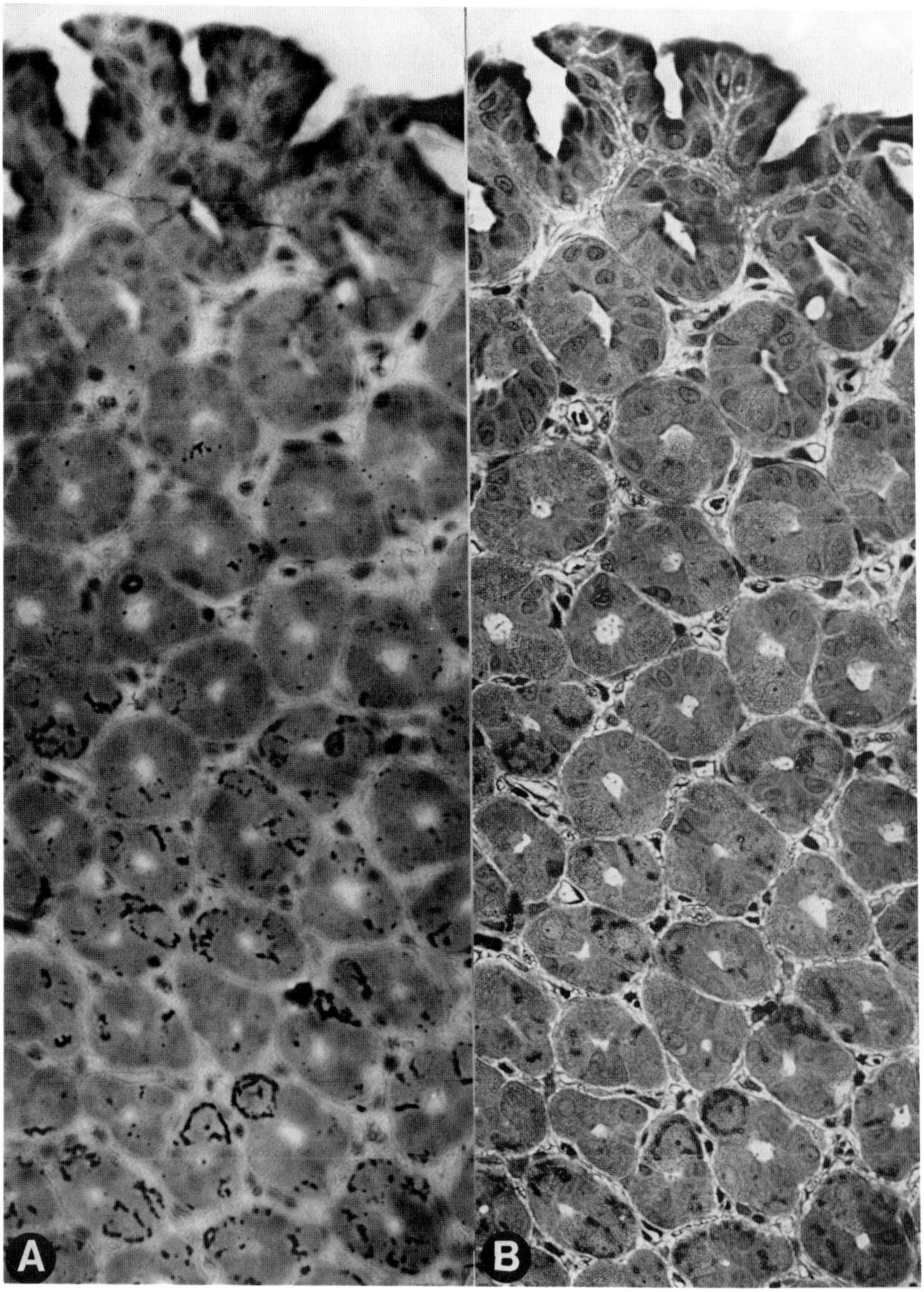


**Fig. 4-8.** Light microscopic radioautograph of the $^{3}$H-PZ-binding sites in the fundic mucosa. The silver grains are mainly seen on the parietal cells. (a) focused on the grain. ×800. (b) focused on the underlying tissue. ×800.

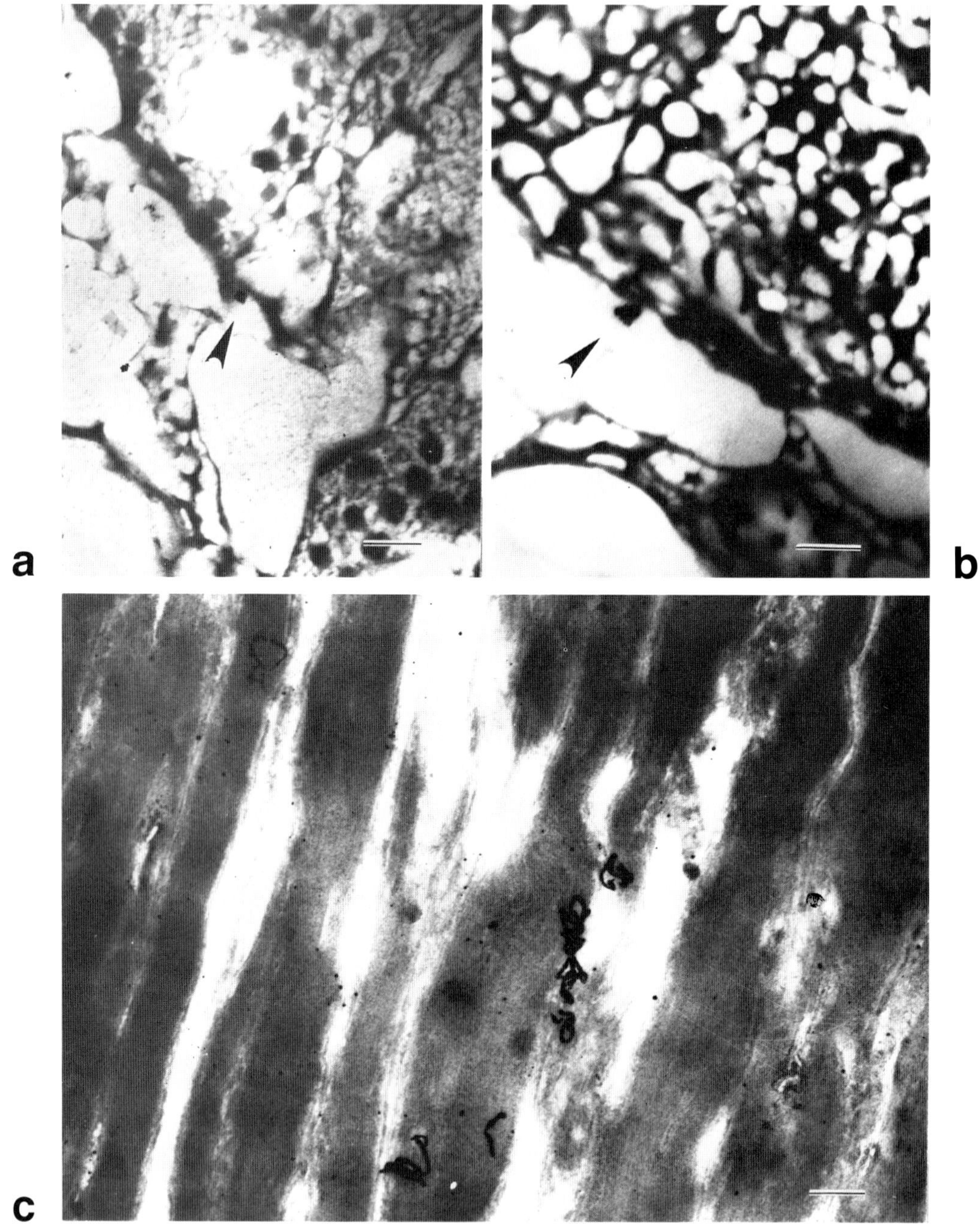

**Fig 4-9.** Electron microscopic radioautographs of the 3H-QNB-binding sites (a), (b). The grains (arrowheads) are found near the plasma membrane of the parietal cells. ×8,000. (c) In the smooth muscle layer, 3H-QNB is found to bind to the smooth muscle cells. The cellular ultrastructure in these radioautographs are not maintained well since the radiographic method for soluble compounds avoids fixation for preventing migration of radiolabelled receptor antagonists. ×8,000

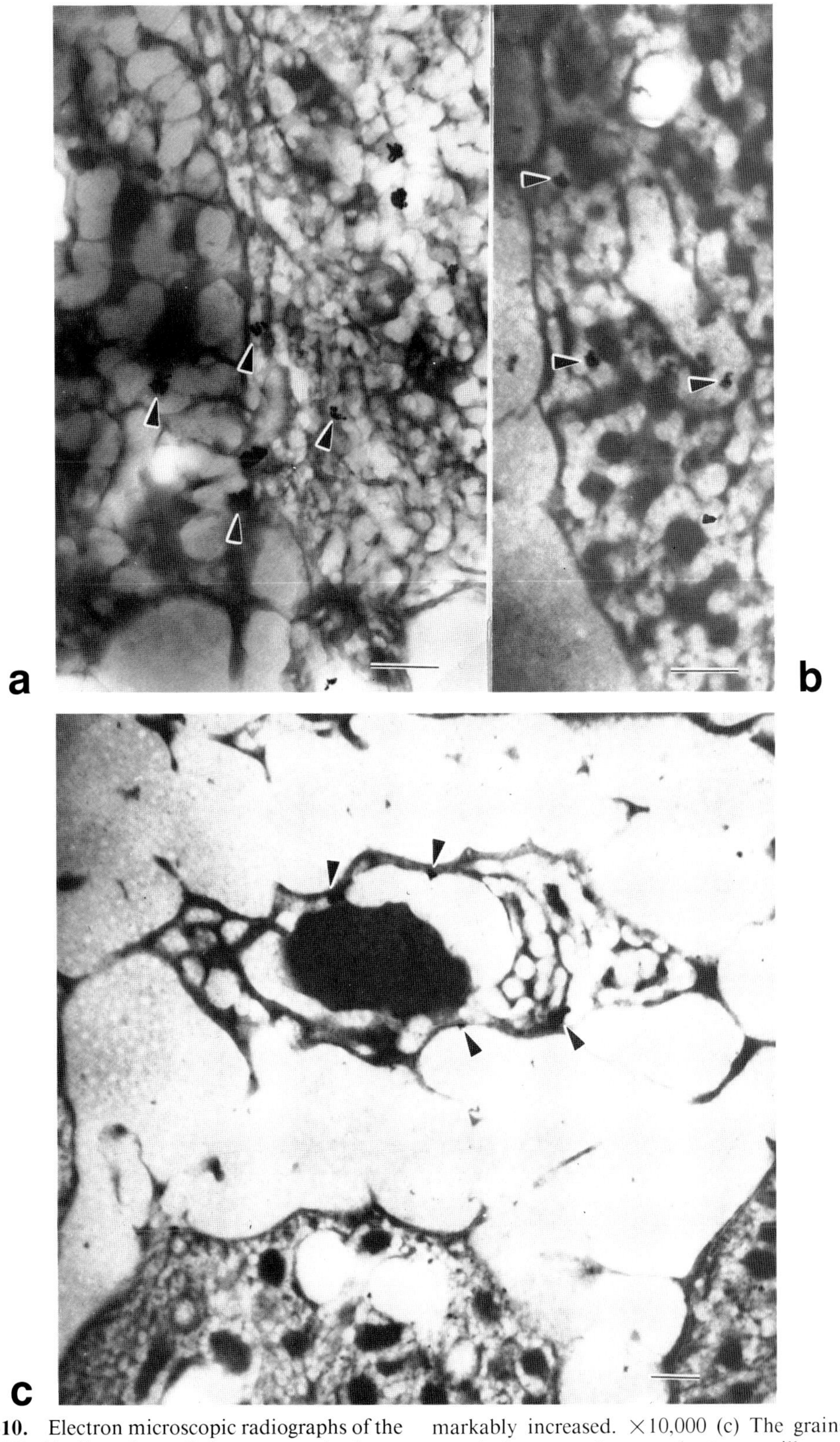

**Fig 4-10.** Electron microscopic radiographs of the 3H-QNB binding sites of the vagotomized rat. (a)(b). The silver grains on the parietal cells are remarkably increased. ×10,000 (c) The grains are seen in large numbers on the true capillary endothelium. ×8,000

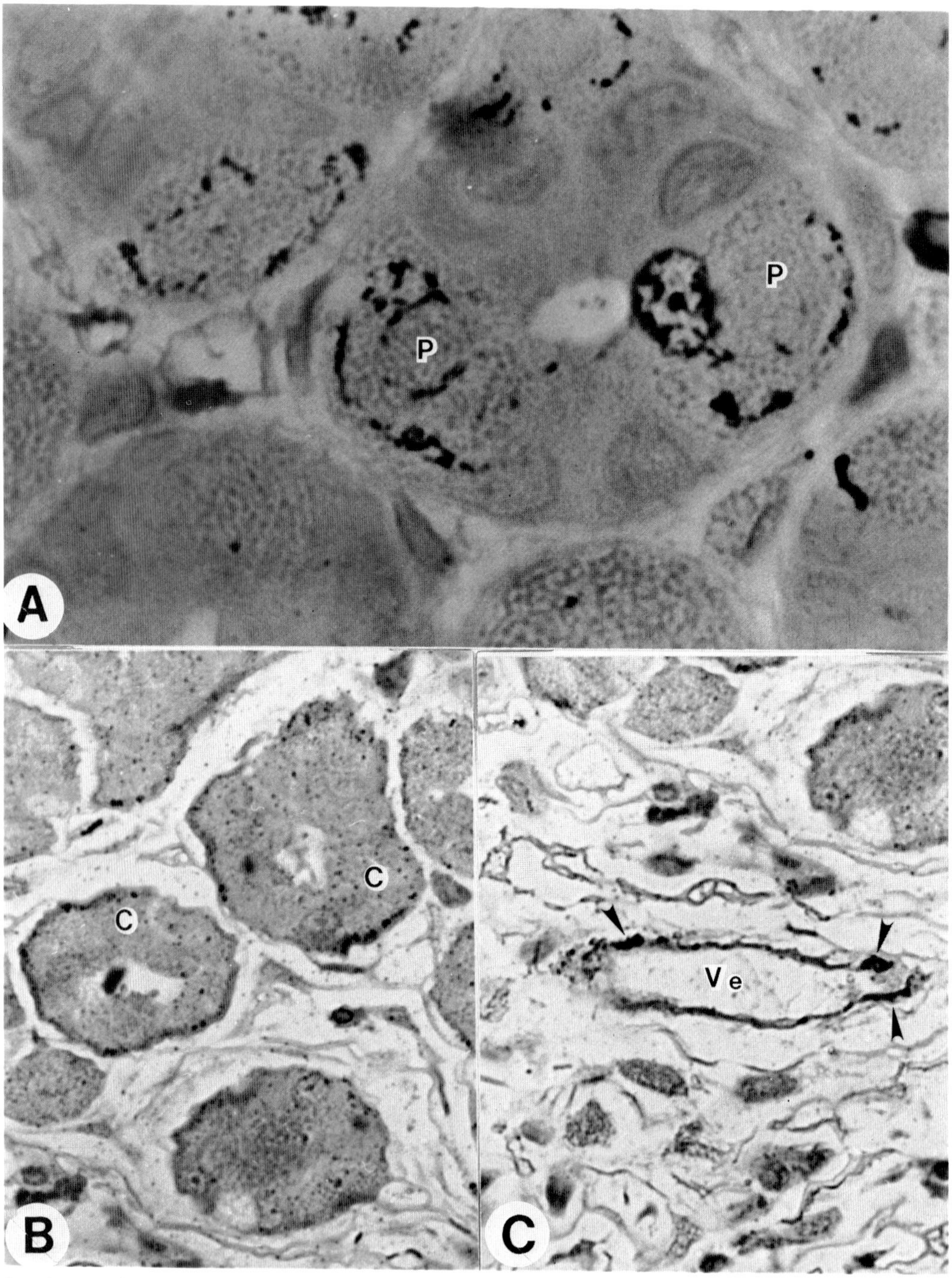


**Fig. 4-11.** Light microscopic radioautographs of the $^{3}$H-PZ binding sites in the gastric mucosa. (a) In the middle portion of the gastric mucosa, a large number of silver grains showing the $^{3}$H-PZ binding sites are deposited on the parietal cells (P). ×800. (b) In the lower portion of the gastric mucosa, the grains are seen on the chief cells (C). ×400. (c) The $^{3}$H-PZ-binding sites are found on the endothelium of the venules (Ve) and the arterioles. ×400.

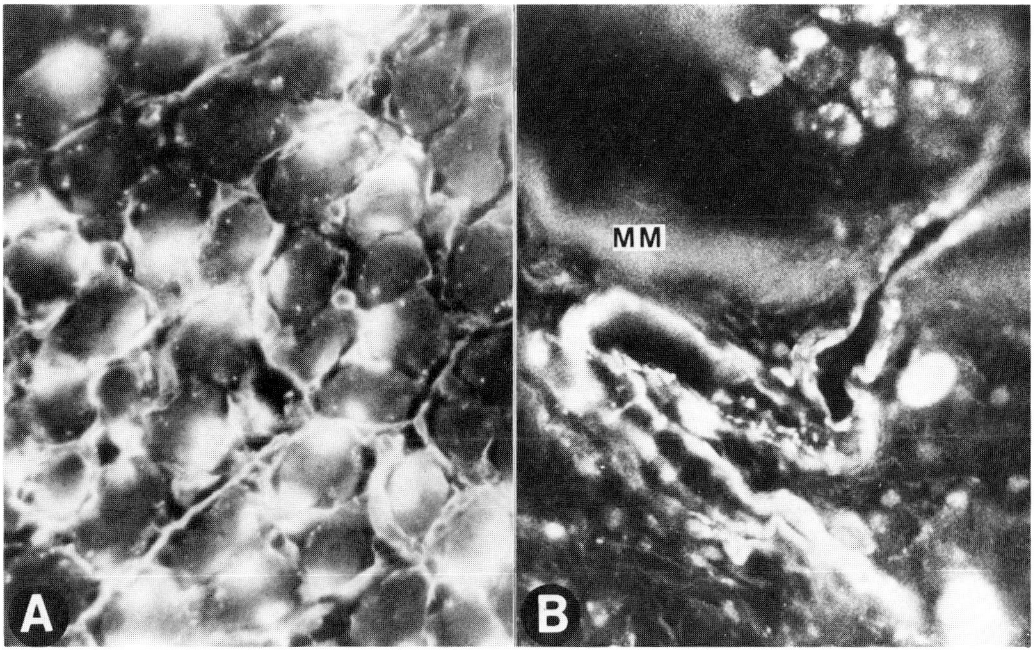


**Fig. 4-12.** Fluorescent micrographs of noradrenaline by the Falck-Hillarp methods. (a) In the mucosal layer, specific fluorescence of noradrenaline, corresponding to the adrenergic nerve fibers, is seen between the epithelial cells. ×400. (b) In the submucosal layer, the arterioles are found to be constricted in the muscularis mucosae (MM). ×400.

dothelial cells, possibly due to contraction of the endothelia and/or enhancement of vesicular and vacuolar transport across the capillary endothelium, leading to an increased permeability of the capillary vessels, concomitant with a variety of vasomotor disturbances in the gastric mucosal microcirculation.[33]

In biopsy specimens of the human gastric mucosa obtained from a patient with gastric ulcer, AChE activity is progressively increased the nearer it is to the hemorrhagic erosions. Using electron microscopy, the increased AChE reaction products are found both on the unmyelinated nerve endings and on the capillary endothelium or on the parietal cell plasma membrane.[33]

According to these studies, it is tentatively speculated that an excessive transmission of ACh to the capillary endothelium would directly cause an increased permeability of the mucosal capillaries around collecting venules, comcomitant with a variety of vasomotor disturbances in the capillary blood flow, leading to ischemic lesions in the gastric mucosa. There is an intimate relation between the autonomic nerve endings and the capillaries in the human gastric mucosa, suggesting that the pathogenesis of acute gastric ulcers (acute gastric hemorrhagic lesions) in humans could be explained, at least in part, by a mechanism similar to that of stress-induced experimental ulcer formation.

## DISTRIBUTION OF THE ADRENERGIC NERVES AND THEIR ACTION ON THE MICROCIRCULATORY SYSTEM

The sympathetic nerve supply to the rat stomach is derived from spinal nerves and terminates in the celiac ganglia. From these ganglia, the postganglionic adrenergic fibers reach the stomach as discrete nerves, as

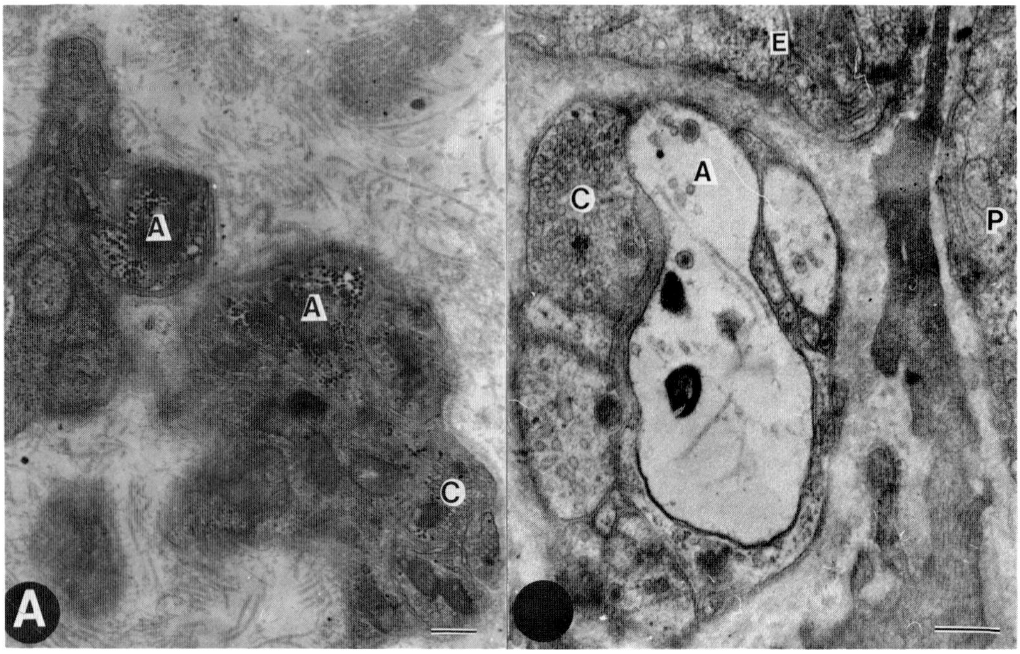


**Fig. 4-13.** Electron micrographs of the adrenergic nerve endings (A) in the mucosa. (a) The granular small synaptic vesicles, specific for noradrenaline, are clearly seen. Chromaffin fixation. ×7,000. (b) Transmission electron micrograph demonstrating the coexistence of the sympathetic and parasympathetic nerve endings in the fundic mucosal layer of rat stomach. The sympathetic nerve endings (A) are selectively degenerated by $\alpha$-hydroxydopamine administration, while parasympathetic nerve endings (C) remain unaltered. P: parietal cell E: true capillary endothelium. ×7,000.

nerves closely associated with vagal nerves or as nerves accompanying the arterial vessels.

Using a fluorescent histochemical method,[40,41] the nerve endings showing the specific noradrenaline fluorescence are located mainly in the perivascular plexuses of the arterioles and some in the myenteric and submucous plexuses of the nerve fibers in the basal portion of the gastric mucosa (Figs. 4-1B, 4-12A&B).[10,42] Electron microscopically, the nerve fibers possessing small electron-dense synaptic vesicles clearly demonstrated in the chromaffin-fixed preparations, probably corresponding to the adrenergic fibers, are found mainly along the terminal arterioles in the basal part of the mucosa as well as along the arterioles in the submucosa (Fig. 4-13A&B), while those in the superficial part of the mucosa are almost devoid of the adrenergic fluorescence.

From the evolutional point of view, a large number of intramural adrenergic neurons are present in the gut of amphibians and reptiles, but few in mammals.[43] In the gut of mammals, peptidergic nerves are thought to act as a counterpart. Therefore, the adrenergic nerves would not be involved in the contraction of the nonvascular smooth muscle layer, but rather in the regulation of the mesenteric blood flow.

The significance of the peripheral dopaminergic nerve has been re-evaluated by a study using anti-dopamine $\beta$-hydroxylase antibody.[23] There are some studies suggesting that most of the adrenergic nerves may belong to the dopaminergic fibers.

To clarify the functional significance of the adrenergic innervation, the effects of noradrenaline, isoproterenol and dopamine on the gastric mucosal microcirculatory system were examined by the infusion of horseradish peroxidase (HRP: Sigma type II) as a marker[44] for microvascular permeability. By the infusion of $\alpha$-agonist noradrenaline, the arterioles in the basal portion of the gastric mucosa are constricted and the permeability of the capil-

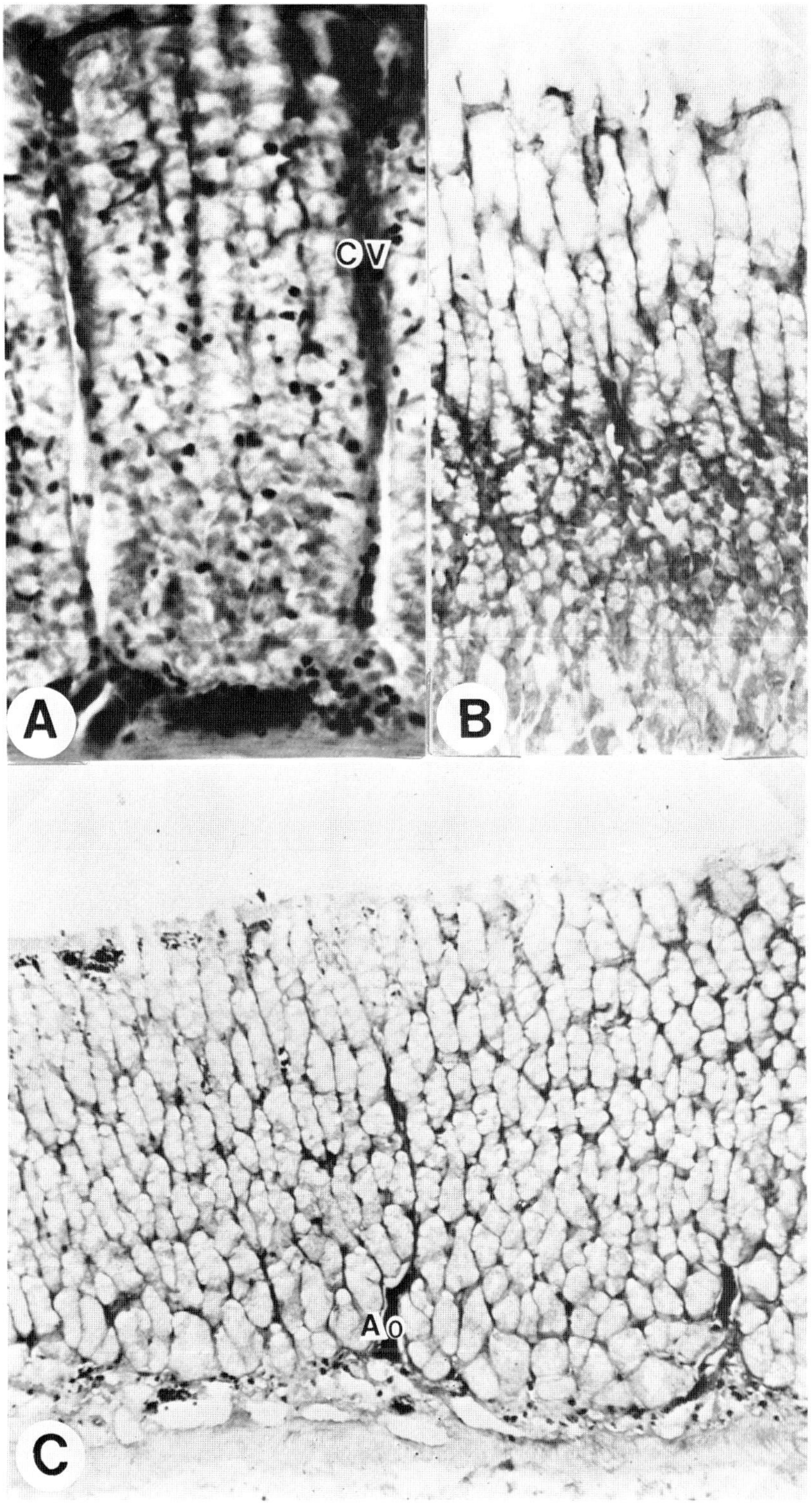


**Fig. 4-14.** The microcirculatory alterations induced by various adrenergic agents. (a) Control group. The upper half of the capillary network and the collecting venules (CV) are seen. ×400. (b) The capillary permeability is clearly increased by noradrenaline infusion. ×400. (c) The arterioles (Ao) in basal portion become enlarged after isoproterenol infusion. ×300.

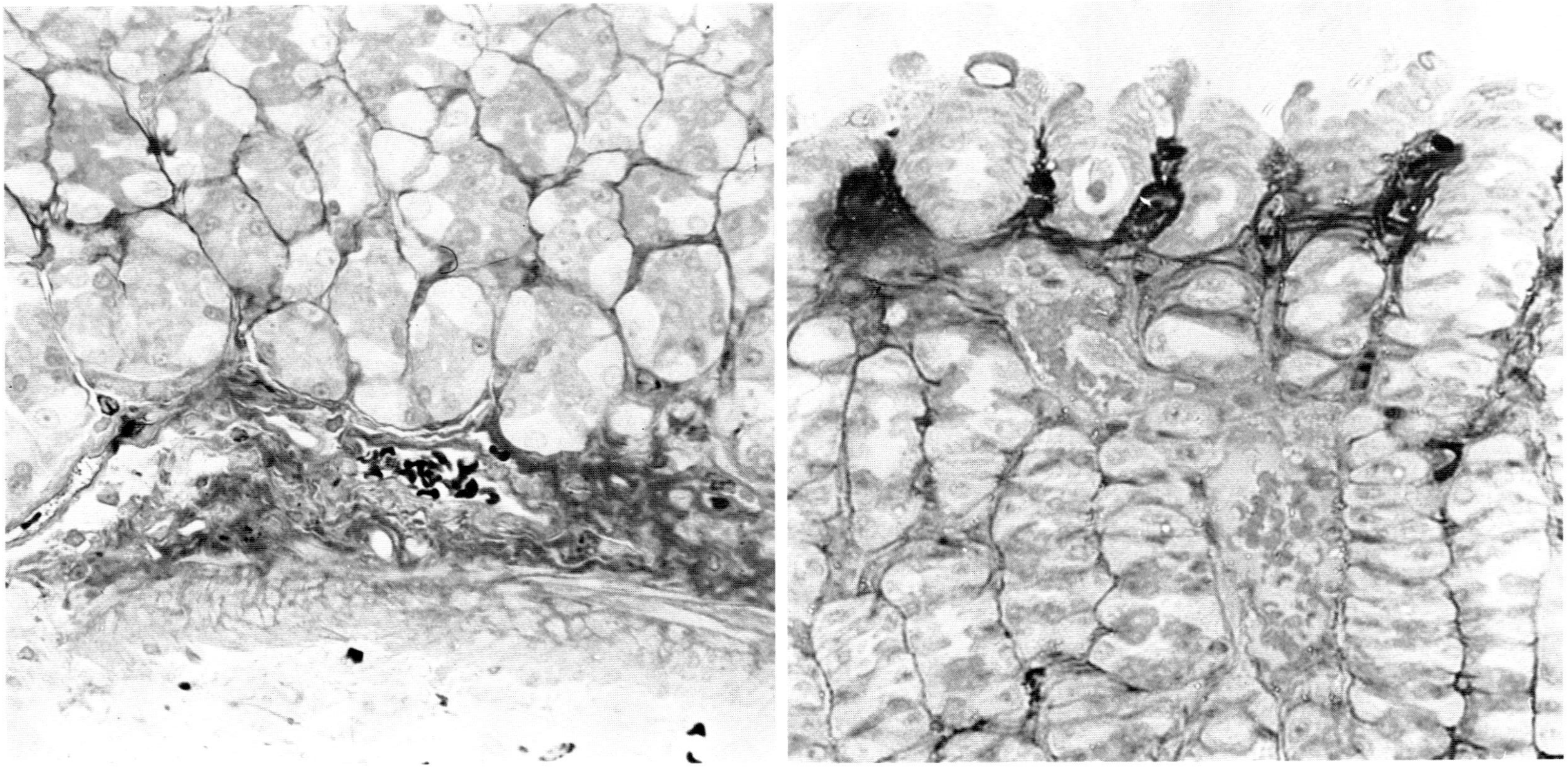

**Fig. 4-15.** Microcirculatory alterations induced by L-dopa administration. The HRP reaction is exclusively found in arterioles and venules (a) $\times 300$ (b) $\times 1{,}200$.

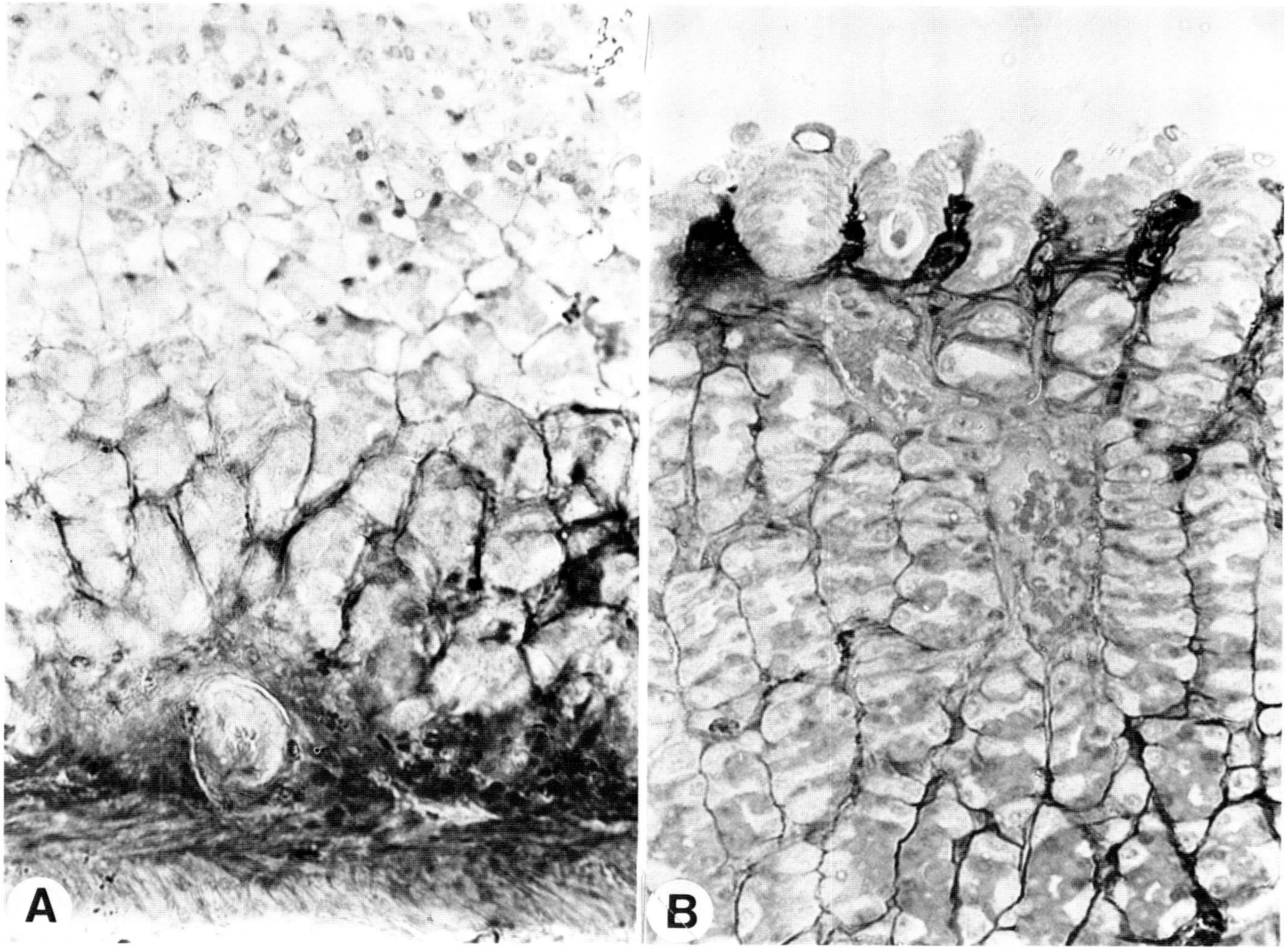


**Fig. 4-16.** Microcirculatory alterations induced by dopamine administration. (a) HRP is present only in the basal portion of the gastric mucosa after dopamine administration. ×1200. (b) In the control group, HRP is found in the top portion of the gastric mucosa. ×1,200.

laries in the middle portion of the gastric mucosa is found to be markedly increased (Fig. 4-14A&B). By the infusion of β-agonist isoproterenol, small arterioles located just above the muscularis mucosae, possibly corresponding to the terminal arterioles or metarterioles, are dilated compared with those in the control group (Fig. 4-14C). By the infusion of L-dopa or dopamine, the upper half of the gastric mucosa becomes ischemic, resembling the mucosal alterations observed in the process of the plaster bandage restraint-induced ulcer formation (Figs. 4-15A&B, 4-16A&B).[34] These observations suggest that dopamine may open the arteriovenous (A-V) anastomoses, causing mucosal ischemia. This would be supported by the report that dopaminergic nerve fibers may regulate the opening of A-V shunts in the dog paw pad.[45]

There is, however, a dispute as to whether A-V anastomosis is present in the gastric microcirculatory system in the rat stomach. It has been postulated that opening the submucosal A-V anastomoses is a important factor for gastric microcirculatory disturbances in stress-induced ulcerogenesis.[46,47] On the contrary, in vivo fluorescence microscopy revealed no A-V anastomosis in normal and sympathetic nerve-stimulated rat stomach,[48,49] implying that A-V shunts play no significant role in the mucosal blood flow responses to sympathetic nerve stimulation. In the restrained rats, the intensity of the specific fluorescence for adrenergic nerves is decreased in the mucosal layer, indicating that cholinergic nerves are excessively overstimulated in the gastric mucosa in the process of restraint-induced ulcerogenesis as described above.[34]

## DISTRIBUTION OF VIP-ERGIC NERVE FIBERS AND THE LOCALIZATION OF VIP RECEPTORS

The VIP-immunoreactivity-positive nerve fibers (i.e., VIP-ergic nerve fibers) show a distribution almost like that of the cholinergic nerve fibers in the gastric mucosa. Electron microscopically, the large cored vesicle-containing nerves are thought to be peptidergic in nature (Fig. 4-17A&B).[17] Some of these nerve fibers are shown to be immunoreactive to VIP in the rat stomach.

The localization of VIP-binding sites in the gastric mucosa was observed by radioautography for soluble compounds, as described above, using $^{125}$I-VIP as a ligand.

The receptors of VIP are found on the parietal cells in the gastric mucosa (Fig. 4-18A). Some VIP receptors are also visualized on the endothelia of the arterioles (Fig. 4-18B), suggesting that VIP may have some direct effects on the mucosal microcirculatory system.

There is a possibility that some of VIP-positive nerve fibers extending to the inferior mesenteric ganglia may correspond to sensory fibers.[50] Some of the nerves like VIP-ergic nerves may act as afferent fibers in the local reflex circuit.

## HISTAMINE-CONTAINING CELLS, HISTAMINERGIC NERVES AND THE LOCALIZATION OF HISTAMINE $H_1$ AND $H_2$ RECEPTORS

There is increasing evidence that histamine functions as a neurotransmitter in the central and peripheral nervous system.[21,51] In recent years, it was revealed that histamine-containing nerves are located mainly in the ganglia in the submucosal layer, not in the mucosal layer of the gastrointestinal tract.[21] Histamine-containing nerve fibers are present in the external muscle layer. In the mucosal layer of the rodent stomach, histamine is synthesized and stored in mast cells and enterochromaffin-like cells, but not in the nerve fibers.[21]

It is generally accepted that histamine $H_1$ receptors[52] located on smooth muscles and blood vessels are involved in the regulation of blood flow, while histamine $H_2$ receptors[53] specifically located on parietal cells are involved in the regulation of acid secretion.

In the stomach histamine is considered not

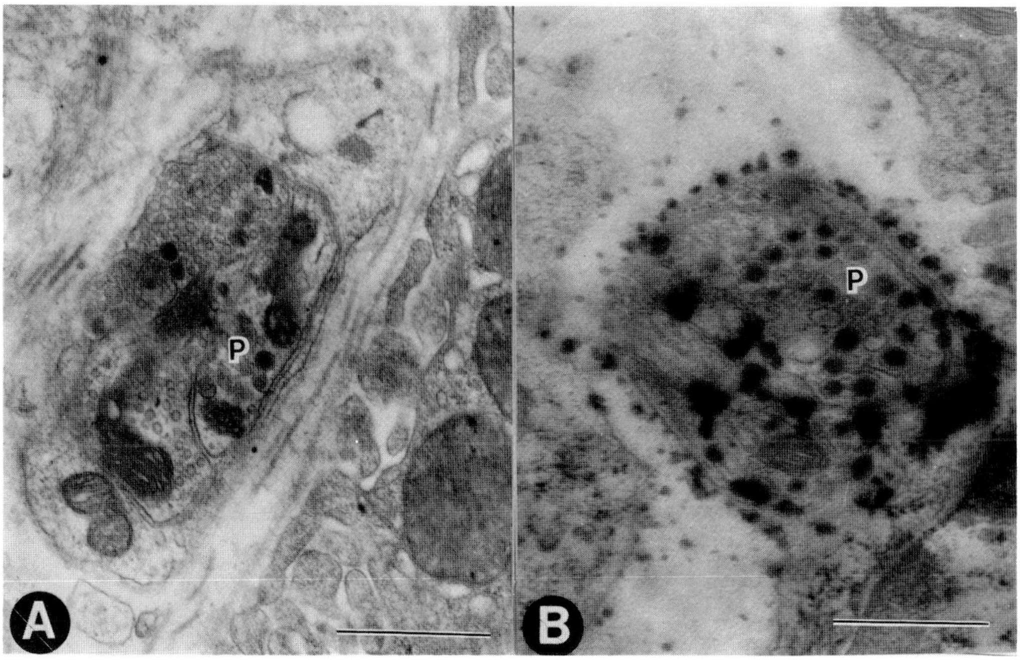


**Fig. 4-17.** Electron micrographs of the nerve endings composed of peptidergic (P) and cholinergic (C) nerve endings. (a) Some nerve fibers contain large granular vesicles probably corresponding to peptidergic nerves. ×25,000. (b) In the AChE staining, few reaction products are found on the axonal membranes of the peptidergic nerve endings. ×25,000

only to induce acid secretion from the parietal cells through $H_2$ receptors,[54] but also to dilate the submucosal arterioles through $H_1$ and $H_2$ receptors.[55]

$H_1$ receptor antagonist, diphenhydramine, decreases the gastric mucosal blood flow enhanced by the specific receptor agonist, 2-methylhistamine, while it hardly increases acid secretion, suggesting that $H_1$ receptors may play a possible physiological role in the control of the mucosal blood flow, regardless of acid secretion.[53] Histamine receptor antagonists suppress an increase in the gastric mucosal blood flow induced by $H_2$ receptor agonist but also inhibit acid secretion.[56] Therefore it still remains equivocal whether $H_2$ receptors directly regulate the mucosal blood flow, or indirectly affect the blood flow via acid secretory responses.[53]

The localization of both types of histamine receptors in the gastric mucosa was clarified by radioautography using the tritium-labelled histamine $H_1$ antagonist, $^3$H-pyrilamine and $H_2$ antagonist, $^3$H-cimetidine, as described above.[57] $H_1$ receptors are distributed mainly on the endothelial cells of the collecting venules, and $H_2$ receptors are chiefly present both on the parietal cells and on the collecting venules (Fig. 4-19A–C).

The presence of both $H_1$ and $H_2$ receptors on the collecting venules and their capillaries implies that direct interaction of both receptors may regulate the gastric mucosal microcirculation.[57] In particular, $H_2$ receptors located on the collecting venules and capillaries would be involved in the regulation of vascular permeability in the mucosal microcirculatory system. This is supported by evidence that $H_2$ receptors may regulate capillary permeability, whereas $H_1$ receptors may control arteriolar dilatation.[58] Increased microvascular permeability induced by histamine in the gastric mucosa is one of the factors causing a variety of vasomotor disturbances in the mucosal microcirculatory system, leading to the impairment of mucosal defensive mechanisms. Histamine is released from mast cells and enterochromaffin-like

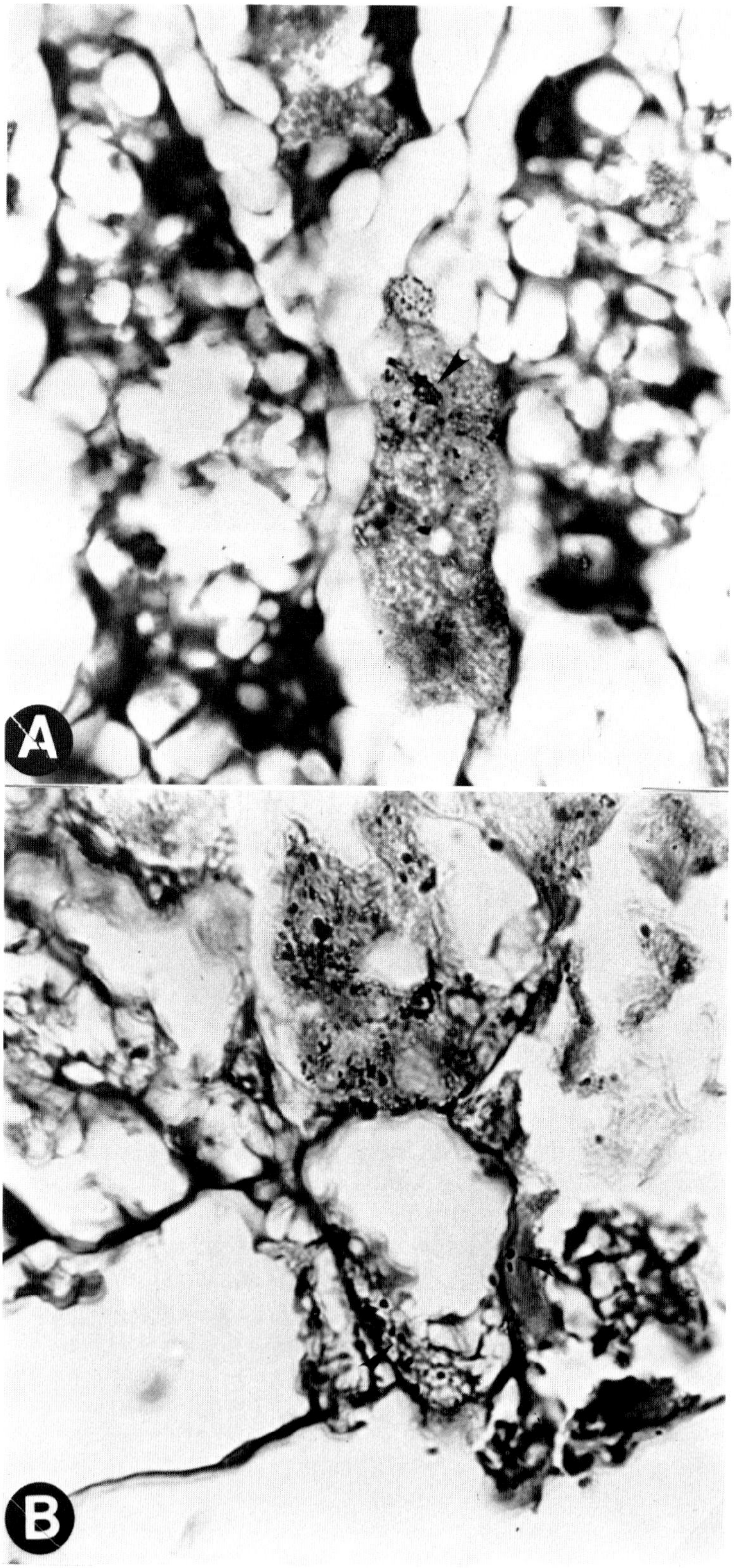

**Fig. 4-18.** Light microscopic radioautographs of the $^{125}$I-VIP binding sites in the gastric mucosa. (a) In the middle portion of the gastric mucosa, the grains are mainly found on the parietal cells (arrowhead). ×2,000. (b) In the basal portion of the gastric mucosa the grains are found on the smooth muscle cells of the arterioles (arrowheads). ×200.

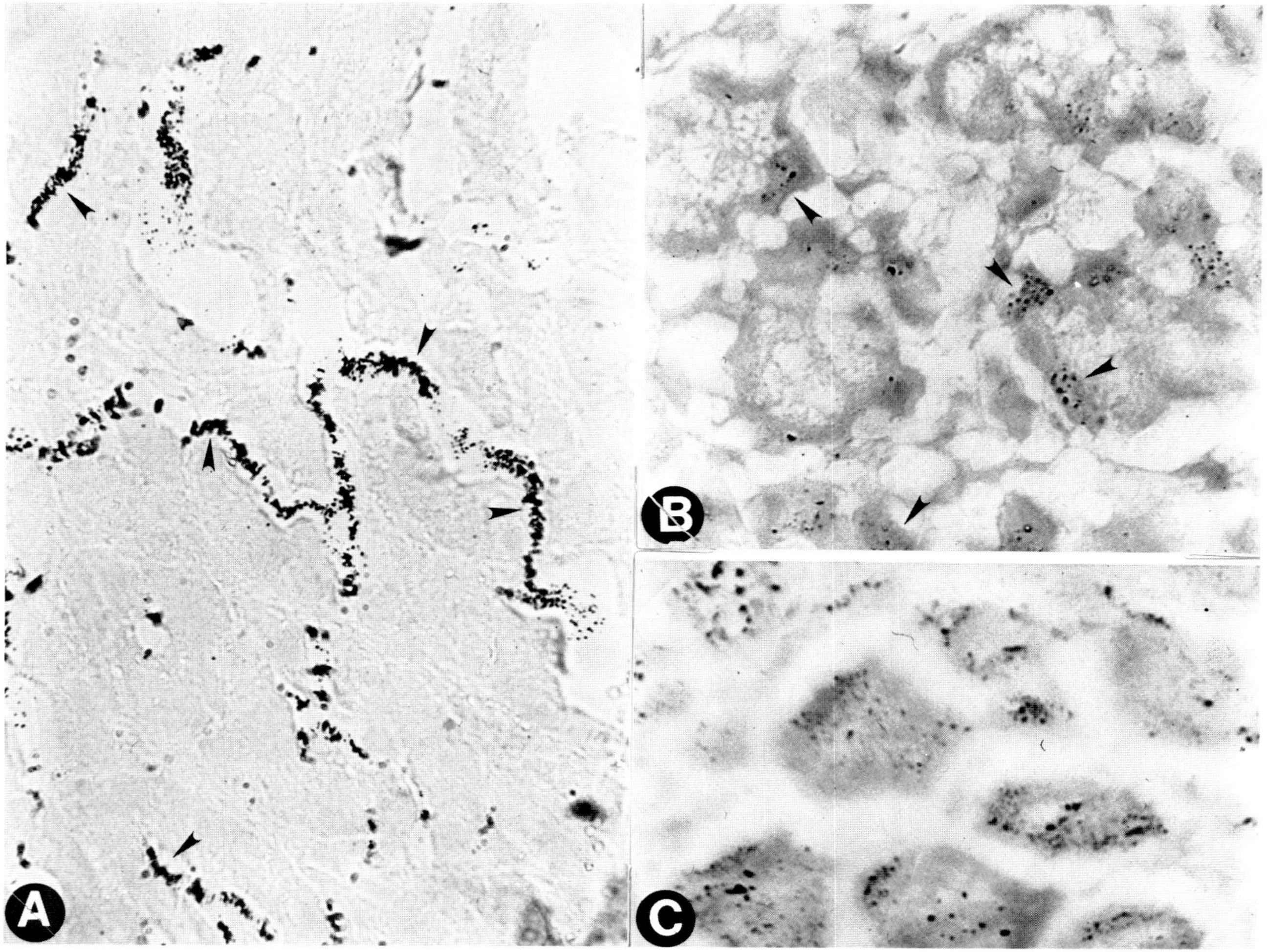


**Fig. 4-19.** Light microscopic radioautographs showing the $H_1$ and $H_2$ receptor antagonists in the gastric mucosa. (a) The $H_1$ receptor antagonist, $^3$H-pyrilamine, is binding to the endothelial cells of the true capillaries and the collecting venules (arrowheads). ×2,000. (b) The $H_2$ receptor antagonist, $^3$H-cimetidine, is binding to the parietal cells in the middle portion of the gastric mucosa (arrowheads). ×2,000. (c) $^3$H-cimetidine is also binding to the endothelial cells of the collecting venule and true capillaries. ×2,000.

# DISTRIBUTION OF AUTONOMIC NERVES AND THEIR RECEPTORS

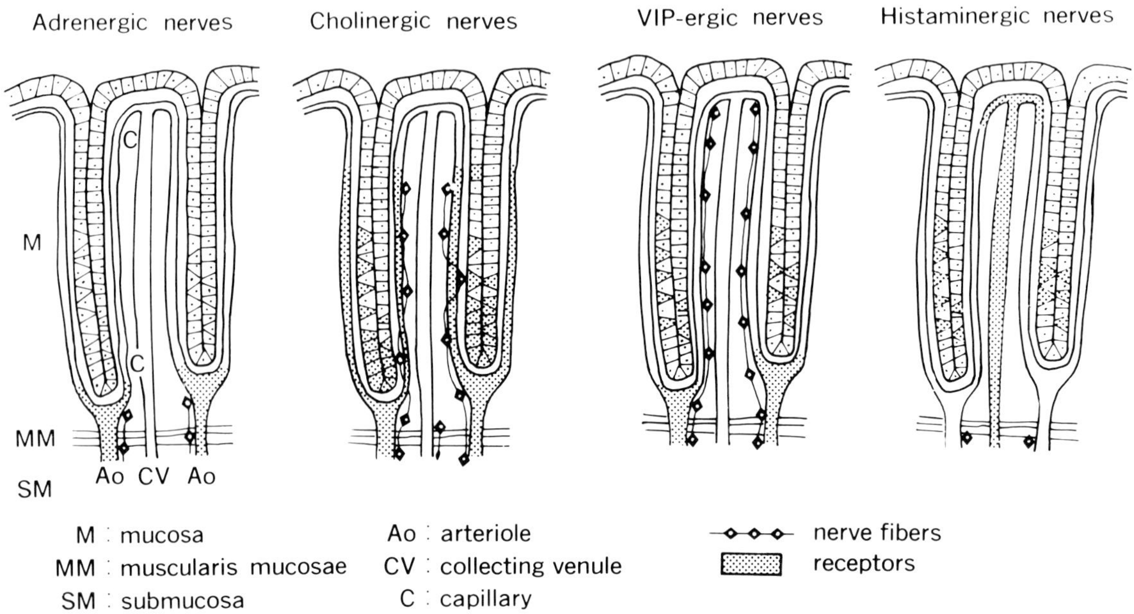


**Fig. 4-20.** Schematic illustration of adrenergic, cholinergic, VIP-ergic and histaminergic innervation of the gastric mucosa in the rat. The dotted area denotes the localization of adrenaline $\alpha$-receptors, muscarinic acetylcholine receptors, VIP receptors or histamine receptors on the effector cells and shows the areas innervated by each type of aminergic nerve fibers.

cells, and possibly from histamine-containing nerves in the gastric wall. Histamine release from mast cells is partly enhanced by cholinergic stimulation.

## SUMMARY

Adrenergic, cholinergic, VIP-ergic, and histaminergic innervation of the gastric mucosa in the rat is schematically illustrated in Fig. 4-20. Adrenergic $\alpha$-receptors, muscarinic acetylcholine receptors and VIP receptors are present on the mucosal effector cells in close vicinity of the autonomic peripheral nerves containing respectively each neurotransmitter noradrenaline, acetylcholine, and VIP. The distribution of cholinergic nerve fibers is similar to that of VIP-ergic nerve fibers, extending up to the upper portion of the mucosa and innervating the mucosal microvessels and epithelial cells such as parietal cells. Cholinergic and VIP-ergic innervation is predominant throughout the mucosa. The adrenergic nerve fibers extend to the basal portion of the mucosa partly in coexistence with cholinergic nerve fibers, also innervating the mucosal microvessels and possibly the epithelial cells. Dopamine would contribute to the opening of arteriovenous anastomoses, just above the muscularis mucosae. Histamine $H_2$ receptors are located mainly in the upper and middle portions of the gastric mucosa, while histaminergic nerve fibers are localized in the submucosa, suggesting that histaminergic fibers may not be directly involved in the regulation of a variety of gastric mucosal functions.

Abnormalities of the above mentioned characteristic innervation of the gastric mucosa are considered to play an important role in impairments of mucosal microcirculation and epithelial cell functions, leading to ulcer formation.

## ACKNOWLEDGMENTS

The present study was supported by the Grant-in-Aid for Scientific Research of the Ministry of Education, Science, and Culture in the year of 1983 (#58370024) and 1984 (#59370025).

## REFERENCES

1. Cushing H.: Peptic ulcers and the interbrain. Surg Gynecol Obstet, **55**:1–34, 1932
2. Bergamann G.: Das spasmogene Ulcus Pepticum. Münch. Med. Wochenschr., **60**:169–174, 1913
3. Sun D.C.H.: Etiology and pathology of peptic ulcer, In: Gastroenterology Vol 1 Edited by H.C. Bockus, Ed. W.B. Saunders Co, Philadelphia, pp 579–610, 1974
4. Tsuchiya M., Oda M., Nakamura M., Watanabe N. and Ohya Y.: Gastric mucosal microcirculation and its disturbances—with special reference to gastric ulcerogenesis; In: Defence Mechanism of Gastrointestinal Mucosa. Mucosal Blood Flow. Proceedings of the 2nd Symposium Defence Mechanism of Gastrointestinal Mucosa, March, 1981, Kyoto, Japan. Ed. K. Kawai. Iryokenkyushinsha, Kyoto, pp 93–99, 1981
5. Syay H.: Stress and gastric secretion. Gastroenterology, **26**:316–319, 1954
6. Hollander F.: The two-component mucous barrier. Its activity in protecting the gastroduodenal mucosa against peptic ulceration. Arch Intern Med, **93**:107–120, 1954
7. Oda M., Nakamura M., Watanabe N., Nagata H. and Tsuchiya M.: Microcirculatory changes in the restraint-induced gastric ulcer formation of the rat—a vital and electron microscopic study. In: Advances in Experimental Ulcer. Proceedings of the 4th International Conference for Experimental Ulcer, October 18–19, 1980, Tokyo, Japan. Eds. S. Umehara and H. Ito. Tokyo Medical College, Tokyo, pp 226–236, 1982
8. Davenport H.W.: Gastric mucosal injury by fatty and acetylsalicylic acids. Gastroenterology, **46**:245–253, 1964
9. Lanciault G. and Jacobson E.D.: Progress in gastroenterology. Gastroenterology, **71**:851–873, 1976
10. Nakamura M., Watanabe N., Tsukada N., Oda M. and Tsuchiya M.: Demonstration of the adrenergic nerves in the rat gastric mucosa—a histofluorescence and electron microscopic study in comparison with the distribution of the cholinergic nerves. Okajima's Folia Anat Jpn, **59**:65–86, 1982
11. Van-Driel C. and Drukker J.: A contribution study of the architecture of the autonomic nervous system of the digestive tract of the rat. J Neural Trans, **34**:301–320, 1973
12. Gabella G.: Innervation of the gastrointestinal tract. Int Rev Cytol, **59**:129–193, 1979
13. Llewellyn-Smith I.J., Furness J.B., Wilson A.J. and Costa M.: Organization and fine structure of enteric ganglia. In: Autonomic Ganglia. Ed. L-G. Elvin. John Wiley & Sons, Chinchester, pp 145–182, 1983
14. Kyösola K., Veijola L. and Rechardt L.: Cholinergic innervation of the gastric wall of the cat. Histochemistry, **44**:23–30, 1975
15. Costa M. and Gabella G.: Adrenergic innervation of the alimentary canal. Z. Zellforsch., **122**:357–377, 1971
16 Pearse A.G.E. and Polak J.M.: Immunocytochemical localization of substance P in mammalian intestine. Histochem., **41**:373–375, 1975
17. Lundberg J.M., Hökfelt T., Schultzberg M., Uvnas-Wallensten K., Kohler C. and Said S.I.: Occurrence of vasoactive intestinal polypeptide (VIP)-like immunoreactivity in certain cholinergic neurons of the cat: evidence from combined immunohistochemistry and acetylcholinesterase staining. Neuroscience, **4**:1539–1559, 1979
18. Lundberg J.M.: Evidence for coexistence of vasoactive intestinal polypeptide (VIP) and acetylcholine in neurons of cat exocrine glands: Morphological, biochemical and functional study. Acta Physiol Scand (suppl), **496**:1–57, 1981
19. Iwanaga T.: Gastrin-releasing peptide (GRP)/bombesin-like immunoreactivity in the neurons and paraneurons of the gut and lung. Biomed Res **4**:93–104, 1983
20. Lundberg J.M. and Hökfelt T.: Coexistence of peptides and classical neurotransmitters. Trends in Neurosci., **6**:325–333, 1983
21. Panula P., Kaartinen M., Macklin M. and Costa E.: Histamine-containing peripheral neuronal and endocrine systems. J Histochem Cytochem, **33**:933–941, 1985
22. Gershon M.D., Sherman D., Erde S.M. and Rothman T.P.: Serotonergic neurons and mammalian gut, In: Functional Disorders of the Digestive Tract, Ed. W.Y. Chey. Raven Press, New York, pp 59–77, 1983
23. Lackovic Z. and Relja M.: Evidence of a widely distributed peripheral dopaminergic system. Fed Proc., **42**:3000–3004, 1983
24. Burnstock G.: Purinergic nerves. Pharmacol Rev, **24**:509–581, 1972
25. Bell C.: Fine structural localization of acetylcholinesterase at a cholinergic vasodilator nerve-arterial smooth muscle synapse. Circ. Res., **24**:61–70, 1969
26. Karnovsky M.J. and Roots L.: A direct coloring thiocholine method for cholinesterases. J Histochem Cytochem, **12**:219–221, 1964
27. Nakamura M.: Studies of the cholinergic innervation in the rat fundic mucosa—with special reference to the gastric mucosal microcirculation. Keio Igaku, **63**:13–28, 1986 (in Japanese)
28. Nakamura M., Watanabe N., Oda M., and Tsuchiya M.: Histochemical, fluorescence and electron microscopic studies on the distribution of autonomic nerve endings in the gastric mucosa. The Autonomic Nervous System, **17**:338–345, 1980 (in Japanese)
29. Bunge R., Johnson M. and Rosse C.D.: Nature and nurture of the autonomic neuron. Science, **199**:1409–1416, 1978
30. Nakamura M., Oda M., Yonei Y., Komatsu H., Tsukada N., Watanabe N. and Tsuchiya M.: Histochemical and electron microscopic cytochemical studies on the autonomic innervation of the gastric mucosa in

rats—embryological differentiation of the parietal cell and acetylcholinesterase activity. The Autonomic Nervous System, **21**:386–398, 1984 (in Japanese)
31. Chamley J.H. and Campbell G.R.: Trophic influence of sympathetic and cyclic AMP on differentiation and proliferation of isolated smooth muscle cell in culture. Cell Tissue Res., **208**:1–19, 1980
32. Nakamura M., Oda M., Watanabe N., Ohya Y., Sekizuka E., Tsukada N., Yonei Y., Komatsu H. and Tsuchiya M.: Dynamic aspects of the gastric mucosal microcirculation in the healthy and stress condition—with special reference to the autonomic nervous control, in: Intravital Observation of Organ Microcirculation. Proceedings of the Tokyo Symposium, June 18, 1983. Eds. Tsuchiya M., Wayland H., Oda M. and Okazaki I.. Excerpta Medica, Amsterdam pp 65–97, 1983
33. Oda M., Nakamura M., Watanabe N., Tsukada N., Yonei Y., Komatsu H., Ohya Y., Sekizuka E. and Tsuchiya M.: Dual action of the parasympathetic nerve in the gastric mucosa—significance of its overactivity in the pathogenesis of gastric ulcer, In: Gastrointestinal Function. Regulation and Disturbances of Gastrointestinal Function, September 18, 1982, Tokyo, Japan. Eds. Kasuya Y., Tsuchiya M., Nagao F. and Matsuo Y. Amsterdam Excerpta Medica, pp 145–173, 1983
34. Oda M., Nakamura M., Watanabe N., Tsukada N., Ohya Y., Sekizuka E. and Tsuchiya M.: Autonomic nerve regulation of gastric mucosal microcirculation—with special reference to the pathogenesis of stress-induced ulcer, In: Basic Aspects of Microcirculation. Proceedings of Tokyo International Symposium on Microcirculation, July 26, 1981, Tokyo, Japan. Eds. Tsuchiya M., Oda M., and Asano M. Amsterdam Excerpta Medica, pp 209–229, 1982
35. Nagata T., Nawa T. and Yokota S.: A new technique for electron microscopic drymounting radioautography of soluble compounds. Histochemie, **18**:241–249, 1969
36. Nakamura M., Oda M., Yonei Y., Tsukada N., Watanabe N., Komatsu H. and Tsuchiya M.: Demonstration of the localization of muscarinic acetylcholine receptors in the gastric mucosa—light and electron microscopic autoradiographic studies using $^3$H-quinuclidinyl benzilate. Acta Histochem Cytochem, **17**:297–309, 1984
37. Nakamura M., Oda M., Yonei Y., Tsukada N., Komatsu H. and Tsuchiya M.: Muscarinic acetylcholine receptors in rat gastric mucosa—a radioautographic study using a potent muscarinic antagonist, $^3$H-pirenzepine. Histochemistry, **83**:479–487, 1985
38. Holm-Rutili L. and Öbrink K.J.: Rat gastric mucosal microcirculation in vivo. Am J Physiol, **248**:G741–746, 1985
39. Guth P.H. and Smith E.: Neural control of gastric mucosal blood flow in the rat. Gastroenterology, **69**:935–940, 1975
40. Ajelis V., Björklund A., Falck B., Lindvall O., Loren J. and Walles B.: Application of the aluminium formaldehyde (ALFA) histofluorescence method for demonstration of peripheral stores of catecholamines and indolamines in freeze-dried paraffin-embedded tissue, cryostat sections and whole-mounts. Histochemistry, **65**:1–15, 1979
41. Falck B. and Hillarp N.: Fluorescence of catecholamine and related compounds condensed with formaldehyde. Histochem Cytochem, **10**:348–354, 1973
42. Furness J.B.: The adrenergic innervation of the vessels supplying and draining the gastrointestinal tract. Z. Zellforsch., **113**:67–82, 1971
43. Read J. and Burnstock G.: Competitive histochemical studies of adrenergic nerves in the enteric plexuses of vertebrate large intestine. Comp. Biochem. Physiol., **27**:505–517, 1968
44. Nakamura M., Ohya Y., Morishita T. and Oda M.: The structure of the gastric mucosal microcirculatory system and its regulatory mechanism—with special reference to autonomic nervous function. J Japanese College of Angiology, **24**:11–18, 1984
45. Bell C., Lang W.J. and Laska F.: Dopamine-cotaining axons supplying the arteriovenous anastomosis of the canine paw pad. J Neurochem, **31**:1329–1333, 1978
46. Hase T. and Moss B.J.: Microvascular changes of gastric mucosa in the development of stress ulcer in rats. Gastroenterology, **65**:224–234, 1973
47. Kitajima M., Wolfe R.R., Trelftadt R.L., Allsop J.R. and Burk J.F.: Gastric mucosal lesion after burn injury: Relationship to $H^+$-back diffusion and the microcirculation. J Trauma, **18**:644–650, 1978
48. Guth P.H. and Rosenberg A.: In vivo microscopy of the gastric microcirculation. Am J Dig Dis, **17**:391–398, 1972
49. Guth P.H.: In vivo microscopy of the gastric microcirculation: anatomical and physiological findings, In: Basic Aspects of Microcirculation. Proceedings of Tokyo International Symposium on Microcirculation, July 26, 1981, Tokyo, Japan. Eds. M Tsuchiya, Oda M. and Asano M. Excerpta Medica, Amsterdam pp 209–229, 1982
50. Szurszewski J.H. and Weems W.A.: A study of peripheral input to and its control by postganglionic neurones of the inferior mesenteric ganglion. J Physiol, **256**:541–556, 1976
51. Schwartz J.C., Pollard H. and Quach T.T.: Histamine as a neurotransmitter in mammalian brain. J Neurochem, **35**:26–33, 1980
52. Ash A.S. and Schild H.O.: Receptors mediating some actions of histamine. Br J Pharmacol Chemother, **27**:427–439, 1966
53. Blach J.W., Duncan W.A.M., Durant C.J., Ganellin C.R. and Parsons E.M.: Definition and antagonism of histamine $H_2$-receptors. Nature, **236**:385–390, 1972
54. Soll A.H.: The interaction of histamine with gastrin and carbamylcholine on oxygen uptake by isolated mammalian parietal cells. J Clin Invest, **61**:381–389, 1978
55. Guth P.H., Smith E. and Moler T.: $H_1$ and $H_2$ receptors in rat gastric submucosal arterioles. Microvasc Res, **19**:320–328, 1980
56. Curwain B.P., Holton P. and Spencer J.: Evidence that the inhibitory effect of burimamide on gastric secretion is not due to decreased gastric mucosal blood flow. J Physiol, **230**:33p–34p, 1973
57. Nakamura M., Oda M., Yonei Y., Kaneko K., Komatsu H., Tsukada N., Tsuchiya M. and Fujishiro Y.: Radioautographic demonstration of localization of histamine $H_1$ and $H_2$ receptors in the gastric mucosa. In: Annual report 1985 Japanese Society for Microcirculation. Eds. Tsuchiya M., Asano M., Oda M. and Okazaki I. Amsterdam Excerpta Medica, pp 217–223, 1985
58. Mortillaro N.A., Granger D.N. and Kvietys P.R.: Effects of histamine and histamine antagonists on intestinal capillary permeability. Am J Physiol **240**:381–386, 1981

# 5

# Non-Hodgkin's Lymphomas of the Gastrointestinal Tract: A Review with Special Reference to the Gut-associated Lymphoid Tissue

P. van der Valk M.D, Ph.D
J. Lindeman M.D, Ph.D
C.J.L.M. Meijer M.D, Ph.D

Non-Hodgkin's lymphomas (NHL) are intriguing tumors for several reasons. First, they show a marked variety of histological pictures. Second, though most common in the lymphoid tissues, they can be found in any tissue or organ of the body; and third, they are related to the immune system, as lymphocytes are the cells composing that system. Our knowledge concerning NHL has increased enormously in the last 20 years, due largely to technical advances, such as immunohistochemistry with monoclonal antibodies and electron microscopy. Basic to our present insights is the realization that normal lymphocyte physiology can be seen mirrored in NHL. Malignant lymphoid cells resemble normal lymphocytes in some state of their development, both morphologically and functionally. As lymphocytes are engaged in reactions in the immune response and malignant lymphoid cells mimic normal lymphocytes in morphology and behavior, NHL can be regarded as neoplastic counterparts of the immune reactions. This concept[1,2,3,4] is the basis of proper understanding of NHL and is reflected in the classification schemes according to Lukes & Collins[2] and Kiel.[3]

This concept is based largely on knowledge of NHL of the (peripheral) lymph nodes. The lymphoid tissue, however, is not confined to the lymph nodes: accumulations are found as watchdogs against antigenic attacks along the epithelia of the gut (gut-associated lymphoid tissue (GALT)) with concentrations in the terminal ileum and appendix,[5] of the bronchi (bronchus-associated lymphoid tissue or BALT),[6] of the genital tract,[7] and some foregut-related appendages, such as thyroid[8] and salivary glands.[9] As these systems have features in common, morphologically[6] and functionally,[10] the term mucosa-associated lymphoid tissue (MALT) was introduced.[11] Here we shall stick to the term GALT as we are concerned with gastrointestinal lymphoid tissue only.

The GALT and the peripheral lymph nodes differ in some essential points. Most important of these is that the GALT acts to prevent extensive reactions against antigens and generally has a dampening influence immunologically,[12] whereas in the lymph nodes, reactions against antigens are meant to augment immune responses. The goal of this "tolerance" for some antigens is to prevent undue reactions against molecules in the gastrointestinal lumen. This is partly achieved by covering these molecules with IgA.[13]

This difference in function between GALT and peripheral lymph nodes is achieved, among others, through a difference in homing of lymphocyte subsets to GALT. Thus, B-cells preferentially home to the GALT, whereas T-lymphocytes tend to favor the peripheral lymph nodes.[14] Of the B-cells, IgA carrying lymphocytes are found in much higher numbers in the GALT compared to the peripheral nodes. In the T-lymphocytes there appear to be subsets preferentially localizing in the GALT,[15] which of course may cause differences in function.[16] The peculiar distribution of suppressor T-cells and helper T-cells found in the GALT, with intraepithelial lymphocytes being of suppressor/cytotoxic phenotype and lamina propria lymphocytes mainly of helper/inducer phenotype[12,17] may explain the tendency towards tolerance innate to the GALT.

Thus, the GALT has its own cellular pool and physiology. In short, cells are brought in contact with antigen in the bowel wall. Here, the epithelium may play a role as GALT localizations are covered by a specialized epithelium containing cells with microfolds on their luminal surface, the so-called M-cells.[5] After antigenic contact B-cells migrate to the mesenteric lymph nodes and via the thoracic duct and the peripheral blood, back to the GALT. During this journey they differentiate towards plasma cells. These plasma cells, finally, are found in the GALT in the lamina propria, while most of their precursors are not, at least under normal conditions. These precursors (e.g., the follicle center cell phase) can be found in other (earlier) locations such as the mesenteric lymph nodes or that part of the bowel wall where contact with the antigen takes place.[5]

Since NHL from peripheral lymph nodes mimic the normal behavior of peripheral lymph node cells, NHL arising in the GALT can be expected to do the same. Therefore, in discussing gastrointestinal NHL, the concept of the GALT has to be considered. Not all GI-tract NHL arise in the GALT, however. According to the GALT concept, the following subdivision can be made:

I. *Primary GI-NHL.* They arise in the GALT and may be confined to the GALT and regional lymph nodes (Ia) or show dissemination beyond the regional lymph nodes (Ib).

II. *Secondary GI-NHL,* in which the GI tract involvement is secondary to wide dissemination.

Approximately 40% would fall into category Ia, primary GI-NHL restricted to GALT,[18] whereas a similar percentage is reported for primary GI-NHL with dissemination beyond the GALT.[19]

Involvement of the GI tract secondary to a "peripheral" NHL is recognized in ± 20% of all NHL,[19] but at autopsy higher percentages are found, ranging from 45–70%.[18,19]

In the next paragraphs we will discuss incidence and localization of GI-NHL. In the part on pathology the significant NHL categories are considered. The importance of marker studies in diagnosis and classification is stressed. Next, prognosis, prognostic factors and implications for staging procedures and treatment are discussed, and finally some remarks on therapy will be made. Where possible reference shall be made to the abovementioned categories (Ia and b and II).

## INCIDENCE

Extranodal NHL are not uncommon: 20–40% arise outside the lymph nodes.[20,21] From these primary extranodal localizations, the GI tract is involved most frequently, followed by Waldeyer's ring, skin, the oribital region, salivary glands, bone, and lungs.[20] Of all NHL 4–10% are primarily located somewhere along the gastrointestinal tract,[20,22,23] while 1–4% of all GI tumors are NHL. That involvement of the GI tract in NHL, regardless of the initial localization, is fairly common was mentioned before (20% of all NHL recognized during life and 45–70% at autopsy).

## CLINICAL DATA

GI tract NHL show no clear age predilection and are found twice more often in men than in women. They usually cause symptoms, such as abdominal pain or discomfort, bleeding with hematemesis or melena, obstruction, intussusception, perforation with or without peritonitis, and/or general symptoms such as fever, weakness, weight loss, etc.[18] Obstruction is seen most frequently in small intestine localizations. Intussusceptions are especially frequent in ileocecal localizations and are thus seen most frequently in children.[22,24] Perforation is a dreaded complication; it is reported in 1–28% of all cases.[22]

## LOCALIZATION

Though accounts tend to vary, the majority of studies show the stomach to be involved most often. Small intestine follows closely. Some studies list the ileocecal region separately. It is involved in approximately 10% of the cases, as is the large intestine. Table 5-1 lists the data of several studies from the literature, as well as the data from our material.

In children most GI tract NHL are located in the ileocecal region.[22] Most studies mentioned concern primary GI-NHL, which makes it likely that these tumors originated in the GALT. However, distinguishing between a GALT lymphoma with extensive dissemination (Ib) and a nodal NHL with involvement of the GI tract (II) is not always possible. Though likely, it is not absolutely certain that GALT-NHL (group I) follow the pattern of localization outlined above. Reports on six GALT-NHL mention the stomach (5×) and the small intestine (1×) as localizations.[25,26,27]

**TABLE 5-1**
Localization of NHL in GI Tract (in percentages).

| Reference | n | Stomach | SI | ICR | LI |
|---|---|---|---|---|---|
| Lewin et al.[22] | 117 | 41 | 32 | 12 | 9 |
| Isaacson et al.[34] | 66 | 36 | 49 | 12 | 3 |
| Saraga et al.[28] | 66 | 55 | 30 | NS | 15 |
| Weingrad et al.[23] | 104 | 73 | 14 | NS | 13 |
| Filippa et al., 1983[31] | 60 | 75 | 7 | NS | 18 |
| Grody et al.[30] | 25 | 68 | 20 | NS | 12 |
| Our material | 51 | 27 | 17 | NS | 7 |

n = number of patients; SI = small intestine; LI = large intestine; ICR = ileocecal region; NS = not stated

## PATHOLOGY

### Macroscopy

There are no specific macroscopic features. Ulceration is fairly common,[22] but is seen in nonmalignant lesions as well.[28] A diffuse thickening of the bowel wall is found in roughly a quarter of the cases and is very suspicious for lymphoma. More commonly, however, lymphomas produce a discrete mass, in some cases polypoid.[28]

### Microscopy

Microscopically, most GI tract-NHL are large-cell lymphomas; there is a predominance of diffuse over follicular NHL.[19,22,28–30] Here we will discuss several categories of NHL separately:

#### B-cell NHL: Follicle Center Cell Lymphomas (FCC)

True follicular NHL in the GI tract are less common, with percentages reported varying from 2.7–10%.[18,19,28–30]

Among all diffuse GI-NHL, there is a predominance of FCC.[23,30–33] Isaacson et al[34] report an FCC origin for all their lymphoid GI-

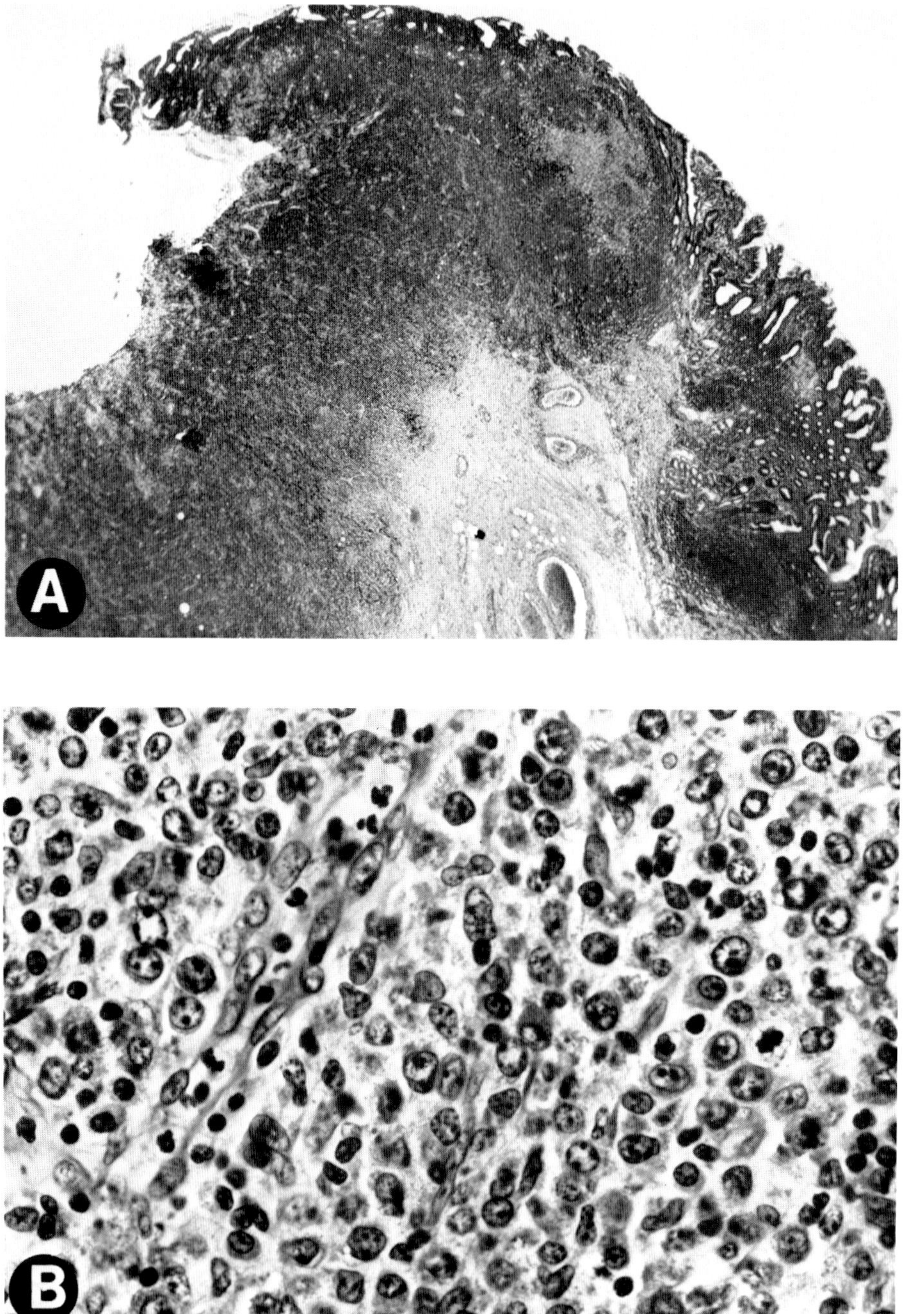

**Fig. 5-1.** Centroblastic lymphoma localized in the antrum of the stomach. (a) Low power view of the tumor. (HE stain ×25). (b) Detail of the tumor cells. (HE stain ×400). (c) Nearly all neoplastic cells stain with a monoclonal antibody against $\kappa$ light chain immunoglobulin.

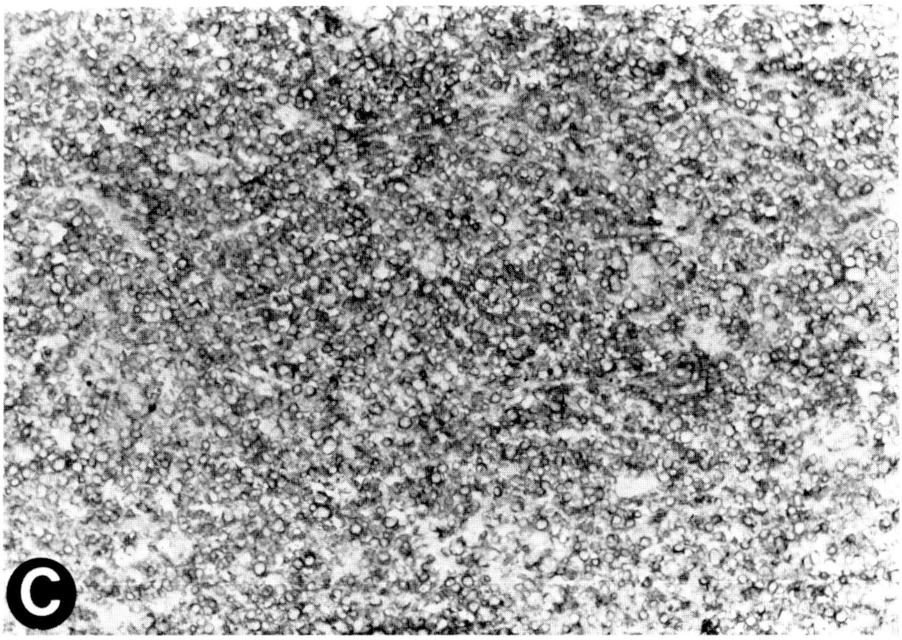

**Fig. 5-1.** *(continued)*

NHL. Most common are the *large non-cleaved* or *centroblastic NHL* (Fig. 5-1). They consist predominantly of large cells with large, vesicular nuclei, 1–3 marginal nucleoli, and little cytoplasm. Usually there is some mixture with cells having single and central nucleoli and ample cytoplasm. (i.e., immunoblast-like cells). If this admixture is pronounced and the number of immunoblasts does not exceed the number of centroblasts, the term polymorphic centroblastic lymphoma is used.

Futhermore, there are always large cells with cleaved nuclei present. Small, dark, and angular/cleaved cells or centrocytes can be seen in varying numbers, usually scant. In centroblastic NHL, macrophages are usually present in high numbers (10–15%).[35] Occasionally, these large cell FCC can resemble carcinomas.

*Centroblastic/centrocytic lymphomas* are often diffuse, though it is not uncommon to find follicular areas. These areas are difficult to differentiate from lymphoid hyperplasia,[28,36] even when applying strict morphological criteria. In resection specimens the diffuse areas will provide the important clue to diagnosis of malignancy, but in a small biopsy specimen these areas may be missing. Marker studies, especially demonstration of monoclonality by immunoglobulin light chain typing, are essential here, as they are in all NHL diagnostics.

*Centrocytic lymphomas* are diffuse. They can be present in a very typical way: as multiple polypoid lesions along large parts of the GI tract.[24] These NHL consist entirely of small cells with angular or cleaved nuclei with moderately dense chromatin and scanty cytoplasm. They show a relative high tendency to become leukemic.

B-cell NHL: B-immunoblastic NHL (B-IB)

B-IB are found somewhat less frequently than centroblastic NHL, but this may vary per localization: Otto et al.[37] report a predominance of B-IB in their *intestinal* large-cell lymphomas. B-IB tends to involve the entire bowel wall. It destroys the muscularis, producing fissures that explain the high rate of perforation in these tumors.[24] The microscopic picture of this NHL is typical. The cells are large, with large nuclei. There is usually one large (para)central nucleolus, though more nucleoli are occasionally seen. The cytoplasm is ample and basophilic. There is some differentiation to plasma cell morphology. Admixed small cells have round nuclei. Macrophages can be numerous.

### B-Cell NHL: (Lympho)plasmacytoid NHL

*Plasmacytomas* show no preference for a certain site,[22,38,39] but lymphoplasmacytoid NHL are somewhat more prevalent in the small intestine.[28,37] Plasmacytomas are usually easily recognized, however, atypical cases occur. Plasmacytomas where the cells have signet ring cell morphology have been described.[27,40] We have seen a plasmacytoma where the nuclei were deformed by immunoglobulin-containing vacuoles in the cytoplasm. The nuclei were angular and/or dented and the cells did not resemble plasma cells at all. Such cases can cause diagnostic problems and immunohistochemistry is necessary.

*Lymphoplasmacytoid NHL* consists of lymphocytes with moderate amounts of cytoplasm, and round to slightly irregular nuclei that show a tendency to a spoke-wheel pattern of chromatin. Plasma cells can be seen, and sometimes a few immunoblasts can be found. In this context mention must be made of the so called *"Mediterranean lymphoma,"* or *immunoproliferative small intestine disease (IPSID)* as it has come to be called. This is a clinicopathologic entity; clinical features are chronic diarrhea, weight loss, and abdominal pain.[41,42] Furthermore, a number of these patients have an abnormal IgA molecule in their serum, which can also be found in the cells of the concomitant mucosal infiltrate in the small intestine,[43] and that has led to the name $\alpha$-chain disease. However, not all patients with IPSID have $\alpha$-chain disease.[44] Pathologically there are two variants of IPSID. One is the classical diffuse (lympho)plasmacytoid infiltration of the duodenal and/or jejunal mucosa, associated with $\alpha$-chain disease. Transformation of this variant into B-immunoblastic lymphomas is frequently found in this setting. In the other there is a follicular lymphoid hyperplasia. Lymphomas developing in this setting are frequently of the undifferentiated type (Rappaport classification).[45] These two types are probably both a reflection of GALT physiology. There is an initial phase (FCC reaction, not necessarily taking place at the site of the lymphoplasmacytoid infiltrate), and a terminal lymphoplasmacytoid phase that develops in the end phase of plasmacytic differentiation. Both phases can take place in separate portions of the gut, but not necessarily so. Under sufficient antigenic pressure, follicles (the initial phase of the reaction) can arise anywhere in the GI tract. Support for this theory is found in marker studies. They have identified an identical immunophenotype on cells of both phases (initial FCC phase, and terminal lymphoplasmacytoid phase) of a lymphoma in a single patient.[46] Thus, IPSID appears to be an example of a GALT-NHL. Classification of a lymphoma with both phases represented in the histology is sometimes difficult. They can best be classified as a pleomorphic immunocytoma. An FCC origin for these lymphomas in the lymph nodes (similar to the GALT situation), was suggested earlier.[35,47]

### B-Cell: B Lymphoblastic NHL (Burkitt or Non-Burkitt Type)

These lymphomas show a characteristic clinicopathologic picture. They are most frequent in children, with boys predominating (M:F = 2:1). The patients often have an acute obstruction, due to intussusception in the ileocecal region where these lymphomas are found most frequently, though not exclusively.[22,37] In fact a clinical presentation like that in a child is highly suggestive for lymphoblastic NHL. Microscopically, the tumor seems to spare the muscularis even when it is disseminated beyond the bowel. Another striking feature is the reluctance to invade the regional lymph nodes. Lymph nodes can be seen, completely encased by tumor, but without infiltration of the lymph node itself.[24] Besides their locally invasive character that leads to fixation of the bowel to adjacent structures, there is a clear tendency to dissemination[48] involving extranodal localizations such as the kidney, the gut, pleura, and central nervous system.[24,48]

The histology of these NHL is monotonous (Fig. 5-2). It is a uniform proliferation of medium-sized cells, with little cytoplasm and some degree of nuclear polymorphism. In cytology the vacuolated aspect of the cytoplasm is especially well appreciated. In many, especially Burkitt-type cases, the abundance of admixed macrophages causes the so-called "starry sky" pattern. It is striking, but not specific (centroblastic lymphomas can also show a starry sky pattern) and not invariably present in our experience.

Occasionally we have seen lymphoblastic NHL where the cells resembled small centroblasts, with 2–3 marginal, though less conspicuous nucleoli, but with the grayish, finely dispersed chromatin characteristic of lymphoblasts. The clinical course of these cases does not appear to be different from other lymphoblastic NHL, Burkitt, or non-Burkitt type.

## T-Cell Lymphomas

Lymphomas of T-lymphocytes in the GI tract are very rare by all accounts, probably reflecting the preference of these cells for the peripheral lymph nodes over the GALT.[14] Grody et al.[30] reported two T-cell lymphomas among their 25 patients (8%), which is the highest number we found in the literature. Classification of T-cell lymphomas is still troublesome, even in the peripheral lymph nodes and with the scarcity of cases, this makes any statement on GI-T-cell lymphomas difficult. Of interest is the report on a T-cell NHL in the gut showing marked epitheliotropism,[49] not unlike the epidermotropism seen in mycosis fungoides. Interestingly, the tumor cells were Leu2a positive (i.e., of suppressor/cytotoxic phenotype). Since intraepithelial lymphocytes have a similar phenotype, this case underlines the similarity between normal and malignant lymphocytes. But many more cases will have to be studied in order to obtain a clear picture of T-cell lymphomas in the GI tract.

## Histiocytic Sarcomas or True Histiocytic Lymphomas

Though as an entity histiocytic sarcoma is established, its frequency among NHL is controversial. The controversy was sparked off by Isaacson et al.[34] who drew attention to this tumor in the gut and reported a frequency of 50% in their 66 primary GI-NHL. Other investigators did not find such high percentages; some even questioned the existence of histiocytic sarcoma as a primary GI-NHL.[30] Other percentages mentioned were 18 (lysozyme positive),[29] 18.4 (lysozyme and/or $\alpha_1$-antitrypsin positive),[50] and 9.[51] In our experience the incidence of histiocytic sarcoma in the GI tract is not essentially different from that of the whole group of histiocytic sarcomas, (i.e. 5–10%).[52,53]

Many of these histiocytic sarcomas were associated with malabsorption states, such as celiac disease.[54,55]

After starting this controversy on incidence, Isaacson and colleagues recently published data indicating a T-cell origin for four cases previously diagnosed as malignant histiocytosis of intestine,[56] suggesting that most celiac disease-associated lymphomas are actually of T-cell origin. The reason for this sudden change was the presence of the 3A1 pan-T-cell antigen on the tumor cells and the finding of lymphoid tumors that were $\alpha_1$-antitrypsin positive,[57] while $\alpha_1$-antitrypsin was considered the most important marker criterion for histiocytic tumors by Isaacson et al.[34] This clearly illustrates that markers alone are not the solution to the problem. Apart from the presence of 3A1 antigen in all four neoplasms the tumor cells of three cases also showed rearrangements of genes for the $\beta$-chain of the T-cell antigen receptor. Questions concerning the specificity of this finding, however, can also arise. Little or nothing is known about gene rearrangements in macrophages/histiocytes and gene rearrangements are not 100% lineage-specific, as T-cell lym-

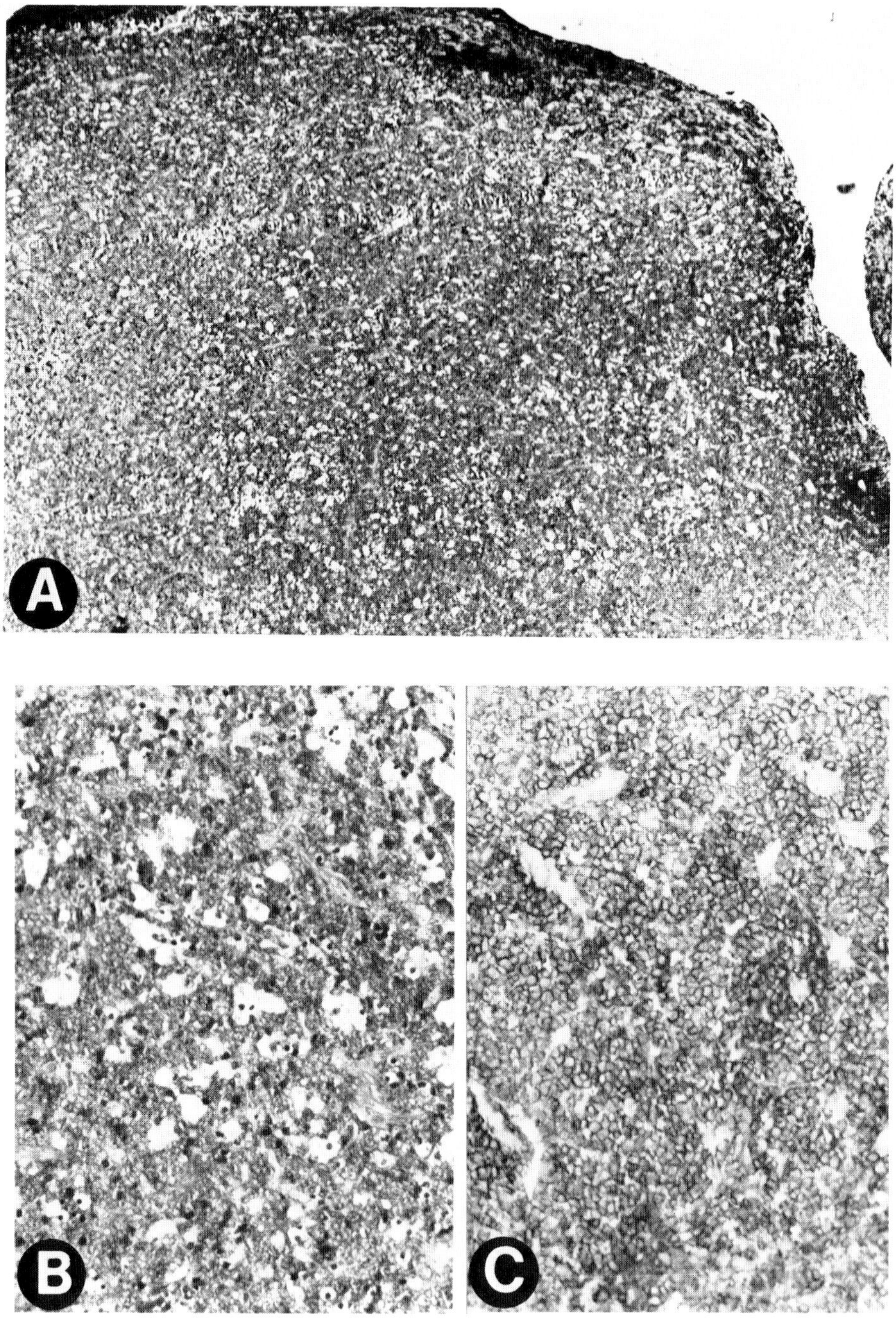

**Fig. 5-2.** Primary localization of lymphoblastic lymphoma, Burkitt type in the ileocoecal region of a 7 year old boy. (a) Low magnification; note starry sky appearance. (HE stain, paraffin embedding. ×25) (b) Higher magnification. Optical empty spaces are filled by nuclei of macrophages with often brushed, very pale staining cytoplasm. (×100). (c) Demonstration of the B cell nature by the pan B cell monoclonal antibody Leu 14. (d) High power view of the lymphoblastic cells. (HE stain ×400).

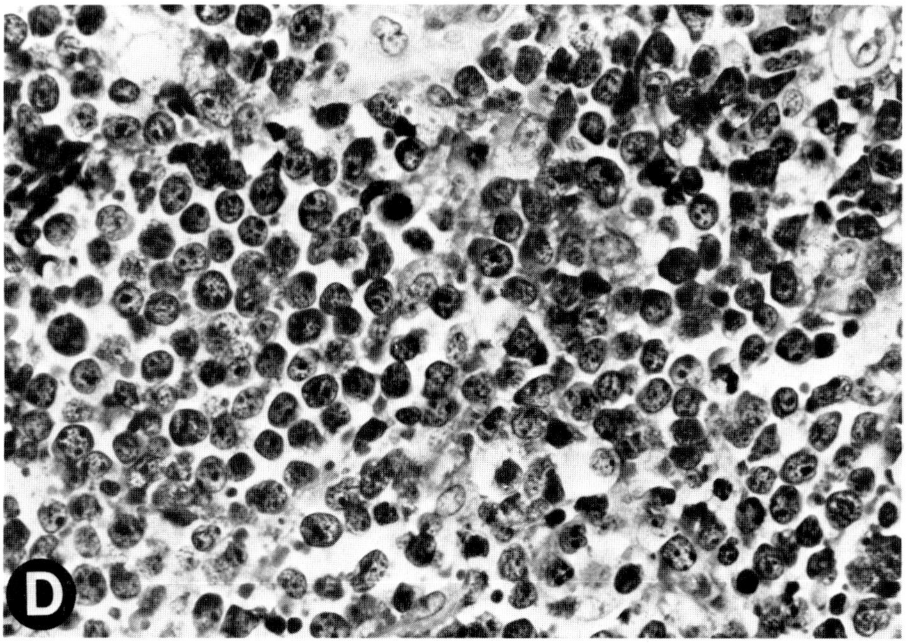

**Fig. 5-2.** *(continued)*

phomas have been described with immunoglobulin gene rearrangements.[58]

Though the findings of Isaacson et al.[56] are certainly suggestive, we feel that this matter is not yet settled and consistent, and that extensive marker studies (including, when possible, gene rearrangement studies) are of vital importance. As an illustration of the diversity in this field, we cite the report of Otto et al.,[37] who claim a B-cell nature for their celiac disease-associated lymphomas, since these NHL show monoclonal cytoplasmic immunoglobulins. It is not unlikely that all three possibilities (for celiac disease-associated NHL) can occur: B-cell, T-cell, and histiocytic origin.

The histology of histiocytic sarcoma has been amply described.[53] The cells are large, with large and mostly (very) irregular nuclei with conspicuous nucleoli and nuclear membranes (Fig. 5-3). Cytoplasm is ample and the cells show signs of phagocytosis. Multinucleated giant cells are virtually always present. Immunologically, lysozyme, $\alpha_1$-antitrypsin and/or $\alpha_1$-antichymotrypsin and nonspecific esterase and acid phosphatase can be demonstrated in the cytoplasm. Furthermore, the tumor cells react with monoclonal antibodies against monocytes/histiocytes[53] and lack T- (Leu4, Leu5, 3A1,) and B-cell (Leu14, B1) markers.

## THE IMPORTANCE OF MARKER STUDIES

From several of the above-mentioned facts, the crucial importance of marker studies emerges. Their role in diagnosis cannot be overestimated: the diagnosis of NHL can hinge on the use of markers.

There are some basic rules that have to be maintained in using markers:[60]

The material should be handled optimally.

Never rely on a single marker. Always use a small panel to avoid confusion because of cross-reactions.

Use markers as an *additional* technique to morphology.

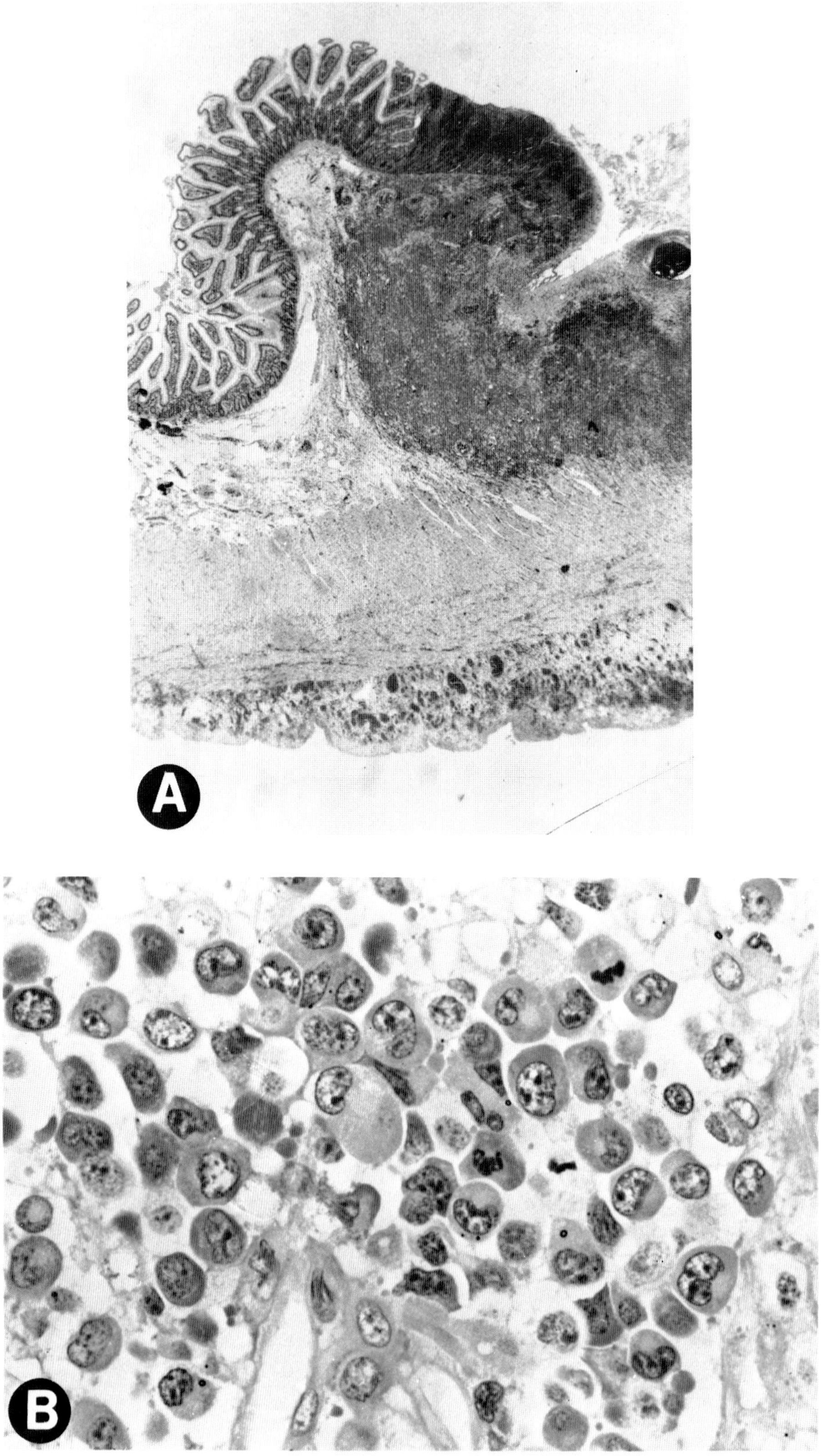

**Fig. 5-3.** True histiocytic lymphoma of the small intestine. (a) Low power view of the tumor. (HE stain ×25). (b)Higher power view of the neoplastic cells. Note the irregular nuclear contour and the ample cytoplasm. (Giemsa staining, glycol methacrylate embedding, ×400)

## Lymphoma versus Carcinoma

Cases of gastrointestinal tumors where a differential diagnosis of carcinoma and lymphoma was considered may not be frequent, but they are by no means rare. Whether this is because carcinoma cells can look like transformed lymphocytes (especially lymphoblasts and centroblasts) or lymphocytes take on (e.g.) a signet ring cell appearance (mentioned above) is irrelevant. In some cases the distinction is impossible on clinical and morphologic grounds. Here markers are a necessity and it has been shown that a small panel of monoclonal antibodies, (i.e., 115D8 directed against the MAM6 antigen, cytokeratins; vimentin; NKI-C3, a melanoma-associated antigen and leucocyte common antigen), can effectively distinguish among carcinoma, lymphoma, sarcoma, and melanoma in cases of undifferentiated tumors.[59–61]

## Lymphoma vs. Pseudolymphoma

Also mentioned above was the difficulty in distinguishing lymphomas from reactive lymphoid lesions. Though criteria have been mentioned to distinguish between benign (pseudolymphomas) and malignant lesions (NHL) in the GALT,[28,36,62] and the BALT,[63] there are an increasing number of reports stating that it is often difficult and sometimes even impossible to diagnose a lesion properly without immunological markers.[28,33,64–66] In practice distinguishing between lymphoma and pseudolymphoma is limited to follicular lesions. If monoclonality for light chain immunoglobulins is demonstrated the lesion is malignant and a lymphoma; if not the lesion is a pseudolymphoma or lymphoid hyperplasia, a term we prefer as it is more apt and less confusing than pseudolymphoma. The clinical relevance of the demonstration of monoclonality has been stressed.[67] Marker studies also are imporant for pathologists with less experience in this difficult field.

Marker studies can and should also be applied to material removed for staging procedures, as staging is very important; especially when on morphological grounds distinction between benign versus malignant processes in lymph nodes removed during staging procedures and showing multiple monotonous follicles cannot be made. Demonstration of monoclonality is crucial here.

### Immunophenotyping of Lymphoma

Additionally, there is the role of markers in diagnosing the type of lymphoma (i.e., B-cell, T-cell, histiocytic). In contrast to node-based NHL, this appears to have limited prognostic value for GI-NHL (see Prognostic Factors). There are, however, only a limited number of large series of GI-NHL classified after really extensive marker studies and the relevance of such typing has yet to emerge fully. Considering the debate generated by the question of the incidence of histiocytic tumors in the GI-tract, marker studies are here to stay.

A marker panel should consist of pan-B-cell markers (B1 and/or Leu14), and anti-light chain antisera to demonstrate monotypic surface and intracytoplasmic immunoglobulin staining and pan-T-cell markers, even if T-cell lymphomas are rare in the GI-tract (e.g., monoclonal antibodies Leu4/OKT3, Leu5/OKT11 and 3A1). Thus a lymphoid origin can be established. If these markers are negative and morphology suggests a histiocytic origin, with histiocytic markers such as lysozyme, $\alpha_1$-antitrypsin, and/or $\alpha_1$-antichymotrypsin the revealed diagnosis is histiocytic sarcoma.

## PROGNOSTIC FACTORS

Overall survival of primary (Group I) GI-NHL is reported to be 44% in two large series.[22,23] Secondary involvement of GI-tract by lymphoma (Group II) usually spells doom for the patient. The median survival is reported to be 9.1 months.[19] There are, however, several factors that influence the prognosis:

*Size of the tumor.* Several investigators report the size to be a prognostically important factor.[31] However, it is probably closely related to other factors, such as stage of disease and infiltration of adjacent structures.[33,68]

*Histology and immunophenotype of the NHL.* Surprisingly this has only limited bearing on prognosis. Follicular lymphomas tend to do better than diffuse ones.[18,68] Lymphoplasmacytoid NHL are reported to have a slightly better prognosis[23,31] perhaps because these cells, reflecting normal GALT physiology, tend to home back to the GALT and thus remain localized there. The group of NHL studied by Evans[69] shows some examples of such cases. Most studies, however, clearly state that histology is not a prognostic factor.[22,24,28]

The marker profile of the neoplastic cells is also of limited importance, but as mentioned above, more data are needed. Nevertheless, absence of immunoglobulin staining on B-cell NHL appears to correlate with an unfavorable prognosis.[28,29]

*Site.* Taken as a group, lymphomas in the stomach do better than small intestinal lymphomas, which do better than NHL from the large intestine.[18,33] This is irrespective of type of NHL. Ileocecal lymphomas are often lymphoblastic; they have a poor prognosis.

*Perforation.* This is an ominous sign,[7] reported with a varying incidence of 1–28%.[22]

*Staging.* Most studies agree that staging is the most important factor prognostically. As with perforation, infiltration of adjacent structures by NHL is a bad sign.[18] It should be looked for. The most important factor, however, is whether the NHL has spread beyond the GALT or not.[18,22,23,28,33] Whether involvement of regional lymph nodes is prognostically unfavorable is controversial, but most authors agree it is not.[22,23,28] These viewpoints have led to alternative staging schemes.[18,70,71] These schemes resemble staging according to the TNM staging scheme for carcinomas, stressing that the histology of NHL is of relatively little relevance for prognosis.

With prognosis dependent on whether or not the NHL is restricted to the confines of the GALT system (including the regional lymph nodes) staging procedures become very important. However, there is no consensus concerning the methods of staging, whether abdominal CT scan with or without lymphangiography is sufficient, or if laparotomy is always indicated. This is more or less dependent on the choice of therapy. If a patient will receive radiation therapy, a radiation field can be chosen to treat potentially involved lymph nodes, an operation can be avoided, and CT scanning will suffice.

Unfortunately no studies are available comparing treatment results in patients receiving radiation therapy and patients who have undergone extensive staging (laparotomy) with surgical treatment plus possibly chemotherapy and/or radiotherapy. Studies like that are needed to settle the question of which staging method (and which therapeutic modality) to choose. In any case special care must be taken to document spread beyond the GALT. Abdominal CT scan/laparotomy and, if indicated, investigation on laparotomy of paraaortic or more distant lymph nodes, with bone marrow aspiration and/or biopsy and, on indication, liver biopsy are important. It must be kept in mind that the lymph nodes can show numerous monotonous follicles, suggestive of NHL. In these cases demonstration of monoclonality by markers ($\kappa$ or $\lambda$ light chains) brings the definitive answer.

## THERAPY

As GI-NHL are not very frequent, experience with different therapeutic regimens is limited. As was stated before, no studies are available comparing survival of patients treated with radiotherapy alone to that of patients treated with surgery with or without additional radiotherapy. In practice most people are treated surgically with or without additional chemo- and/or radiotherapy. While awaiting the results of such a comparative study, the current data from the literature are as follows: For group I patients (GI-NHL restricted to GALT) resection of the stomach or bowel specimen with regional lymph nodes is usually effective.[18,23,24,33] Additional radiotherapy does not appear to influence survival,[18,23] though Herrmann et al.[19] do find a beneficial effect on relapse-free survival time.

"Complete" resection, (i.e., bowel and nodal disease and invaded adjacent structures), gives superior results compared to incomplete removal.[18] Investigation by frozen sections of the resection edges can give important information on radicality of the resection. Though complete resection is the obvious goal, it is best not to be tempted to perform heroic surgery such as thoraco-abdominal explorations since they have high risk at operation. Moreover, in lymphomas, absolute certainty about "completeness" of a resection is never obtained, given the fact that lymphoma cells recirculate. Thus for GALT-restricted NHL a laparotomy with removal of the affected part of the bowel and sampling of regional lymph nodes as well as non-contiguous lymph nodes, investigated if possible with marker studies, is indicated for both proper staging (prognosis) and therapy. (Of course staging will also have to include bone marrow biopsy, palpation, and investigation of peripheral lymph nodes, if necessary).[33]

For the group Ib and II patients, systemic therapy seems to be indicated. Resection may still play a part as many patients develop local complications (12 of 31 patients (39%!) reported by Herrmann et al.)[19] Otherwise, radiotherapy may be helpful, especially in patients where an operation is unattractive (older and/or debilitated patients). Maybe for some patients from group Ib, especially those with not too extensive a spread of lymphoma, radiation therapy alone will give satisfactory results, but as stated before, this awaits prospective studies.

## CONCLUSIONS

GI-NHL are mostly derived from the GALT.

Approximately 10% of all NHL are located primarily in the GI-tract. The most common type of lymphoma is the diffuse large-cell NHL, with those of FCC origin predominating. The majority of GI-NHL are of B-cell origin. Histiocytic sarcomas occur, but their incidence is uncertain. T-cell lymphomas are rare.

Immunophenotyping is important for: (a) distinguishing pseudolymphoma from NHL; and (b) distinguishing between lymphoid and nonlymphoid lesions. And, to a lesser degree, it has prognostic implications. Nearly half of the patients with GI-NHL have regional lymph node involvement at diagnosis.

Prognosis depends more on the extent of the disease than on the histology of the neoplasm. NHL restricted to the GALT (including the regional lymph nodes) have a much better prognosis than those NHL that have disseminated beyond the confines of the GALT, or those in which GI tract involvement is part of a widely disseminated "nodal" NHL.

Staging procedures are important and should include investigation for peripheral lymphadenopathy and splenomegaly, bone marrow aspiration and/or biopsy, and either abdominal CT-scan or laparotomy. This last point is not yet settled. If there are enlarged nonregional nodes, histologic and immunologic investigation is indicated.

## REFERENCES

1. Lennert K.: Follicular lymphoma. A tumor of the germinal centers. Malignant Disease of the Hematopoietic System. GANN monograph on Cancer Research, vol 15. University of Tokyo Press, Tokyo, pp. 217–231, 1973
2. Lukes R.J., Collins R.D.: A functional approach to the classification of malignant lymphoma. Recent Results Cancer Res. **46**:18–30, 1974
3. Lennert K: Malignant lymphomas, other than Hodgkin's disease. Handbuch der speziellen pathologischen Anatomie und Histologie. Band I, Teil 3B, Springer-Verlag 1978
4. Mann R.B., Jaffe E.S., Berard C.W.: Malignant lymphomas: A conceptual understanding of morphologic diversity. Am J Pathol **94**:104–191, 1979
5. Parrott D.M.V.: The gut as a lymphoid organ. Clin. Gastroenterol. 5:211–228, 1976
6. Bienenstock J., Johnston N., Perey D.Y.E.: Bronchial lymphoid tissue I. Morphologic characteristics. Lab Invest **28**:686–698, 1973
7. Morris H., Edwards J., Tiltman A., Emms M.: Endometrial lymphoid tissue: An immunohistological study. J Clin Pathol **38**:644–652, 1985

8. Anscombe A.A., Wright D.H.: Primary lymphoma of the thyroid, a tumour of mucosa-associated lymphoid tissue: Review of seventy-six cases. Histopathology **9**:81–97, 1985
9. Segatto O., Giacomini P., Santoro L., Perrino A., Natali P.G.: Lymphoid stroma of Warthin's tumour: Phenotypic analogies with gut-associated lymphoid tissue. Clin Immunol Immunopathol **34**:39–47, 1985
10. MacDermott M.R., Bienenstock J.: Evidence for a common mucosal immunologic system. I. Migration of B-immunoblasts into intestinal, respiratory, and genital tissues. J Immunol **122**:1892–1898, 1979
11. Bienenstock J., Befus A.D., McDermott M.: Mucosal immunity. From: Monographs in Allergy, vol 16: Essays on the anatomy and physiology of lymphoid tissues. Karger S.: Basel pp 1–18, 1980
12. Brown W.R.: Immunology. Chapter 7 from the Gastro-enterology Annual/2 eds., Kermÿn F., Blum A.L.: Elsevier, Amsterdam, pp. 190–213, 1984
13. Thompson R.A.: Immunological mechanisms. From: Immunology of the gastrointestinal tract. Ed: P. Asquith. Churchill Livingstone, Edinburgh, pp 14–22, 1979
14. Stevens S.K., Weissman I.L., Butcher E.C.: Differences in the migration of B and T lymphocytes: Organ-selective localization in vivo and the role of lymphocyte-endothelial cell recognition. J Immunol **128**:844–851, 1982
15. Cahill R.N.P., Poskitt D.C., Frost H., Trnka Z.: Two distinct pools of recirculating T lymphocytes: Migratory characteristics of nodal and intestinal T lymphocytes. J Exp Med **145**:420–428, 1977
16. Elson C.O., Heck J.A., Strober W.: T-cell regulation of murine IgA synthesis. J Exp Med **149**:632–643, 1979
17. Selby W.S., Janossy G., Bofill M., Jewell D.P.: Intestinal lymphocyte subpopulations in inflammatory bowel disease: an analysis by immunohistological and cell isolation techniques. Gut **25**:32–40, 1984
18. Blackledge G., Bush H., Dodge O.G., Crowthers D.: A study of gastrointestinal lymphoma. Clin Oncol **5**:209–219, 1979
19. Herrmann R., Panahon A.M., Barcos M.P., Walsh D., Stutzman L.: Gastrointestinal involvement in non-Hodgkin's lymphoma. Cancer **46**:215–222, 1980
20. Freeman C., Berg J.W., Cutler S.J.: Occurrence and prognosis of extranodal lymphomas. Cancer **29**:252–260, 1972
21. Haak H.L., Kluin Ph.M, Meijer C.J.L.M., Otter R., Steijnen Th.: Population-based registration of non-Hodgkin's lymphoma in the region covered by the Comprehensive Cancer Centre West. Neth. J. Med. **29**:105–110, 1987
22. Lewin K.J., Ranchod M., Dorfman R.F.: Lymphomas of the gastrointestinal tract. A study of 117 cases presenting with gastrointestinal disease. Cancer **42**:693–707, 1978
23. Weingrad D.N., DeCosse J.J., Sherlock P., Straus D., Lieberman P.H., Filippa D.A.: Primary gastrointestinal lymphoma: A 30-year review. Cancer **49**:1258–1265, 1982
24. Blackshaw A.J.: Non-Hodgkin's lymphomas of the gut. Recent Advances in Gastrointestinal Pathology. Wright R. (Ed). Philadelphia, Wm. Saunders 1980 pp 213–240
25. Isaacson P. Wright D.H.: Malignant lymphoma of mucosa-associated lymphoid tissue. A distinctive type of B-cell lymphoma. Cancer **52**:1410–1416, 1983
26. Isaacson P. Wright D.H.: Extranodal malignant lymphoma arising from mucosa-associated lymphoid tissue. Cancer **53**:2515–2524, 1984
27. Hernandez J.A., Sheehan W.W.: Lymphomas of the mucosa-associated lymphoid tissue. Signet ring cell lymphomas presenting in mucosal lymphoid organs. Cancer **55**:592–597, 1985
28. Saraga P., Hurlimann J., Ozzello L.: Lymphomas and pseudolymphomas of the alimentary tract. An immunohistochemical study with clinicopathologic correlations. Hum Path **12**:713–723, 1981
29. Seo I.S., Binkley W.B., Warnez T.F.C.S., Warfel K.A.: 442 A combined morphologic and immunologic approach to the diagnosis of gastrointestinal lymphomas: I Malignant lymphoma of the stomach (22 cases). Cancer **49**:493–501, 1982
30. Grody W.W., Magidson J.G., Weiss L.A., Hu E., Warnke R.A., Lewin K.J.: Gastrointestinal lymphomas. Immunohistochemical studies on the cell of origin. Am J Surg Pathol **9**:328–337, 1985
31. Filippa D.A., DeCosse J.J., Lieberman P.H., Bretsky S.S., Weingrad D.N.: Primary lymphomas of the gastrointestinal tract. Analysis of prognostic factors with emphasis on histological type. Am J Surg Pathol **7**:363–372, 1983
32. Wright D.H., Isaacson P.G.: Extranodal malignant lymphomas. From: Biopsy Pathology of the Lymphoreticular System. Chapman & Hall, London, pp 267–309, 1983
33. Appelman H.D., Schnitzer B., Hirsch S.D., Loon W.W.: Clinicopathologic overview of gastrointestinal lymphomas. Am J Surg Pathol **9**:71–83, 1985
34. Isaacson P. Wright D.H., Judd M.A., Mepham B.L.: Primary gastrointestinal lymphomas. A classification of 66 cases. Cancer **43**:1805–1819, 1979
35. Valk P. van der, Jansen J., Daha M.R., Meijer C.J.L.M.: Characterization of B-cell Non-Hodgkin's lymphomas. Virchows Arch. A 401:289–305, 1983.
36. Ranchod M., Lewin K.J., Dorfman R.F.: Lymphoid hyperplasia of the gastrointestinal tract. A study of 26 cases and review of the literature. Am J Surg Pathol **2**:383–400, 1978
37. Otto H.F., Bettman I., Weltzien J.V., Gebbers J.O.: Primary intestinal lymphoma. Virchows Arch A **391**:9–31, 1981
38. Kotner L.M., Wang C.C.: Plasmacytoma of the upper air and food passages. Cancer **30**:414–418, 1972
39. Asselah F., Crow J., Slavin G., Sheldon C., Asselah H.: Solitary plasmacytoma of the intestine. Histopathology **6**:631–645, 1982
40. Tweel J.G. van der, Taylor C.R., Parker J.W., Lukes R.J.: Immunoglobulin inclusions in non-Hodgkin's lymphomas. Am J Clin Pathol **69**:306–313, 1978
41. Rappaport H., Ramot B., Hulu N., Part J.K.: The pathology of the so-called Mediterranean abdominal lymphoma with malabsorption. Cancer **29**:1502–1511, 1972
42. Khojasteh A., Haghshenass M., Haghighi P.: Immunoproliferative small intestinal disease. A "Third-World lesion." N Eng J Med **308**:1401–1405, 1983
43. Isaacson P.: Middle-East lymphoma and $\alpha$-chain disease. An immunohistochemical study. Am J Surg. Pathol. **3**:431–441, 1979
44. Gilinsky N.H., Mee A.S., Beatty D.W., Novis B.H., Young G., Price S., Purves L.R., Marks I.L.: Plasmacell infiltration of the small bowel: Lack of evidence for a non-secretory form of alpha-heavy chain disease. Gut **26**:928–934, 1985
45. Nassar V.H., Salem P.A., Shadid M.J., Alami S.Y., Balikian J.B., Salem A.A., Nasrallah S.M.: Mediter-

ranean abdominal lymphoma" or immunoproliferative small intestinal disease. Part II. Pathological aspects. Cancer **41**:1340–1354, 1978
46. Isaacson P., Price S.K.: Light chains in Mediterranean lymphoma, J Clin Pathol **38**:601–677, 1978
47. Wright D.H.: The identification and classification of non-Hodgkin's lymphomas: A review. Diagn Histopathol **5**:73–111, 1982
48. Banks A.M., Arseneau J.C., Gralnick H.R., Canellos G.P., De Vita V.T., Berard C.W.: American Burkitt's lymphoma: A clinicopathologic study of 30 cases. II Pathologic correlations. Am J Med **58**:322–329, 1975
49. Foucar K., Foucar E., Mitros F., Clamon G., Goeken J., Crossett J.: Epitheliotropic lymphoma of the small bowel. Report of a fatal case with cytotoxic/suppressor T-cell immunotypes. Cancer **54**:54–60, 1984
50. Mir R., Kahn L.B.: Immunohistochemistry of primary gastrointestinal lymphomas: A study of 38 cases. Lab Invest **48**:59A, 1983
51. MacLennan K.A., Bennett M.H., Tu A.: The pathology of primary gastrointestinal lymphoma (report no. 10). Clin Radiol **32**:513–518, 1982
52. Valk P. van der, Meijer C.J.L.M., Willemze R., Oosterom A.T. van, Spaander P.J., Velde T. te: Histiocytic sarcoma (true histiocytic lymphoma): A clinicopathological study of 20 cases. Histopathology **8**:105–123, 1984
53. Valk P. van der, Meijer C.J.L.M: Histiocytic sarcoma. Clinical picture, morphology, markers, differential diagnosis. Pathol Annu **20**(Part 2):1–28, 1985
54. Isaacson P., Wright D.H.: Malignant histiocytosis of the intestine. Its relationship to malabsorption and ulcerative jejunitis. Hum Pathol **9**:661–677, 1978
55. Isaacson P., Wright D.H., Jones D.B.: Malignant lymphoma of true histiocytic (monocytic/macrophage) origin. Cancer **51**:80–91, 1983
56. Isaacson P.G., O'Connor N.T.J., Spencer J., Bevan D.H., Conolly C.E., Kirkham H., Pollock D.J., Wainscoat J.S., Stein H., Mason D.Y.: Malignant histiocytosis of the intestine: A T-cell lymphoma. Lancet **2**:688–691, 1985
57. Stein H., Lennert K., Feller A.C., Mason D.Y.: Immunohistological analysis of human lymphoma: Correlation of histological and immunological categories. Adv. Cancer. Res. **42**:67–73, 1984
58. Knowles II D.M., Dodson L., Burke J.S., Ming Wang J., Bonetti F., Pelicci P.G., Flug F., Favera R., Wang C.Y.: SIg -, E - ("null-cell") non-Hodgkin's lymphomas. Multiparametric determination of their B- or T-cell lineage. Am J Pathol **120**:356–370, 1985
59. Meijer C.J.L.M., Willemze R., Henzen-Logmans S.C., vàn der Valk P.: Monoclonal antibodies in the histopathological diagnosis of non-Hodgkins's lymphomas. Neth J Med **20**:138–141, 1985
60. Meijer C.J. L.M., vàn der Valk P., Poppema S.: Markers of malignant lymphomas. Diagnostic implications. In: Tumor Immunology—Mechanisms, Diagnosis, Therapy. Eds. Wolen Otter, E. J. Ruiteabey, Elseviers Science Publ Chap 12, pp, 187–226, 1987
61. Meijer C.J.L.M., Mulliak M., Hearen-Rogmans S.C.: Practical application of monoclonal antibodies to diagnostic tumor pathology and sòme future perspectives. In: Application of monoclonal antibodies in tumor pathology. Eds D. J. Raiter et. al. Martinus Nyhoff Publ Chap 17, pp 299–318, 1987
62. Faris T.D., Saltzstein S.L.: Gastric lymphoid hyperplasia: A lesion confused with lymphosarcoma. Cancer **17**:207–212, 1964
63. Saltzstein S.L.: Pulmonary malignant lymphomas and pseudolymphomas. Classification, therapy, and prognosis. Cancer **16**:928–955, 1963
64. Greenberg S.D., Heisler J.G., Gyorkey F., Jenkins D.E.: Pulmonary lymphoma versus pseudolymphoma: A perplexing problem. South Med J **65**:775–784, 1972
65. Julsrudd P.R., Brown L.R., Li G-Y., Rosenow III E.C., Crowe J.K.: Pulmonary processes of mature-appearing lymphocytes: Pseudolymphoma, well differentiated lymphocytic lymphoma, and lymphocytic interstial pneumonitis. Radiology **127**:289–296, 1978
66. Lerman-Sagie T., Zio Y., Rubin M., More C., Dintsman M.: Gastric lymphoma versus pseudolymphoma: The importance of immunological differentiation. Am J Gastroenterol **80**:763–707, 1978
67. Vimadalal S.D., Said J.W., Voyles III H.: Gastric lymphoreticular neoplasms: An immunologic study of 36 cases. Am J Clin Pathol **80**:792–799, 1983
68. Brooks J.J., Enterline H.T.: Primary gastric lymphomas: A clinicopathologic study of 58 cases with long-term follow-up and literature review. Cancer **51**:701–711, 1983
69. Evans H.L.: Extranodal small lymphocytic proliferation: A clinicopathologic and immunocytochemical study. Cancer **49**:84–96, 1982
70. Lim F.E., Hartman A.S., Tan E.G.C., Cody B., Meissner W.A.: Factors in the prognosis of gastric lymphomas. Cancer **39**:1715–1720, 1977
71. Musshoff K.: Klinische Stadieneinteilung der Nicht-HodgkinLymphome. Strahlentherapie **153**:218–221, 1977

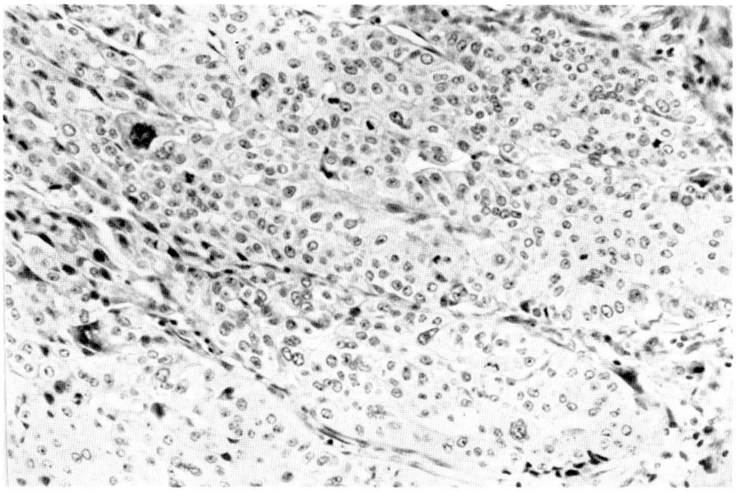

**Fig. 6-4.** *Well differentiated type* of medullary ECC of the stomach. Tumor cells have numerous mitoses and pleomorphism. H&E, ×300.

carcinoids. Expression of S-100 protein, however, is less common than that of NSE, and its incidence is about 25% of all GI carcinoids. $Alpha_1$-antitrypsin (AAT)-immunoreactivity is also noted, its incidence being 15% of all GI carcinoids.

Biological Behavior

All GI carcinoids are regarded as malignant tumors on pathologic and biologic grounds, but their malignancy is generally of a low grade. More than 70% of gastric carcinoids, however, show metastases to local lymph nodes and liver. Figure 6-3 shows a comparison of the 7-year cumulative survival rates between gastric carcinoid and colon-rectum carcinoid. For gastric carcinoid, the 7-year cumulative survival rate is about 50%, while that for colon-rectum carcinoid is about 80%. The prognosis for gastric carcinoid thus is worse than that for colon-rectum carcinoid.

## Endocrine Cell Carcinoma

Carcinoma fulfilling the following two criteria should be diagnosed as endocrine cell carcinoma (ECC): (1) The vast majority of tumor cells are endocrine cells with atypia, pleomorphism, and many mitoses, and (2) these endocrine cells are present with diffuse distribution throughout the tumor tissue. ECC can be divided into medullary type and scirrhous type according to the amount of stromal connective tissue. Moreover, according to the cellular and structural atypicality of tumor cells, medullary ECC is subdivided into well differentiated, poorly differentiated, and undifferentiated types. Most of the ECC cells show a positive reaction to Grimelius' stain.

Subclassification of ECC

1. Medullary ECC
   a. Well Differentiated Type
      Medullary ECC of well differentiated type frequently occurs in the stomach, being especially more common in the fundus than in the antrum. Macroscopically, gastric tumors usually show polypoid carcinomatous growth corresponding to Borrmann's type 1. By light microscopy these tumors have solid islands or trabecular patterns, resembling carcinoid but remarkable mitoses and pleomorphism are often seen (Fig. 6-4).

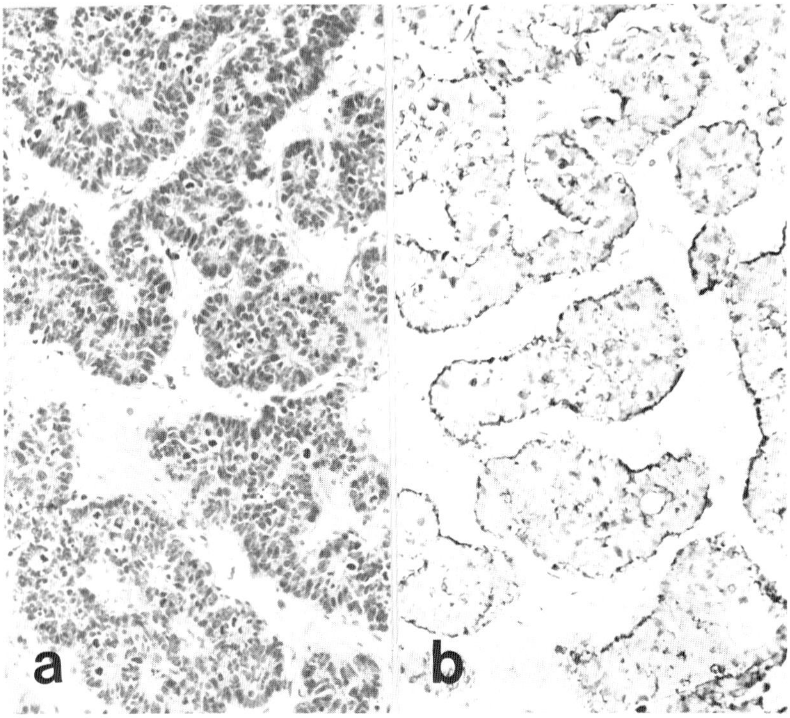


**Fig. 6-5 a and b.** *Poorly differentiated type* of medullary ECC of the stomach. (a) Tumor cells with remarkable mitoses form tubular structures, resembling adenocarcinoma. H&E, ×300. (b) Tumor cells are diffusely positive with argyrophil reaction. Grimelius stain, ×300.

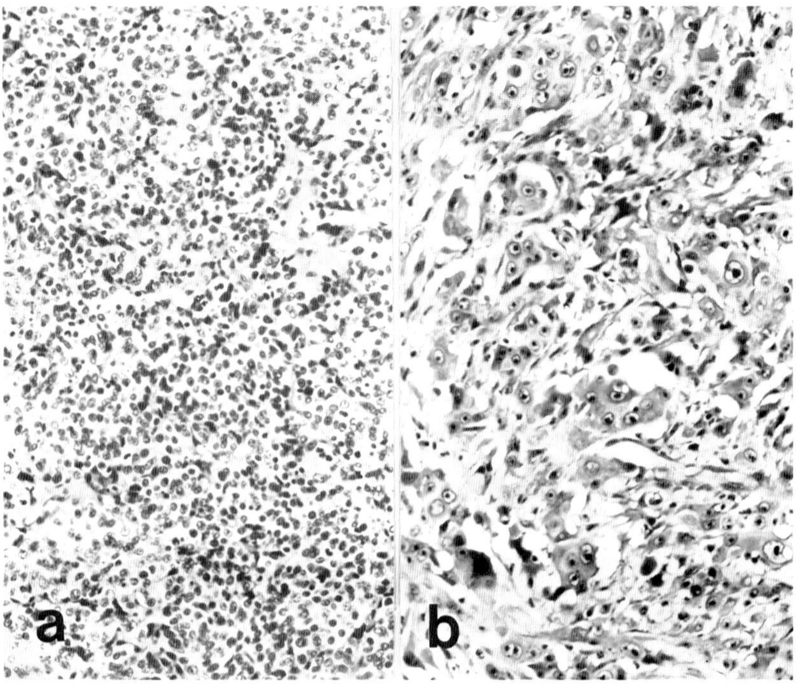

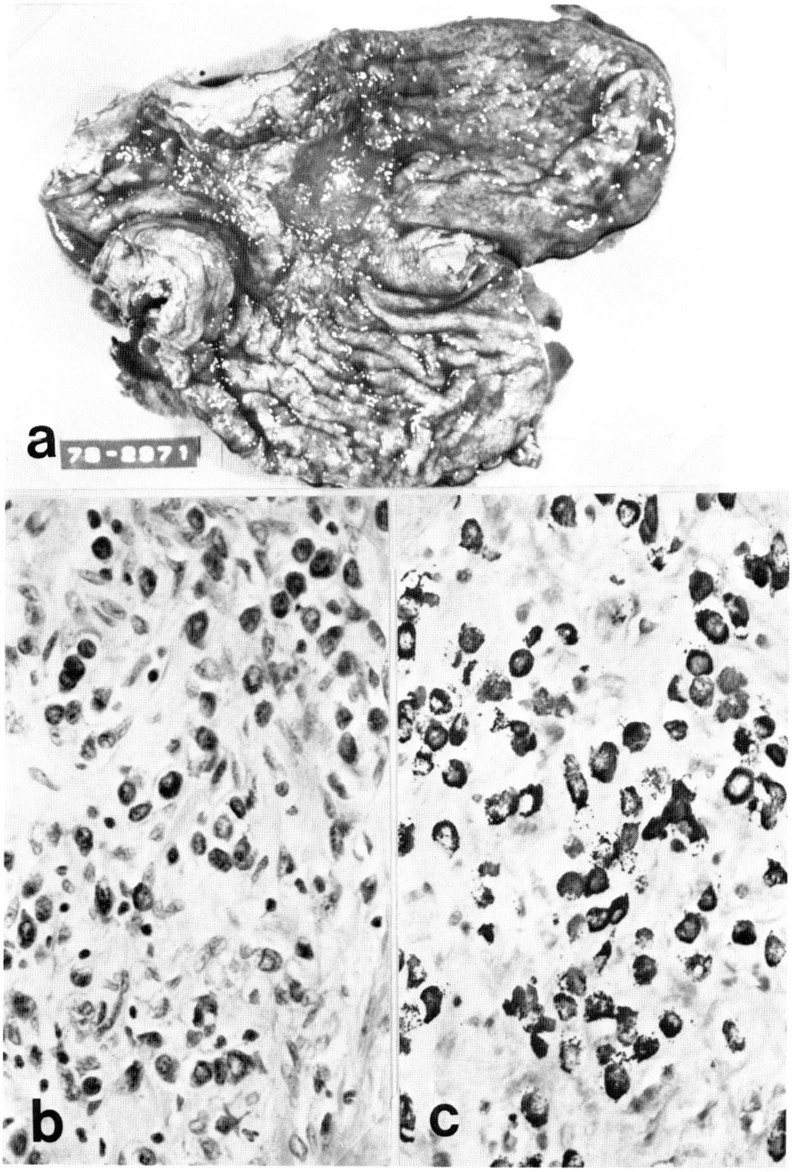


**Fig. 6-7 a, b and c.** *Scirrhous ECC* of the stomach from a 44-year-old woman, showing diffusely infiltrative carcinoma or Borrmann's type 4 carcinoma (a). (b) The tumor has abundant fibrosis. H&E, ×500. (c) Tumor cells with fine eosinophilic granules are diffusely positive with Grimelius stain. ×500.

←

**Fig. 6-6 a and b.** *Undifferentiated type* of medullary ECC of the esophagus (a) and the colon (b). (a) Tumor cells are of small cell type. (b) Tumor cells are of giant cell type with prominent nucleoli. H&E, ×300.

b. Poorly Differentiated Type

This type of medullary ECC frequently occurs in the colon and rectum. The tumor usually cannot be distinguished from ordinary carcinoma macroscopically. By light microscopy the tumor cells form glandular or tubular structures, resembling ordinary adenocarcinoma (Fig. 6-5a,b). Carcinoid pattern may be occasionally seen in a part of the tumor.

c. Undifferentiated Type

This type of tumor frequently develops in the esophagus and stomach and shows the same macroscopic appearance as in ordinary solid carcinoma. The tumor cells vary in size, including such varieties as small cell or oat cell type, intermediate cell type, and large cell type (Fig. 6-6a,b). The tumor may show very rapid growth and remarkable vascular invasion.

2. Scirrhous ECC

Scirrhous ECC usually occurs in the stomach, especially in the fundus, and often grossly manifests as a diffusely infiltrative carcinoma or Borrmann's type 4 carcinoma (Fig. 6-7a). It may be rarely seen in the rectum. Microscopically, the tumor resembles poorly differentiated adenocarcinoma with abundant fibrosis (Fig. 6-7b,c). Many tumor cells have fine or strongly stained eosinophilic granules in the cytoplasm. Signet ring cells may be rarely noted.

## Function

ECC as well as carcinoid produce serotonin, and its incidence is about 75% of scirrhous ECC. Moreover, the number of serotonin-immunoreactive cells is greater in ECC than in carcinoid (Fig. 6-8a,b,c,d,e). Vanillylmandelic acid, 5-hydroxy-3-indoleacetic acid and catecholamine also are biochemically detected within the tumor.[8] It is yet unknown, however, whether ECC produces histamine.

On one hand, ECC shows a broad array of peptide-immunoreactivity, such as gastrin, CCK, somatostatin, glucagon, glicentin, PP, ACTH, calcitonin, β-endorphin, and GRP. Synchronous production of these peptides is not a rare phenomenon and is frequently associated with serotonin. Particularly, in young patients under the age of 30 scirrhous ECC of the stomach has a tendency to produce multiple peptides synchronously (Fig.6-9a,b,c,d). The number or distribution density of peptide-immunoreactive cells is greater in ECC than in carcinoid (Fig. 6-10a,b). Ultrastructurally, various endocrine granules are usually seen in the tumor cells (Fig. 6-11a,b,c).[4]

Medullary ECC of the esophagus may on occasion produce ACTH and calcitonin.[10] Gastrin, PP, calcitonin, and glicentin-immunoreactive cells are detected in from 25% to 50% of gastric scirrhous ECC.[4,26] ECC of the colon may have a fair number of gastrin-immunoreactive cells.[27] Compared with carcinoid, ECC appears capable of producing a broader spectrum of peptide hormones. The incidence of peptide-immunoreactivity in ECC examined by the author is summarized in Table 6-2.

Endocrine disturbance due to hyperproduction of peptide hormones in ECC as well as in carcinoid is not usually seen. Hypergastrinemia may on occasion occur in gastric scirrhous ECC.[4]

A variable number of glycoproteins and enzymes is also detected in ECC and the inci-

**Fig. 6-8 a, b, c, d and e.** *Scirrhous ECC* of the stomach from a 31-year-old man. (a) Ulcerative lesion (arrow) in the intermediate zone (b, cut section of the ulcer). Diffuse fibrosis is seen around the deep ulcer. (c) The tumor shows productive fibrosis. H&E, ×150. (d) Many tumor cells have positive immunoreactivity for serotonin. ABC stain, ×150. (e) They are also positive with argentaffin reaction. Masson-Fontana stain, ×150.

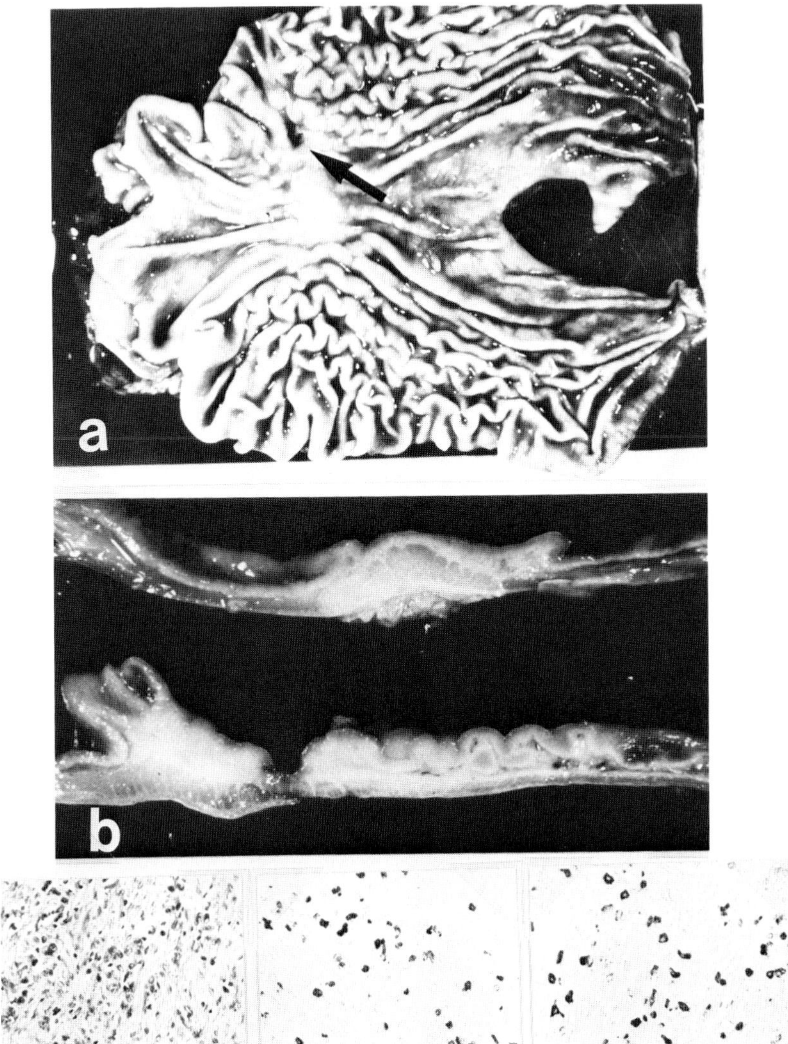
a
b
c
d
e

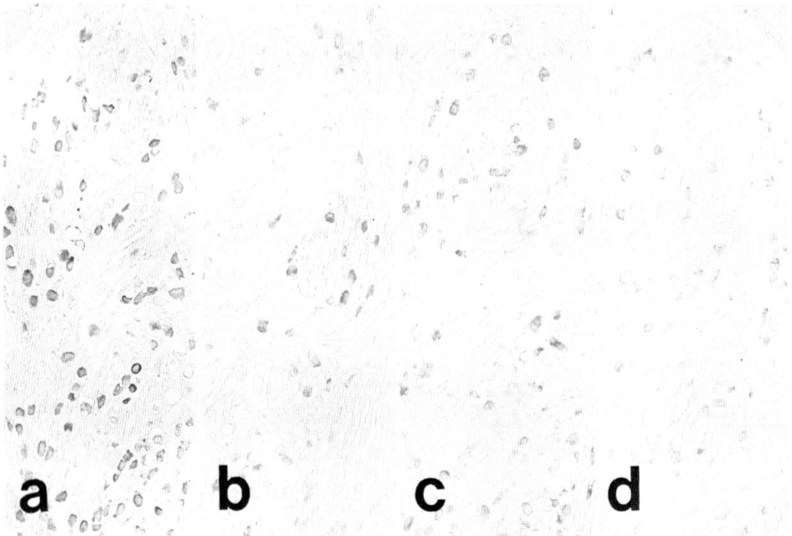


**Fig. 6-9 a, b, c and d.** *Scirrhous* ECC of the stomach from a 29-year-old man, with synchronous production of six polypeptides, CEA, SC and lysozyme. Tumor cells showed gastrin- (a), glicentin- (b), glucagon (c), calcitonin- (d), somatostatin- and pancreatic polypeptide-immunoreactivity synchronously. PAP stain, ×160.

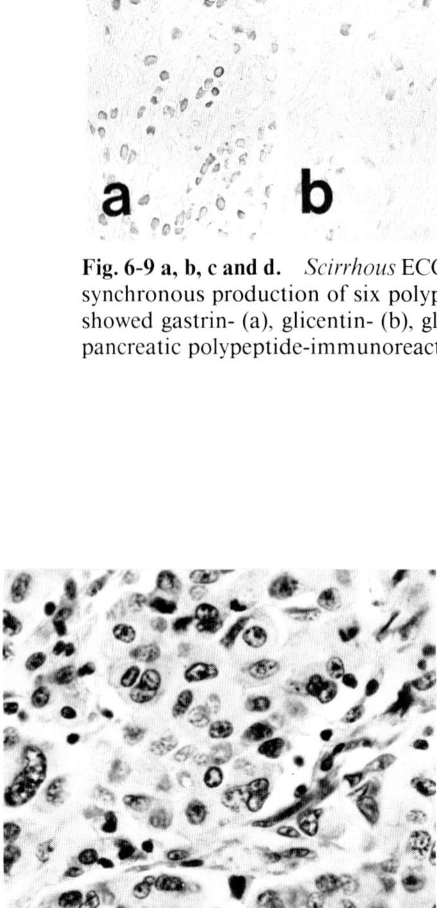


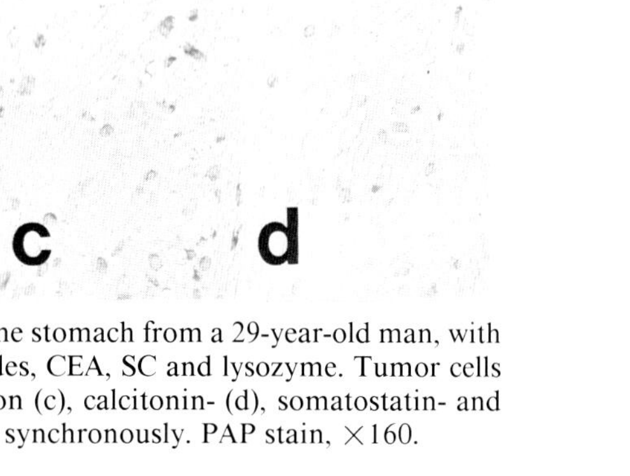

**Fig. 6-10 a and b.** *Medullary* ECC (*undifferentiated type*) of the stomach. (a) Tumor cells are of large cell type. H&E stain, ×600. (b, color) Most of the tumor cells show strong immunoreactivity for glicentin. PAP stain, ×500.

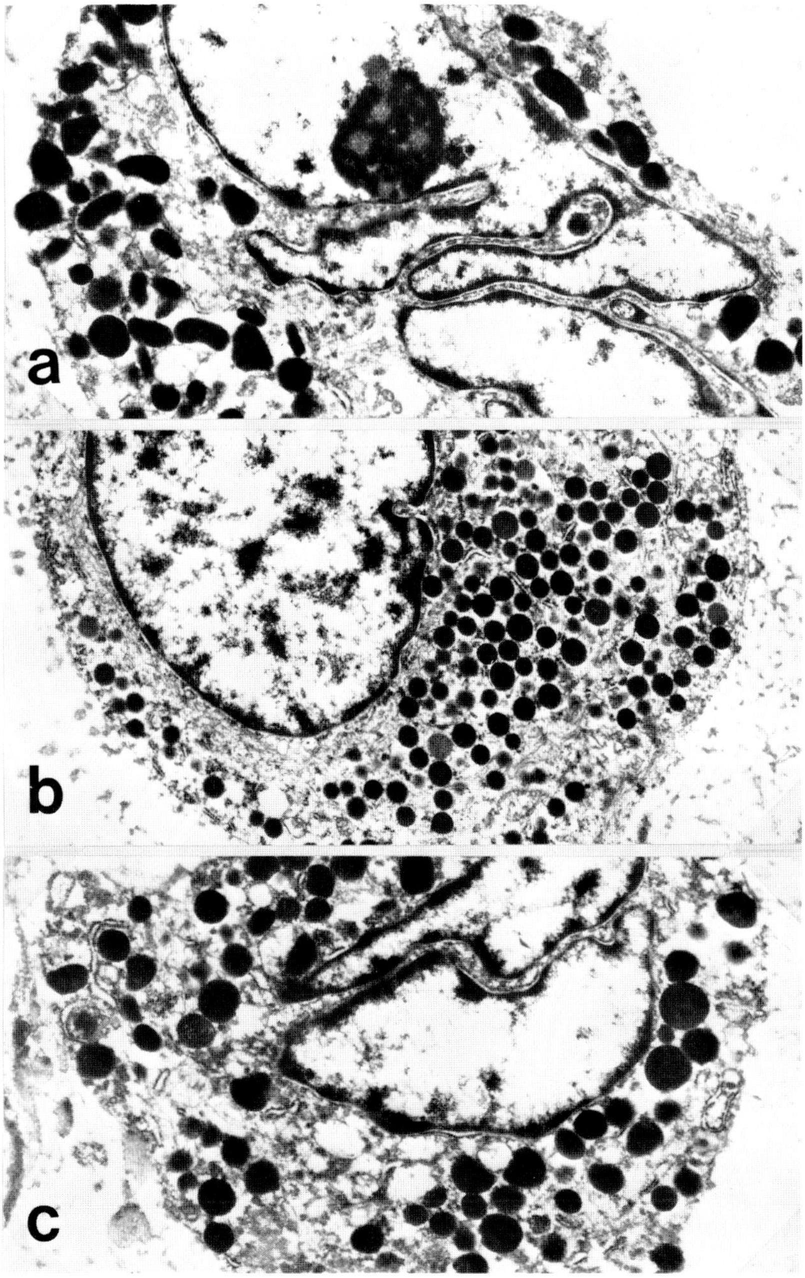

**Fig. 6-11 a, b and c.** Ultrastructure of the same tumor as in Fig. 7. Tumor cells have three types of secretory granules. (a) Pleomorphic and highly osmophilic granules (400-480 nm). ×11,000. (b) Round and electron dense granules (240-320 nm). ×11,000. (c) Round and large granules (440-480 nm). ×11,000.

**TABLE 6-2**
Peptide-Immunoreactivity in ECC of the Gastrointestinal Tract

| Localization | Subclassification | Number of Cases | Peptide-immunoreactivity[a] G | S | Glu | Gli | PP | Ca | ACTH | Serotonin-immunoreactivity |
|---|---|---|---|---|---|---|---|---|---|---|
| Esophagus | Medullary | 2 | 0 | 0 | 0 | 0 | 0 | 0 | 0 | 0 |
| Stomach | Medullary | 16 | 1 | 1 | 0 | 3 | 0 | 0 | 0 | 6 |
| | Scirrhous | 14 | 4 | 5 | 2 | 5 | 2 | 4 | 0 | 9 |
| Colon | Medullary | 4 | 1 | 0 | 0 | 0 | 2 | 1 | 0 | 1 |

[a] G, gastrin; S, somatostatin; Glu, glucagon; Gli, glicentin; PP, pancreatic polypeptide; Ca, calcitonin; ACTH, adrenocorticotropic hormone.

dence of these markers is greater than in carcinoid. CEA-related antigen and SC are seen in the majority of ECC (Fig. 6-12a,b). hCG is found in from 6% to 43% of gastric and colonic ECC. S-100 protein and NSE expression does not differ between ECC and carcinoid (Fig. 6-13a,b). Over 60% of gastric ECC have lysozyme-immunoreactivity (Fig. 6-14a). AAT expression in ECC is greater than that in carcinoid and over 50% of gastric medullary ECC are characterized by AAT expression (Fig. 6-14b). Table 6-3 shows the incidence of glycoprotein and enzyme-immunoreactivity in ECC.

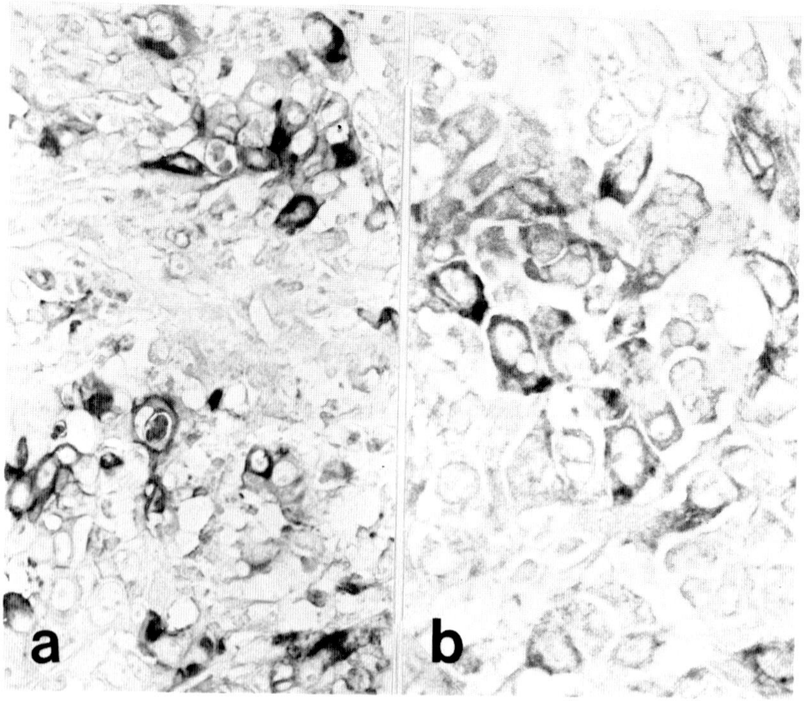


**Fig. 6-12 a and b.** (a) The same tumor as in Fig. 6b. Tumor cells are partially positive with CEA. PAP stain, ×600. (b) The same tumor as in Fig. 10. Tumor cells show SC-immunoreactivity. ABC stain, ×600.

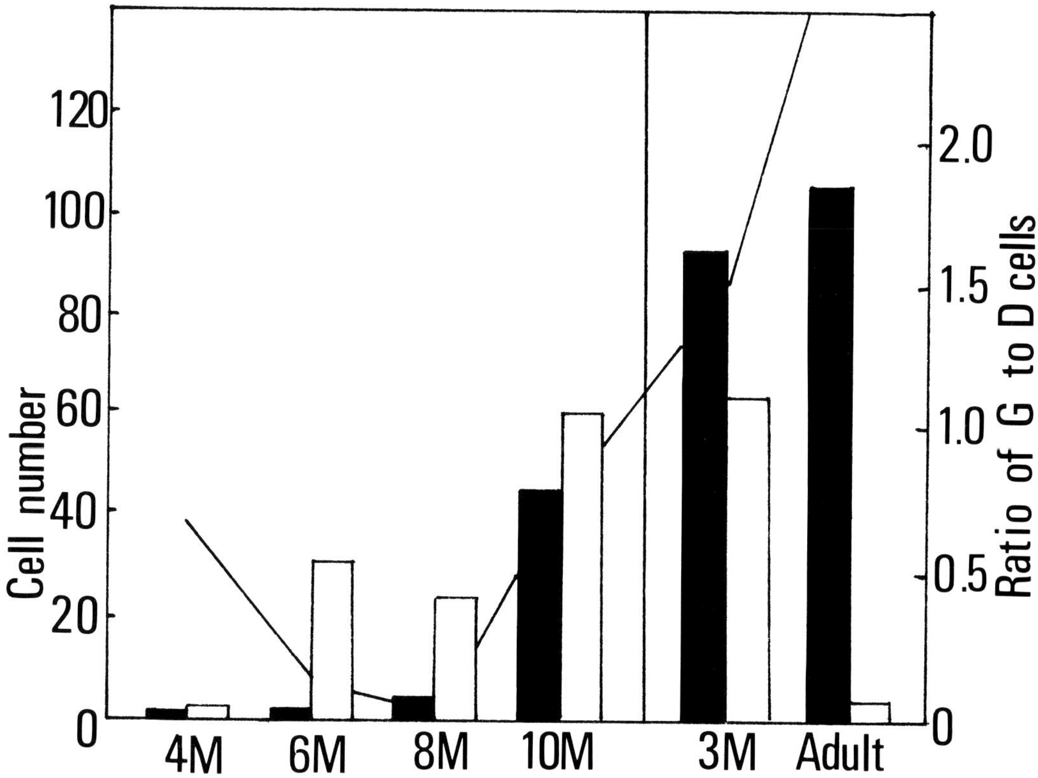


**Fig. 6-17.** The number of G cells and D cells in human fetal and newborn antral mucosa. Open column: The number of D cells among 1000 cells. Closed column: The number of G cells among 1000 cells. Diagonal line: The ratio of the number of G cells to D cells.

mean age 27.1 years, female 10 cases, male 18 cases) and older patients (over 70 years old, mean age 75.8, female 11 cases, male 13 cases), the frequency of somatostatin is significantly higher in aged patients than in young patients, whereas that of gastrin, glicentin and calcitonin is evidently higher in young patients (Table 6-6).

ECC was observed in five (17.9%) of the young patients, but only in one (4.2%) of the aged patients. Moreover, the simultaneous production of over two peptides is seen in six

**TABLE 6-6**
Comparison of the Incidence of Endocrine Cells in Poorly Differentiated Gastric Adenocarcinoma Between Young Patients and Older Patients

| Age | Number of Cases | Peptide-immunoreactivity | | | | Argyrophil Cells | ECC |
|---|---|---|---|---|---|---|---|
| | | Gastrin | Somat[a] | Glicentin | Calcitonin | | |
| Young Patients (under 30 years old) | 28 | 4(14.3)[b] | 5(17.9)[c] | 6(21.4) | 5(17.9) | 18(64.3)[c] | 5(17.9) |
| Older Patients (over 70 years old) | 24 | 1(4.2) | 9(37.5)[c] | 2(8.3) | 1(4.2) | 7(29.2)[c] | 1(4.2) |

[a] Somat: somatostatin.

[b] Values in parentheses represent incidence of cases with peptide-immunoreactivity, argyrophil cells and ECC (percentages).

[c] Significantly different ($P<0.05$).

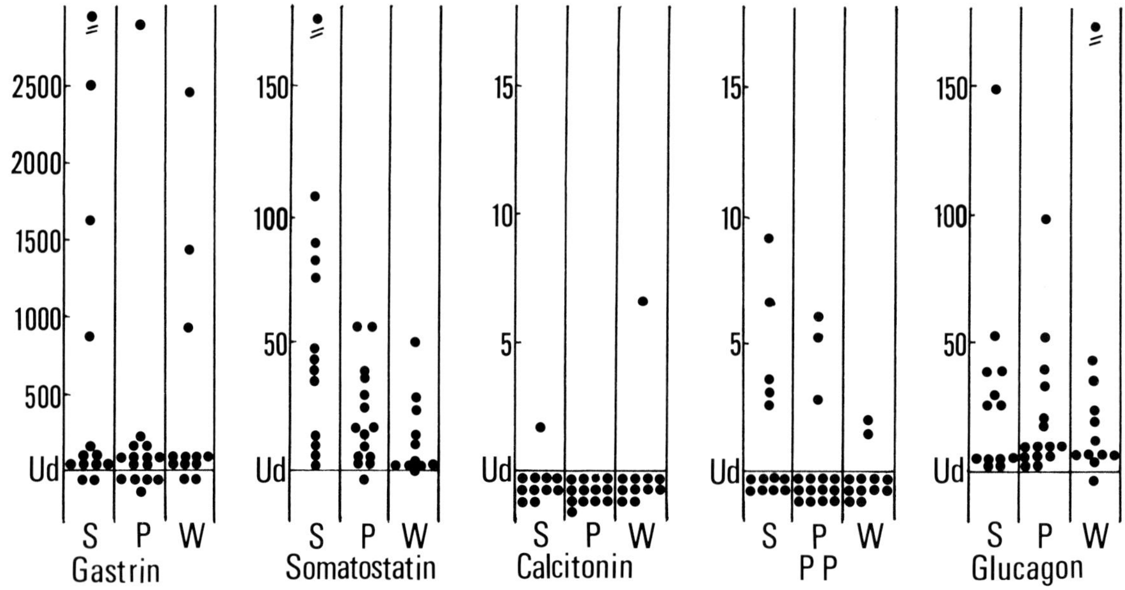


**Fig. 6-18.** Content of peptide hormones in gastric adenocarcinoma by radioimmunoassay.
Values are represented by ng/g wet weight. Ud: Undetectable. S: Scirrhous type. P: Poorly differentiated type. W: Well differentiated type.

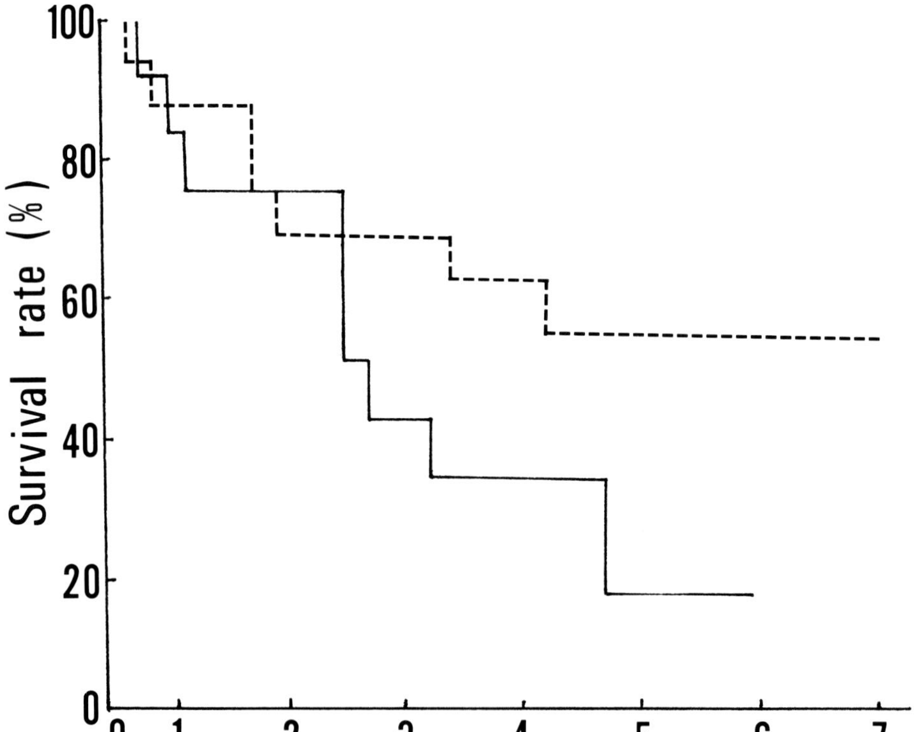


**Fig. 6-19.** Comparison of 7-year survival rates of Stages II and III gastric adenocarcinoma (poorly differentiated type) between patients with peptides and without peptides.
Continuous lines: 13 cases with peptide-producing cells (mean age, 69.1 yr). Dotted line: 17 cases without peptide-producing cells (mean age, 64.5 yr).

**TABLE 6-7**
Endocrine Cells in Adenocarcinoma of the Colon and Rectum

| Localization | Number of Cases | Peptide-immunoreactivity[a] G | S | Glicentin | PP | Ca | Serotonin-immunoreactivity | Argyrophil Cells |
|---|---|---|---|---|---|---|---|---|
| Right Colon | 8 | 0 | 0 | 1(12.5%) | 0 | 0 | 1(12.5%) | 2(25.0%) |
| Trans. Colon[b] | 15 | 0 | 0 | 2(13.3%) | 0 | 0 | 0 | 5(33.3%) |
| Sigmoid Colon | 27 | 0 | 0 | 0 | 0 | 0 | 1(3.7%) | 5(18.5%) |
| Rectum | 28 | 0 | 0 | 2(7.1%) | 0 | 0 | 2(7.1%) | 21(75.0%) |
| Total | 78 | | | 5(6.4%) | | | 4(5.1%) | 33(42.3%) |

[a] G: gastrin; S: somatostatin; PP: pancreatic polypeptide; Ca: calcitonin.
[b] Trans. colon: transverse colon.

(21.4%) of the young patients, but in only two (8.3%) of the older patients (Table 6-5). These findings suggest the possibility that rapid growth of gastric carcinoma in young patients is in part correlated with peptide expression within the tumor. By radioimmunoassay, various hormones such as gastrin, somatostatin, calcitonin, PP, and glucagon are detected. Gastrin and somatostatin content is higher in scirrhous carcinoma than in other histological types (Fig. 6-18).

When the 7-year survival rates of stages II and III advanced carcinomas (excluding scirrhous carcinomas) are compared for patients with peptide-positive and those negative for peptide hormones, the survival rate is 20% for the former, while that for latter is 50% (Fig. 6-19). Patients with peptide hormones evidently have a significantly poorer prognosis than those without peptide hormones ($P < 0.05$).

## Adenocarcinoma of the Colon and Rectum

Colorectal adenocarcinomas as well as gastric adenocarcinomas have a variable number of endocrine cells.[31,32] The incidence of argyrophil cells is about 40% among all colorectal cancer.

Endocrine cell incidence is higher in rectal carcinoma than in colonic carcinoma and is also higher in well differentiated adenocarcinoma than in poorly differentiated adenocarcinoma.

Immunohistochemically, glicentin- and serotonin-positive tumor cells are found in 6.4% and 5.1%, respectively (Table 6-7). There is a case report of an ACTH-producing colon cancer.

No evident correlation exists between peptide expression within the tumor and prognosis of the patients.

## Adenoma of the Stomach

Gastric tubular adenoma also has a marked heterogeneity, comprising SC producing epithelial cells, lysozyme-containing cells, CEA-producing cells, and endocrine cells. The incidence and distribution density of endocrine cells in gastric tubular adenoma are higher than those in gastric adenocarcinoma.

Serotonin-positive EC cells, often showing hyperplasia, occur most frequently (73.5%) throughout the tubular adenoma, followed by glicentin-(67.3%), somatostatin-(30.6%), motilin-(14.3%) and gastrin-(12.2%) positive tumor cells (Table 6-8). Glucagon-positive tumor cells are not seen in the gastric tubular adenoma. Most of these endocrine cells are located in deeper adenomatous glands. The number of endocrine cells markedly decreases with increase in the degree of atypicality of tubular adenomas, and there are no endocrine cells in the foci of carcinoma within some tu-

**TABLE 6-8**
Relationship between Histological Grade and Distribution Density of Endocrine Cells in Tubular Adenomas

| Histological Grade | Number of Cases | Cases with Endocrine Cell (%) Distribution Density of Endocrine Cells | | | | |
|---|---|---|---|---|---|---|
| | | EC-cell[a] | L-cell | D-cell | Mo-cell | G-cell |
| Mild Atypia | 18 | 15(83.3%)<br>222.6 ± 88.1[b,c] | 15(83.3%)<br>97.3 ± 28.8 | 7(38.9%)<br>16.6 ± 13.9 | 5(27.8%)<br>7.4 ± 4.3 | 6(33.3%)<br>0.5 ± 0.2 |
| Moderate Atypia | 24 | 19(79.2%)<br>101.7 ± 40.6 | 15(62.5%)<br>78.3 ± 33.7 | 6(24.0%)<br>7.3 ± 6.3 | 2(8.3%)<br>0.1 ± 0.01 | 0 |
| Severe Atypia | 7 | 2(28.6%)<br>2.7 ± 2.3 | 2(28.6%)<br>12.0 ± 6.7 | 2(28.6%)<br>2.3 ± 1.7 | 0 | 0 |
| Total | 49 | 36(73.5%) | 33(67.3%) | 15(30.6%) | 7(14.3%) | 6(12.2%) |

[a] EC-cell: serotonin-containing cell; L-cell: glicentin-containing cell; D-cell: somatostatin-containing cell; Mo-cell: motilin-containing cell; G-cell: gastrin-containing cell.

[b] Distribution density of each endocrine cell was obtained as follows: Total number of endocrine cells in tubular adenoma × 5 mm/diameter of adenoma (mm).

[c] Results are expressed as mean ± S.E.

bular adenomas. Similar changes are seen in lysozyme- and SC-positive cells as well.

Glicentin-containing L cells, which are not present in normal gastric mucosa, but preferentially appear in intestinal metaplasia, first occur in the gastric mucosa of the transitional area between metaplastic and intact gastric glands. They frequently show hyperplasia or micronoduli in the budding area of the deeper metaplastic glands (Fig. 6-20a,b,c),[26] but in completely intestinalized mucosa these endocrine cells decrease remarkably. In view of the localization of glicentin-positive cells in tubular adenoma and the physiological function of glicentin, which has a trophic action on intestinal epithelia and inhibits gastric acid secretion, the selective increase of glicentin-containing L cells in intestinal metaplasia may be correlated with the development of gastric tubular adenoma.

## Adenoma of the Colon and Rectum

Colorectal adenoma also has a good number of endocrine cells, of which glicentin- and serotonin-positive cells are dominant, as in gastric adenoma. PYY producing cells are present in the colorectal mucosa and PYY and PP-immunoreactivity is also detected within L cells. There is a possibility that colorectal adenoma has PYY- or PP-positive cells. The occurrence of endocrine cells has the tendency to increase in adenomas of the lower large intestine rather than in those of the upper large intestine. Malignant changes in colorectal adenoma induce a decrease in the number of endocrine cells within the tumor.

## Hyperplasia of Endocrine Cells

Hyperplasia of G cells is seen in the antrum of patients with Zollinger-Ellison syndrome type I or duodenal ulcer showing hypergastrinemia.

Micronoduli, which are composed of 4 to 5 endocrine cells, frequently occur not only in chronic atrophic gastritis, but also in the gastric mucosa adjacent to gastric ulcer, carcinoma, and adenoma. Endocrine cell types of micronoduli include G cells, EC cells, and L cells. Hyperplasia of D cells is not seen and D

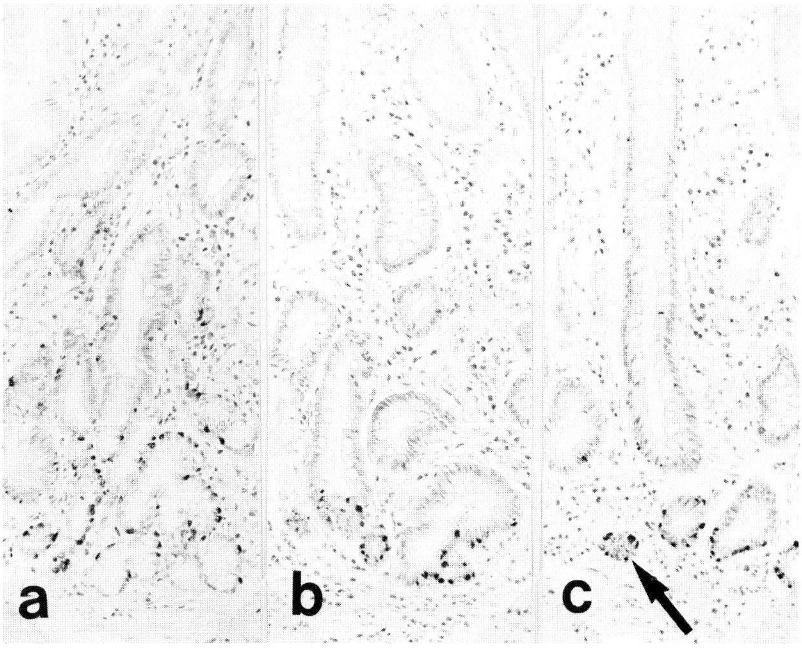


**Fig. 6-20 a, b and c.** (a) and (b) significant numbers of glicentin-immunoreactive cells are found in the deeper portion of intestinal metaplasia, showing budding, PAP stain, ×160. (c) Micronodule composed of glicentin-positive cells (arrow). PAP stain, ×160.

cells rapidly decrease with extension of intestinal metaplasia. In pernicious anemia and severe atrophic gastritis associated with hypergastrinemia, multifocal hyperplasia of ECL cells frequently occurs and may on occasion develop into carcinoid.[15,33] Micronoduli of endocrine cells are derived not from "neuroendocrine cells"[34] or "stromal endocrine cells"[35] in the lamina propria mucosae, but from endocrine cells of gastric glands.

In the colorectal mucosa, micronoduli of endocrine cells are rare, compared with those in gastric mucosa. In familial polyposis, multiple micronoduli of endocrine cells and microcarcinoid may on occasion occur.

## HISTOGENESIS OF ENDOCRINE TUMORS

The relationship between endocrine cells in the GI tract and endocrine or other tumors can be analyzed as follows: (1) classical carcinoids of endocrine cell origin, (2) ECC, and (3) endocrine cell clones scattered in the tumor (Fig. 6-21).[36,37] As for its origin ECC has several possibilities, such as epithelial stem cells, endocrine cells, carcinoid, and endocrine cell clones within adenocarcinoma. In view of the morphological and functional heterogeneity of ECC, totipotent stem cells and endocrine cell clones in adenocarcinoma may be the most closely related to the development of ECC. Endocrine cell clones in the tumor may not originate from endocrine cells, but may be based on differentiation of some tumor cells into endocrine cells. There is an interesting theory of "cell hybridization," which postulates that hybridization of tumor cells with endocrine cells will progress into a tumor with mixed cell populations.[5]

Production processes of peptide hormones by tumor cells essentially seem to be the same as those of normal endocrine cells but larger molecule types of hormones or fragments are detected more frequently in the tumors than

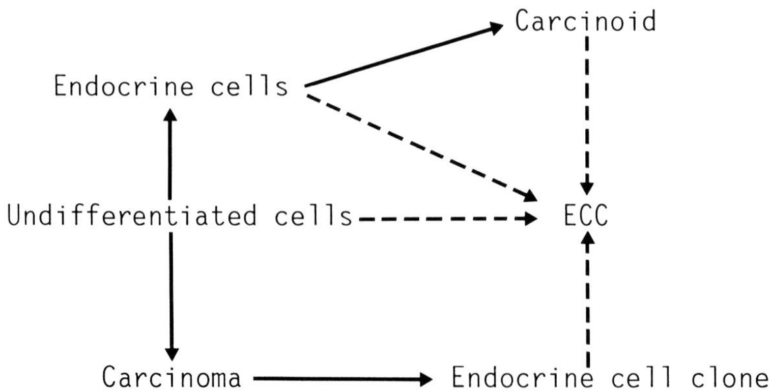


**Fig. 6-21.** Relation between GI endocrine cells and tumors.

in normal endocrine tissue.[38] This may be accounted for by the abnormal processing of prohormone after translation, involving a deficiency of processing enzymes or enhancement of processing within tumor cells. The differences in regulatory gene expression between peptide hormone-producing tumors and normal endocrine tissues should be elucidated in the future.

## PEPTIDE HORMONES, GROWTH FACTORS AND ONCOGENE PRODUCTS

Gut hormones as well as growth factors regulate the growth and differentiation of GI epithelial cells through endocrine and paracrine mechanisms. Gastrin, CCK, glicentin, and glucagon have growth-trophic actions on target cells specifically and they can be regarded as "growth factors." These peptides also stimulate the growth of tumor cells of GI carcinomas both in vitro and in vivo.[39-42] The growth of human gastric carcinoma cell line TMK-1, which shows parietal cell differentiation (Fig. 6-22), is promoted by gastrin in a dose-dependent manner (Fig. 6-23).[42] These data suggest that some of the GI carcinomas have peptide hormone receptors and that their growth is stimulated by peptides derived from tumor cells themselves through endocrine, paracrine or autocrine secretion in vivo.

Many biological events caused by peptide hormones are linked to cAMP metabolism. cAMP production and cAMP-dependent protein kinase are responsible for the growth-promoting effect of gastrin on TMK-1 and xenotransplantable human gastric carcinoma SC-6-JCK.[40,42] cAMP-dependent protein kinase is classified into type I and type II isoenzymes according to differences in the molecular form of the regulatory subunits. Type I isoenzyme is involved in cell growth and transformation, while type II isoenzyme is involved in differentiation and inhibition of cell growth. The proportion of type I isoenzyme is significantly elevated in human gastric carcinoma in comparison with normal gastric mucosa (Table 6-9).[43] Moreover, type I cAMP-dependent protein kinase can play an important role in the enhanced effect of gastrin on rat stomach carcinogenesis induced by N-methyl-N′-nitro-N-nitrosoguanidine.[44] cAMP-dependent protein kinase and oncogenic tyrosine kinase comprise a single divergent gene family, owing to the homology of amino acid sequences.[45] In addition, G protein regulating cAMP metabolism shares a limited sequence homology with *ras* oncogene product p21.[46]

On one hand, gastrin and the transforming protein (middle T-antigen) of polyoma virus may have evolved from a common ancestor because of their highly homologous amino acid sequences.[47] Furthermore, epidermal growth factor (EGF) receptor has a close se-

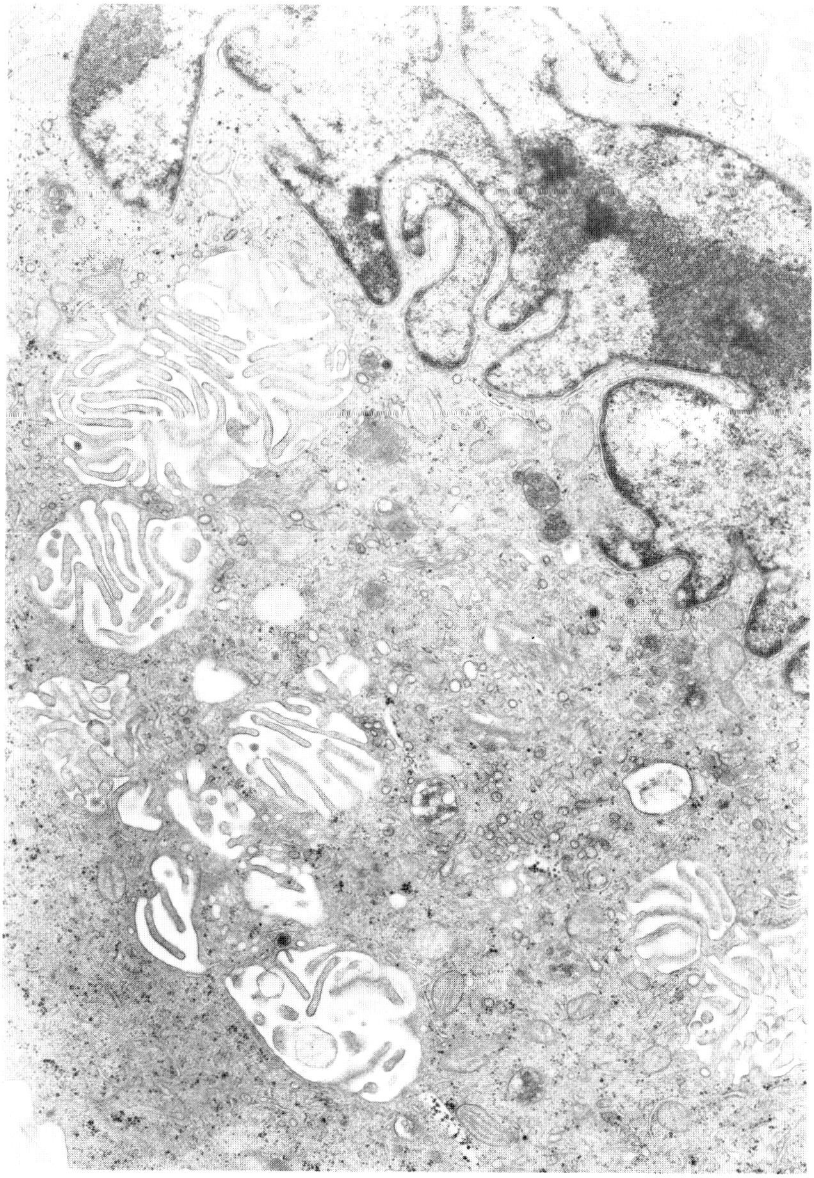

**Fig. 6-22.** Ultrastructure of TMK-1 cells. The tumor cell shows parietal cell differentiation characterized by abundant mitochondria, tubulovesicles and intracellular canaliculi filled with numerous microvilli. ×20,000.

quence homology with erythroblastosis virus oncogene protein (*erb*-B). The relation between "growth factors" or their receptors and oncogenes or oncogene products provides a clue in clarifying "autocrine secretion" for self-stimulation, whereby a tumor cell secretes peptides for which the tumor cell itself has peptide receptors.

Endocrine tumors of the GI tract as well as ordinary carcinomas produce human EGF (Fig. 6-24a).[49] It is detected in 11% of gastric carcinoid and in 21% of gastric scirrhous ECC (Table 6-10). The incidence of human EGF expression in gastric carcinoid is clearly lower than that in advanced gastric carcinomas. Transforming growth factor (TGF)$\alpha$, which

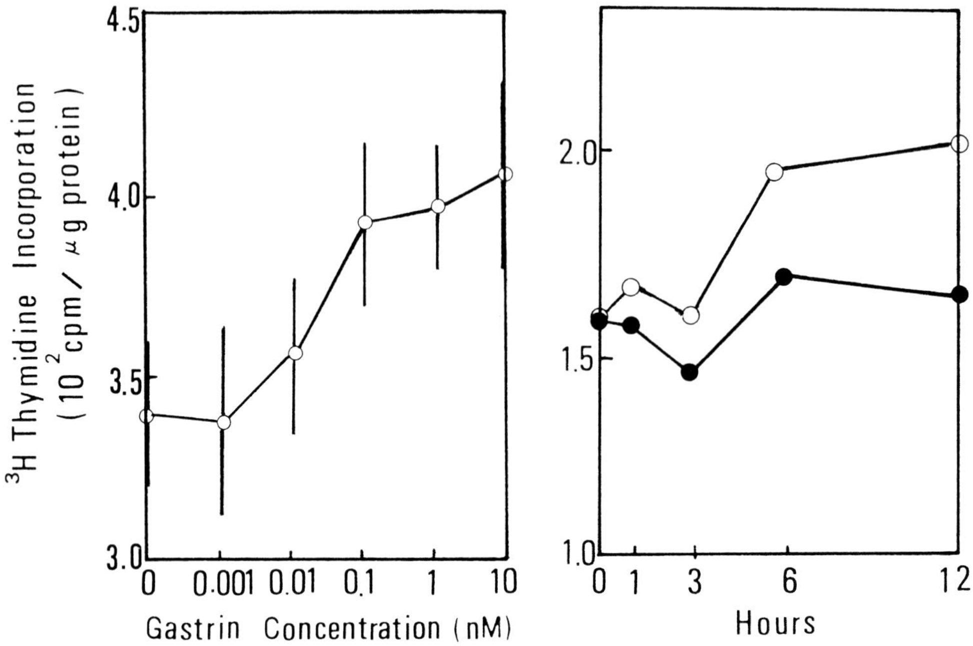


**Fig. 6-23.** Gastrin stimulated DNA synthesis of TMK-1 cells.[42] (Left) Gastrin dose-dependent curve. Points: Mean of 3 experiments. Bars: S.D. (Right) Time course of gastrin stimulated DNA synthesis. Open circle: Addition of 10 nM human gastrin. Closed circle: Addition of phosphate buffered saline. Points: Mean of 3 experiments.

## TABLE 6-9

The Proportion of Types I and II cAMP-Dependent Protein Kinase in Human Gastric Mucosa and Carcinoma[43]

| | Relative Activity[a](%) | | |
|---|---|---|---|
| | Type I | Type II | Type I: Type II |
| Normal Mucosa | 16.2 ± 1.21[b] | 78.5 ± 2.03 | 5.01 ± 0.59 |
| Fundus | 14.9 | 80.7 | 5.60 |
| Antrum | 18.2 | 75.2 | 4.13 |
| Gastric Carcinoma | | | |
| Well[c] | 24.7 ± 3.00 | 64.0 ± 1.57 | 2.75 ± 0.38 |
| Poorly[c] | 22.9 ± 1.00 | 70.4 ± 2.10 | 3.04 ± 0.17 |
| SC-6-JCK[d] | 34.0 ± 3.00[e] | 55.2 ± 4.83[e] | 1.70 ± 0.30[e] |
| St-15[d] | 30.6 ± 1.73[e] | 54.3 ± 3.97[e] | 1.81 ± 0.21[e] |

[a] The proportion of Types I and II in total cAMP-dependent protein kinase activity eluted from DEAE-cellulose column.

[b] Mean ± S.E. from at least 4 experiments.

[c] Well: well differentiated adenocarcinoma, Poorly: poorly differentiated adenocarcinoma.

[d] Xenotransplantable human gastric carcinomas in nude mice.

[e] Significantly different from normal gastric mucosa ($P<0.05$).

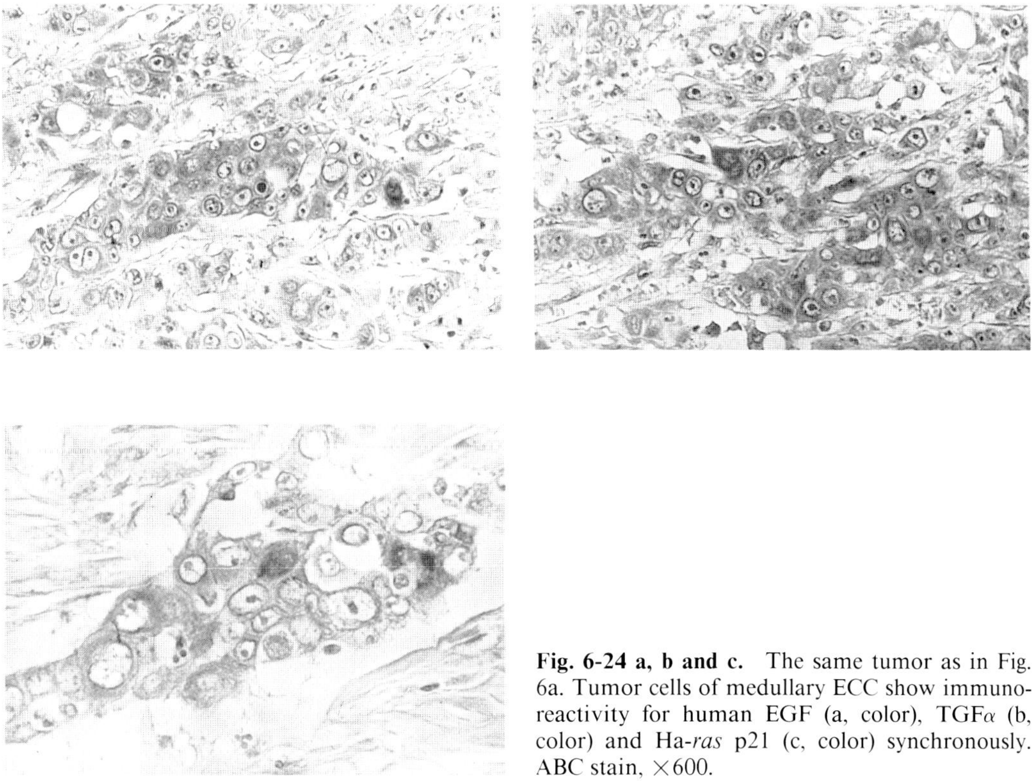

**Fig. 6-24 a, b and c.** The same tumor as in Fig. 6a. Tumor cells of medullary ECC show immunoreactivity for human EGF (a, color), TGF$\alpha$ (b, color) and Ha-*ras* p21 (c, color) synchronously. ABC stain, $\times$600.

**TABLE 6-10**
Growth Factors- and Ha-*ras* p21-Immunoreactivity in Endocrine Tumors of the Stomach

| Endocrine Tumors | Number of Cases | Immunoreactivity[a] EGF | TGF$\alpha$ | p21 |
|---|---|---|---|---|
| Carcinoid | 9 | 1 (11.1%) | 1 (11.1%) | 1 (11.1%) |
| ECC | | | | |
| Medullary | 16 | 1 (6.2%) | 6 (37.5%) | 4 (25.0%) |
| Scirrhous | 14 | 3 (21.4%) | 6 (42.8%) | 1 (30.6%) |

[a] EGF: epidermal growth factor; TGF$\alpha$: transforming growth factor $\alpha$.

has sequence homology to EGF and competes with EGF for binding to the EGF receptor,[50] is detected in 11% of gastric carcinoid and in 40% of gastric ECC (Fig. 6-24b). Expression of Ha-*ras* oncogene product p21 in gastric medullary ECC (25%) is also higher than that in gastric carcinoid (11%) (Table 6-10, Fig. 6-24c). GI hormones, growth factors or their receptors and *ras* oncoprotein may be closely interrelated with growth and invasiveness of ECC. Moreover, calcium-activated, phospholipid-dependent protein kinase (protein kinase C), which is activated by many growth factors and phorbol esters, is considered to play an important role in cellular proliferation. Protein kinase C activity in the soluble fraction in human gastric carcinoma is significantly higher than that in nonneoplastic gas-

## TABLE 6-11

Distribution of Protein Kinase C in Soluble and Particulate Fractions of Gastric Mucosa and Carcinoma[51]

| | Protein Kinase C Activity[a] | | | | |
|---|---|---|---|---|---|
| | Soluble Fraction | | Particulate Fraction | | |
| Tissue | units/g tissue | units/g protein | units/g tissue | units/g protein | Total Activity in Soluble Fraction (%) |
| Gastric Mucosa (8)[b] | 11.19 ± 1.12[c] | 215.3 ± 23.5 | 2.40 ± 0.41 | 111.5 ± 15.7 | 81.4 ± 39.5 |
| Fundus (4) | 10.61 | 224.0 | 2.34 | 110.5 | 81.0 |
| Antrum (4) | 11.77 | 206.5 | 2.45 | 112.6 | 81.8 |
| Gastric Cancer (8) | 18.13 ± 1.92[d] | 357.7 ± 57.5[e] | 2.16 ± 0.52 | 86.7 ± 20.8 | 89.5 ± 19.3 |
| Well[f] (4) | 19.53 | 396.9 | 1.29 | 41.7 | 93.8 |
| Poorly (4) | 16.74 | 318.5 | 3.03 | 131.7 | 85.3 |

[a] Each tissue was homogenized and centrifuged. The supernatant was employed as soluble fraction and the precipitate was resuspended, sonicated and treated with Triton X-100.

[b] Numbers in parentheses are numbers of experiments.

[c] Mean ± S.E.

[d] Value is significantly higher than that in nonneoplastic mucosa ($P<0.01$).

[e] Value is significantly higher than that in nonneoplastic mucosa ($P<0.05$).

[f] Well: well differentiated adenocarcinoma; Poorly: poorly differentiated adenocarcinoma.

tric mucosa (Table 6-11).[51] Further study is necessary to clarify the interaction between protein kinase C and gut hormones in the growth of ECC.

## REFERENCES


1. Solcia E., Polak J.M., Larsson L.I., et al: Update on Lausanne classification of endocrine cells, in Bloom S.R., Polak J.M. (eds): Gut Hormones. London, Churchill Livingstone, 1981, pp 96–100
2. Azzopardi J.G., Pollock J.M.: Argentaffin and argyrophil cells in gastric carcinoma. J Pathol Bacteriol **86**:443, 1963.
3. Kubo T., Watanabe H.: Neoplastic argentaffin cells in gastric and intestinal carcinomas. Cancer **27**:447, 1971
4. Tahara E., Ito H., Nakagami K., et al: Scirrhous argyrophil cell carcinoma of the stomach with mutliple production of polypeptide hormones, amines, CEA, lysozyme and HCG. Cancer **49**:1904, 1982
5. Tahara E., Ito H., Shimamoto F., et al: Argyrophil cells in early gastric carcinoma: An immunohistochemical and ultrastructural study. J Cancer Res Clin Oncol **103**:187, 1982
6. Soga J., Tazawa K., Aizawa O., et al: Argentaffin cell adenocarcinoma of the stomach. Cancer **28**:999, 1971
7. Sweeney E.C., McDonnell L.: Atypical gastric carcinoids. Histopathology **4**:215, 1980
8. Chejfec G., Gould V.E.: Malignant gastric neuroendocrinomas: Ultrastructural and biochemical characterization of their secretory activity. Human Pathol **8**:433, 1977
9. Gould V.E., Memoli V.A., Sobel H.J., et al.: Neuroendocrine carcinomas with multiple immunoreactive peptides and melanin production. Ultrastructural Pathol **2**:199, 1981
10. Reyes C.V., Chejfec G., Jao W., Gould V.E.: Neuroendocrine carcinomas of the esophagus. Ultrastructural Pathol **1**:367, 1980
11. Soga J., Tazawa K.: Pathologic analysis of carcinoids: Histologic reevaluation of 62 cases. Cancer **28**:990, 1971
12. Williams E.D., Siebenmann R.E., Sobin L.H.: Histological classification of tumors of the diffuse endocrine system, in Histological Typing of Endocrine Tumors No. 23. Geneva, World Health Organization, 1980
13. Soga J.: Carcinoid syndrome. Surgery (Tokyo) **45**:1359, 1983
14. Capella C., Polak J.M., Frigerio B., Solcia E.: Gastric carcinoids of argyrophil ECL cells. Ultrastructural Pathol **1**:411, 1980
15. Taniyama K., Tahara E., Yamamoto M., Harada T.: A case of multiple microcarcinoids of the stomach. Pathol Clin Med **3**:554, 1985
16. Alumets J., Hakanson R., Ingemansson S., Sundler F.: Substance P and 5-HT in granules isolated from an intestinal argentaffin carcinoid. Histochemistry **52**:217, 1977
17. Wilander E., El-Salhy M., Lundzvist M., et al: Polypeptide YY (PYY) and pancreatic polypeptide (PP) in rectal carcinoids. Virchow Arch Pathol Anat **401**:67, 1983
18. Solt J., Kadas I., Polak J.M., et al.: A pancreatic polypeptide-producing tumor of the stomach. Cancer **54**:1101, 1984
19. Tsutsumi Y.: Neuroendocrine and related substances. Pathol Clin Med **2**:1610, 1984

20. Sano T., Hizawa K., Shimoda T.: Demonstration of peptide hormone-immunoreactive cells in classical carcinoids and allied tumors: A histological and immunohistochemical study. Pathol Clin Med **1**:1315, 1983
21. Yang K., Ulich T., Cheng L., Wewin K.J.: The neuroendocrine products of intestinal carcinoids: An immunoperoxidase study of 35 carcinoid tumors stained for serotonin and eight polypeptide hormones. Cancer **51**:1918, 1983
22. Creutzfeldt W., Arnold R., Creutzfeldt C., Track N.S.: Pathomorphologic, biochemical and diagnostic aspects of gastrinomas (Zollinger-Ellison syndrome). Human Pathol **6**:47, 1975
23. O'Neal L.W., Kipnis D.M., Luse S.A., et al.: Secretion of various substances by ACTH-secreting tumors—gastrin, melanotropin, norepinephrine, serotonin, parathormone, vasopressin, glucagon, Cancer **21**:1219, 1968
24. Hata J., Taniyama K., Tahara E., et al.: Functional differentiation of gastrointestinal carcinoids. In Proceedings 42nd Annual Meeting Japanese Cancer Association, Nagoya, Japan, p 358, 1983
25. Hata J., Ito H., Tahara E., et al.: Immunohistochemical study of human gastrointestinal carcinoid: Special reference to the distribution of NSE and S-100 protein. In Proceedings 43rd Annual Meeting Japanese Cancer Association, Fukuoka, Japan, p 381, 1984
26. Ito H., Yokozaki H., Tahara E., et al.: Glicentin-containing cells in intestinal metaplasia, adenoma and carcinoma of the stomach. Virchow Arch Pathol Anat **404**:17, 1984
27. Thomas R.U., Lorna C., Henry G., et al.: A colonic adenocarcinoma with argentaffin cells: An immunoperoxidase study demonstrating the presence of numerous neuroendocrine products. Cancer **51**:1483, 1983
28. Warner T.F.C.S., Seo I.S.: Goblet cell carcinoid of appendix: Ultrastructural features and histogenetic aspects. Cancer **44**:1700, 1979
29. Olsson B., Ljungberg O.: Adenocarcinoid of the vermiform appendix. Virchow Arch Pathol Anat **386**:201, 1980
30. Ito H., Hata J., Tahara E., et al.: Immunohistochemical localization of calcitonin in human gastric mucosa and tumor tissue. IGAKU NO AYUMI **131**:315, 1984
31. Iwashita A.: Argentaffin and argyrophil cells in colonic carcinomas. Fukuoka J Med **70**:370, 1979
32. Smith D.M., Haggitt R.C.: The prevalence and prognostic significance of argyrophil cells in colorectal carcinomas. Am J Surg Pathol **8**:123, 1984
33. Grigioni W.F., Caletti G.C., Gabrielli M., Marrano D.: Gastric carcinoids of ECL cells: Pathological and clinical analysis of eight cases. Acta Pathol Jpn **35**:361, 1985
34. Rode J., Dhillon A.P., Papadaki L., Griffiths D.: Neurosecretory cells of the lamina propria of the appendix and their possible relationship to carcinoids. Histopathology **6**:69, 1982
35. Stachura J., Kause W.J., Jivey K.: Ultrastructure of endocrine-like cells in lamina propria of human gastric mucosa. Gut **22**:534, 1981
36. Tahara E., Haizuka S., Kodama T., Yamada A.: The relationship of gastrointestinal endocrine cells to gastric epithelial changes with special reference to gastric cancer. Acta Pathol Jpn **25**:161, 1975
37. Black W.C.: Enterochromaffin cell types and corresponding carcinoid tumors. Laboratory Invest **19**:473, 1968
38. Yamaguchi K., Abe K.. Clinical and endocrinological aspects of pancreatic endocrine tumors. Pathol Clin Med **2**:467, 1984
39. Kobori O., Vuillot M.T., Martin F.: Growth response of rat stomach cancer cells to gastro-entero-pancreatic hormones. Int J Cancer **30**:65, 1982
40. Sumiyoshi H., Yasui W., Ochiai A., Tahara E.: Effects of gastrin on tumor growth and cyclic nucleotide metabolism in xenotransplantable human gastric and colonic carcinomas in nude mice. Cancer Res **44**:4276, 1984
41. Murakami H., Masui H.: Hormonal control of human colon carcinoma cell growth in serum-free medium. Proc Natl Acad Sci USA **77**:3464, 1980
42. Ochiai A., Yasui W., Tahara E.: Growth promoting effect of gastrin on human gastric carcinoma cell line TMK-1. Jpn J Cancer Res (Gann) **76**:1064, 1985
43. Yasui W., Sumiyoshi H., Tahara E., et al: Type I and II cyclic adenosine 3′:5′-monophosphate-dependent protein kinase in human gastric mucosa and carcinomas. Cancer Res **45**:1565, 1985
44. Yasui W., Tahara E.: Effects of gastrin on gastric mucosal cyclic adenosine 3′:5′-monophosphate-dependent protein kinase activity in rat stomach carcinogenesis induced by N-methyl-N′-nitro-N-nitrosoguanidine. Cancer Res **45**:4767, 1985
45. Baldwin G.S.: Gastrin and the transforming protein of polyoma virus have evolved from a common ancestor. FEBS Lett **137**:1, 1982
46. Hurley J.B., Simon M.I., Gilman A.G., et al.: Homologies between signal transducing G proteins and *ras* gene products. Science **226**:860, 1984.
47. Kamps M.P., Taylor S.S., Sefton B.M.: Direct evidence that oncogenic tyrosine kinase and cyclic AMP-dependent protein kinase have homologous ATP-binding sites. Nature (London) **310**:589, 1984
48. Downward J., Yarden Y., Waterfield M.D., et al: Close similarity of epidermal growth factor receptor and v-*erb* B oncogene protein sequences. Nature (London) **307**:521, 1984
49. Tahara E., Sumiyoshi H., Sakamoto S., et al: Human epidermal growth factor in gastric carcinoma as a biologic marker of high malignancy. Jpn J Cancer Res (Gann) (in press), 1986
50. Reynolds F.H., Todaro G.J., Fryling C., Stephenson J.R.: Human transforming growth factors induce tyrosine phosphorylation of EGF receptors. Nature (London) **292**:259, 1981
51. Yasui W., Sumiyoshi H., Ochiai A., Tahara E.: Calcium-activated, phospholipid-dependent protein kinase in human gastric mucosa and carcinoma. Jpn J Cancer Res (Gann) **76**:1164, 1985

# 7

# Immunohistochemical Localization of Chromogranin and Neuron Specific Enolase in Gastroenteropancreatic Tumors

Ricardo V. Lloyd M.D., Ph.D.

Chromogranin and neuron specific enolase (NSE) are present in most neuroendocrine cells and tumors of the diffuse neuroendocrine system (DNES). Silver stains such as argyrophil and argentaffin stains can be used to determine if a certain cell or tumor belongs to the DNES. However, the use of well characterized polyclonal antisera or monoclonal antibodies for the immunohistochemical study of neuroendocrine cells and tumors offers the advantages of greater specificity, reproducibility, and sensitivity intrinsic to immunohistochemical procedures. The combination of chromogranin and NSE immunostaining in examining cells and tumors for neuroendocrine features has many advantages. Among these are (1) the use of two or more markers in immunohistochemical procedures, which increases the sensitivity of the method and the reliability of a positive result, especially if both markers are positive; (2) demonstration that the intracytoplasmic target structures of chromogranin and NSE are different, so a cell may express at least one of these two markers, if not both; and (3) evidence of some gastroenteropancreatic (GEP) cells and tumors that are producing peptides and other products, which have not been characterized as yet, so specific antisera are not available to examine these lesions. The use of chromogranin and NSE can be extremely helpful in revealing the neuroendocrine features of such lesions.

## IMMUNOHISTOCHEMICAL PROCEDURES

As with most other procedures, familiarity with all aspects of the techniques is essential for correct interpretation. Knowledge about the distribution and chemical composition of the antigens used to produce the antibodies, the specificity, cross-reactivity, and other features of the antibodies are critical for proper interpretation of immunohistochemical staining.

## NEURON SPECIFIC ENOLASE

Moore and his co-workers[1,2] isolated two proteins S-100 and 14-3-2 from bovine brain. Antibodies developed against 14-3-2 showed that this protein was present predominantly in neurons, while S-100 protein was found mostly in glial cells. Marangos et al[3–6] characterized the 14-3-2 protein, which was initially called neuron-specific protein. It was subsequently shown that protein 14-3-2 was localized in neuronal cells within the brain and in peripheral nervous tissue with the use of specific antisera to this protein, and neuron-specific protein was designated as neuron specific enolase (NSE).[7] Subsequent studies revealed that NSE was an isoenzyme of the glycolytic enzyme enolase.[8] Further work indicated that NSE was present in most tissues of the DNES.[9,10] There are several forms of enolase that exist in the brain and other tissues. NSE has a molecular weight of 78,000 daltons and is composed of two subunits designated as $\gamma\gamma$. This form of enolase is present in neurons, peripheral nerves and cells of the DNES.

Nonneuronal enolase (NNE) is composed of two $\alpha$ subunits and has a molecular weight of 87,000 daltons. It is present in glial cells in the brain and in liver cells. A hybrid enolase of molecular weight 82,500 is composed of a $\alpha$ and a $\gamma$ subunit.[6,8] The distribution of the $\alpha$ isoenzyme has not been well characterized in the brain. The $\beta\beta$ isoenzyme of enolase is present predominantly in muscle tissues. Because of the overlapping subunit structures between NSE and the hybrid enolase it becomes critical to characterize anti-NSE antisera rigorously before they can be used as a specific marker for NSE.

A few commercial laboratories have produced antisera against NSE. These and other polyclonal antisera have been used by many investigators as research and as diagnostic tools. Several reports indicate that some antisera presumed to be specific for NSE reacted with many nonendocrine tissues, and this raised many questions about the specificity of NSE as a marker for the DNES.[10–15] However, well characterized antisera against NSE were used by several investigators to study neuroendocrine cells and tumors, and only occasional instances of reactivity were observed.[16–20] NSE is also a valuable serum marker for small cell carcinoma of the lung and neuroblastomas.[21–22] Patients with these neoplasms often have elevated serum levels of NSE, especially with metastatic disease, and the serum elevation of NSE may be related to the patient's prognosis.[6]

To avoid some of the problems with the specificity of polyclonal antisera, some investigators are producing monoclonal antibodies against NSE. A recent report indicated that a highly specific monoclonal antibody that did not cross-react with NSE reacted with frozen sections of normal brain tissues and small cell carcinomas of the lung.[23] A preliminary report also suggested that a monoclonal antibody against NSE was more specific than a heterologous antiserum tested for the diagnosis of neuroendocrine and other tumors.[24] If these reports can be corroborated, monoclonal antibodies against NSE may eliminate some of the problems with cross reactivity that are sometimes encountered when immunostaining is done with polyclonal antisera against NSE.

The ultrastructural localization of NSE in rat and mouse brain has shown that this enzyme is present in neuronal perikarya and is associated with ribosomes, granular rough endoplasmic reticulum and microtubules.[25]

## Chromogranin

The chromogranins, a family of acidic protein molecules, have been known to be present in the adrenal medulla for some time.[26–31] Chromogranin A comprises about 40–50% of the total soluble proteins of fractionated granules. It has a molecular weight between 68,000–81,000 daltons, depending on the species of animals and the electrophoretic system used to analyze the proteins.[28] Other chromogranin molecules of different molecular weights have also been identified.[27] Human chromogranin A has a molecular weight of 68,000 daltons. Other chromogranins with higher molecular weights have also been recently described.[31]

The ubiquitous distribution of this family of proteins in most endocrine cells with secretory granules was described recently with the development of polyclonal antisera and monoclonal antibodies against chromogranin.[32–40] A recent study suggested that chromogranin immunoreactivity is also present in lymphoid cells in the spleen, lymph node, thymus, and fetal liver of rats in addition to the cells of the DNES.[41]

The immunohistochemical localization of chromogranin in some cells of the central nervous system that forms part of the DNES varied depending on the antiserum used. While some investigators found chromogranin immunoreactivity in the CNS with the use of polyclonal antisera against bovine chromogranins,[37,38] others did not observe such immunoreactivity with other polyclonal antisera against bovine chromogranin,[33] with a polyclonal antiserum against human chromogranin,[31] or with a monoclonal antibody against human chromogranin.[34,35]

Immunoreactivity in different cells of the pituitary and the GEP axis also varied with the antibody being used.[33–36,39,42,43] Ultrastructural immunohistochemical localization of chromogranin showed that it is associated with endocrine secretory granules in the adrenal medulla,[35] pituitary,[44] and pancreas.[40] Chromogranin A has also been detected in the serum of normal patients and in patients with pheochromocytomas, so it may also be a potential serum marker for patients with neuroendocrine tumors.[45]

## IMMUNOHISTOCHEMICAL LOCALIZATION OF NSE AND CHROMOGRANIN IN NORMAL GASTROENTEROPANCREATIC TISSUES

NSE has been localized in all of the normal islet cells of the pancreas (Fig. 7-1).[16,18] NSE has also been found in all currently identifiable endocrine cell types and in nerves of the gut and pancreas.[16,18,42] The simultaneous localization of NSE in both endocrine cells and nerves can thus provide a rapid way of demonstrating the relationship between these two groups of tissues (Fig. 7-2).[16] The exocrine cells of the pancreas and the nonendocrine cells in the gastrointestinal tract do not react with highly specific antisera against NSE.

The localization of chromogranin within the pancreas varies with the antibody used. O'Connor et al localized chromogranin primarily of the insulin-producing cells of the islet with the polyclonal antiserum against bovine chromogranin,[46] while Cohn et al localized chromogranin A in the somatostatin and pancreatic polypeptide-producing, but not in insulin or glucagon-producing cells of the rat pancreas with polyclonal antisera against bovine parathyroid SP-I and porcine adrenal medulla chromogranin.[39] Others found chromogranin immunoreactivity predominantly in glucagon-producing cells and only weakly in insulin-producing cells of human pancreas in formalin fixed tissues with the use of a monoclonal antibody (LK2H10) against human chromogranin (Fig.7-1B).[34,35,42] Chromogranin immunoreactivity, however, was found in insulin, glucagon, somatostatin, and pancreatic polypeptide-producing cells with the same monoclonal antibody (LK2H10) using freeze-dried tissue vapor-fixed with benzoquinone by Facer et al.[43] These latter observations indicate that fixation and processing are critical to obtain optimal immunoreactivity when using antibodies against chromogranin within the GEP axis. Chromogranin immunoreactivity was found in all GEP endocrine cells examined, including cells producing gastrin, somatostatin, gastrin inhibiting polypeptide, secretin, cholecystokinin, motilin, neurotensin, enteroglucagon, peptide YY, and serotonin (Fig. 7-3).[43] Other investigators also localized chromogranin in the enterochromaffin cells of the intestine.[34,35]

## NSE AND CHROMOGRANIN LOCALIZATION IN GASTROENTEROPANCREATIC CELL HYPERPLASIA

Lloyd, et al found that both NSE and chromogranin were helpful markers in re-

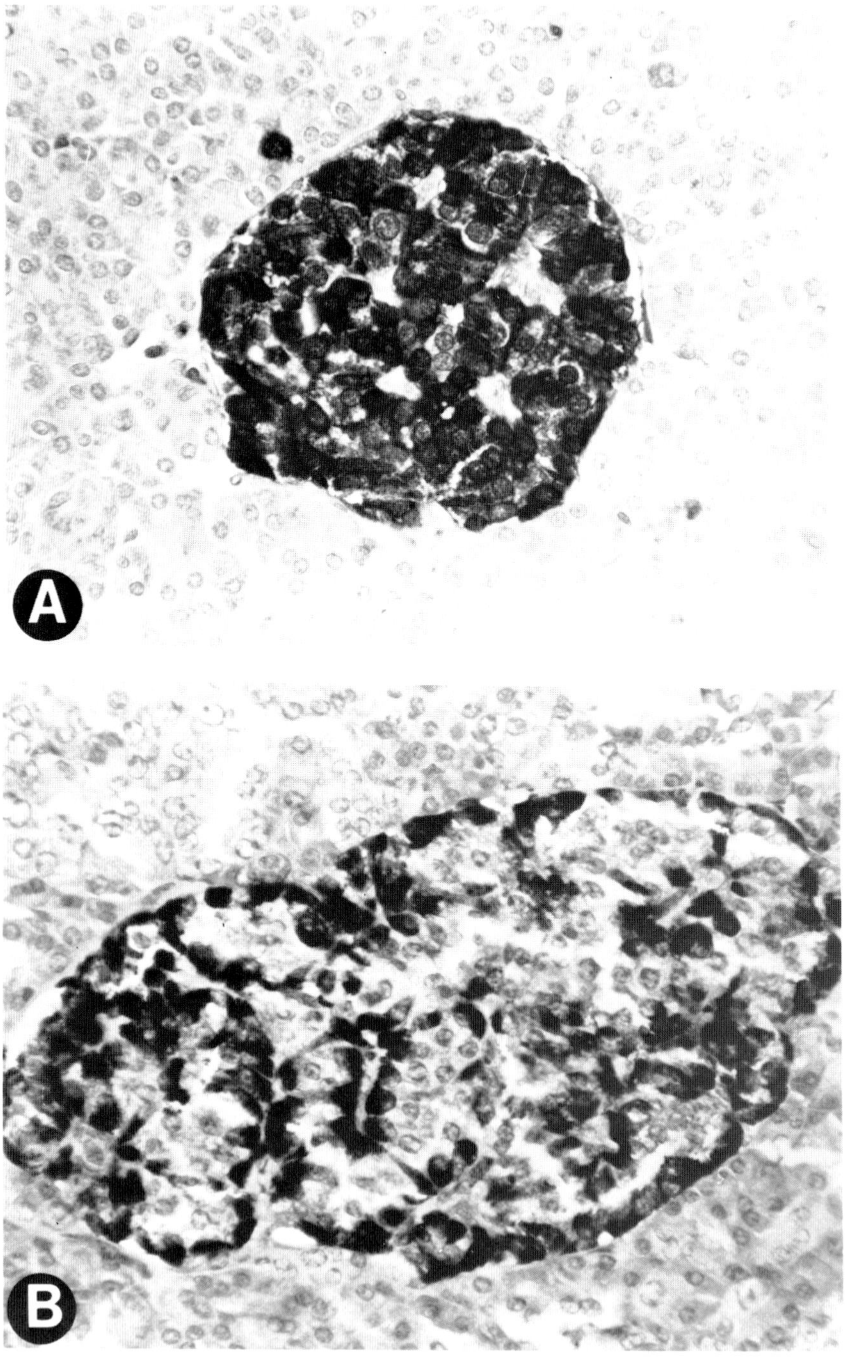

**Fig. 7-1A.** Pancreatic islet showing positive immunoreactivity for NSE. There is diffuse positive immunoreactivity in all of the islet cells (Immunoperoxidase ×208).
**Fig. 7-1(B).** Pancreatic islet showing positive immunoreactivity for chromogranin. The cells at the periphery of the islets, which are predominantly glucagon-producing cells, show the strongest immunoreactivity (Immunoperoxidase ×330).

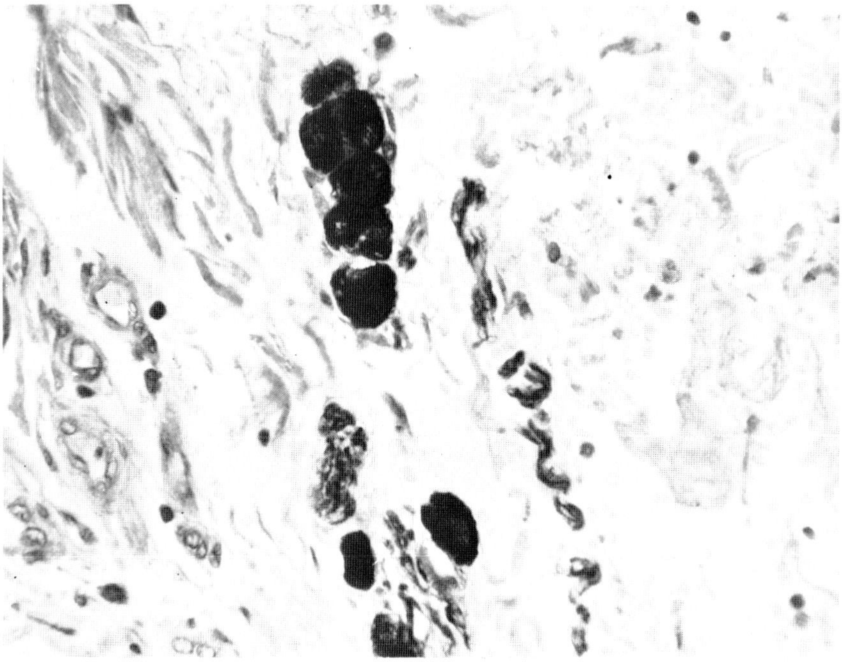

**Fig. 7-2.** Ganglion cells and nerve fibers from the duodenum showing positive immunoreactivity for NSE while the adjacent fibrous and vascular tissues are negative (Immunoperoxidase ×330).

**Fig. 7-3.** Chromogranin immunostaining in duodenum reveals abundant endocrine cells in the villi (Immunoperoxidase ×132).

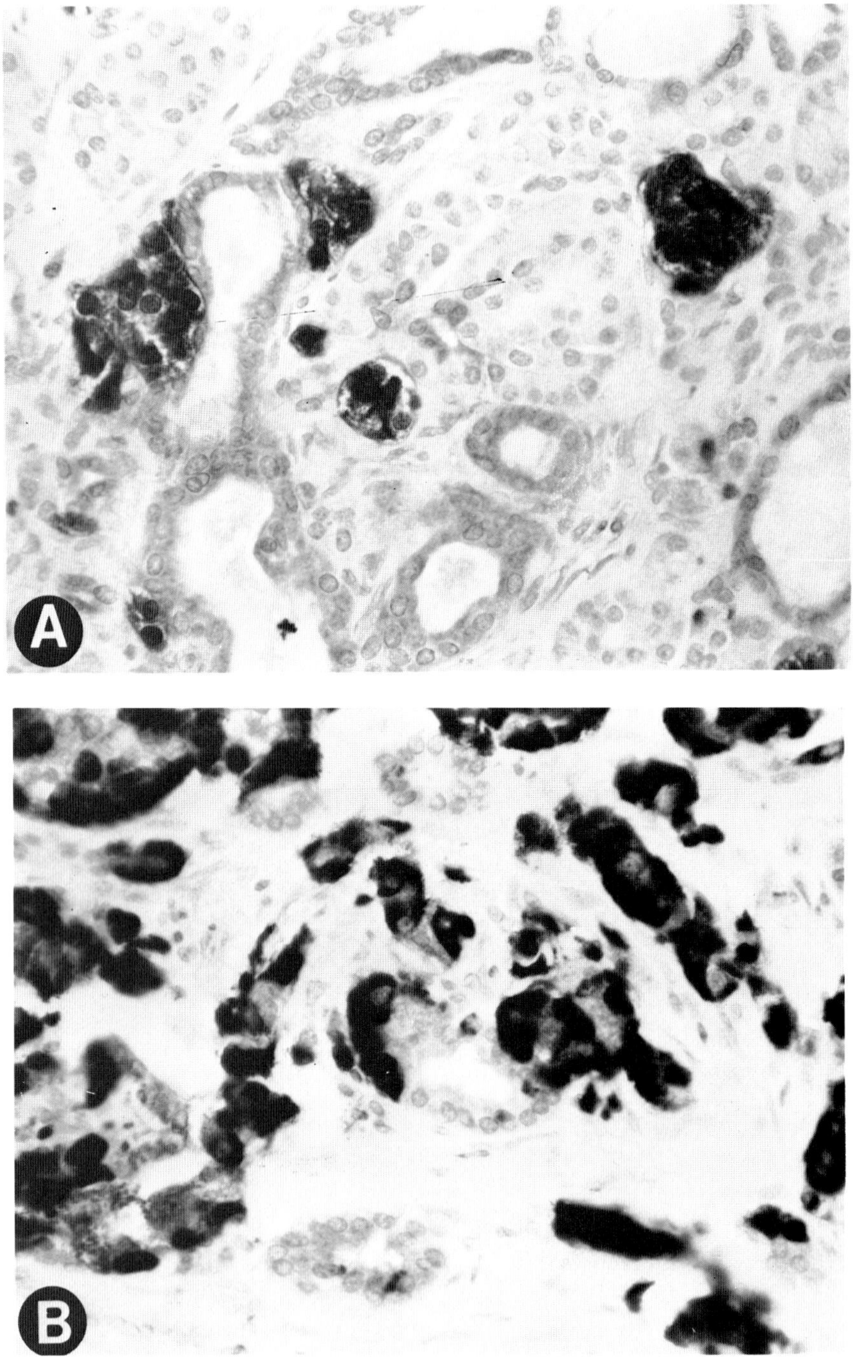

**Fig. 7-4A.** Pancreatic tissues showing nesidioblastosis with islet cells in close association with pancreatic ducts after immunostaining for NSE. (Immunoperoxidase × 208).

**Fig. 7-4(B).** Pancreatic islet tissue from a patient with multiple endocrine neoplasia type 1 showing nesidioblastosis and many small nests of islet cells after immunostaining for chromogranin. (Immunoperoxidase ×330).

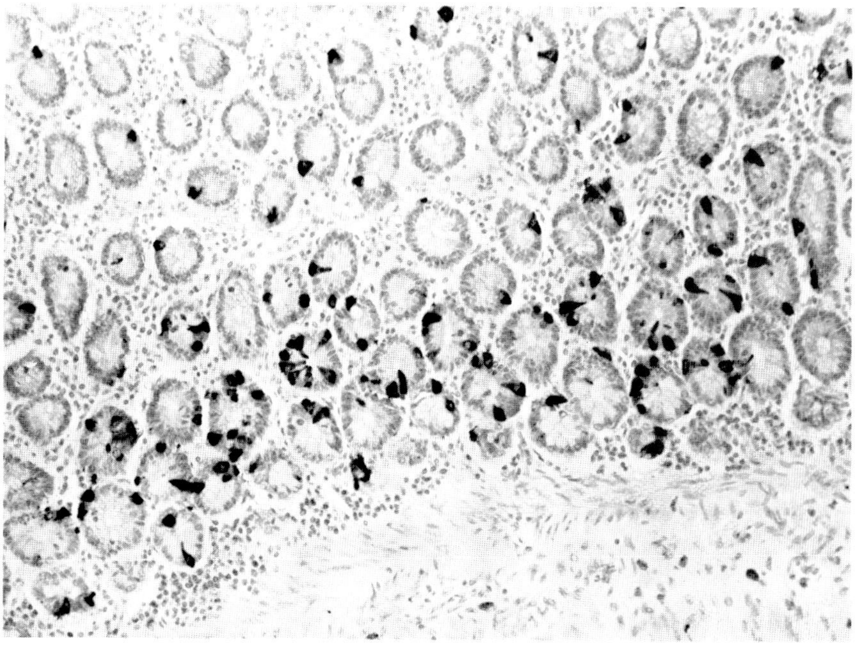

**Fig. 7-5.** Gastric biopsy from a patient with G-cell hyperplasia. Endocrine cells which are positive for chromogranin and for gastrin are revealed after chromogranin staining (Immunoperoxidase ×132).

vealing islet cell hyperplasia and nesidioblastosis (Figs. 7-4A and 7-4B).[42] We also observed increased staining of gastrin-producing cells in four cases of G-cell hyperplasia of the stomach with chromogranin (unpublished observations) (Fig. 7-5). NSE and chromogranin should be helpful markers in the morphometric evaluation of endocrine cell hyperplasia of the stomach and pancreas, but very little work has been done in this area to date.

## NSE AND CHROMOGRANIN IN PANCREATIC ENDOCRINE TUMORS

The use of NSE and chromogranin as broad spectrum markers for pancreatic endocrine tumors is extremely helpful, especially in cases of nonfunctioning tumors that are not producing any known polypeptide hormones.[42] Since NSE stains the cytoplasm of most cells diffusely, while chromogranin stains the secretory granules, the combined use of these markers reveals different staining patterns, and the intensity of chromogranin staining can give an estimate of the numbers of secretory granules within the tumor cells if ultrastructural studies are not available (Figs. 7-6,7-7). Glucagonomas showed intense staining in a recent study of pancreatic endocrine tumors, while insulinomas were generally negative for chromogranin.[42] Other workers detected chromogranin immunoreactivity in pancreatic endocrine tumors.[47] Walts et al recently reported on the use of chromogranin as a neuroendocrine marker for the detection of pancreatic endocrine tumors in cytologic specimens.[48] Our recent studies of normal pancreatic islets and pancreatic endocrine tumors strongly suggest that the mechanism of action of argyrophilic silver stains such as the Grimelius stain might involve binding to chromogranin.[42] This observation has also been noted by other investigators.[40]

Although the serum levels of NSE have

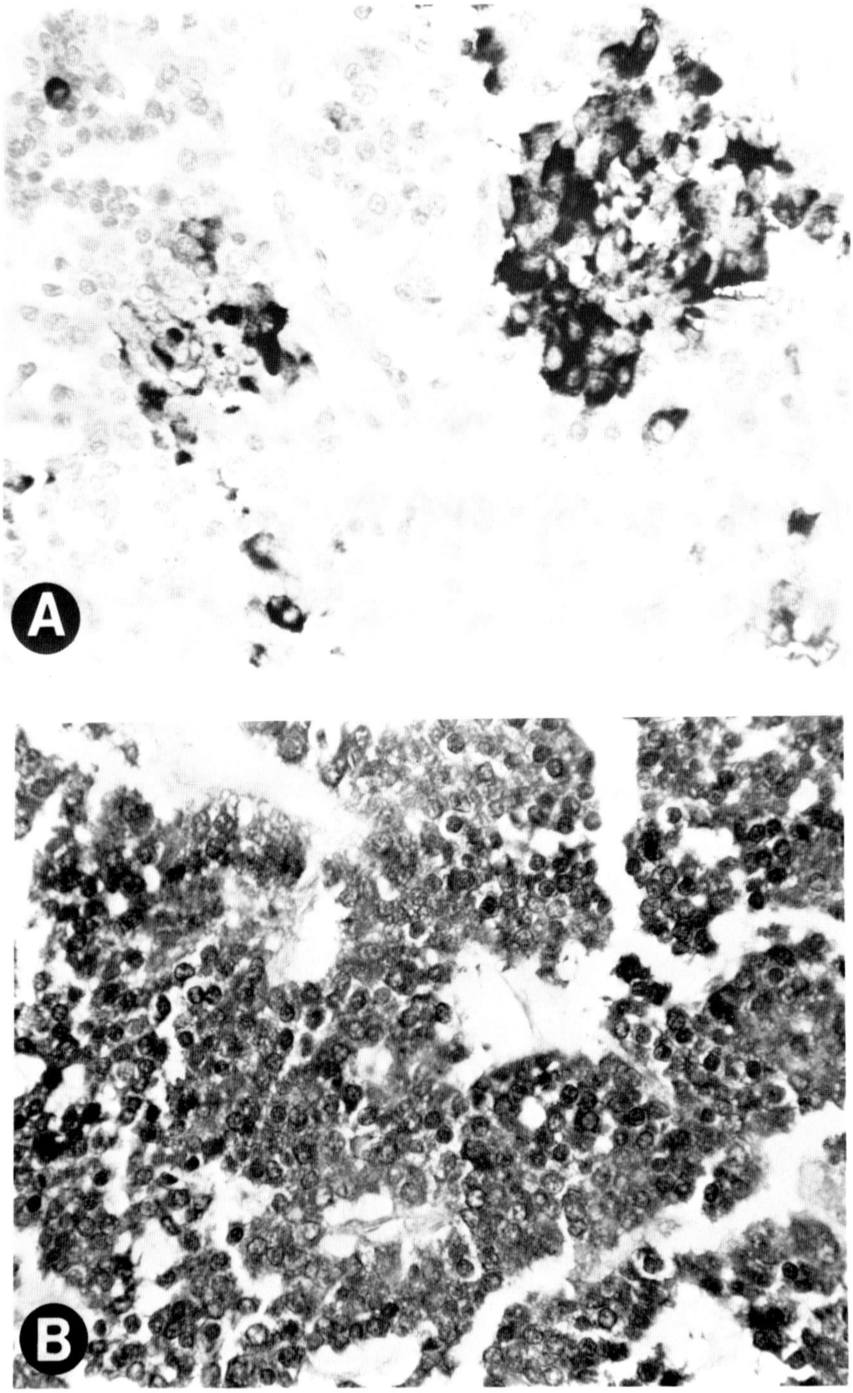


**Fig. 7-6A.** Pancreatic gastrinoma showing focal areas of tumor cells positive for chromogranin. These areas probably contain many endocrine granules while the chromogranin negative areas of the tumor probably contain very few endocrine granules (Immunoperoxidase $\times 330$).

**Fig. 7-6B.** The same tumor as in 6A shows diffuse immunostaining for NSE. NSE immunostains the cytoplasm of endocrine cells diffusely and is not dependent on the presence of secretory granules (Immunoperoxidase $\times 330$).

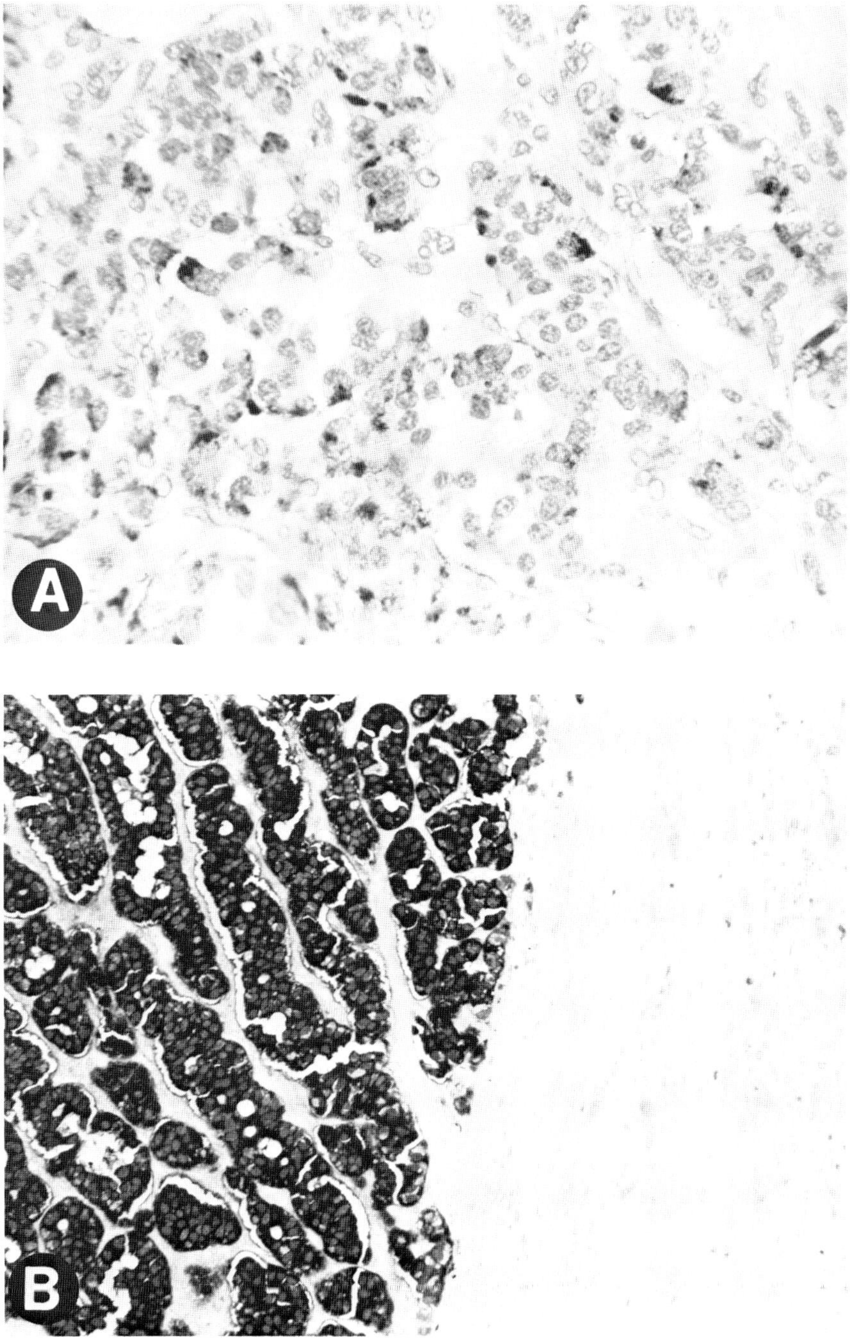

**Fig. 7-7A.** Metastatic pancreatic endocrine tumor to liver showing a distinct pattern of immunostaining for chromogranin in many tumor cells (Immunoperoxidase × 208).

**Fig. 7-7B.** The same metastatic pancreatic endocrine tumor to the liver as in 7A showing a diffuse pattern of immunostaining for NSE. (Immunoperoxidase ×132).

**TABLE 7-1**
Immunoreactivity for Chromogranin and Silver Staining With the Grimelius and Fontana-Masson Stains in Gastrointestinal Carcinoid Tumors.

| Tumor Location | No. of Cases | Positive Reactivity Chromogranin | Grimelius | Fontana |
|---|---|---|---|---|
| Gastric | 3 | 3 | 3 | 2 |
| Small Intestine | 5 | 5 | 5 | 5 |
| Appendix | 4 | 4 | 4 | 4 |
| Colon | 6 | 5 | 4 | 2 |

been examined in GEP tumors and have been found to be elevated accompanying some neoplasms,[49,50] only a few studies correlated serum levels of NSE with the immunohistochemical localization of NSE.[18] In a recent publication that examined serum levels of NSE along with immunohistochemical staining for NSE and tissue extracts analyzed by radioimmunoassay for NSE, only one of ten patients had slightly elevated serum NSE levels. This patient had a metastatic gastrinoma to the liver. The tissue levels were markedly elevated in eight of the ten patients with pancreatic tumors.[18]

## NSE AND CHROMOGRANIN IN CARCINOID TUMORS

Carcinoids are usually designated as foregut, midgut, or hindgut tumors according to their anatomical location.[51] The use of specific antisera to polypeptide hormones and amines in the study of carcinoid tumors has shown that such tumors may produce a predominant polypeptide and/or amine depending on their anatomic location. Thus intestinal foregut carcinoids commonly produce somatostatin and gastrin;[52] midgut carcinoids commonly produce serotonin[52] and hindgut carcinoids often produce immunoreactive pancreatic polypeptide.[53]

The silver stains are commonly used as diagnostic tools for GEP tumors including carcinoids.[49,50] Argyrophilic stains, including the Grimelius method, are usually more sensitive than argentaffin stains in revealing endocrine cells or tumors. In a recent study, comparison of chromogranin immunoreactivity, with the Grimelius and Masson-Fontana silver stains in a study of carcinoid tumors from the gastrointestinal tract revealed that chromogranin reactivity was the most sensitive method of identifying carcinoid tumors and was only slightly more sensitive than the Grimelius technique. (Table 7-1).[57] Chromogranin was much more sensitive than the Masson-Fontana stain in identifying carcinoid tumors from various locations in the intestine (Table 7-1) (Figs. 7-8,7-9).

NSE is also produced by carcinoid tumors (Fig. 7-10). We have found elevated tissue levels of NSE in carcinoid tumors, although the serum levels were not significantly elevated.[56] Prinz et al found a slightly elevated serum level of NSE in one of five patients with intestinal carcinoid tumors.[50] The concentration of serum levels of NSE may also be related to the presence of metastatic disease.[20,56]

## NSE AND CHROMOGRANIN IN OTHER GEP TUMORS

We have localized NSE and chromogranin in goblet cell carcinoid tumors of the appendix and in duodenal paragangliomas (unpublished observations). Other workers have found chromogranin immunoreactivity in pancreatic ductal adenocarcinomas, indicating a mixed endocrine and ductal differentia-

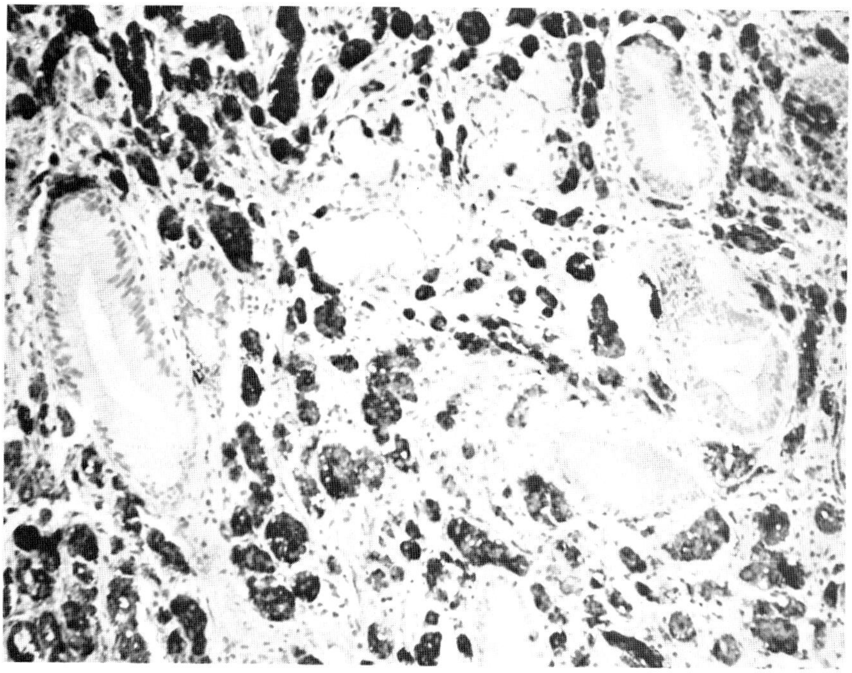

**Fig. 7-8.** Gastrin-producing carcinoid tumor from stomach showing positive immunostaining for chromogranin in the infiltrating nests of tumor cells (Immunoperoxidase × 208).

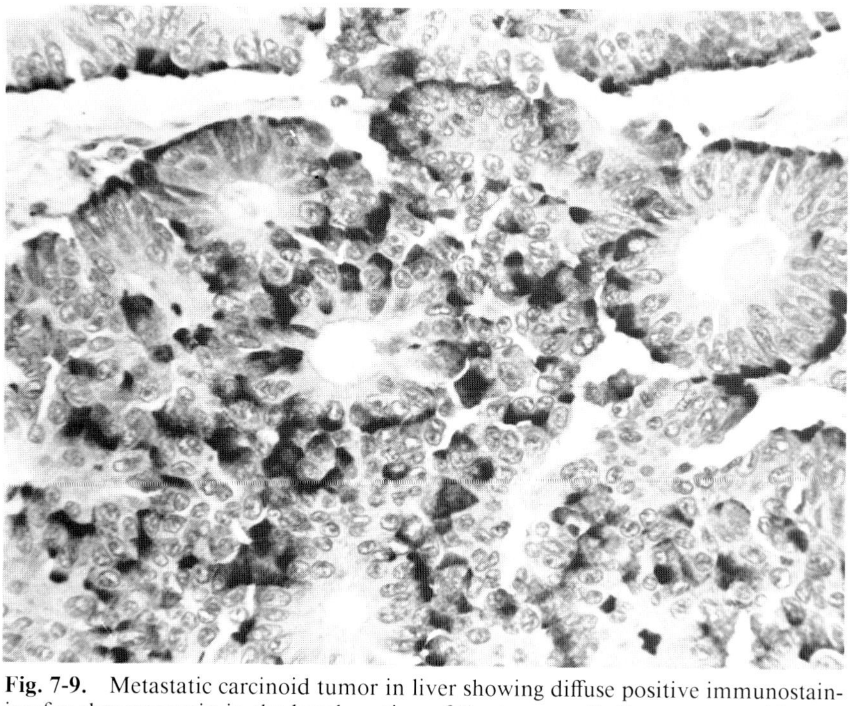

**Fig. 7-9.** Metastatic carcinoid tumor in liver showing diffuse positive immunostaining for chromogranin in the basal portion of the tumor cells (Immunoperoxidase × 330).

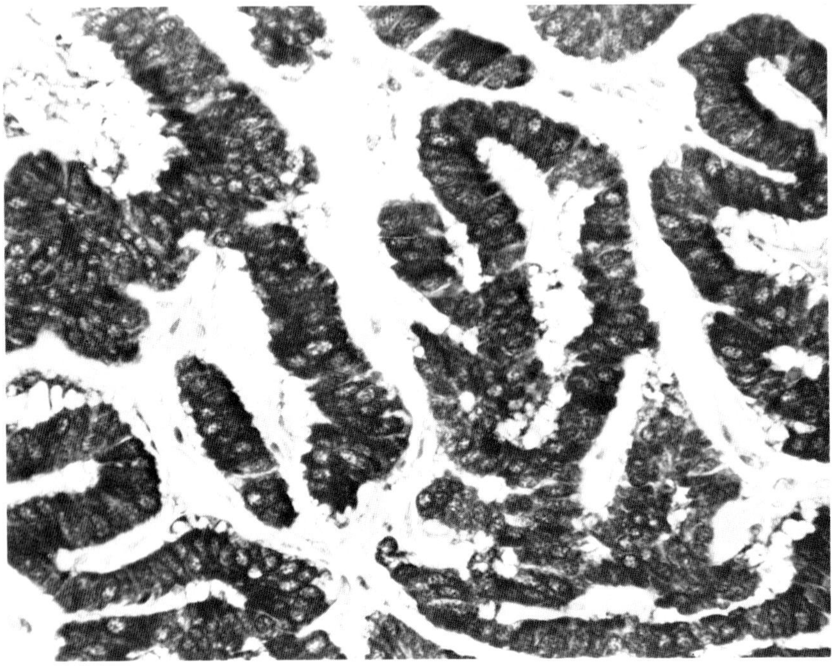

**Fig. 7-10.** Colonic carcinoid showing intense diffuse positive immunostaining for NSE. (Immunoperoxidase ×330).

tion in these tumors.[58] Chromogranin immunostaining was also more sensitive than the Grimelius technique in localizing neuroendocrine cells in mixed exocrine and endocrine pancreatic tumors.[58]

## FUTURE PROSPECTS

The use of NSE and chromogranin to analyze differentiation of endocrine cells, mixed endocrine-exocrine GEP tumors, and hyperplasia of various endocrine cells has not been fully explored. The unique advantage of these broad spectrum markers in studying GEP neuroendocrine tumors is that one can detect endocrine differentiation even if a specific antibody against certain peptides is not available. Thus, the systematic study of normal and neoplastic GEP endocrine cells with NSE and chromogranin may lead to the detection of novel endocrine cells that would not have been discovered with the use of antisera that react only with known peptides.

## SUMMARY

The use of well characterized antibodies against NSE and chromogranin as general markers of endocrine differentiation offers many advantages. Because NSE is a diffuse cytoplasmic marker and chromogranin is localized in secretory granules, these markers are complementary to each other. The use of chromogranin can give some general information about the granule content of endocrine cells and tumors. Chromogranin immunoreactivity and the Grimelius silver stain appear to be closely related, but chromogranin immunoreactivity appears to represent a more sensitive marker for the detection of endocrine differentiation. NSE can be used to study the localization of endocrine cells and nerves within the same tissue, so that the relationship between these two tissues can be visualized simultaneously. The use of NSE and chromogranin as immunohistochemical markers can contribute to the study of endocrine cell and tumor development and differentiation. They also serve as helpful diagnostic aids in pathology.

## REFERENCES


1. Moore B.W.: Chemistry and biology of two proteins, S-100 and 14-3-2, specific to the nervous system, in International Review of Neurobiology, Vol 15 C.C. Pfeiffer and J.R. Smythies, (eds) New York, Academic Press, 1972, pp 215–225
2. Moore B.W., McGregor D: Chromatographic and electrophoretic fractionation of soluble proteins of brain and liver. J Biol Chem **146**:1647–1653, 1965
3. Marangos P.J., Zomzely-Neurath C., Luk D.C.M., York C.: Isolation and characterization of the nervous system specific protein 14-3-2 from rat brain. J Biol Chem **250**:1884–1891, 1975
4. Marangos P.J., Parma A.M., Goodwin F.K.: Functional properties of neuronal and glial isoenzymes of the glycolytic enzyme enolase in brain. J Neurochem **31**:727–737, 1978
5. Marangos P.J., Zis A.D., and Clark R.L., Goodwin F.K.: Neuronal, non-neuronal and hybrid forms of enolase in brain: Structural, immunological and functional comparisons. Brain Res **150**:113–117, 1978
6. Marangos P.J.: Clinical utility of neuron-specific enolase as a neuroendocrine tumour marker, in Endocrine Tumours. The Pathobiology of Regulatory Peptide-producing Tumours. J.M. Polak and S.R. Bloom (eds). Churchill Livingstone, Edinburgh, 1985, pp 181–192
7. Marangos P.J., Schmechel D.: The neurobiology of the brain enolases, in Essays in Neurochemistry and Neuropharmacology Vol IV. M.B.H. Youdim, W. Lovenberg, D.F. Sharman, Jr. and J.R. Lagnado (eds), Wiley, New York, 1980, pp 211–247
8. Schmechel D.E., Marangos P.J., Zis A.P., Brightman M., Goodwin, F.K.: The brain enolases as specific markers of neuronal and glial cells. Science **199**:313–315, 1978
9. Schmechel D.E., Marangos P.J., Brightman M.W.: Neuron specific enolase is a marker for peripheral and central neuroendocrine cells. Nature **276**:834–836, 1979
10. Tapia F.J., Barbosa A.J.A., Marangos P.J., Polak J.M., Bloom S.R., Dermody C.: Neuron-specific enolase is produced by neuroendocrine tumours. Lancet **i**:808–811, 1981
11. Haimoto H., Takahashi Y., Koshikawa T., Nagra H., Kaito K.: Immunohistochemical localization of $\gamma$-enolase in normal human tissues other than neurons and neuroendocrine tissues. Lab Invest. **52**:257–263, 1983
12. Schmechel D.E.: $\gamma$-subunit of the glycolytic enzyme enolase: nonspecific or neuron specific. (Editorial) Lab Invest **52**:239–242, 1985
13. Vinores S.A., Bonnin J.H., Rubinstein L.S., Marangos P.J.: Immunohistochemical demonstration of neuron-specific enolase in neoplasms of the CNS and other tissues. Arch Pathol Lab Med **108**:536–540, 1984
14. Wick M.R., Scheithauer B.W., Kovacs K.: Neuron specific enolase in neuroendocrine tumors of the thymus, bronchus and skin. Am J Clin Pathol **79**:703–707, 1983
15. Tsokos M., Linoila R.I., Chandra R.S., Triche T.J.: Neuron specific enolase in the diagnosis of neuroblastomas and other small round cell tumors in children. Human Pathol **15**:575–584, 1984
16. Bishop A.E., Polak J.M., Facer P., Ferri G.L., Marangos P.J., Pearse A.G.E.: Neuron specific enolase: A common marker for the endocrine cells and innervation of the gut and pancreas. Gastroenterol **83**:902–915, 1982
17. Asa S.L., Ryan N., Kovacs K., Singer W., Marangos P.J.: Immunohistochemical localization of neuron-specific enolase in the human hypophysis and pituitary adenomas. Arch Pathol Lab Med **108**:40–43, 1984
18. Simpson S., Vinik A., Marangos P.J., Lloyd R.V.: Immunohistochemical localization of neuron-specific enolase in gastroenteropancreatic neuroendocrine tumors. Correlation with tissue and serum levels of neuron-specific enolase. Cancer **54**:1364–1369, 1984
19. Lloyd R.V., Sisson J.C., Marangos P.J.: Calcitonin, carcinoembryonic antigen and neuron-specific enolase in medullary thyroid carcinomas. An immunohistochemical study. Cancer **51**:2234–2239, 1983
20. Lloyd R.V., Warner T.F.: Immunohistochemistry of neuron-specific enolase. In Advances in Immunohistochemistry. R.A. DeLellis (ed), Masson Publishing USA, Inc., 1984, pp 127–140
21. Carney D.D., Ihde D.C., Cohen M.H., Marangos P.J., Bunn P.A., Jr., Minna J.D., Gazder A.F.: Serum neuron-specific enolase: A marker for disease extent and response to therapy of small-cell lung cancer. Lancet **i**:583–585, 1982
22. Zelter P.M., Marangos P.J., Parma A.M., Sather H., Dalton A., Hammond D., Siegel S.B., Seeger R.C.: Raised neuron specific enolase in serum of children with metastatic neuroblastoma. Lancet **ii**:361–363, 1983
23. Seshi B., Bell C.E.: Preparation and characterization of monoclonal antibodies to human neuron-specific enolase. Hybridoma **4**:13–25, 1985
24. Thomas P., Battifora H., Mandenno C.: Is neuron-specific enolase specific? An immunohistochemical comparison of a monoclonal and a polyclonal antibody against neuron specific enolase. Lab Invest **54**:63A, 1986 (Abstract)
25. Vinores S.A., Herman M.M., Rubinstein L.J., Marangos P.J.: Electron microscopic localization of neuron-specific enolase in rat and mouse brain. J Histochem Cytochem **32**:1295–1302, 1984
26. Blaschko H., Comline R.S., Schneider F.H., Silver M., Smith A.D.: Secretion of a chromaffin granule protein, chromogranin, from the adrenal medulla after splanchnic nerve stimulation. Nature **215**:58–59, 1967
27. Winkler H.: The composition of adrenal chromaffin granules. An assessment of controversial results. Neurosciences **1**:65–80, 1976
28. Smith A.D., Winkler H.: Purification and properties of an acidic protein from chromaffin granules on a large scale. Biochem J **103**:480–482, 1967

29. Kirschner A.G., Kirschner N.: A specific soluble protein from the catecholamine storage vesicles of bovine adrenal medulla. Biochem Biophys Acta **181**:219–225, 1969
30. O'Connor D.T., Frigon R.P., Sokoloff R.L.: Human chromogranin A. Purification and characterization from catecholamine storage vesicles of human pheochromocytoma. Hypertension **6**:2–12, 1984
31. Hagn C., Schmid K. W., Fischer-Colbvie R., Winkler H. Chromogranin A, B, and C in human adrenal medulla and endocrine tissues. Lab Invest **55**:405–411, 1986.
32. Aunis D., Hesketch J.E., Devilliens G.: Immunohistochemical and immunocytochemical localization of myosin, chromogranin A and dopamine β-hydroxylase in nerve cells in culture and adrenal glands. J Neurocytol **9**:255–274, 1980
33. O'Connor D.J.: Chromogranin: widespread immunoreactivity in polypeptide hormone producing tissues and in serum. Regulatory Peptides **6**:263–280, 1983
34. Lloyd R.V., Wilson B.S.: Specific endocrine marker defined by a monoclonal antibody. Science **222**:628–630, 1983
35. Wilson B.S., Lloyd R.V.: Detection of chromogranin in neuroendocrine cells with a monoclonal antibody. Am J Pathol **115**:458–468, 1984
36. O'Connor D.T., Burton P., Deftos L.J.: Immunoreactive human chromogranin A in diverse polypeptide hormone producing human tumors and normal endocrine tissues. J Clin Endocrinal **57**:1084–1087, 1983.
37. Nolan J.A., Trojanowski J.Q., Hogue-Angeletti R.: Neurons and neuroendocrine cells contain chromogranin: Detection of the molecule in normal bovine tissues by immunochemical and immunohistochemical methods. J Histochem Cytochem **33**:791–798, 1985
38. Somogyi P., Hodgson A.J., Depotter R.W., Fischer-Colbrie R., Schober M., Winkler H., Chubb I.W.: Chromogranin immunoreactivity in the central nervous system. Immunochemical characterization, distribution and relationship to catecholamine and enkephalin pathways. Brain Res Reviews **8**:193–230, 1984
39. Cohn D.V., Elting J.J., Frick M., Elde, R.: Selective localization of the parathyroid secretory protein-I/adrenal medulla chromogranin. A protein family in a wide variety of endocrine cells of the rat. Endocrinology **113**:1963–1974, 1984
40. Varndell I.M., Lloyd R.V., Wilson B.S., Polak J.M.: Ultrastructural localization of chromogranin: A protential marker for the electron microscopical recognition of endocrine cell secretory granules. Histochem J **17**:981–992, 1985
41. Hogue-Angeletti R., Hicker W.F.: A neuroendocrine marker in tissues of the immune system. Science **230**:89–96, 1985
42. Lloyd R.V., Mervak T., Schmidt K., Warner T.F.C.S., Wilson B.S.: Immunohistochemical detection of chromogranin and neuron-specific enolase in pancreatic endocrine neoplasm. Am J Surg Pathol **8**:607–614, 1984
43. Facer P., Bishop A.E., Lloyd R.V., Wilson B.S., Hennessy R.J., Polak J.M.: Chromogranin: A newly recognized marker for endocrine cells of the human gastrointestinal tract. Gastroenterol **89**:1366–1373, 1985
44. DeStephano D.B., Lloyd R.V., Pike A.M., Wilson B.S.: Pituitary adenomas. An immunohistochemical study of hormone production and chromogranin localization. Am J Pathol **116**:464–472, 1984
45. O'Connor D.T., Bernstein K.N.: Radioimmunoassay of chromogranin A in plasma as a measure of exocytotic sympathoadrenal activity in normal subjects and patients with pheochromocytomas. N Engl J Med **311**:764–776, 1984
46. O'Connor D.T., Burton D., Deftos L.J.: Chromogranin A: Immunohistology reveals its universal occurrence in normal polypeptide hormone producing endocrine glands. Life Science **33**:1657–1663, 1983
47. O'Connor D.T., Burton D.W., Parmer R.J., Deftos L.J.: Human chromogranin A: Detection by immunohistochemistry in C cells and diverse polypeptide hormone producing tumors, in Endocrine Control of Bone and Calcium Metabolism. Cohn D.V., Fugita T., Potts, Jr J.J.,Talmage, R.V. (eds). Elsevier Scientific Publications B.V., 1984, pp 187–190
48. Walts A.E., Said J.E., Shintaker P., Lloyd R.V.: Chromogranin as a marker of neuroendocrine cells in cytologic material—an immunocytochemical study. Am J Clin Pathol **84**:273–277, 1985
49. Prinz R.A., Marangos P.J.: Use of neuron-specific enolase as a serum marker for neuroendocrine neoplasms. Surgery **92**:887–889, 1982
50. Prinz R.A., Berme E.W., Kimmel J.R., Marangos P.J.: Serum markers for pancreatic islet cell and intestinal carcinoid tumors: A comparison of neuron-specific enolase, β-human chorionic gonadotropin and pancreatic polypeptide. Surgery **94**:1019–1023, 1983
51. Williams E.D., Sandler M.: The classification of carcinoid tumours, Lancet **1**:238–239, 1963
52. Dayal Y.: Endocrine cells of the gut and their neoplasms. Contemp Issues Surg Pathol **2**:267–302, 1983
53. O'Brian D.S., Tischler A.S., Dayal Y., Beudon R., DeLellis R.A., Wolfe H.J.: Rectal carcinoids as tumors of the hindgut endocrine cells. A morphological and immunohistochemical analysis. Am J Surg Pathol **6**:131–142, 1982
54. Grimelius L., Wilander E.: Silver stains in the study of endocrine cells of the gut and pancreas. Invest Cell Pathol **3**:3–12, 1980
55. Solcia E., Capella C., Buffa R., Frigerio B.: Histochemical and ultrastructural studies on the argentaffin and argyrophil cells of the gut. Chromaffin, Enterochromaffin and Related Cells. Coupland, R.E., Fujita T., (eds) Elsevier Scientific Publishing Company. The Netherlands, 1976, pp 209–225
56. Vinik A.J., Strodel W.E., Lloyd R.V., Thompson N.W.: Unusual gastroenteropancreatic (GEP) tumors and their hormones. In Thompson N.W., Vinik A.I. (eds) Endocrine Surgery Update. Grune & Stratton, New York, 1983, pp 293–320
57. Kumar N.B., Cookingham C.L., Lloyd R.V., Appelman H.: Detection of human chromogranin with a monoclonal antibody in carcinoid secretory granules and its comparison with the generic silver stains and with serotonin. Lab Invest **50**:33A, 1984 (Abstract)
58. Kay D., DeLellis R.A., Dayal Y., Lloyd R.V., Duggan M.A., Tallberg K., Sternberg S.S., Wolfe H.J.: Ductal adenocarcinomas of the pancreas with neuroendocrine cells. An immunohistochemical study. Lab Invest. **52**:33A, 1986 (Abstract).

# 8

# Protein-losing Enteropathy Including Intestinal Lymphangiectasia and Ménétrier's Disease

Hitoshi Asakura M.D.
Akira Morita M.D.
Soichiro Miura M.D.
Masaharu Tsuchiya M.D.
Yasuyoshi Enomoto Ph.D.
Yoonosuke Watanabe M.D.

Protein-losing gastroenteropathy, characterized by an excessive loss of plasma protein into the gastrointestinal lumen, is caused by a wide variety of gastrointestional disorders, which may be classified into three categories:[1] The first category includes disorders that cause an obstruction of intestinal lymphatics. Direct leakage of intestinal lymph into the intestinal lumen is thought to be the mechanism of protein loss. Primary intestinal lymphangiectasia is a typical example of this group.[2,3] Secondary intestinal lymphangiectasia may occur in certain cardiac diseases such as constrictive pericarditis[4] and congestive heart failure, lymphoma, Whipple's disease, Crohn's disease,[5] intestinal tuberculosis, and retroperitoneal fibrosis.[6]

The second group consists of mucosal diseases with erosion or ulceration including ulcerative colitis,[7] Crohn's disease, radiation enteritis, pseudomembranous enterocolitis, and malignant tumors of the gastrointestinal tract.[8] Inflammatory exudation may be the primary cause of protein loss.

The last group includes mucosal disorders without ulceration such as Ménétrier's disease (giant hypertrophy of the gastric rugae),[9] allergic gastroenteropathy,[10] eosinophilic gastroenteritis, sprue syndrome,[11] intestinal bacterial overgrowth[12] and parasitic infections. Loss of proteins into the gastrointestinal lumen is thought to be due to an increased mucosal permeability[13] to protein because of surface cell damage, increased cell loss, and local release of mediators. Vascular permeability may also be an important factor in the gastrointestinal loss of plasms proteins.[14,15] Causes of protein-losing gastroenteropathy are listed in Table 8-1.

## DIAGNOSIS OF PROTEIN-LOSING GASTROENTEROPATHY

A major clinical manifestation of protein-losing gastroenteropathy is edema caused by lowered colloidal pressure of plasma and increased transudation of fluid from the capillaries. In addition to the low plasma levels of albumin, the plasma concentrations of

**TABLE 8-1**
Causes of Protein-losing Gastroenteropathy.

| |
|---|
| 1. Esophagus |
| Esophageal carcinoma |
| 2. Stomach |
| Giant hypertrophic gastritis |
| Ménétrier's disease |
| Gastric polyposis (polyp) |
| Gastric carcinoma |
| Postgastrectomy syndrome |
| 3. Small intestine |
| Tropical sprue, nontropical sprue |
| Regional enteritis (Crohn's disease) |
| Whipple's disease |
| Nonspecific granulomatous disease |
| Gastrointestinal tuberculosis |
| Acute gastrointestinal infection |
| Hookworm infection, Trichinosis |
| Allergic gastroenteropathy |
| Eosinophilic gastroenteritis |
| Intestinal lymphangiectasia |
| Blind loop syndrome |
| Lymphosarcoma, Hodgkin's disease |
| Intestinal lymphoma |
| Stenosis |
| 4. Colon |
| Ulcerative colitis |
| Colonic neoplasm |
| Polyposis (Cronkhite-Canada syndrome) |
| 5. Heart |
| Congestive heart failure |
| Constrictive pericarditis |
| Interatrial septal defect |
| Primary myocardial disease |
| 6. Miscellaneous |
| Nephrotic syndrome |
| Liver cirrhosis |
| Chronic pancreatitis |
| Kwashiorkor |
| Amyloidosis |
| Acute transient gastrointestinal protein loss |
| Idiopathic retroperitoneal fibrosis |
| Anaphylactoid purpura |

gamma globulin, fibrinogen, lipoproteins, alpha 1-antitrypsin, transferrin, and ceruloplasmin are found to be decreased. It is, however, rare that the enteric loss of plasma proteins other than albumin causes clinical problems. Secondary hypogammaglobulinemia and the loss of blood coagulating factors are rarely sufficient, and the depletion of hormone-binding proteins is well compensated by the presence of free hormones. In patients with obstruction of intestinal lymphatics, the leakage and/or impaired absorption of long chain triglyceride and fat-soluble vitamins may be associated with the enteric loss of protein.

The possibility of protein-losing gastroenteropathy should be considered in patients who exhibit hypoproteinemia with or without edema, when other causes for hypoproteinemia, such as liver disease, malabsorption syndrome, and proteinuria are ruled out. Attempts to measure the excretion of protein into the gastrointestinal lumen by direct analysis of aspirated gastrointestinal fluid have been limited by the rapid proteolytic digestion of plasma protein. Therefore, a variety of labeled substances that resist proteolytic digestion and reabsorption have been used for the diagnosis of protein-losing gastroenterpathy. Those include $^{131}$I-human serum albumin,[16] $^{131}$I-PVP,[17] $^{59}$Fe-dextran, $^{95}$Nb-albumin, $^{67}$Cu-ceruloplasmin and $^{51}$Cr-albumin.[18] These are still not ideal, however, since they are nonphysiological substances and have a considerably shorter half life in the circulation when compared to that of $^{131}$I-albumin. Recently, alpha 1-antitrypsin, a natural plasma protein, has been found to be useful in studying enteric protein loss.[19] Although it is digested in acid gastric juice, it resists proteolytic digestion in the intestinal lumen. It is not selectively secreted into the intestine and its level in plasma and stool can be easily measured. Moreover, the use of radioisotope is not needed in assessment of alpha 1-antitrypsin loss. In addition to the direct methods stated above to detect the loss of plasma protein into the gastrointestinal lumen, kinetic study using radioiodinated human plasma albumin has been widely used to determine if the hypoproteinemia is due to hypercatabolism.

## Intestinal Lymphangiectasia of the Small Intestine

Intestinal lymphangiectasia is a disease characterized by a generalized disorder of the lymphatic channels including dilated lym-

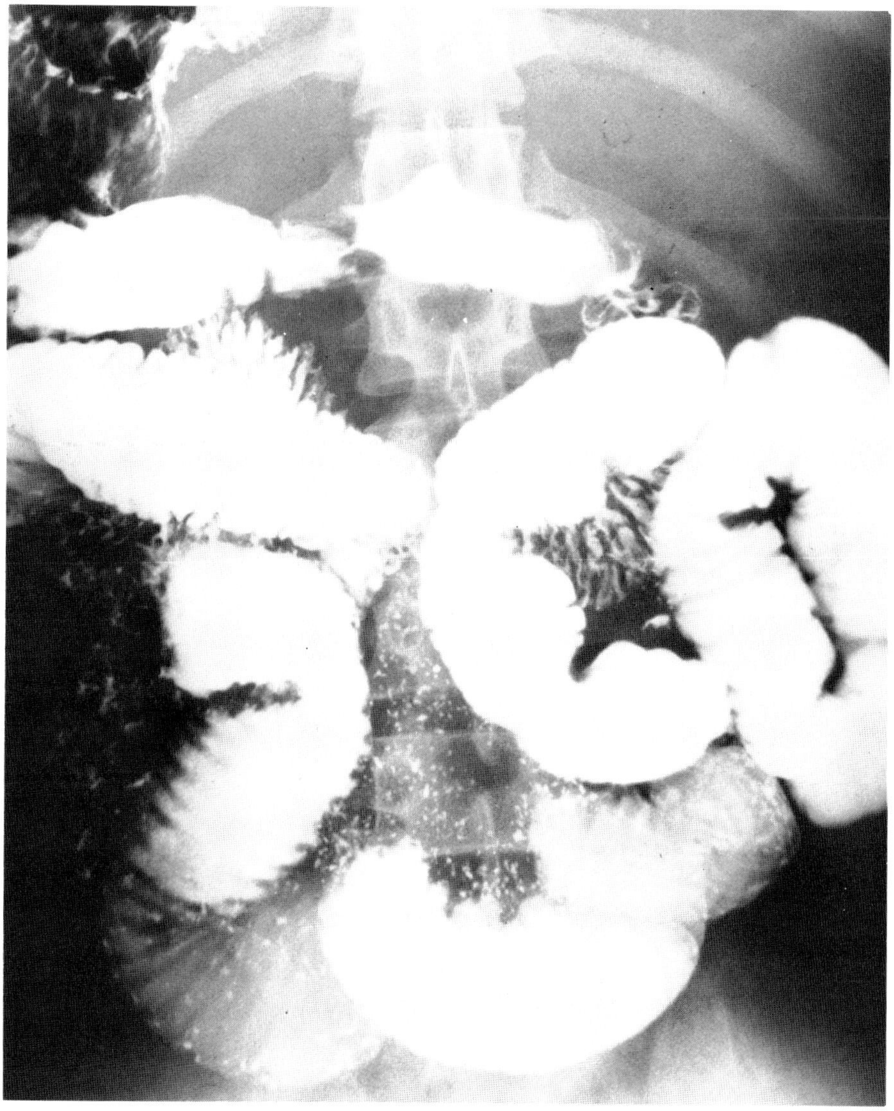

**Fig. 8-1.** X ray picture of the small intestine in a patient with primary intestinal lymphangiectasia showed thickening of Kerckring's folds and dilatation of bowel lumen.

phatic vessels of the intestinal mucosa and excessive enteric loss of plasma proteins.[2,3] Other important features are hypocalcemia, lymphedema, chyluria, chylothorax, chylous ascites, growth retardation, and lymphocytopenia.[20] This disorder is thought to be caused by mechanical and/or functional obstruction to the flow of lymph from the intestinal lymphatics to the junction of the thoracic duct and subclavian vein. In 1961, Waldmann et al[2] first demonstrated that by using intestinal biopsy and lymphangiography hypoalbuminemia in patients with idiopathic hypoproteinemia was due to the enteric loss of plasma protein and associated with dilated and presumably blocked lymphatic vessels of the intestinal mucosa.

Primary intestinal lymphangiectasia is the manifestation of a generalized disorder in the development of the lymphatic system, which may occur congenitally or by acquired mechanisms. Early onset of peripheral lymphatic edema is often seen in patients with primary intestinal lymphangiectasia. The exact cause

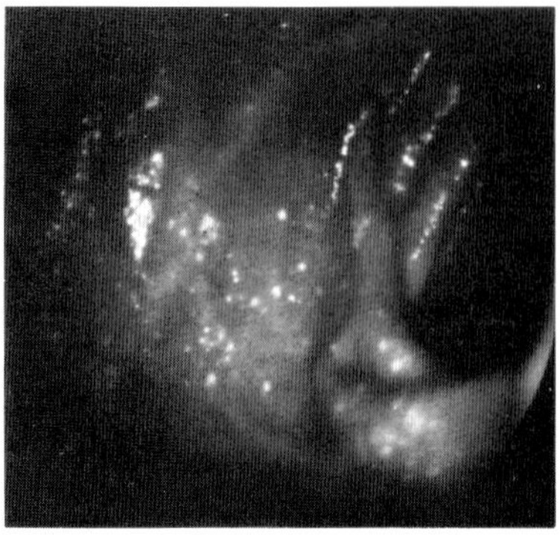

**Fig. 8-2.** Jejunal endoscopic picture showed scattered white spots and white villi in the jejunal mucosa.

of the lymphatic abnormality, however, has not been fully elucidated. Secondary intestinal lymphangiectasia may occur by obstruction of intestinal and/or mesenteric lymphatic channels and by disturbed drainage of intestinal lymph into the venous system. In case of cardiac diseases such as constrictive pericarditis, it seems that the drainage of lymph into the venous system is deranged by an increased venous pressure.[21]

Thickening of the Kerckring's folds, dilution of the barium column, dilatation of bowel lumen and mucosal nodularity or punctate lucency are the major abnormal findings in the radiographic examination of the small bowel in patients with small intestinal lymphangiectasia (Fig. 8-1).[22] Thickening of the Kerckring's folds appears to be due to the presence of edema and dilated lymphatics in the intestinal mucosa and submucosa. Upper GI X-ray series are usually normal. Diffuse nodular thickening of the intestinal wall with no adenopathy or hepatosplenomegaly and ascites with occasional coexistence of pleural effusion have been noted in body computed tomography (CT) examination in a patient with primary intestinal lymphangiectasia.[23] These small intestinal X-ray and CT findings, however, are not specific for this disorder.

Lymphangiographic studies performed by Kinmonth's method[24] have revealed a variety of abnormalities in intestinal lymphangiectasia. These abnormalities are divided into two conditions; hyperplasia and hypoplasia. Lymphatic blockage at the level of the cisterna chyli, tortuous lymphatic channels, hypoplasia of abdominal lymph nodes in the paraaortic area and obstruction of the thoracic duct may be observed.

With the development of small intestinal endoscopy, it has recently become possible to observe the jejunal mucosa that is 10–40 cm distal to the ligamentum of Treitz.[25] The major small intestinal endoscopic findings in patients with intestinal lymphangiectasia are scattered white spots, white villi and chyle-like substance covering the mucosa.[26] Tiny scattered white spots with a clear margin can be noted on the duodenal and jejunal mucosa (Fig. 8-2). The number of spots observed varied in each case. Those spots are not stained with methylene blue, by which normal intestinal epithelial cells are stained. In addition, they can not be washed or rubbed away. When a magnifying endoscope, Olympus GIF-HM, with the maximal magnifying power of 35 times was used to observe the intestinal mucosa, two types of distribution of white spots, (i.e., solitary or grouped type), were noted (Fig. 8-3). In addition, some villi with white spots were distended and showed an appearance like crabbed fingers. Dissecting microscopic study of biopsied specimens revealed the presence of milky white spots in the stroma of the villi. Further histopathological study demonstrated that the formation of white spots appeared to be due to the markedly dilated lymphatics. Scanning electron microscopic study in Norwegian Lundehunds (puffin dogs) with intestinal lymphangiectasia revealed that some villi were markedly expanded and appeared as coalesced pyramid-shaped structures with a crater-shaped lesion at the villous tip.[27]

In cases of intestinal lymphangiectasia, the degree of dilatation of intestinal lymphatics varies considerably (Fig. 8-4). Dilated lymphatics can be observed in the lamina propria, submucosa and also in the serosa. They may be noted in many villi in some cases or in others only in a few. Edema was observed

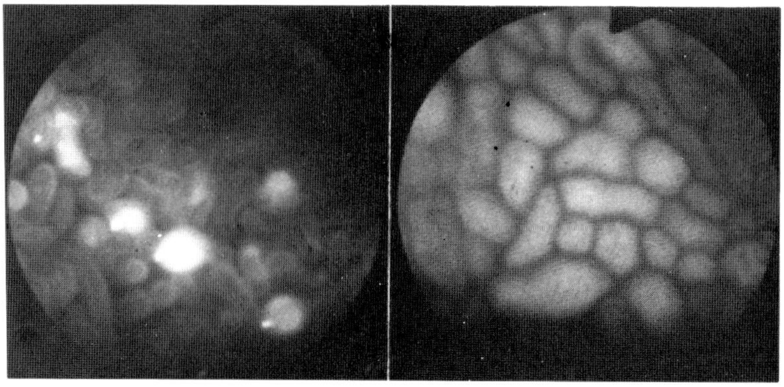

**Fig. 8-3.** Magnified endoscopic picture revealed each of the mucosal villi white spot (left) and white villi (right) in back of the mucosal villi.

in upper portion of the lamina propria between the epithelial lining and dilated lymphatics (Fig. 8-5). Electron microscopic study revealed that the cavity of the dilated lymphatic vessel was filled with chylomicrons and precipitated lymphprotein (Fig. 8-6). Pinocytotic vesicles containing chylomicron-like substance were noted in the endothelial cells of lymphatic vessel (Fig. 8-7). When the cavity was filled with chylomicron-like substance and precipitated lymphprotein, the thickness of the endothelial cells of intestinal lymphatics in the lamina propria decreased. According to Dobbins, the basal lamina supporting cells, collagen fibers around the lymphatic endothelium and endothelial fibrils were more prominently observed in intestinal lymphangiectasia than in normal subjects (Fig. 8-8).[28]

Since the electron microscopic study demonstrated that the interepithelial spaces and

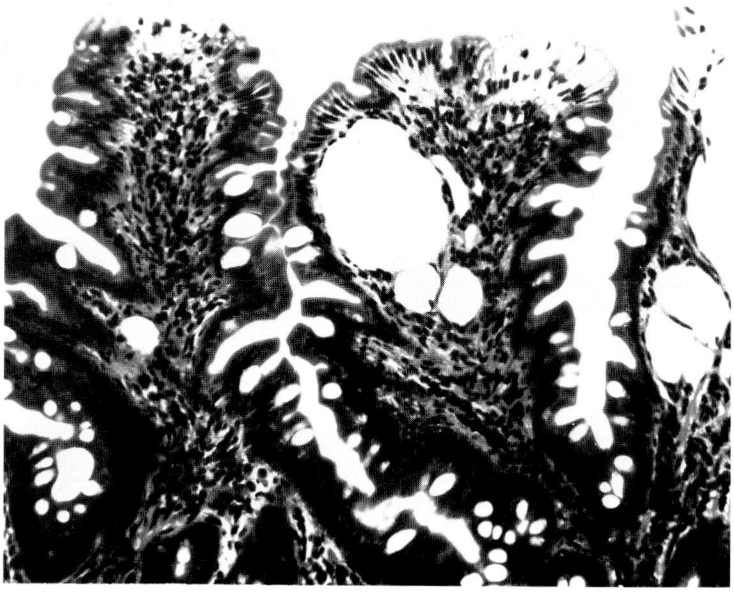

**Fig. 8-4.** Microscopic picture showed markedly dilated lymphatics in the lamina propria of the jejunal mucosa. ×100, H & E

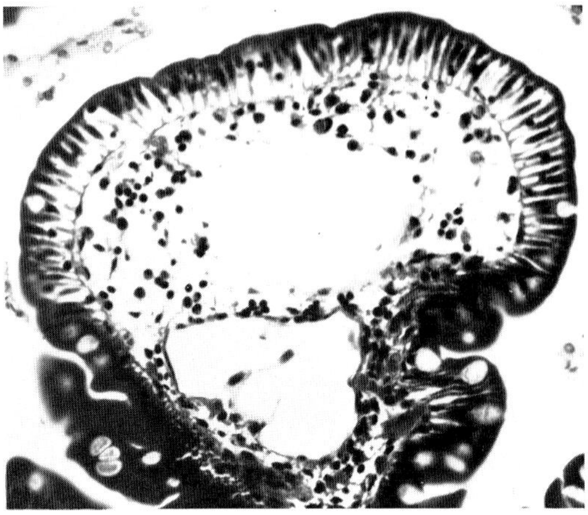

**Fig. 8-5.** Microscopic picture showed marked edema in the subepithelial space and dilatation of interepithelial spaces. ×200, H & E

stroma were filled with chylomicrons (Figs. 8-9, 8-10) and that the lipoprotein-like substance can be observed in the cavities of endoplasmic reticulum and Golgi apparatus (Fig. 8-11), it is likely that the white color of the villi is due to the mucosal deposition of fats. In the upper portions of villi, a gap between the basal portions of epithelial cells has been observed. Although some enterocytes had prominent microvilli, those of other cells were blunted and decreased in number.[29] Vacuoles containing protein-like material and fat were observed in the cytoplasm of enterocytes and at the intercellular space.

Intestinal lymphangiectasia is frequently seen among Norwegian Lundehunds.[27] In these dogs, vacuolated epithelial cells in the

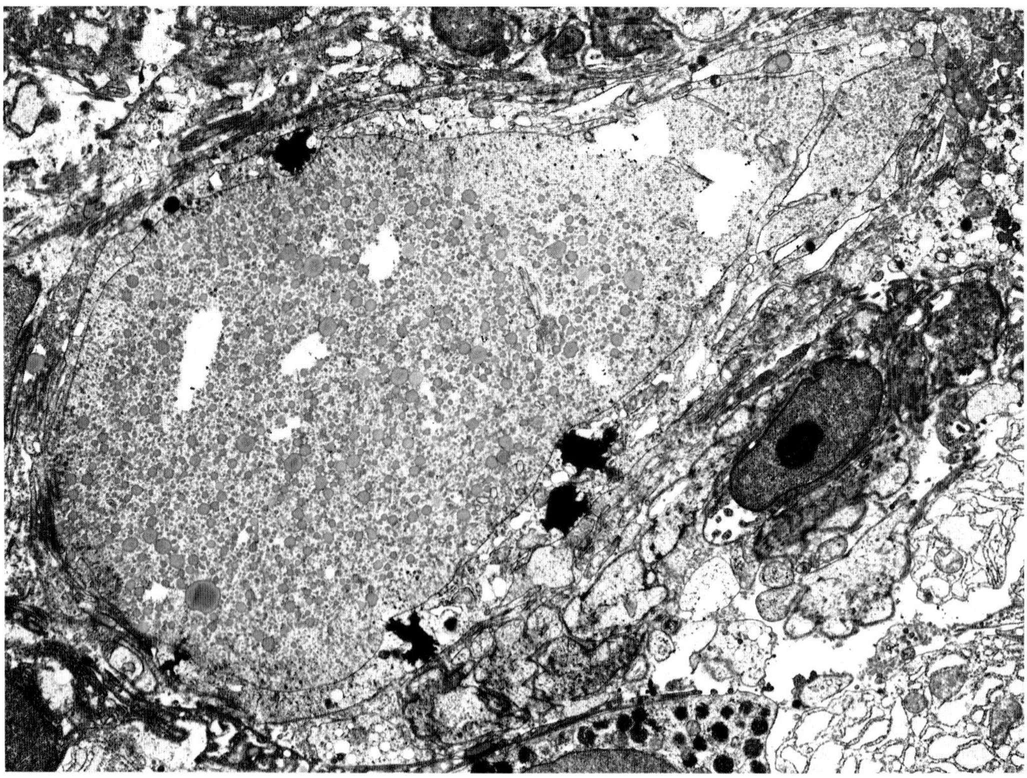

**Fig. 8-6.** Electron microscopic picture showing large cavity of a dilated lymphatic vessel which was filled with chylomicrons and precipitated lymph proteins. ×5,500

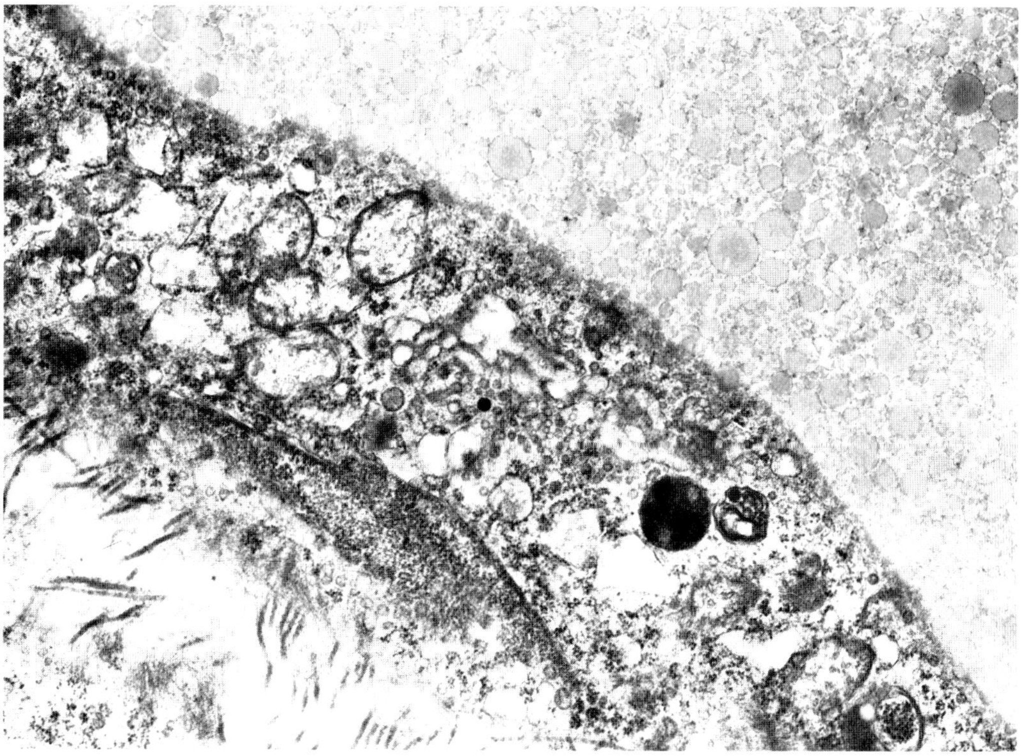

**Fig. 8-7.** Electron microscopic picture of a lymphatic vessel showed many pinocytotic vesicles containing chylomicron-like substances in its endothelial cells. ×21,000

proximal small intestine have been shown to contain fat detected by oil red staining. The separation of the epithelial cells from the tip of the villi accompanied by a bulging of the epithelial layer is likely to be due to the subepithelial fluid accumulation. Moreover, a snow-white duodenum or white villi was observed in a patient with hypobetalipoproteinemia[30] and in a patient with Whipple's disease.[31]

The diagnosis of intestinal lymphangiectasia is usually established by demonstrating the presence of dilated lymphatics in the intestinal biopsy specimen. Care should be taken, however, since the marked dilatation of intestinal lymphatic vessels has been observed in patients with liver cirrhosis and Behçet's disease who do not exhibit protein-losing gastroenteropathy.[32] It seems important to prove directly the loss of plasma protein into the gut lumen, since it appears that the dilatation of lymphatic vessels of the small intestine is not a sufficient finding to indicate the presence of protein-losing enteropathy.

Chyle-like substances covering the surface of mucosa have been observed at endoscopy examination and surgery (Fig. 8-12) in some cases of intestinal lymphangiectasia. Electron microscopic study has revealed that this substance contains chylomicron-like substances (Fig. 8-13).

Since immunoglobulins and lymphocytes also may be lost into the gut lumen, it is possible that an immunodeficiency state is provoked in patients with this disorder. Serum immunoglobulin levels are decreased in approximately 50% of the patients. We have shown that the number of immunoglobulin-containing cells in the lamina propria of the upper jejunum is markedly decreased in patients with protein-losing enteropathy. Although a count of white blood cells in the peripheral blood is usually normal, the number

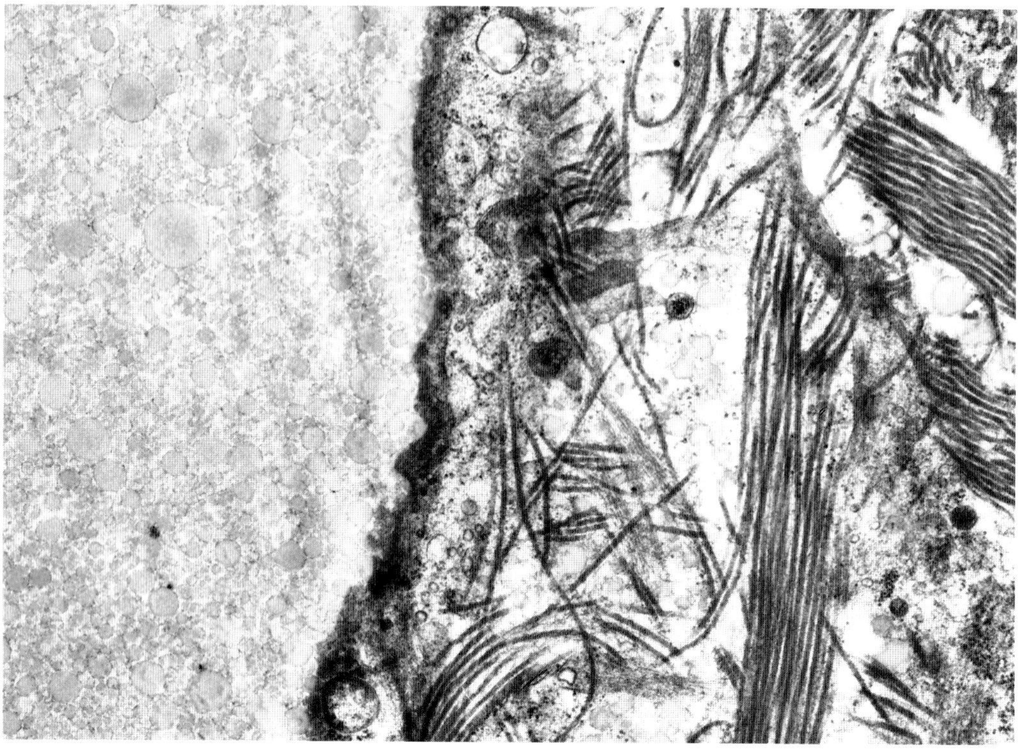

**Fig. 8-8.** Electron microscopic picture of a lymphatic vessel showed numerous collagen fibers around it. ×21,000

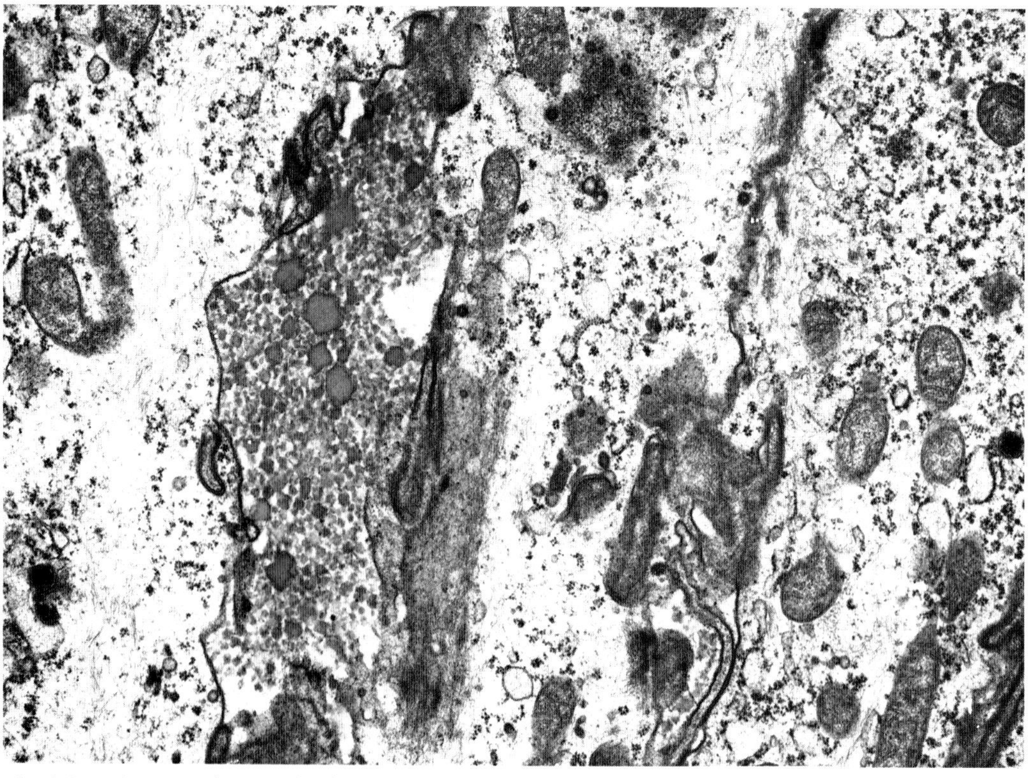

**Fig. 8-9.** Electron microscopic picture showing lipoprotein-like substances in the interepithelial spaces. ×21,000

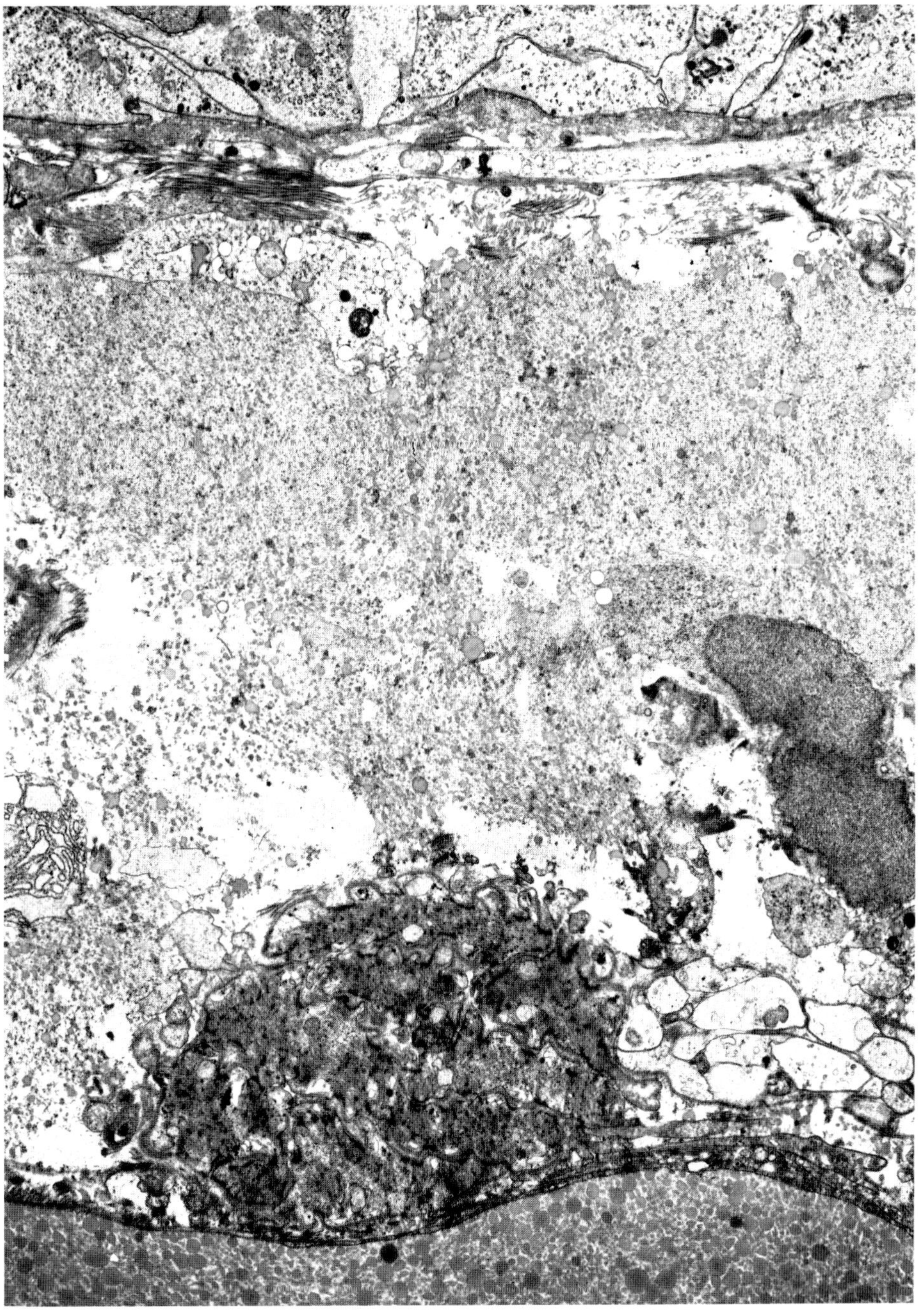

**Fig. 8-10.** Electron microscopic picture showing numerous chylomicrons and precipitated proteins in the lamina propria of villi of specimens obtained on fasting. ×5,400

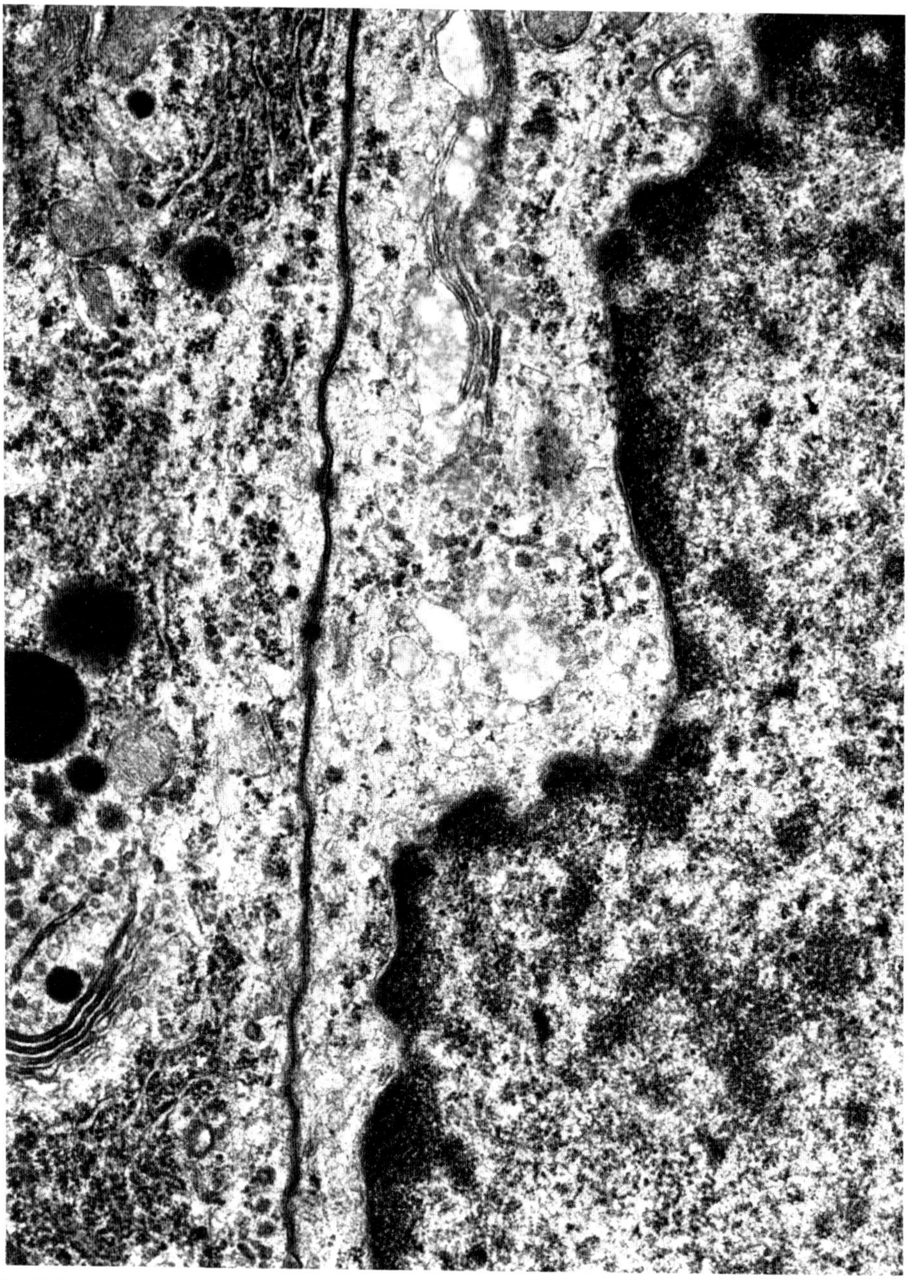

**Fig. 8-11.** Electron microscopic picture showing lipoprotein-like substances in endoplasmic reticulum and Golgi apparatus. Specimens were obtained in fasting state. ×25,000

of lymphocytes is markedly decreased in many cases. When the subpopulation of lymphocytes is examined, it has been observed that T-cells are decreased, with a relative increase of B-cells (Fig. 8-14). In addition, allergy to skin test antigens and impaired homograft rejection are often noted in patients with intestinal lymphangiectasia.[20,33]

The exact mechanism of the excessive enteric loss of plasma protein in this disease has not been fully elucidated. It is likely that an increased hydrostatic pressure and lymphatic dilatation resulting from the functional or mechanical obstruction of lymph flow may cause a rupture of lacteals concomitant with a loss of chyle into the intestinal lumen.[34] Although this concept is supported by lymphangiographic and endoscopic findings, direct evidence to confirm this hypothesis is not available. According to Landsverk et al,[27] the alteration in the subepithelial hydrostatic tissue pressure may be more important than the mechanism stated above, since an increased tissue pressure may affect the paracellular shunt pathway and permeability of tight junctions. It is thought, however, at this time, that the cellular route is an important pathway for the loss of plasma protein, since epithelial cells have been shown to contain a large number of vacuoles filled with protein-like substance and fat in their cytoplasm.

Low-fat diet is usually effective in treating intestinal lymphangiectasia. This is probably due to a decrease in the pressure within the intestinal lymphatics, since it has been shown that the absorption of long-chain triglycerides increases the flow of intestinal lymph. Medium-chain triglycerides, which are transported to the portal vein, are a good substitute for long-chain triglycerides. A specific drug to treat this disease is not available. However, administration of steroids may be effective in certain cases. Surgical treatment is of limited value, although lymph-enteric fistulas may be resected and lymphatic-venous anastomosis may decrease the pressure within intestinal lymphatics. In cases of secondary intestinal lymphangiectasia, specific treatment should be directed at the primary disease.

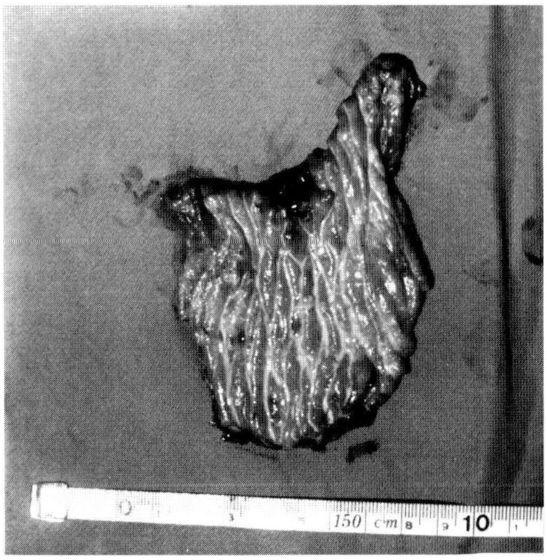

**Fig. 8-12.** Gross picture of resected specimens obtained from a patient with primary intestinal lymphangiectasia. Milky white material covered the surface of the small intestinal mucosa.

## Intestinal Lymphangiectasia of the Large Intestine.

To date, only a few cases of lymphangiectasia of the colon associated with protein-losing enteropathy have been reported by Schaefer et al[35] in 1968, by Ivey et al[36] in 1969, by Griffen et al[37] in 1972, and by Kingham et al[38] in 1982. Cardinal symptoms of this disorder are watery diarrhea, weight loss and edema. Recently we have observed a case of colonic lymphangiectasia with enteric protein loss.[39] In this case, however, edema was not evident for 17 years. Although the mechanism of enteric loss of plasma proteins in this disorder has not been fully understood, it has been shown that the effect of partial colectomy is dramatic in all reported cases. It appears that the treatment and prognosis of this disease are considerably different from those of small intestinal lymphangiectasia.

Slightly different histopathological findings have been obtained in each case. The gross specimens had a pale, glistening and ulcer-free mucosa that contained clear fluid when cut. In other cases, multiple sessile polyps

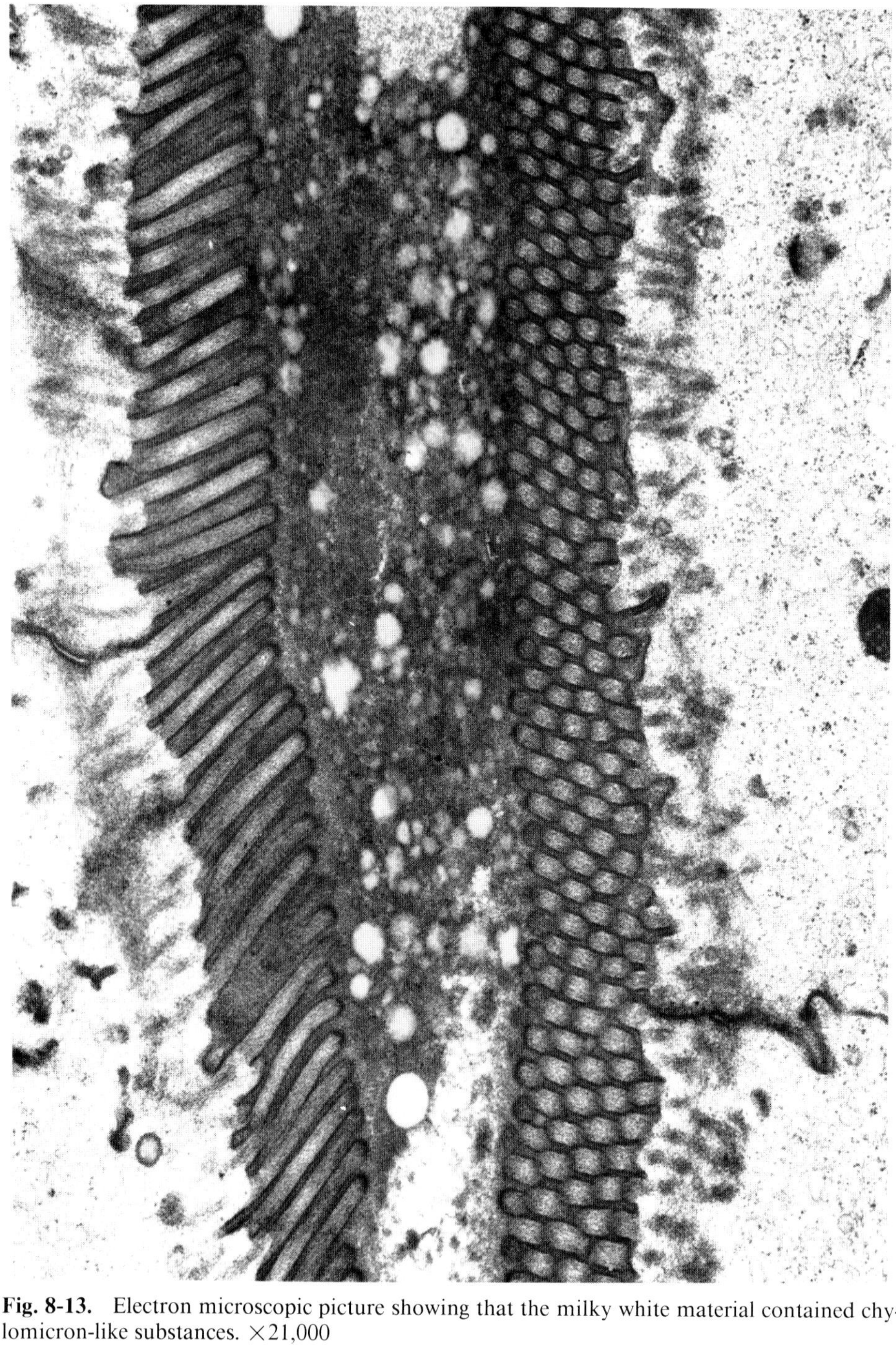

**Fig. 8-13.** Electron microscopic picture showing that the milky white material contained chylomicron-like substances. ×21,000

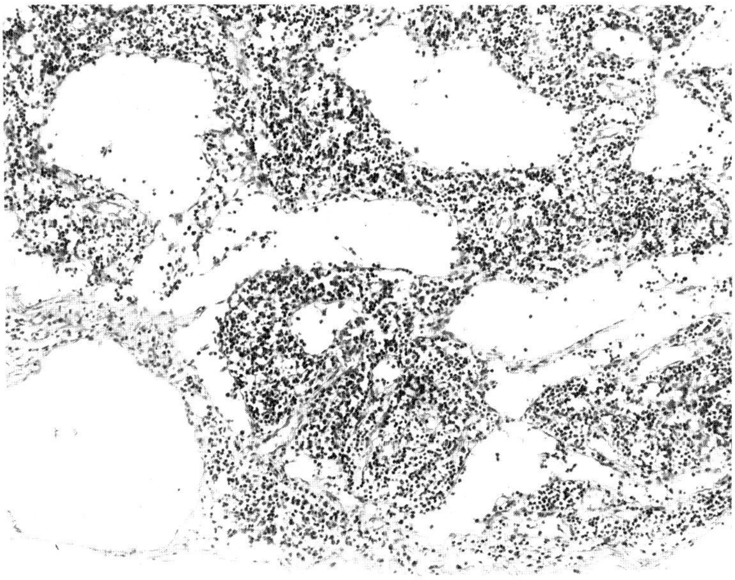

**Fig. 8-14.** Mesenteric lymph node obtained from a patient with protein-losing enteropathy. Note that paracortical areas (T cell areas) were depleted of lymphocytes. ×100, H & E

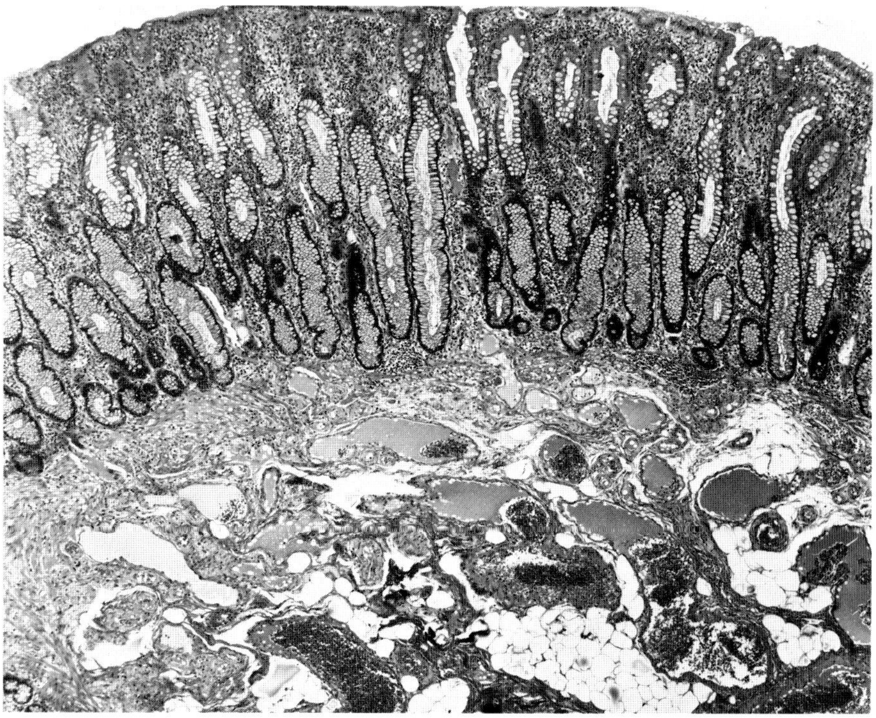

**Fig. 8-15.** Microscopic picture of resected specimen from a patient with intestinal lymphangiectasia of the large intestine which showed dilated lymphatic vessels in the submucosa and muscularis mucosae. ×40, H & E

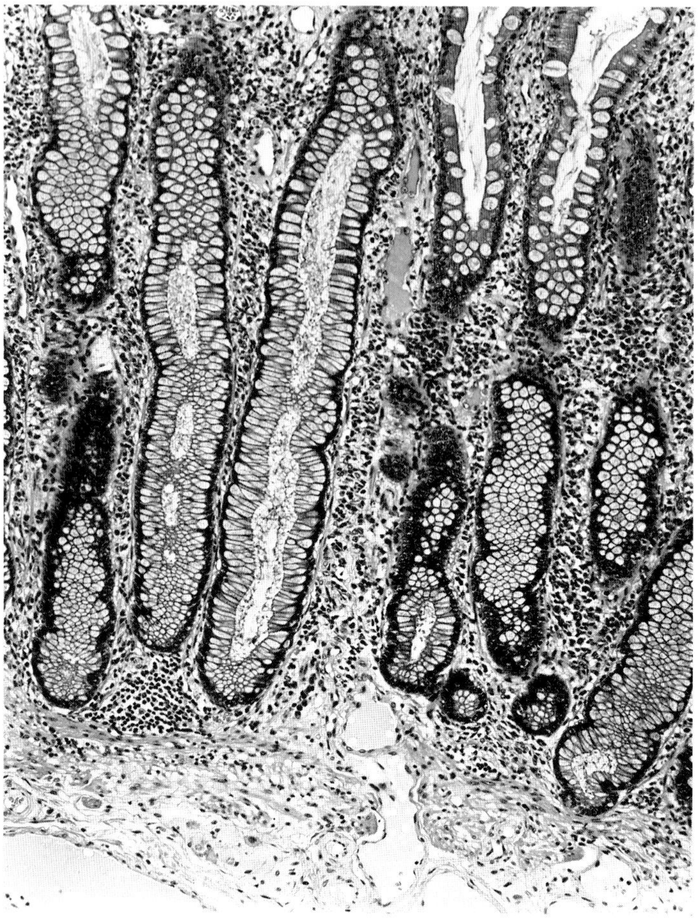

**Fig. 8-16.** Microscopic picture of lymphangiectasia of the large intestine showing the high location of lymphatics in the lamina propria of the colon. ×100, H & E

were observed in the rectosigmoid area by colonoscopy. Scattered white spots, white villi, and chyle-like substance covering the mucosa, which can be observed in small intestinal lymphangiectasia, are not found in colonic lymphangiectasia. This is probably because fat absorption is not taking place in the colon. Under microscopic examination, commonly observed findings were generalized edema and dilated lymphatic vessels in the submucosa and muscularis mucosae (Fig. 8-15). It has been reported that normally lymphatics are not present in the colonic mucosa except in the lowermost portion next to the muscularis mucosae.[40] In our case, however, the lymphatics could be observed in the higher portion of lamina propria of the colon (Fig. 8-16). Electron microscopic study revealed that there was a dilated lymphatic-like vessel in the lamina propria of the colonic mucosa (Fig. 8-17). There was, however, no chylomicron-like substance except for precipitated lymph protein in its cavity. This finding may support the basic lesion of protein-losing enteropathy.

Schaefer et al[35] observed a fair amount of clear fluid covering the diseased colonic mucosa but failed to detect significant amounts

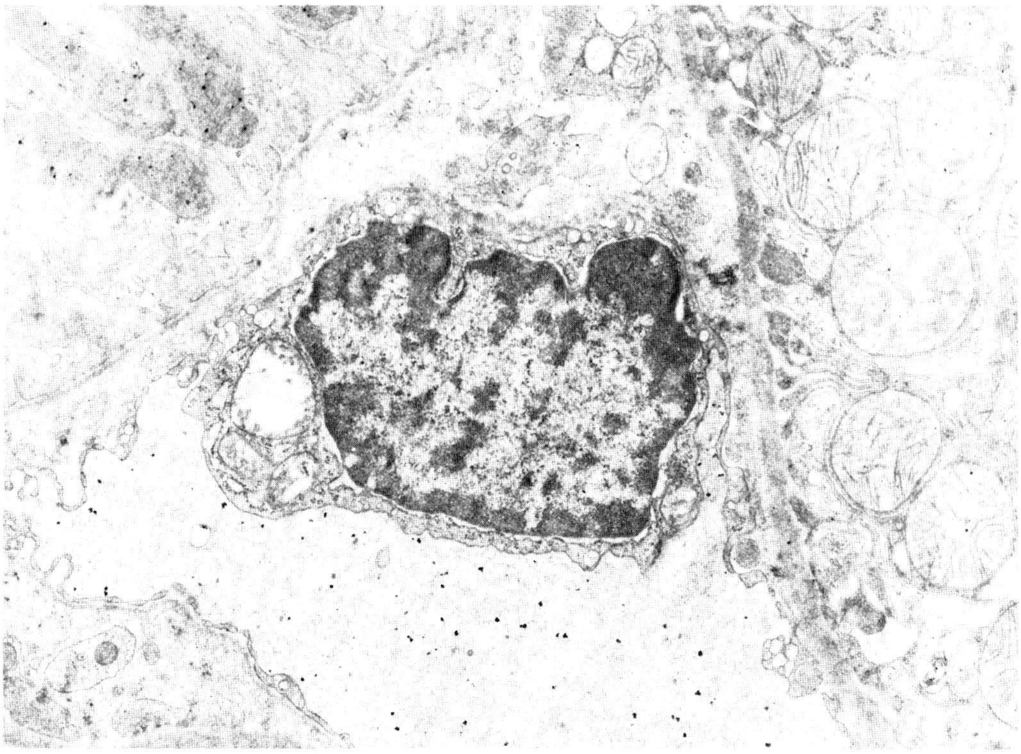

**Fig. 8-17.** Electron microscopic picture revealed a lymphatic-like vessel in the lamina propria of the colonic mucosa. ×7,000

of protein. Analysis of rectal fluid in our case revealed that the proteins in the fluid were both qualitatively and quantitatively similar to those in the patient's serum, suggesting leakage of serum protein into the colonic lumen.

## MÉNÉTRIER'S DISEASE

Giant folds of the stomach can be observed in various diseases including hypertrophic glandular gastritis, Ménétrier's disease, Zollinger-Ellison syndrome, and Bormann type IV gastric cancer.

Diffuse thickening of the gastric wall caused by marked proliferation of the mucosa was first described by Ménétrier[9] in 1888. A number of synonyms for this rare disorder have been used in the literature. These include giant hypertrophic gastritis,[41] tumor-simulating hypertrophic gastritis, gastric polyposis, cystic gastritis, and giant rugal hypertrophy (Fig. 8-18). Ménétrier described two different conditions in his original monograph, namely polyadenomes polypeux and polyadenomes en nappe (sheet-like polyadenomes).[42]

According to Schindler,[43] hypertrophic gastritis can be classified into three forms: chronic hypertrophic interstitial gastritis, chronic hypertrophic proliferative gastritis, and chronic hypertrophic glandular gastritis. The term giant hypertrophic gastritis has been used to describe a variety of microscopic pictures. Detailed histopathological characteristics varied among fourteen cases of giant hypertrophic gastritis reported by Butz.[44] Schindler emphasized that "Ménétrier's disease" should be used only for cases with destruction of glands, tubular overgrowth of

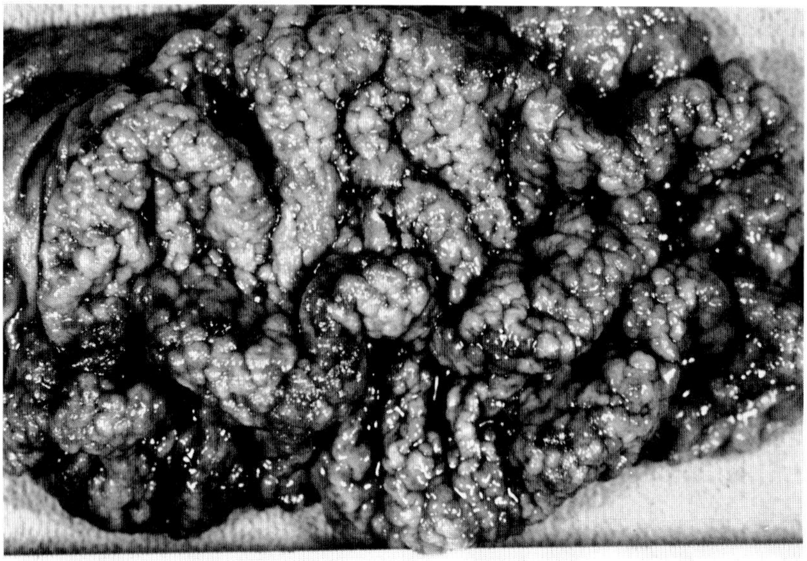

**Fig. 8-18.** Gross specimen of resected stomach obtained from a patient with Ménétrier's disease.

the surface epithelium, low acid output, and hypoproteinemia.

We have examined six patients with giant gastric folds and/or polyposis with protein-losing gastropathy. Gastroscopy revealed varying degrees of tortuous giant folds that were not obliterated by insufflation (Figs. 8-19, 8-20). The surface of the folds showed irregular and nodular appearances in some cases, but it was rather smooth in one patient. Large amounts of white sticky mucus covering the mucosa were noted in all patients. The active and continuous secretion of gastric juice, which we call hypersecretion (stalactite grotto phenomenon), was also observed.

The major histopathological finding in Ménétrier's disease is hyperplasia of the surface mucous cells, which causes deepening and

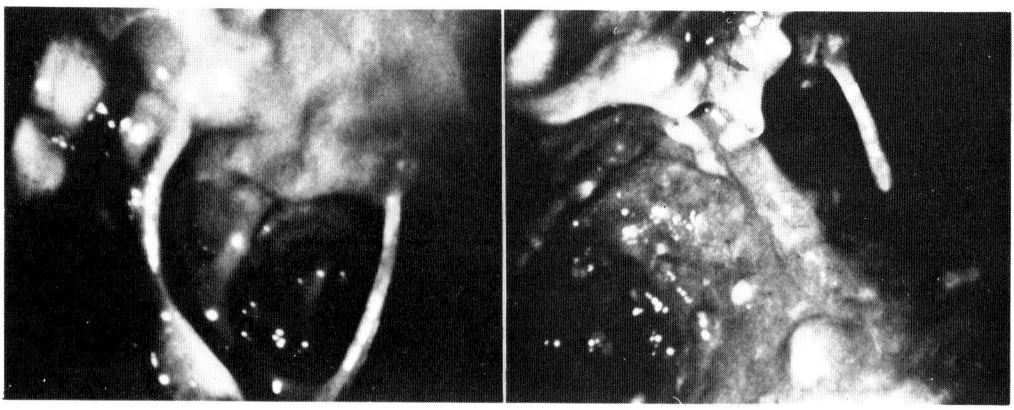

**Fig. 8-19.** Gastroendoscopy showing giant folds of the stomach. Note hypersecretion and mucus covering the mucosal surface.

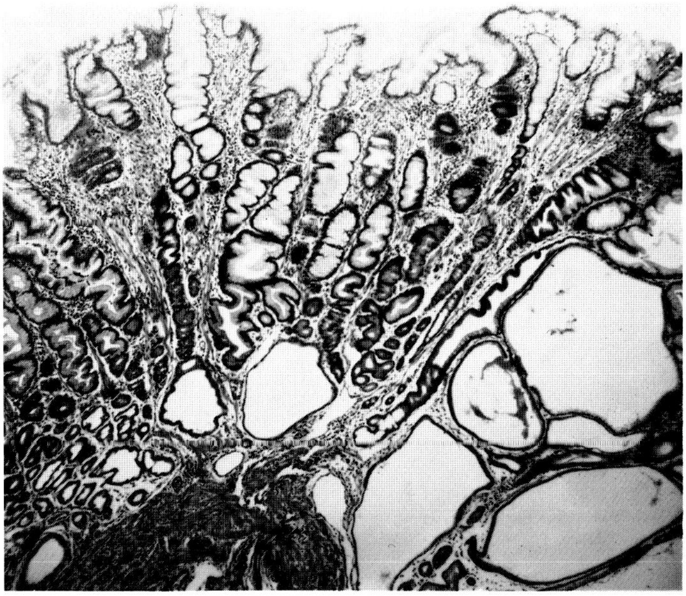

**Fig. 8-20.** Microscopic picture of the giant folds showed marked proliferation of surface epithelium like a corkscrew. Cystic dilatation of gastric glands was observed. ×40, H & E

tortuosity of the gastric pits. Microscopic pictures of giant folds can be classified into two categories. In one group, the decreased fundic glands with hyperplasia of surface mucous cells are noted. This is accompanied by a complete replacement of parietal cells by mucus-secreting cells (Fig. 8-20). Another type is a hyperplasia of the fundic glands.[45] A varied degree of cystic dilatation of the glands containing eosinophilic substance is observed. Surface epithelial cells of gastric pits secrete a large amount of mucus that is positive for double staining using alcian blue and PAS (Fig. 8-21). In some cases, moderate lymphangiectasia is seen in the submucosa and/or in the lamina propria.[46] It was observed electron microscopically that surface mucous cells were secreting mucous granules into the gastric lumen (Fig. 8-22).

In 1957, Citrin and coworkers[16] first demonstrated loss of plasma protein into the gastric lumen in a patient with giant hypertrophy of gastric mucosa. Although many routes for loss of plasma protein have been postulated in protein-losing gastroenteropathy, the exact

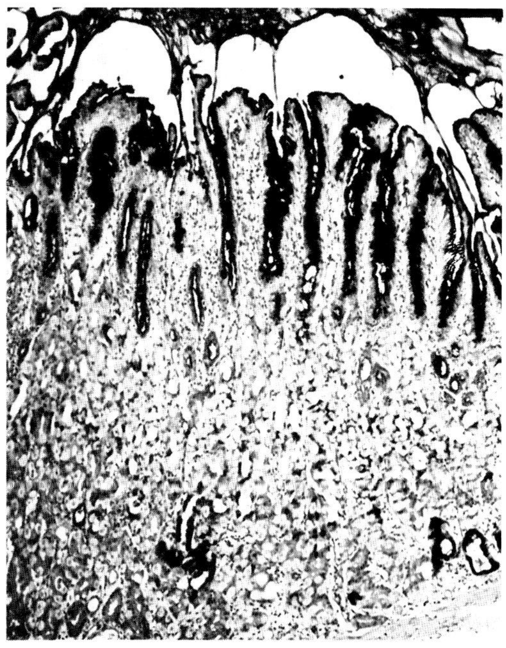

**Fig. 8-21.** Microscopic picture of gastric giant folds stained with Alcian-blue and PAS showed hyperplasia of mucin-secreting cells and a large amount of mucus. ×120, AB-PAS

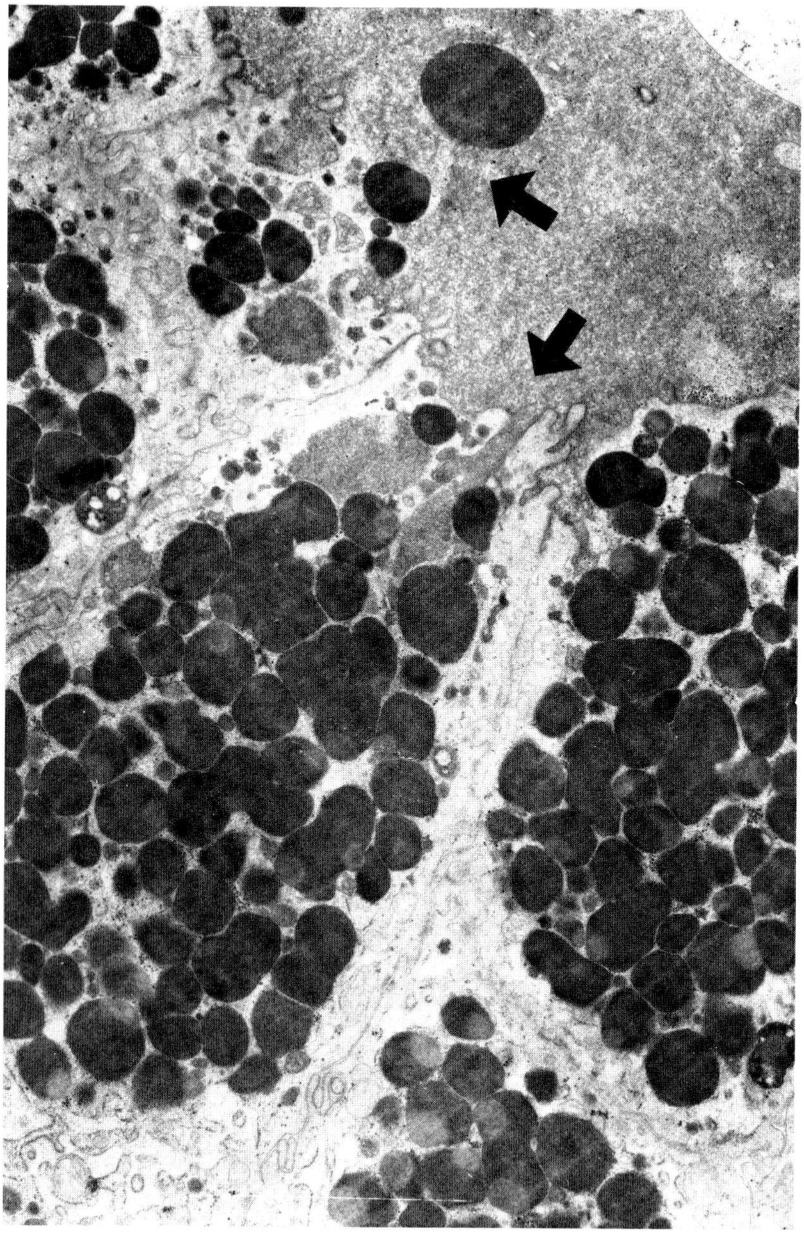

**Fig. 8-22.** Electron microscopic picture showing that surface mucous cells were secreting their mucus granules into the gastric lumen (arrows). ×3,000

pathway of protein loss through the gastric mucosa has not been clarified. According to Lev and Brus,[47] the transcellular pathway may be a major route for transmucosal efflux of plasma protein, since many intracellular vacuoles containing protein could be observed histochemically in mucosal biopsy specimens obtained from patients with protein-losing gastroenteropathy. However, the importance of an intercellular pathway has been emphasized in experimental protein-losing gastropathy.[48]

In seven patients with hypertrophic gastropathy, Kelly and coworkers performed gastric perfusion and electron microscopic study attempting to elucidate the route of protein loss.[49] Under electron microscopy, tight junctions appeared to be wider than normal in all patients. In addition, acute administration of propantheline bromide reduced leakage of albumin into the gastric lumen and decreased the width of tight junctions. Another antisecretory agent, cimetidine, failed to demonstrate a consistent effect on protein loss and on the width of tight junctions. However, administration of ranitidine, a histamine $H_2$ receptor antagonist, significantly reduced the gastric protein loss in a few patients with Ménétrier's disease.[50] These results indicate that the paracellular pathway through tight junctions plays an important role in transmucosal efflux of plasma protein. The coexistence of a transcellular pathway, however, cannot be ruled out.

Therapy of hypertrophic gastropathy is still controversial. Total gastrectomy has been reported to be very effective, and an increase in serum albumin level is observed after surgery.[51] Long term administration of anticholinergic agents appeared to be effective for the protein-losing gastropathy.[52]

## CRONKHITE-CANADA SYNDROME

In Cronkhite-Canada syndrome,[53] the extensive polyposis in the stomach and intestine may be involved, with ectodermal symptoms and hypoproteinemia due to gastrointestinal protein loss. Ectodermal symptoms are alopecia, hyperpigmentation, and dystrophy of the fingernails and toenails. The mechanism of the excessive protein loss in this syndrome is not known. The early reports by Cronkhite and Canada described the polyps as adenomatous in appearance, but recently these polyps were thought to be of the juvenile type. The polyps had cystically dilated glands and an extensive inflammatory reaction similar in some respects to juvenile polyps (Fig. 8-23).

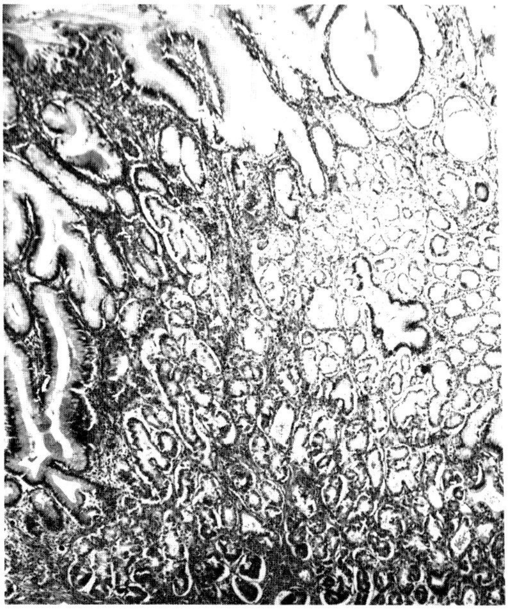

**Fig. 8-23.** Microscopic picture of gastric lesions from a patient with Cronkhite-Canada syndrome. ×120, H & E

Surface epithelial cells of gastric pits secrete a large amount of mucus that is positive with double staining using alcian blue and PAS (Fig. 8-24). One may think that the mechanism of gastric protein loss in this lesion is similar to that in Ménétrier's disease. The prognosis is poor, but several cases have been reported in which hyperalimentation and prednisolone were effective in clinical improvement.

## CONCLUSION

Protein-losing gastroenteropathy is caused by various gastrointestinal disorders. Examination of primary intestinal lymphangiectasia has clarified that the protein loss was caused by direct leakage of intestinal lymph into the intestinal lumen. An increased hydrostatic pressure within the lymphatics may be considered to cause a rupture of lecteals, or an alteration in the subepithelial hydrostatic tissue

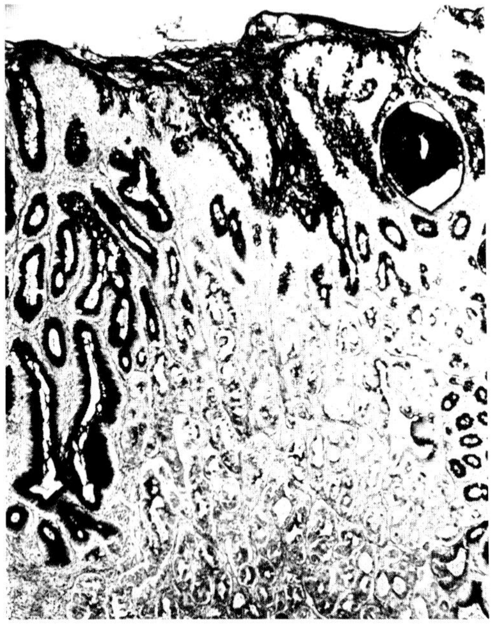

**Fig. 8-24.** Microscopic picture of the gastric lesions stained with Alcian-blue and PAS. ×120, AB-PAS

pressure, which may be more important. However, ultrastructural study in the present work suggested that the cellular route is an important pathway for the loss of plasma protein.

Rare related disorders, such as lymphangiectasia of the large intestine, Ménétrier's disease, and Cronkhite-Canada syndrome also were briefly described.

## REFERENCES


1. Strober W.: Protein-losing enteropathy, In Textbook of Gastroenterology Bouchier I.A.D., Allan R.N., Hodgson H.J.F., et al (eds.). Baillière Tindall, 1984, p 598
2. Waldmann T.A., Steinfeld J.L., Dutcher T.F., Davidson J.D., Gordon R.S.: The role of the gastrointestinal system in idiopathic hypoproteinemia. Gastroenterology **41**:197, 1961
3. Pomerantz M., Waldmann T.A.: Systemic lymphatic abnormalities associated with gastro-intestinal protein loss secondary to intestinal lymphangiectasia. Gastroenterology **45**:703, 1963
4. Petersen V.P., Hastrop J.: Protein-losing enteropathy in constrictive pericarditis, Acta Med Scand **173**:410, 1963
5. Beeker W.L., Busch H.J., Sylvester D.L.: Intestinal protein loss in Crohn's disease. Gastroenterology **62**:207, 1972
6. Chew C.K., Jarzylo S.V., Valberg L.S.: Idiopathic retroperitoneal fibrosis with protein-losing enteropathy and duodenal obstruction successfully treated with corticosteroids. Can Med Assoc J **95**:1183, 1963
7. Steinfield J.L., Davidson J.D., Gordon R.S. Jr., Greene F.E.: The mechanism of hypoproteinemia in patients with regional enteritis and ulcerative colitis. Am J Med **29**:405, 1960
8. Waldmann T.A., Broder S., Strober W.: Protein-losing enteropathies in malignancy. Ann New York Acad Sci **230**:306, 1974
9. Ménétrier P.: Des polyadenomes gastriques et de leurs rapports avec le cancer de l'estomac. Arch Physiol Normale Pathol **4**:32, 1888
10. Waldmann T.A., Wochner R.D., Laster L., Gordon R.S. Jr.: Allergic gastroenteropathy. A cause of excessive gastrointestinal protein loss. New Engl J Med **276**:761, 1967
11. Parkin R.A.: Protein-losing enteropathy in the sprue syndrome. Lancet **ii**:1366, 1968
12. King C.E., Toskes P.P.: Protein-losing enteropathy in the human and experimental rat blind-loop syndrome. Gastroenterology **80**:504, 1981
13. Kondo M., Bamba T., Hosokawa K., Hosoda S., Kawai K., Masuda M.: Tissue plasminogen activator in the pathogenesis of protein-losing gastroenteropathy. Gastroenterology **70**:1045, 1976
14. Wood J.G., Davenport H.W.: Measurement of canine gastric vascular permeability to plasma proteins in the normal and protein-losing states. Gastroenterology **82**:725, 1982
15. Tsuchiya M., Oshio C., Asakura H., Ishii H., Aoki I., Miyairi M.: Budd-Chiari syndrome associated with protein-losing enteropathy. Gastroenterology **75**:114, 1978
16. Citrin Y., Sterling K., Halsted J.A.: The mechanism of hypoproteinemia associated with giant hypertrophy of the gastric mucosa. N Engl J Med **257**:906, 1957
17. Gordon R.S.: Exudative enteropathy, Abnormal permeability of the gastrointestinal tract demonstrable with labelled P.V.P. Lancet **1**:325, 1959
18. Waldmann T.A., Wochner R.D., Strober W.: The role of the gastrointestinal tract in plasma protein metabolism studies with $^{51}$Cr-albumin. Am J Med **46**:775, 1969
19. Florent C., L'Hirondel C., Desmàzures C., Aymes C., Bernier J.J.: Intestinal clearance of $\alpha_1$-antitrypsin. A sensitive method for the detection of protein-losing enteropathy. Gastroenterology **81**:777, 1981
20. Strober W., Wochner R.D., Carbone P.P., Waldmann T.A.: Intestinal lymphangiectasia: a protein losing enteropathy with hypogammaglobulinemia, lymphopenia and impaired homograft rejection. J Clin Invest **46**:1643, 1967
21. Nelson D.L., Blaese R.M., Strober W., Bruce R.M., Waldmann T.A.: Constrictive pericarditis, intestinal lymphangiectasia, and reversible immunologic deficiency. J Pediatrics **86**:548, 1975
22. Vardy P.A., Lebenthal E., Schwachman H.: Intestinal lymphangiectasia, A reappraisal. Pediatrics **55**:842, 1975
23. Fakhri A., Fishman E.K., Jones B., Kuhajda F., Siegelman S.S.: Primary intestinal lympangiectasia: clinical and CT findings. J Comput Assist Tomogr **9**:767, 1985

24. Kinmonth J.B., Taylor G.W., Harper R.K.: Lymphangiectasia lymphangiography: A technique for its clinical use in the lower limb. Br Med J **1**:940, 1955
25. Morishita T., Hibi T., Asakura H., Tsuchiya M., Pescante M., Uylangco C.: Endoscopy of the jejunal mucosa in human cholera. Gastrointest Endosc **24**:284, 1978
26. Asakura H., Miura S., Morishita T., Aiso S., Tanaka T., Kitahora T., Tsuchiya M., Enomoto Y., Watanabe Y.: Endoscopic and histopathological study on primary and secondary intestinal lymphangiectasia. Dig Dis Sci **26**:423, 1982
27. Landsverk T., Gamlem H.: Intestinal lymphangiectasia in the Lundehund. Acta Path Microbiol Immunol Scand (Sect A)**92**:353, 1984
28. Dobbins W.O.: Electron microscopic study of the intestinal mucosa in intestinal lymphangiectasia. Gastroenterology **51**:1004, 1966
29. Bujanover Y., Liebman W.M., Goodman J.R., Thaler M.M.: Primary intestinal lymphangiectasia. Case report with radiological and ultrastructual study. Digestion **21**:107, 1981
30. Mitchell C.J., Scott B.B., Bullen A.W., Lonowsky M.S.: Snow-white duodenum. A new endoscopic sign in a patient with hypobetalipoproteinemia. Gastrointest Endosc **24**:123, 1978
31. Volpicelli N.A., Salyer W.R., Milligan F.D., Bayless T.M., Yardley J.H.: The endoscopic appearance of the duodenum in Whipple's disease. Johns Hopkins Med J **138**:19, 1976
32. Asakura H., Morita A., Morishita T., Tsuchiya M., Watanabe Y., Enomoto Y.: Histopathological and electron microscopic studies of lymphangiectasia of the small intestine in Behçet's disease. Gut **14**:196, 1973
33. Weiden P.L., Blaese R.M., Strober W., Block B.J., Waldmann T.A.: Impaired lymphocyte transformation in intestinal lymphangiectasia: Evidence for at least two functionally distinct lymphocyte populations in man. J Clin Invest **51**:1319, 1972
34. Mistilis S.P., Skyring A.P., Stephen D.D.: Intestinal lymphangiectasia: Mechanism of enteric loss of plasma-protein and fat. Lancet, **1**:77, 1965
35. Schaefer J.W., Griffen W.O., Dubilier L.D.: Colonic lymphangiectasis associated with a potassium depletion syndrome. Gastroenterology **55**:515, 1968
36. Ivey K., DenBesten L., Kent T.H., Clifton J.A.: Lymphangiectasia of the colon with protein loss and malabsorption. Gastroenterology **57**:709, 1969
37. Griffen W.O., Belin R.P., Furman R.W., Lieber A., Schaefer J.W., Dubilier L.D.: Colonic lymphangiectasia: Report of two cases. Dis Col Rect **15**:49, 1972
38. Kingham J.G.C., Moriarty K.J., Furness M., Levison D.A.: Lymphangiectasia of the colon and small intestine. Brit J Radiol **55**:774, 1982
39. Asakura H., Tsuchiya M., Katoh S., Kobayashi K., Yonei Y., Yoshida T., Hamada Y., Miura S., Morita A., Kuramochi S., Teramoto T.: Pathological findings of lymphangiectasia of the large intestine in a patient with protein-losing enteropathy. Gastroenterology **91**:719, 1986
40. Fenoglio C.M., Kaye G.I., Lane N.: Distribution of human colonic lymphatics in normal, hyperplastic, and adenomatous tissue. Gastroenterology **64**:51, 1973
41. Fieber S.S.: Hypertrophic gastritis. Report of two cases and analysis of fifty pathologically verified cases from the literature. Gastroenterology **28**:39, 1955
42. Palmer D.: What Ménétrier really said. Gastrointest Endosc **15**:83, 1968
43. Schindler R.: On hypertrophic glandular gastritis, hypertrophic gastropathy, and parietal cell mass. Gastroenterology **45**:77, 1963
44. Butz W.C.: Giant hypertrophic gastritis. A report of fourteen cases. Gastroenterology **39**:183, 1960
45. Brooks A.M., Isenberg J., Goldstein H.: Giant thickening of the gastric mucosa with acid hypersecretion and protein losing gastropathy. Gastroenterology **58**:73, 1970
46. Miura S., Asakura H., Tsuchiya M.: Lymphatic abnormalities in protein-losing gastropathy, especially in Ménétrier's disease. Angiology **32**:345, 1981
47. Lev R., Brus I.: Morphological and histochemical demonstration of protein in gastric surface epithelium in protein losing gastropathies. Am J Dig Dis **16**:589, 1971
48. Munro D.R.: Route of protein losing during a model protein losing gastropathy in dogs. Gastroenterology **66**:960, 1974
49. Kelly D.G., Miller L.J., Malagelada J-R., Huizenga K.A., Markowitz H.: Giant hypertrophic gastropathy (Ménétrier's disease): Pharmacologic effects on protein leakage and mucosal ultrastructure. Gastroenterology **83**:58, 1982
50. Reinhart W.H., Weigand K., Kappeler M., Roesler H., Halter F.: Comparison of gastrointestinal loss of alpha-1-antitrypsin and chromium-51-albumin in Ménétrier's disease and the influence of ranitidine. Digestion **26**:192, 1983
51. Balfour D.C., Hightower N.C., Gambill E.E., Waugh J.M., Dockerty M.B.: Giant hypertrophy of the gastric rugae (Ménétrier's disease) associated with severe hypoproteinemia relieved only by total gastrectomy: report of case. Gastroenterology **16**:773, 1950
52. Smith R.L., Powell D.W.: Prolonged treatment of Ménétrier's disease with an oral anticholinergic drug. Gastroenterology **74**:903, 1978
53. Cronkhite L.W., Canada W.J.: Generalized gastrointestinal polyposis: An unusual syndrome of polyposis, pigmentation, alopecia and onychotrophia. N Engl J Med **252**:1011, 1955

# 9

# Secretory IgA and Mucosal Immune Responses

H. Nagura M.D.
Y. Sumi M.D.

Mucosal immunity is characterized predominantly by a secretory antibody response, involving immunoglobulins of the IgA class. They provide an immunological barrier to foreign matter by preventing absorption of such materials into the mucosal epithelium and penetration into the body. The humoral responses in nonmucosal sites are largely of the IgG class. The cell-mediated immune mechanism is also distinctive in mucosal and nonmucosal lymphoid organs. During the past decade, significant advances have been made in understanding the mucosal immune system. Ontological and physiological relationships between immunocompetent cells in mucosal and nonmucosal sites have been characterized, and the postulation of a common mucosal immune system[1,2] involving the intestinal tract, biliary tract, mammary glands, salivary glands, lacrimal glands, and female genital tract has led to new insights.

The mucosal surface is exposed to a myriad of antigenic substances that have readily demonstrable immunostimulatory or immunomodulatory properties, such as microbes, chemicals, and food, and contact between these antigens, and the mucosal immunological apparatus initiates a diverse series of immunologic events. These include the production of antibodies that are secreted into extracellular body fluids and, in striking contrast, induce hyporesponsiveness of certain nonmucosal (systemic) immunologic reactions.[3,4] The importance of the mucosal immune system in the host-environment interaction and in the pathogenesis of certain diseases of mucosal and nonmucosal tissues has received much appreciation in recent years. A deficiency in mucosal IgA, for example, can severely impair mucosal barrier function, resulting in uptake of noxious substances that could contribute to the pathogenesis of intestinal or systemic diseases.[5] In this review we have summarized the wealth of information about the mucosal immune system, with emphasis on the role of liver in the regulation of the immune responses involving IgA.

## PARTICIPATION OF SECRETORY IgA IN THE MUCOSAL IMMUNE SYSTEM IN THE NEONATE

IgG is the only class of antibodies in rat or mouse breast fluid to be transported intact into the offspring circulation across the intestine in substantial quantities, even though these fluids also contain IgA and IgM antibodies.[6,7] The transfer of IgG, however, is sharply limited in time to the first 18 to 21 days of life in the rat.[6,7] Colostrum IgG is

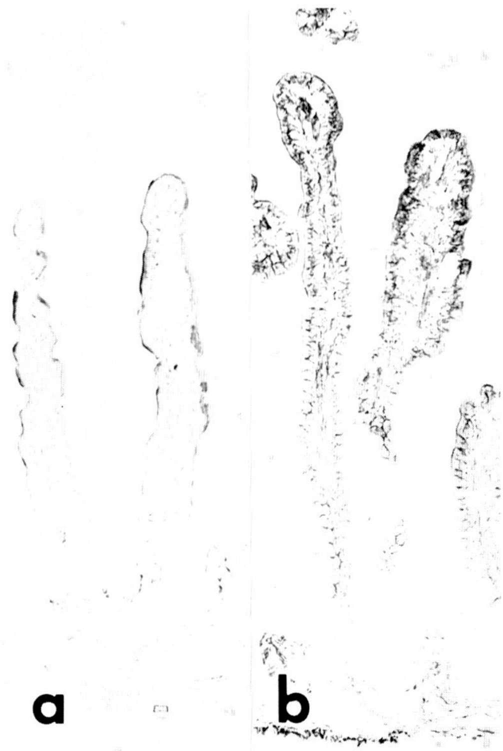


**Fig. 9-1.** Immunohistochemical localization of IgA (a) and IgG (b) in the proximal intestine of breast-fed neonatal rats. IgA is found on the surface of enterocytes, whereas IgG is localized on the basolateral plasma membranes in addition to the apical surface. No plasma cells are present in the lamina propria.

found in the lower portion of microvilli and intervening apical plasma membranes of proximal enterocytes of breast-fed neonatal rats (Figs. 9-1, 9-2), and is internalized and transported through the cells in cytoplasmic vesicles.[7,8] In the distal small intestine, however, IgG is found in cytoplasmic vacuoles of enterocytes without evidence of transference through the cells.[7,9] Luminal proteolysis is depressed at this age to give the absorptive epithelium in the proximal intestine a chance to remove intact IgG from the other milk proteins and for IgG to be transferred by receptor mediated endocytosis into the circulation. Large quantities of the intact maternal IgG in the circulation may provide passive systemic immunity for the neonates.

In these early days of life in the rat, neither IgA plasma cells in the lamina propria nor IgA in serum can be detected.[7] From the onset of suckling to some time between the 15th and 21st days of life, enterocytes in the proximal small intestine selectively bind colostral IgA (secretory IgA, sIgA) to their surface, and enterocytes in the distal small intestine nonselectively absorb and digest IgA.[7] In suckling calves and piglets, however, much IgA in colostrum is transported into the circulation during the first 24 hours of life, and in man a small amount of breast fluid IgA is transferred across enterocytes for 18 to 24 hours after birth.[10]

Studies of the antibodies in breast milk have shown secretory IgA antibodies against viruses, including polio virus and retrovirus, a series of microbial antigens, such as from E. coli, Salmonella O, Shigella and Vibrio cholerae, and various food proteins such as cow's milk.[11] It is probable that these secretory IgA antibodies on the surface of proximal enterocytes play important roles in the defense of the breast-fed baby against diarrheal infections. It is well documented that such infections are more common in artificially fed than in breast-fed infants.[12] An active response of sIgA antibodies to food proteins also seems to be important as an antigen-exclusion mechanism to prevent allergic diseases in infants.[13]

Breast milk contains many anti-infectious properties other than immunoglobulins, such as lactoferrin, lysozyme, phagocytes, and T- and B-lymphocytes.[12,14,15] When tested separately, lactoferrin or sIgA shows only slight bacteriostatic activity against commensal or enteropathogenic strains of E. coli.[16] Thus the bacteriostatic activity seems to be due to the combined effects of lactoferrin and sIgA, and it was proven that some amounts of lactoferrin are naturally bound to sIgA.[17] Phagocytes in breast milk are composed of lipid-laden neutrophils and macrophages, and they contain large amounts of sIgA. Recently the sIgA secretion from the phagocytes was proven to be initiated by surface membrane stimuli, and to play a role in the immunologic protection of the neonate.[18]

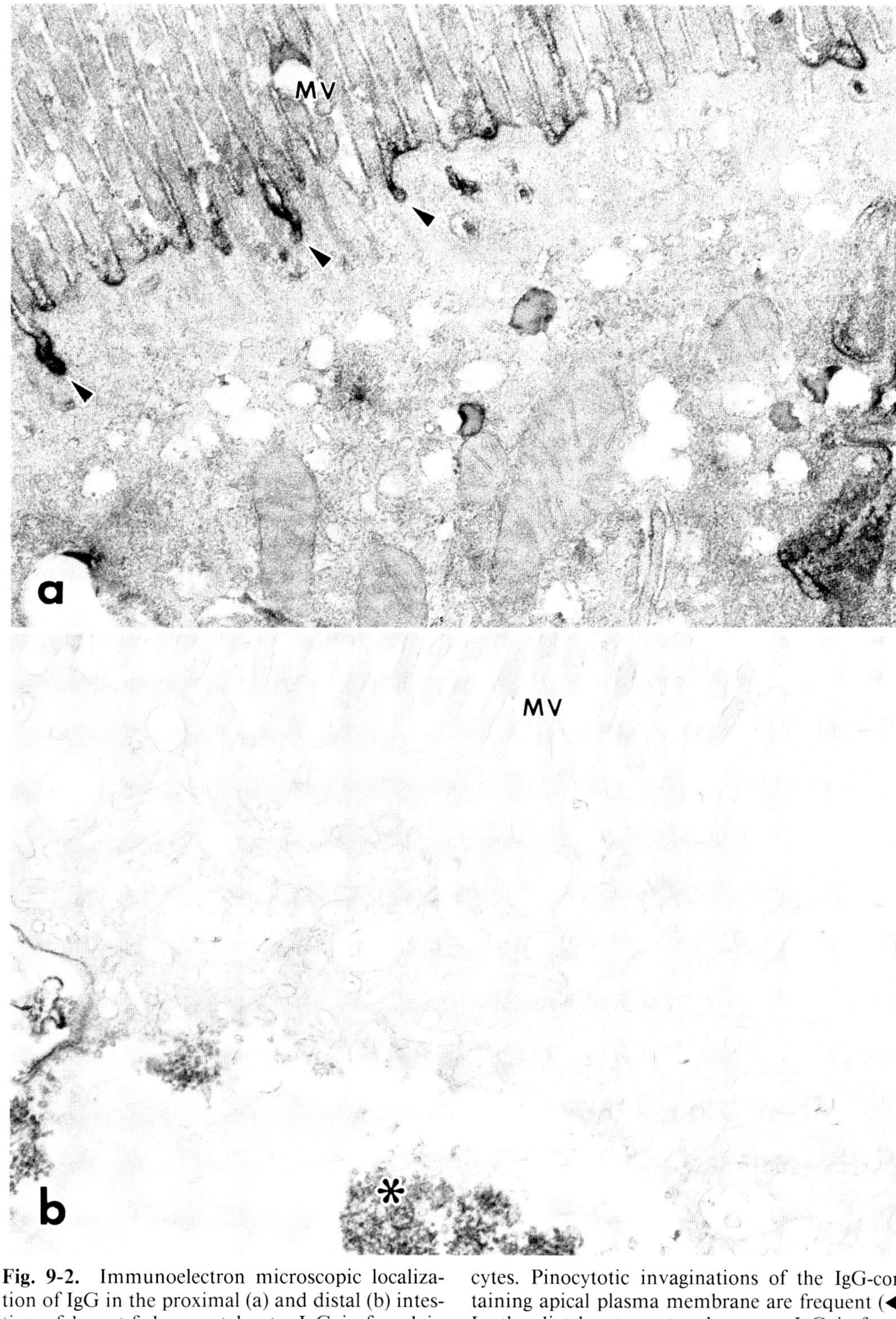


**Fig. 9-2.** Immunoelectron microscopic localization of IgG in the proximal (a) and distal (b) intestine of breast-fed neonatal rats. IgG is found in the lower portion of microvilli (MV) and apical and lateral plasma membranes of proximal enterocytes. Pinocytotic invaginations of the IgG-containing apical plasma membrane are frequent (◀). In the distal enterocytes, however, IgG is found only in cytoplasmic vacuoles (*) (a, ×30,000 ; b, ×18,000)

# DEVELOPMENT AND STRUCTURE OF GUT-ASSOCIATED LYMPHOID TISSUE—ROLE OF ENVIRONMENTAL ANTIGENS IN THE ONTOGENY OF THE MUCOSAL IMMUNE RESPONSES

## Structure of Gut-Associated Lymphoid Tissue

The gut-associated lymphoid tissue (GALT) consists of the organized mucosal lymphoid tissues of the gut that comprise Peyer's patches and solitary lymphoid follicles, diffuse collections of lymphocytes and plasma cells within the lamina propria, and the separated lymphocytes between villous epithelial cells. Peyer's patches consist of a collection of lymphoid follicles that occupy the full thickness of the intestinal mucosa and have the specialized patch-associated lymphoepithelium over them. It is now well established that they contain large numbers of B lymphocytes committed to synthesis of IgA antibodies.[19] Peyer's patches consist of a subepithelial dome of comparatively low cell density, follicles that are areas of closely packed small lymphocytes (corona) containing the germinal center with large blast cells, and the interfollicular areas that have been established as thymus-dependent areas with large concentrations of T lymphocytes. The villi overlying the interfollicular areas are known as patch-associated villi (PAV), which have specialized characters and functions for the lymphatic circulation in GALT.

The epithelial cells, which derive from the crypt of the PAV and overlie the Peyer's patch lymphoid tissue, are quite distinct from the absorptive columnar cells. They are more cuboidal and intermingled with specialized cells bearing only a few microvilli on the luminal surface. These cells called "M" cells appear to be specialized to sample the antigenic material present in the lumen of the gut.[20,21] Lymphocytes, mainly T lymphocytes, are abundant in the interepithelial spaces, and some of these lymphocytes may receive antigenic substances from "M" cells and function to process them.[21] Thus the antigen sampling by "M" cells is supposed to play an important role in the first step of the afferent limb of the mucosal immune response.[22]

The dome region immediately beneath the specialized lymphoepithelial cell layer contains a heterogeneous population of cells,[23] such as large and medium-sized lymphocytes of helper/inducer and suppressor/cytotoxic phenotypes, B lymphocytes, and plasma cells secreting IgM, IgG, and IgA, and macrophages with cell debris and bacterial remnants. Ia antigen-positive dendritic cells are also seen in the dome and the overlying epithelium,[24] and are speculated to function as antigen-presenting cells or as accessory cells for antigen presentation.

The follicles beneath the dome comprise B lymphocyte areas. Most of the recirculating B lymphocytes enter the small lymphocyte zone of the corona.[25,26] Primary follicles without germinal centers are found in the Peyer's patches of neonates and germfree animals, and with stimulation by an antigen, germinal centers develop within the follicle.[27,28] This suggests that the follicle contains cells engaged in specific immune responses. The germinal centers are discrete, well-defined areas where lymphoid blastogenesis takes place. They are composed of large and medium-sized lymphocytes[29] bearing IgM or IgA on their surfaces.[30] IgM and J chain are appreciated in the perinuclear spaces, Golgi complexes, and the scant endoplasmic reticulum in some lymphocytes.[31] Mitotic figures are common. It is speculated that the germinal center is the site of antigen-specific immune responses and of class switching from IgM to IgA.[32] The processes of follicular dendritic cells are prominent in the germinal center,[29,33] and they might play a role in antigen-trapping. Considerable numbers of T lymphocytes of the helper phenotype[33] and Leu 7-positive human natural killer cells are scattered throughout the corona and germinal centers in human Peyer's patches and solitary lymphoid follicles.[34,35] These cells might collaborate with B lymphocytes in immune responses.

The interfollicular areas, thymus-dependent areas analogous to the paracortex of lymph nodes, contain many venules with unique, tall endothelial cells termed postcapillary venules (PCV),[36] which take origin from venules in the PAV.[37,38] The PCV have been well documented as the sites for traffic of recirculating lymphocytes, as mentioned later. The T lymphocytes are mainly small cells that are in close contact with processes of Ia antigen-positive interdigitating cells.[24] The major populations of T lymphocytes there express the helper phenotype.[34] IgA-secreting plasmablasts are also present in this area.[23] Solitary lymphoid follicles look like small Peyer's patches. They are numerous and distributed in the lamina propria throughout the gastrointestinal tract. The epithelium overlying these structures and the follicles themselves show a similar cellular composition to those of the Peyer's patch.[34,39] Thus, these follicles are supposed to have the same functional abilities as those of the Peyer's patch, and their effect on mucosal immunity must be considerable (Fig. 9-3).

There is a diffuse scattering of immunologically competent cells throughout the lamina propria of villi and crypts, and betwen the epithelial cells where they are known as intraepithelial lymphocytes (Fig. 9-4).[40] The mononuclear cells in the lamina propria consist of mixed populations of T lymphocytes and IgA plasma cells. A majority of T cells there express the helper/inducer phenotype,[41] and are either scattered in the lamina propria or gathered into clusters, mainly along the basement membrane of the epithelium. More than 90% of plasma cells are IgA producers, and the number of IgA plasma cells per unit area of tissue is greater in the lamina propria than anywhere else in the body. Normally, small numbers of plasma cells containing IgM, IgG and IgE can be found. The lamina propria of the PAV surrounding the Peyer's patches contains a higher concentration of plasma cells than is found in villi elsewhere.[23] In addition the PAV have been reported to be selective sites for lodging of alloactivated T lymphocytes.[42] In contrast, most intraepithelial lymphocytes were T cells and expressed the phenotype associated with suppressor/cytotoxic T cells rather than helper/inducer T cells.[43,44] They are located between and near the basal portion of the epithelial cells,[43,44] and are capable of expressing mitogen-induced cellular cytotoxity, antibody-dependent cellular cytotoxity and natural killer activity.[45]

## Development of Gut-Associated Lymphoid Tissue

It is well known that morphologic alterations and distribution of immunologically competent cells in GALT have been correlated with the response to orally presented antigens. The study of germfree mice or rats over the period of conventionalization[46,47] reveals that the exposure of the adult animal to abundant microorganisms resulted in prompt and potent immune responses, which are first observed in the intestinal mucosa and mesenteric lymph nodes at the end of the first week. There exists abundant literature on the hypogammaglobulinemia of germfree animals and the scarcity of secondary lymphoid follicles in the lamina propria of the villi.[46–50] It is of interest to notice that intraepithelial T lymphocytes and those in the lamina propria are also scanty. By the end of the 3rd or 4th week of conventionalization, these animals have the structure and immunocyte distribution in Peyer's patches or intestinal villi that resemble those of adult conventional animals.[47] This suggests that adult germfree animals are able to respond to external microbial antigens by developing an immunoglobulin-synthesizing tissue, such as GALT, with a potency and a rapidity at least equal to those of conventional animals (Fig. 9-5).

In the study by Hummel,[51] the microscopic anlage of the Peyer's patch first appeared in the wall of fetal rat intestine at 19 to 20 days of gestation. At that time clusters of Ia antigen-positive cells are present beneath the epithelium.[24] In newborn conventional animals, no immunoglobulin-bearing cells are detected in the intestinal lamina propria where aggregates of small lymphocytes have been present. These early lymphocytes are mainly T cells, and Ia antigen-positive dendritic cells are in-

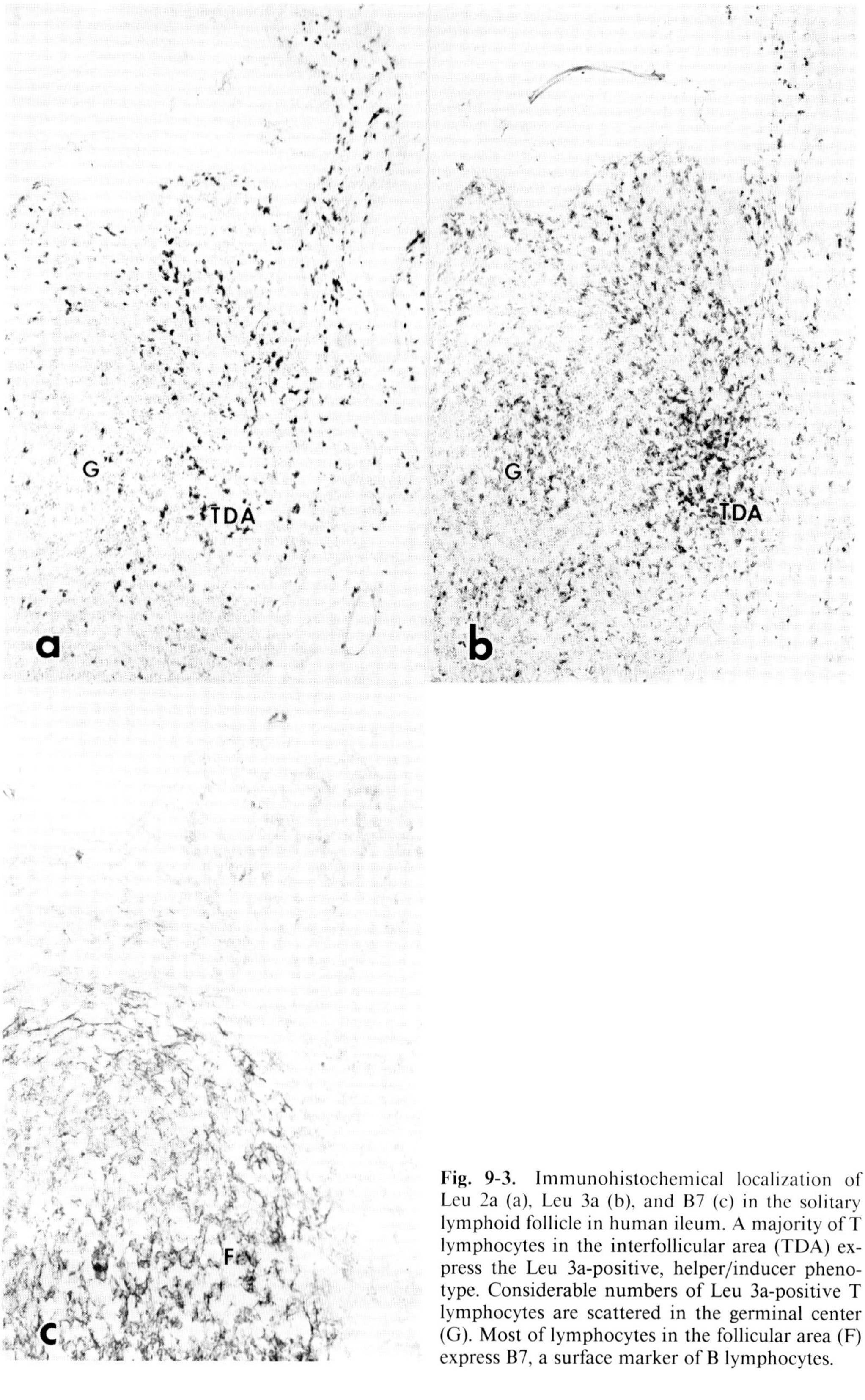


**Fig. 9-3.** Immunohistochemical localization of Leu 2a (a), Leu 3a (b), and B7 (c) in the solitary lymphoid follicle in human ileum. A majority of T lymphocytes in the interfollicular area (TDA) express the Leu 3a-positive, helper/inducer phenotype. Considerable numbers of Leu 3a-positive T lymphocytes are scattered in the germinal center (G). Most of lymphocytes in the follicular area (F) express B7, a surface marker of B lymphocytes.

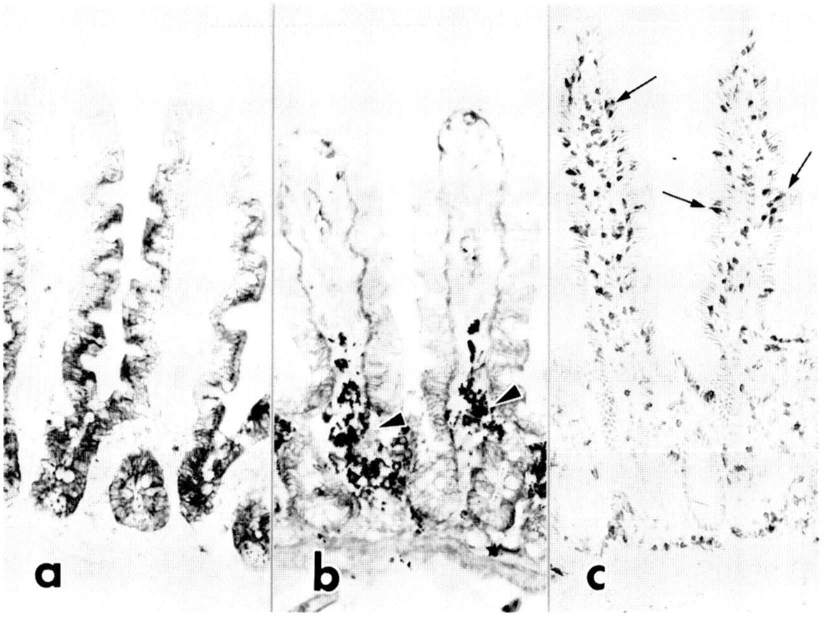


**Fig. 9-4** Immunohistochemical localization of SC (a), IgA (b), and Leu 1 (c) in the human ileum. Staining for SC is most prominent in epithelial cells in the crypts with diminished expression by cells on the villi. IgA-staining is also prominent in the epithelial cells in the crypts along the baso-lateral surfaces. There are numerous IgA plasma cells at the base of villi (◀), and numerous Leu 1-positive lymphocytes throughout the lamina propria of villi and crypts and between the epithelial cells (→).

terspersed within the lymphoid aggregates. Mayrhofer et al [24] speculate that it is the prior congregation of Ia antigen-positive cells in the Peyer's patch anlagen, which induces subsequent congregation of lymphocytes at these sites. More recently Spalding et al[52] demonstrated that dendritic cell-T cell mixtures induce polyclonal IgA secretion by Peyer's patch B cells. The first immunoglobulin-bearing cells in young mice and rats are recognized within the first week of life and belong to the IgM class with J chain.[46,47] At that time the Peyer's patch is not yet visible, and the Peyer's patch in the adult develops first between 10 and 14 days after birth in rats.[47]

Cells of the IgA class are first found in significant numbers on day 21 in the intestinal villi and their numbers increase rapidly.[7,46,47] The germinal center develops at four weeks after birth. At six weeks of age, when the rats have been weaned, and the feeding environment is the same as that of adults, the types and counts of bacteria are almost the same as those in adults.[53] It seems possible that the arrival of IgA plasma cells in the lamina propria and the establishment of microbial flora are intimately related.

## DIFFERENTIATION AND MIGRATION OF MUCOSAL LYMPHOID CELLS

It has been well documented that the germinal center of Peyer's patches consists predominantly of B lymphoblasts, and also contains interspersed macrophages, antigen presenting follicular dendritic cells, and small numbers of T lymphocytes of helper phenotype, as mentioned previously. The recent study of Kawanishi et al[32] suggests that the germinal center microenvironment of the

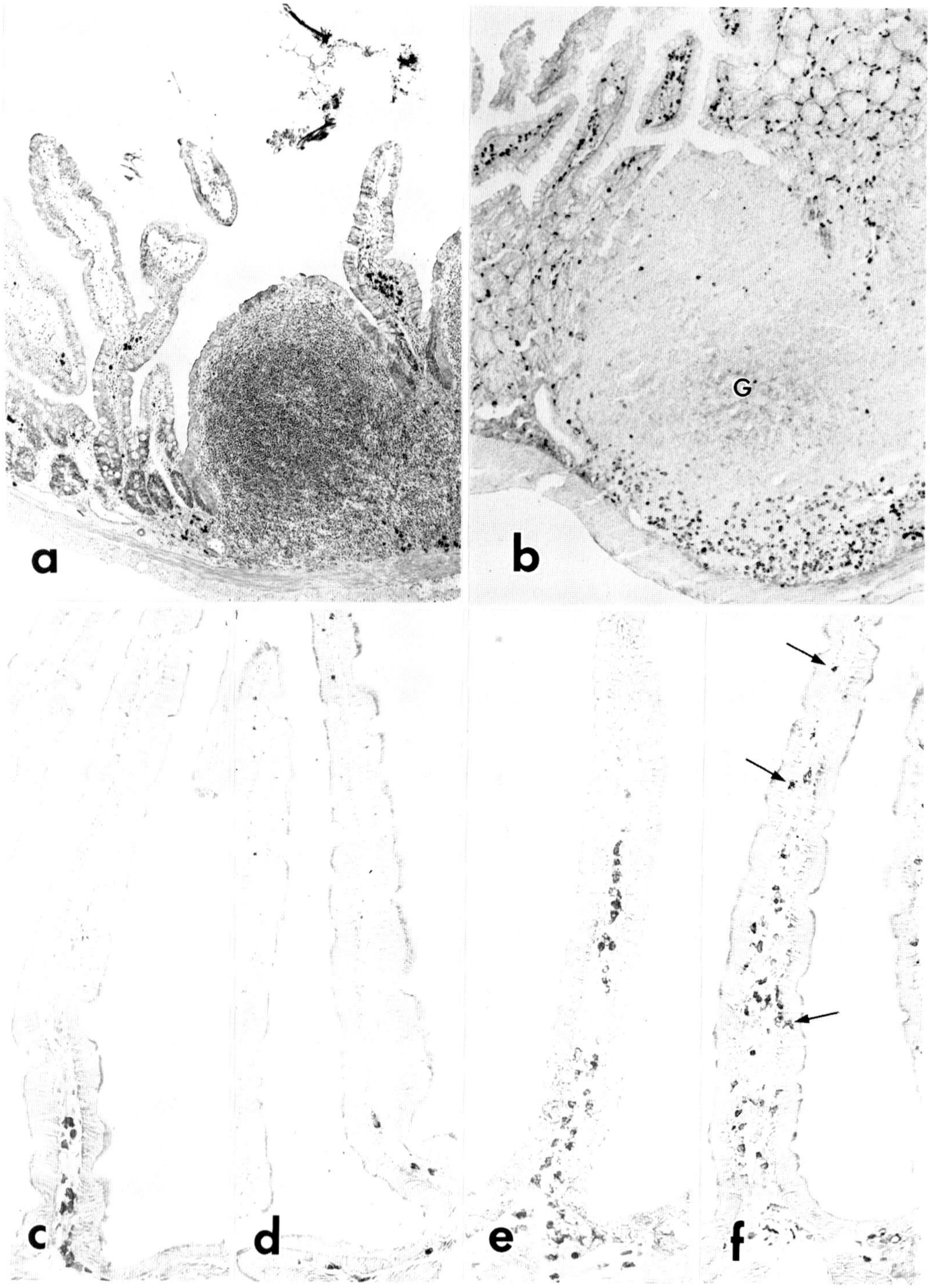


**Fig. 9-5.** Immunohistochemical localization of IgA plasma cells (a, b, c, e) and T lymphocytes (d, f) in the jejunal mucosa of adult germfree and conventional rats. In the conventional rats lymphoid follicles are well developed, and IgA plasma cells are abundant in the lamina propria of villi and crypts (b, e). Numerous intraepithelial T lymphocytes (→) and others in the lamina propria are also present (f). In germfree rats, however, IgA plasma cells and T lymphocytes are scanty (a, c, d). G:germinal center

Peyer's patch plays an important role in activation, proliferation, and heavy chain class switching during B cell responses, which are largely regulated by several subpopulations of immunoregulatory T lymphocytes and their secreted factors. The primed or activated B lymphoblasts, immediate IgA precursor cells,[19] migrate to the mesenteric lymph nodes, and via the thoracic duct to the general circulation, homing to several external-secreting organs. Some of the cells repopulate the intestinal mucosa, others migrate to the bronchial mucosa, salivary glands, biliary tract, urogenital organs, mammary glands, lacrimal glands, and several other sites in mucous membranes or exocrine glands.[2] Gut T lymphocytes also have migration patterns similar or identical to those described for B cells.

Of particular interest is the suggestion that the organ specificity of lymphocyte migration is determined largely by selective interaction of circulating lymphocytes with endothelial cells of PCV.[54] Parrott and Ferguson[55] described that recirculating lymphocytes also enter PAV from Peyer's patches via anastomosing lymphatic channels, and that this may provide a direct route for migration of lymphoblasts. As previously mentioned, the lamina propria of PAV contains higher concentrations of IgA plasma cells or IgA plasmablasts and is supposed to be a selective site for lodgement of alloactivated T lymphocytes.[42] We have recently made the interesting observation that these mucosal endothelial cells in PCV and PAV share antigens with a peripheral blood monocyte or macrophage subset,[56] capable of presenting soluble antigens and triggering autologous mixed lymphocyte reactions or allogenic T lymphocyte proliferation, associated with HLA-DR and OK-M5 (Fig. 9-6).[57]

Butcher et al[54] suggested that endothelial cells in mucosal and peripheral lymphoid tissues express distinctive determinants or factors for lymphocyte recognition and that lymphocyte migration patterns are programmed by lymphocyte surface receptors complementary to those organ-specific endothelial determinants. Such an organ-specific lymphocyte migration mechanism is largely responsible for the unique feature of the mucosal immune responses.

Figure 9-7 is a schema illustrating the cellular traffic in the mucosal immune system.

## TRANSEPITHELIAL TRANSLOCATION OF IMMUNOGLOBULINS INTO EXTERNAL BODY FLUIDS—SC-MEDIATED TRANSPORT MECHANISM

sIgA in the external secretions consists of two molecules of IgA linked by J chain (dimeric IgA, dIgA) in complex with secretory component.[58] These components of sIgA are derived from two different types of cells: plasma cells in the intestinal lamina propria and glandular epithelial cells. Many studies of sIgA origin in mucosal secretions emphasize the role of local production of dIgA molecules by plasma cells underlying the epithelium of mucous membranes and secretory glands.[58–60] The IgA-producing plasma cells in the mucosal sites are responsible for the synthesis of the component proteins of dIgA (the IgA heavy and light chains and the J chain) as well as for the assembly of the components into a dIgA molecule before secretion. However, a significant proportion of IgA in breast milk and bile is serum-derived,[60–62] and in many species the intestine is a site of manufacture of much of the IgA found in blood.[63]

On the other hand, secretory component (SC) is synthesized and expressed on the glandular epithelial cells throughout the entire intestines and biliary ducts as well as in various exocrine glands[34] and, under certain circumstances,[64] the gastric epithelium. The route taken by the IgA across the epithelium has been examined repeatedly by immunohistochemical techniques, most of them involving the gut (Fig. 9-8).[58,65] SC is normally exposed on the basolateral plasma membrane of these epithelial cells. It has been well established that the SC binds dIgA at the basolateral cell surface by noncovalent interactions. The SC-

a
b
c

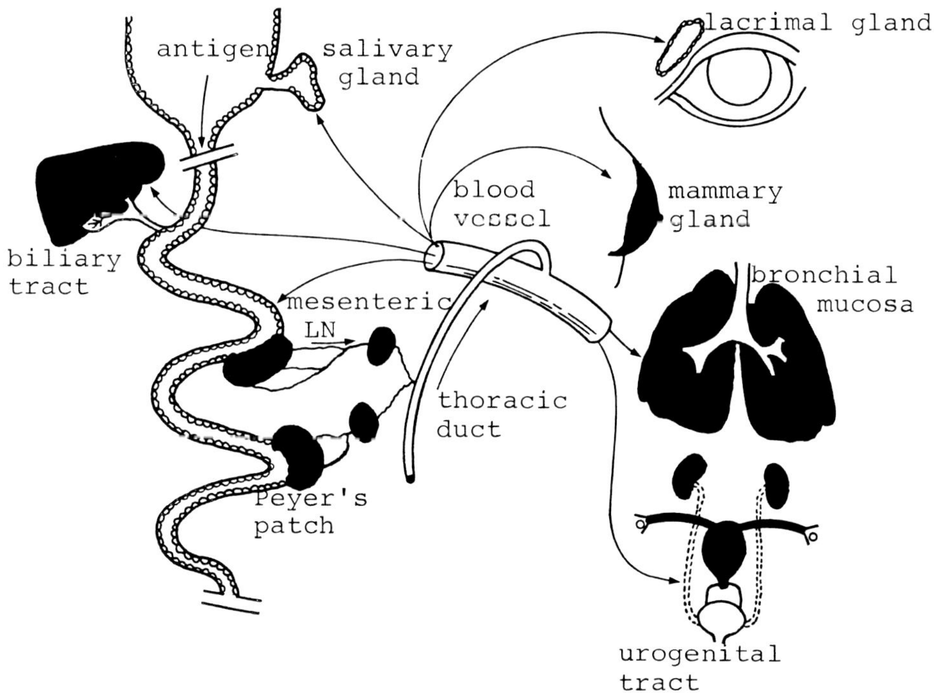


**Fig. 9-7.** A schematic illustration of the cellular traffic of precursors of IgA plasma cells and T lymphocytes leaving the Peyer's patches after antigenic stimulation (revised from reference 3). The cells home to mucosal sites via mesenteric lymph nodes, thoracic duct and blood circulation.

dIgA complex then undergoes endocytosis, and the complex is transported across the cell to the gland lumen by a microtubule-dependent vesicular transport mechanism and exocytosed at the apical cell surface along with some free SC.

At some point during the transport and secretion, the complex is rendered soluble by proteolytic cleavage of the membrane-associated SC molecule to release the soluble sIgA into the gland lumen. Such a model proposed for SC-mediated epithelial IgA reception and translocation gained strong support from observations made on normal[66] and neoplastic living cells.[67] Pentameric IgM also binds SC. Brandtzaeg[66] reported that a stronger noncovalent interaction was found between pentameric IgM and SC than between dIgA and SC. J chain is detected in dIgA and pentameric IgM,[68] and a role for the J chain is postulated in the SC-binding process. Monomeric IgA and IgG lacking J chain, or sIgA, however, do not bind to the membrane SC. Thus, SC appears to be the cell surface receptor for polymeric immunoglobulins associated with J chain. More recently, Mostov and colleagues[69] clearly demonstrated that SC is not synthesized as a secreted protein but as a much larger transmembrane precursor, and is the proteolytically cleaved, extracellular ligand-binding domain of the polymeric immunogloblin receptor.

←

**Fig. 9-6.** Immunohistochemical localization of Factor VIII related antigen (F VIII-RAg) (a), OK-M5 (b), and HLA-DR (c) in the solitary lymphoid follicle of human ileum. Mucosal endothelial cells of capillaries and venules share antigens with peripheral blood monocytes, such as OK-M5 and HLA-DR, as well as an antigen with vascular endothelial cells, F VIII-RAg (◀). Numerous HLA-DR-positive cells are present near the PCV (*).

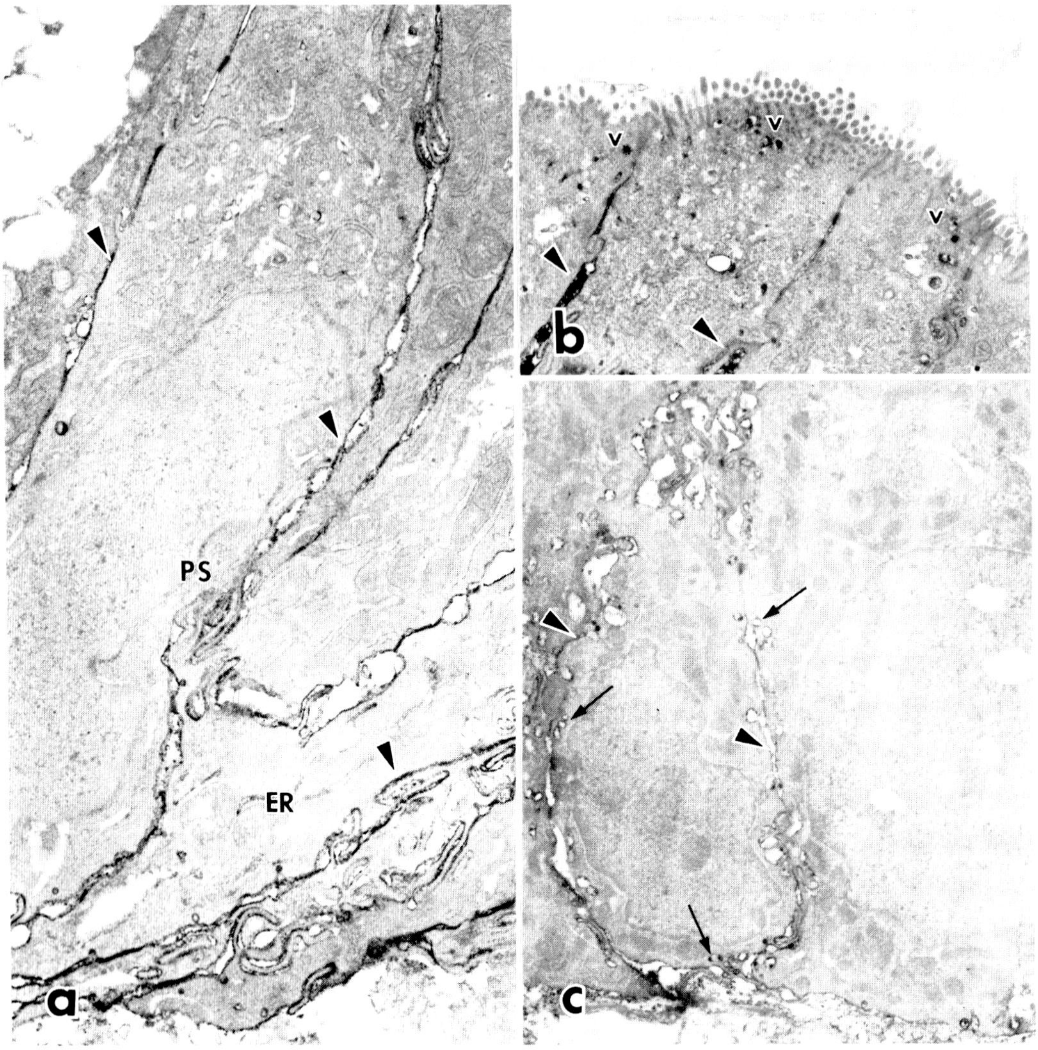


**Fig. 9-8.** Immunoelectron microscopic localization of SC (a) and IgA (b, c) in human enterocytes. SC is found in the perinuclear spaces (PS), rough endoplasmic reticulum (ER), and along the basolateral plasma membranes (◀). IgA is seen on the external surfaces of the basolateral plasma membranes (◀), which are frequently invaginated by pinocytosis (→). IgA-containing vesicles (V) are numerous in the supranuclear regions. (a, ×8.000 ; b, ×10.000; c, ×9.000)

Moreover, the SC-dIgA pathway diverges from most of other receptor-mediated endocytic pathways. Ahnen et al[58] clearly reviewed the distinctions: (1) the ligand (dIgA) is not ultimately degraded by lysosomes; (2) the receptor on the extracellular membrane (SC) is not recycled to the cell surface for reutilization; (3) the receptor-ligand complex membrane (SC-dIgA) is not dissociated after internalization; (4) the ligand (dIgA) is released from the cell in complex with its receptor (membrane SC) as sIgA. The cellular mechanism responsible for the transport of sIgA is schematically illustrated in Figure 9-9.

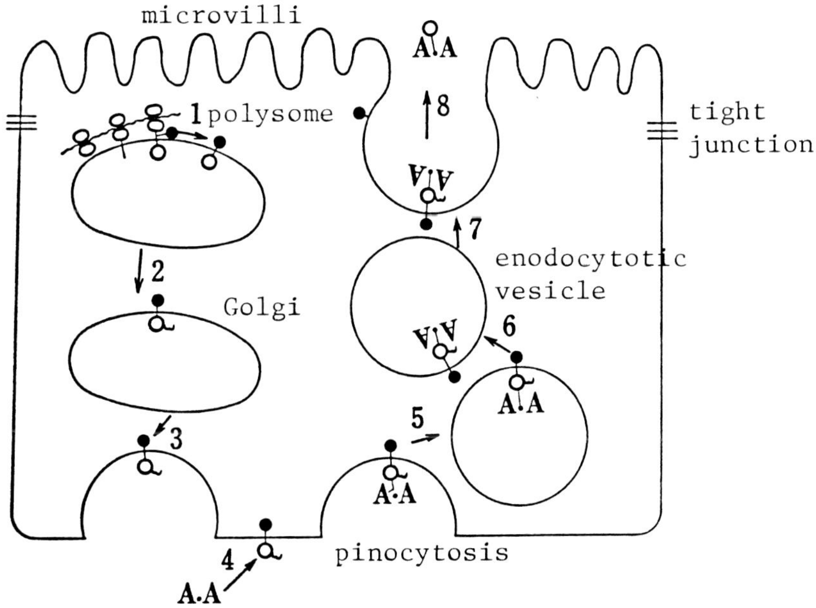


**Fig. 9-9.** A schematic illustration of the SC-dimeric IgA transport system. See text for explanation of the step numbers.
O:SC (70,000–75,000) — large SC, free SC
●:transport protein (15,000–20,000)
A.A:dimeric IgA
W:terminal sugar

## IgA IN LIVER AND BILE—LIVER IS AN INTEGRAL PART OF THE MUCOSAL IMMUNITY

The demonstration of sIgA in normal rat bile has focused attention on the possible relationship of the liver to the mucosal immune system,[70] and the immunological significance of the transport of dimeric IgA by the liver was established soon thereafter. Hepatic bile of man and some other species also contains large amounts of sIgA and perhaps monomeric IgA and dIgA, lacking SC as well.[62,71] In rats, the biliary sIgA is accounted for largely through active transport of dIgA from the circulation to bile. The mechanism is that dIgA combines with SC on the sinusoidal plasma membrane of hepatocytes and the SC-dIgA complexes migrate across the cells by endocytic, vesicular transport to be discharged at the border of the hepatocytic cells that forms the bile canaliculus.[71,72] In man, however, the earlier authors suggested that translocation of IgA in the liver occurs only across biliary epithelial cells; only these cells, not hepatocytes, contain both SC and IgA (Fig. 9-10).[62]

In addition to the transport of free dIgA, it has been shown that the liver can also function in the removal of antigen from the circulation, in the form of IgA immune complexes.[73–75] The mechanism for transport of IgA immune complexes is the same as that for free dIgA, and therefore SC plays a major role.[73,74] Thus, it is speculated that the hepatic transport of IgA immune complexes from the circulation to the bile represents a unique, noninflammatory mechanism for the disposal of antigens, distinct from the phagocyte-mediated mechanisms that clear conventional complexes.[73] It appears that the function of the hepatic transport mechanism is not only to recover free dIgA from serum and pass it

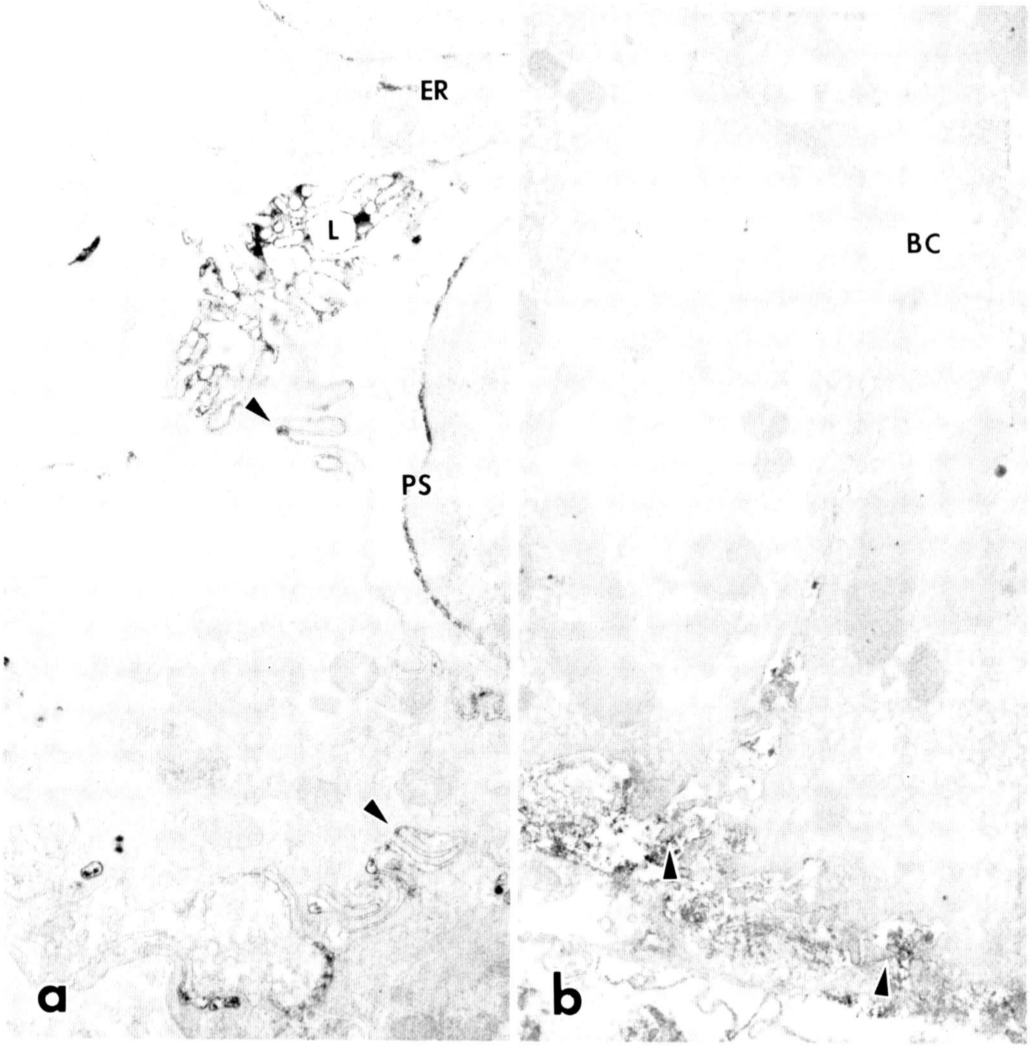


**Fig. 9-10.** Immunoelectron microscopic localization of SC (a) and IgA (b) in the human liver. SC is seen in the perinuclear spaces (PS), the rough endoplasmic reticulum (ER), the ductal lumen (L), and along the lateral plasma membranes (◀) of ductal epithelial cells. In the case of chronic hepatitis, the external surfaces of the plasma membranes of hepatocytes faced toward the sinusoid and Disse's space have deposits of IgA (◀). No IgA is present in the cytoplasm. (a, ×15,000; b, × 11,000) BC: bile canaliculi

**Fig. 9-11.** Immunohistochemical localization of OK-M1 (a), OK-M5 (b), HLA-DR (c), and factor VIII related antigen (F VIII-RAg) (d) in the human liver. Sinusoidal endothelial cells show membrane staining for OK-M5 and HLA-DR, but not for OK-M1 and F VIII-RAg. Endothelial cells in the portal areas fail to express OK-M5, but are positively stained for F VIII-RAg (◀) P: portal area

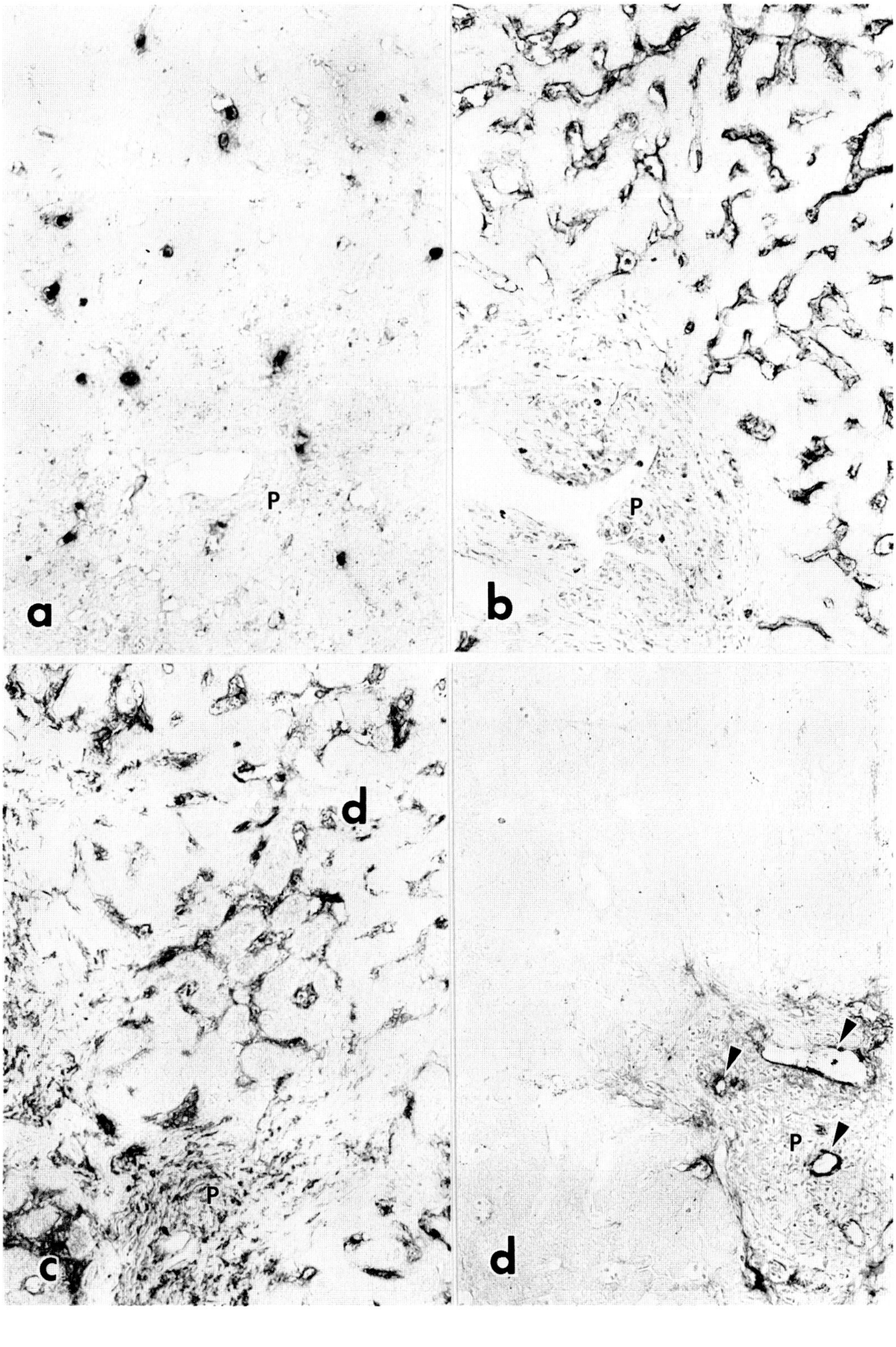
P
a
P
b
d
P
c
P
d

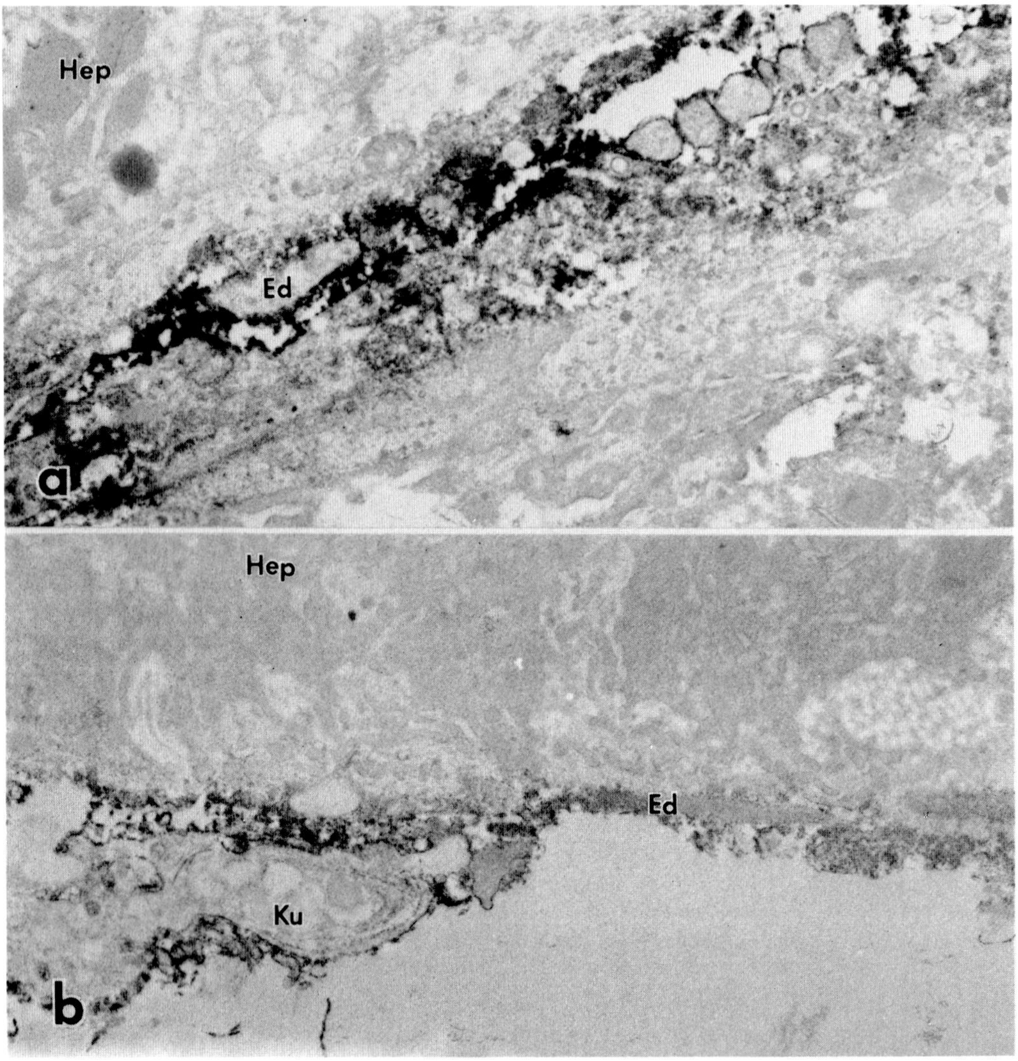


**Fig. 9-12.** Immunoelectron microscopic localization of OK-M5 (a) and HLA-DR (b) in the human liver. OK-M5 is seen along the plasma membrane of the sinusoidal endothelial cells (Ed). HLA-DR is found on the surface of both endothelial cells and Kupffer cells (Ku). Hep: hepatocytes. (a, ×15,000; b, ×15,000)

into the intestine via the biliary system as an "IgA pump,"[76] but also to clear the circulation of immune complexes that may arise in the gut by the interaction of absorbed food or microbial antigens with locally synthesized IgA antibody as a "scavenger."[53] The latter may be a possible mechanism for returning the IgA immune complexes to the intestine before activating a cascade of immune-mediated inflamatory reactions that occasionally results in tissue damage.

Disruption of the hepatobiliary transport of sIgA and sIgA immune complexes may be implicated in the pathogenesis of several human diseases. A number of diseases have been found in which IgA or IgA immune complexes are deposited in tissues; among these are Berger IgA nephropathy, Henoch-Schoenlein purpura, and dermatitis herpetiformis,[77] as well as alcoholic liver disease and chronic active hepatitis.[78,79] Although the property of the bound IgA has not been fully elucidated, the authors obtained immunohistochemical evidence that IgA and J chain can be found concurrently at the same site of tissues in these diseases, but no SC is identified there (Fig. 9-10).[79] In the liver, IgA and J chain are also found in phagosomes in hepatocytes and Kupffer cells simultaneously with acid phosphatase activity. These results are consistent with the known ability of these cells to bind, take up, and digest dIgA and dIgA immune complexes. Thus, the heavy deposition of IgA on the hepatocytes in alcoholic liver disease and chronic active hepatitis might represent excess IgA in the liver as a result of possible alterations in the sequestering and transport functions of the cells, but it could also be due to increased IgA synthesis.

Impairment of hepatic clearance of IgA by any of these routes could contribute to elevated serum sIgA and/or dIgA. Elevated serum sIgA levels are reported in patients with a broad spectrum of liver diseases, which paralleled classical markers of cholestasis such as serum alkaline phosphatase and biliary polymeric sIgA in blood.[73,80,81] Our recent immunoelectron microscopical observations suggest two routes of regurgitation, first through bile canaliculi, and adjacent hepatocytes into sinusoidal blood; second by extravasation from bile ductules into surrounding portal tract tissues and thence into portal blood vessels.[82] Elevated serum sIgA in patients with surgical portacaval shunts and cirrhosis might be attributable to bypassing both routes of clearance. IgA immune complexes in blood are also found in these diseases.[83]

Recently the authors showed that only the hepatic sinusoidal endothelial cells carry antigens with a peripheral blood macrophage subset capable of presenting soluble antigens and triggering autologous mixed lymphocyte reactions. They showed membrane staining for HLA-DR and OK-M5, but not for OK-M1 (Figs. 9-11,9-12).[84] This suggests that the sinusoidal endothelial cells may play an important role in immune responses or regulations in the liver. Although Kupffer cells are also known to constitute a group of Ia antigen-positive fixed macrophages, and to be responsible for the uptake of circulating antibodies and immune complexes, and for antigen presentation,[85–87] Kupffer cells fail to express OK-M5. Richman et al[88] showed that purified Kupffer cells pulsed with antigen in vitro are fully capable of inducing T cell proliferation. It has been well documented, however, that the liver is an important factor in oral tolerance; food and microbial antigens going to the liver via the portal system induce specific unresponsiveness, and the phagocytic function of Kupffer cells is supposed to be critical to the induction of suppressor responses.[89] Thus, failure by Kupffer cells as well as the sIgA system of an impaired liver to clear such enteric antigens and immune complexes formed in the blood circulation, which may themselves be pathogenic, could result in immune-mediated diseases. Thus, Kleinman et al[83] and the present authors have recognized that the liver is an integral part of the enteric mucosal immune system.[53]

## IMMUNOREGULATORY ROLE OF THE MUCOSAL IMMUNE SYSTEM

It is well recognized that the systemic immune response to a specific antigen can be suppressed after the introduction of antigens via the gastrointestinal tract.[89] Recently the mechanism responsible for such important regulatory interactions taking place between the systemic and mucosal systems was extensively explored.[3,4] The anergic state induced by luminal antigens is supposed to be necessary to prevent the occurrence of injurious systemic reactions to antigens that inadvertently cross the mucosal barrier. Although recent studies of the suppression mechanism provide increasing evidence that systemic suppression is due to cellular and/or humoral products of the mucosal immune system, no unifying mechanism responsible for this phenomenon has been elucidated. It is possible that different mechanisms are responsible in different systems. One of the best defined mechanisms for the induction of systemic hyporesponsiveness to orally administered antigens is the introduction of a class-specific regulatory T cell for IgA.[89,90] That reflects the concurrent appearance of T helper cells specific for IgA and T suppressor cells for IgA responses to the antigen fed. Under this condition, oral stimulation may lead to IgG suppression (systemic suppression) associated with IgA enhancement (mucosal enhancement) as stated by Strober et al.[89]

In addition, sIgA antibody is capable of reducing antigen absorption across mucosal surfaces,[91] and hepatobiliary transport of IgA immune complexes provides a means of eliminating antigens that pass the IgA mucosal barrier.[74,75,92] The mucosal antibodies, therefore, may have an important immunoregulatory role. For example, it is well known that patients with selective IgA deficiency have a high incidence of antifood antibodies and an atopic disposition,[93] and patients with chronic liver disease have high titers of antibodies to intestinal microorganisms.[94,95] Experimentally, portacaval shunting in dogs abolishes the tolerogenic effect of feeding dinitrochlorobenzene.[96] Thus, antigen stimulation in the gut can have highly specific and dual immunogenic and/or tolerogenic influence on host immune responses in both intestinal and extraintestinal sites, and the systemic immune unresponsiveness might be very important in the prevention of damaging reactions to antigens that escape the exclusion mechanism at the mucosal surface.

## CONCLUSION

The intestinal mucosa provides an extensive surface on which potentially pathogenic microorganisms and food antigens make their initial contact with the body, and the intestine is richly populated with lymphoid tissues capable of initiating and affecting various immune reactions. Of particular interest is the fact that the mucosal lymphoid tissue initiates a diverse series of immunologic events including the production of secretory antibodies at mucosal sites and, in striking contrast, an unresponsiveness of systemic immunological reactions. On the other hand we have focused on the significance of the liver in the immunoregulatory system, particularly the hepatic transport mechanism of sIgA and IgA immune complexes.

As for the movement of the cells within the mucosal immune system, T and B lymphocytes arising in mucosal follicles rapidly leave the follicle and return only to mucosal sites. This leads to the postulation of a common mucosal immune system, involving whole mucosal and exocrine organs. Thus, we have speculated that the mucosal immune system may play a central role in the maintenance of the homeostasis of the total immune system in the body, as well as in the regulation of the systemic immune system.

Until recently, however, mucosal immunity received relatively little attention from both basic and clinical scientists. The challenge for further research in mucosal immune responses is that it may offer the prospect of improved understanding of the immune mechanisms and the pathogenesis of several gastrointestinal and systemic diseases.

## ACKNOWLEDGMENTS

The author is very grateful to Professors Keiichi Watanabe and Paul K. Nakane of Tokai University School of Medicine, and to Professor William R. Brown of University of Colorado Health Science Center for helpful discussions.

## REFERENCES

1. Bienenstock J.: The physiology of the local immune response and the gastrointestinal tract. In Progress in Immunology 11, vol 4, Brent L, Holborow J. ed. Amsterdam, North-Holland, 1974, p197

2. McDermott M.R., Bienenstock J.: Evidence for a common mucosal immunologic system. I. Migration of B immunoblasts into intestinal, respiratory, and genital tissues. J Immunol **122**:1892, 1979
3. Brown W.R.: The central role of the gastrointestinal tract in immunological reactions. Tokai J Exp Clin Med **8**:1, 1983
4. Stokes C.R.: Induction and control of intestinal immune responses, in Local Immune Responses of the Gut, Newby T.J., Stokes C.R. (eds). Boca Raton, CRC Press, 1984, p97
5. Hong R., Ammann A.J.: Selective absence of IgA. Autoimmune phenomena and autoimmune disease. Am J Pathol **69**:491,1972
6. Morris B., Morris R.: The absorption of $^{125}$I-labelled immunoglobulin G by different regions of the gut in young rats. J Physiol (Lond) **241**:761,1974
7. Nagura H., Nakane P.K., Brown W.R.: Breast milk IgA binds to jejunal epithelium in suckling rats. J Immunol **120**:1333,1978
8. Rodewald R., Kraehenbuhl J.P.: Receptor-mediated transport of IgG. J Cell Biol **99**:159s,1984
9. Rodewald R.: Intestinal transport of antibodies in the newborn rat. J Cell Biol **58**:189,1973
10. Ogra S.S.D., Weintraub D., Ogra P.L.: Immunological aspects of human colostrum and milk. III. Fate and absorption of cellular and soluble components in the gastrointestinal tract of the newborn. J Immunol **119**:245,1977
11. Hanson L.Å., Ahlstedt S., Andersson B., Carlsson B., Dahlgren U., Lidin-Janson G., Mattsby-Baltzer M., Svanborg-Eden C.: The biologic properties of secretory IgA. J Reticuloendothel Soc **28**:1s,1980
12. Hanson L.Å., Winberg J.: Breast milk and defense against infection in the newborn. Arch Dis Child **47**:845,1972
13. Walker W.A.: Antigen penetration across the immature gut: effect of immunologic and maturational factors in colostrum. In Immunology of Breast Milk. Ogra P.L., Dayton D. eds. New York, Raven Press, 1979,p227
14. Diaz-Jouanen E., Williams R.C. Jr.: T and B lymphocytes in human colostrum. Clin Immunol Immunopathol **3**:248,1974
15. Reddy V., Bhaskaram C., Raghuramulu N., Jagadeesan V.: Antimicrobial factors in human milk. Acta Paediatr Scand **66**:229,1977
16. Stephen S., Dolby J.M., Montreuil J., Spik G.: Differences in inhibition of the growth of commensal and enteropathogenic strains of Escherichia coli by lactotransferrin and secretory immunoglobulin A isolated from human milk. Immunology **41**:597,1980
17. Watanabe T., Nagura H., Watanabe K., Brown W.R.: The binding of human milk lactoferrin to immunoglobulin A. FEBS Letters **168**:203,1984
18. Weaver E.A., Rudloff H.E., Goldblum R.M., Davis C.P., Goldman A.S.: Selection of immunoglobulin A by human milk leukocytes initiated by surface membrane stimuli. J Immunol **132**:684,1984
19. Craig S.W., Cebra J.J.: Peyer's patches: an enriched source of precursors for IgA-producing immunocytes in the rabbit. J Exp Med **134**:188,1971
20. Owen R.L., Jones A.L.: Epithelial cell specialization within Peyer's patches: an ultrastructural study of intestinal lymphoid follicles. Gastroenterology **66**:189,1974
21. Owen R.L.: Sequential uptake of horseradish peroxidase by lymphoid follicle epithelium of Peyer's patches in the normal unobstructed mouse intestine. An ultrastructural study. Gastroenterology **72**:440,1977
22. Bockman D.E., Cooper M.D.: Early lymphoepithelial relationship in human appendix. A combined light and electron-microscopic study. Gastroenterology **68**:1160,1975
23. Simina T., Plesch B.E.C.: An immunohistochemical study of cells with surface and cytoplasmic immunoglobulins in situ in Peyer's patches and lamina propria of rat small intestine. Virchow's Arch B **40**:181,1982
24. Mayrhofer G., Pugh C.W., Barclay A.N.: The distribution, ontogeny and origin in the rat of Ia positive cells with dendritic morphology and Ia antigen in epithelia, with special reference to the intestine. Eur J Immunol **13**:112,1983
25. Howard J.C., Hunt S.V., Gowans J.L.: Identification of marrow-derived and thymus-derived small lymphocytes in the lymphoid tissue and thoracic duct lymph of normal rats. J Exp Med **135**:200,1972
26. Meuwissen H.J., Kaplan G.T., Perey D.Y., Good R.A.: Role of rabbit gut-associated lymphoid tissue in cell replication. The follicular cortex as a primary germinative site. Proc Soc Exp Biol Med **130**:300,1969
27. Cooper G.N., Thonard J.C., Crosby R.L., Dalbow M.H.: Immunological responses in rats following antigenic stimulation of Peyer's patches. II. Histological changes in germ-free animals. Aust J Exp Biol Med Sci **46**:407,1968
28. Pollard M., Sharon N.: Responses of the Peyer's patches in germ-free mice to antigenic stimulation. Infect Immun **2**:96,1970
29. Sobhan P.: The light and electron microscopic studies of Peyer's patches in non-germfree adult mice. J Morphol **135**:457,1971
30. Moore A.R., Hall J.G.: Evidence for a primary association between immunoblast and small gut. Nature (Lond) **239**:161,1972
31. Nagura H., Kohler P.F., Brown W.R.: Immunocytochemical characterization of the lymphocytes in nodular lymphoid hyperplasia of the bowel. Lab Invest **40**:66,1979
32. Kawanishi H., Saltzman L.E., Strober W.: Mechanisms regulating IgA class-specific immunoglobulin production in murine gut-associated lymphoid tissues. I. T cells derived from Peyer's patches that switch sIgM B cells to sIgA B cells in vitro. J Exp Med **157**:433,1983
33. Simina T., Janse E.M., Wilders M.M.: Antigen-trapping cells in Peyer's patches of the rat. Scand J Immunol **16**:481,1982
34. Nagura H., Tsutsumi Y., Shimamura K., Shioda Y., Hasegawa H., Tamaoki K.: Immunohistochemical observation of human solitary lymphoid follicles. Digestive Organ and Immunology **12**:89,1984
35. Shioda Y., Nagura H., Tsutsumi Y., Shimamura K., Tamaoki N.: Distribution of Leu7 (HNK-1) antigen in human digestive organs: an immunohistochemical study with monoclonal antibody. Histochem J **16**:843,1984
36. Gowans J.L., Knight E.J.: The route of recirculation of lymphocytes in the rat. Proc Roy Soc Lond Ser B **159**:257,1964
37. Barclay A.N.: Different reticular elements in rat lymphoid tissue identified by localization of Ia, Thy-1 and MRC OX2 antigens. Immunology **44**:727,1981
38. Bhalla D.K., Murakami T., Owen R.L.: Microcirculation of intestinal lymphoid follicles in rat Peyer's patches. Gastroenterology **81**:481,1981

39. Keren D.F.: Immunology and Immunopathology of the Gastrointestinal Tract. Chicago, American Society of Clinical Pathologists, 1980, p10
40. Ferguson A.: Intraepithelial lymphocytes of the small intestine. Gut **18**:921,1977
41. Cerf-Bensussan N., Schneeberger E.E., Bhan A.K.: Immunohistologic and immunoelectron microscopic characterization of the mucosal lymphocytes of human small intestine by the use of monoclonal antibodies. J Immunol **130**:2615,1983
42. Sprent J.: Fate of H2-activated T-lymphocytes in syngeneic host. I. Fate in lymphoid tissues and intestines traced with $^{3}$H-thymidine, $^{125}$I-deoxyuridine and $^{51}$chromium. Cell Immunol **21**:278,1976
43. Selby W.S., Janossy G., Goldstein G., Jewell D.P.: T lymphocyte subsets in human intestinal mucosa: the distribution and relationship to MHC-derived antigens. Clin Exp Immunol **44**:453,1981
44. Shioda Y., Nagura H., Tsutsumi Y., Saito H., Tamaoki K.: Immunohistochemical analysis of intraepithelial lymphocytes of human intestine. Digestive Organ and Immunology **10**:149,1983
45. Flexman J.P., Shellam G.R., Mayrhofer G.: Natural cytotoxicity, responsiveness to interferon and morphology of intraepithelial lymphocytes from the small intestine of the rat. Immunology **48**:733,1983
46. Crabbe P.A., Nash D.R., Bazin H., Eyssen H., Heremans J.F.: Immunohistochemical observations on lymphoid tissue from conventional and germ-free mice. Lab Invest **22**:448,1970
47. Nagura H., Hasegawa H., Yoshimura S., Aihara K., Watanabe K., Ozawa A.: Comparative studies on conventional and germfree rat intestinal mucosa: with special reference to microbial flora and secretory IgA; in Recent Advances in Germfree Research. Sasaki S., Ozawa A., Hashimoto K. (eds). Tokyo, Tokai Univ Press, 1982, p511
48. Gustafsson B.E., Laurell C.B.: Gamma-globulins in germ-free rats. J Exp Med **108**:251,1958
49. Miyakawa M., Iijima S., Kobayashi R., Tajima M.: Observations on the lymphoid tissue of the germ-free guinea pig. Acta Pathol Jpn **7**:183,1957
50. Wastmann B.S.: Recent studies on the serum proteins of germfree animals. Ann NY Acad Sci **94**:272,1961
51. Hummel K.P.: The structure and development of the lymphatic tissue in the intestine of the albino rat. Am J Anat **57**:907,1972
52. Spalding D.M., Williamson S.I., Koopman W.J., McGhee J.R.: Preferential induction of polyclonal IgA secretion by murine Peyer's patch dendritic cell-T cell mixture. J Exp Med **160**:941,1984
53. Nagura H., Watanabe K.: Mucosal immune system and immune responses in the intestine. In Gastrointestinal Function Regulation and Disturbances, vol.2, Kasuya Y., Tsuchiya M., Nagao F., Matsuo Y. eds. Amsterdam, Excerpta Medica, 1984, p147
54. Butcher E.C., Stevens S.K., Reichert R.A., Scollay R.G., Weissman I.L.: Lymphocyte-endothelial cell recognition in lymphocyte migration and the segregation of mucosal and nonmucosal immunity. In Recent Advances in Mucosal Immunity, Strober W., Hanson L.A., Sell K.W. eds, New York, Raven Press, 1982, p3
55. Parrott D.M., Ferguson A.: Selective migration of lymphocytes within the mouse small intestine. Immunology **26**:571,1974
56. Nagura H., Koshikawa T.: Immunocytochemical analysis of the structure and function of Peyer's patches. Jap J Gastroenterol **82**:2312,1985
57. Shen H.H., Talle M.A., Goldstein G., Chess L.: Functional subsets of human monocytes defined by monoclonal antibodies: a distinct subset of monocytes contains the cells capable of including the autologous mixed lymphocyte culture. J Immunol **130**:698,1983
58. Ahnen D.J., Brown W.R., Kloppel T.M.: Secretory component: the polymeric immunoglobulin receptor. What's in it for the gastroenterologist and hepatologist? Gastroenterology **89**:667,1985
59. Nagura H., Brandtzaeg P., Nakane P.K., Brown W.R.: Ultrastructural localization of J chain in human intestinal mucosa. J Immunol **123**:1044,1979
60. Nagura H., Tsutsumi Y., Hasegawa H., Watanabe K., Nakane P.K., Brown W.R.: IgA plasma cells in biliary mucosa: a likely source of locally synthesized IgA in human hepatic bile. Clin Exp Immunol **54**:671,1983
61. Halsey J.F., Johnson B.H., Cebra J.J.: Transport of immunoglobulin from serum into colostrum. J Exp Med **151**:767,1980
62. Nagura H., Smith P.D., Nakane P.K., Brown W.R.: IgA in human bile and liver. J Immunol **126**587,1981
63. Heremans J.F.: Immunoglobulin A. In The Antigens, vol II, Sela Med, New York, Academic Press, 1974, p365
64. Nagura H., Tsutsumi Y., Shioda Y., Watanabe K.: Immunohistochemistry of gastric carcinomas and associated diseases: novel distribution of carcinoembryonic antigen and secretory component on the surface of gastric cancer cells. J Histochem Cytochem **31**:193,1983
65. Brandtzaeg, P.: Transport models for secretory IgA and IgM. Clin Exp Immunol **44**:221,1981
66. Brandtzaeg P.: Polymeric IgA is complexed with secretory component (SC) on the surface of human intestinal epithelial cells. Scand J Immunol **8**:39,1978
67. Nagura H., Nakane P.K., Brown W.R.: Translocation of dimeric IgA through neoplastic colon cells in vitro. J Immunol **123**:2359,1979
68. Koshland M.E.: Structure and function of the J chain. Adv Immunol **20**:41,1975
69. Mostov K.E., Kraehenbuhl J.P., Brobel F.: Receptor-mediated transcellular transport of immunoglobulin: synthesis of secretory component as multiple and larger transmembrane forms. Proc Natl Acad Sci USA **77**:7257,1980
70. Lemaitre-Coelho I., Jackson G.D.F., Vaerman J-P.: Rat bile as a convenient source of secretory IgA and free secretory component. Eur J Immunol **8**:588,1977
71. Vaerman J-P., Lemaitre-Coelho, I.M., Limet J.N., Delacroix D.L.: Hepatic transfer of polymeric IgA from plasma to bile in rats and other mammals: a survey. In Recent Advances in Mucosal Immunity. Strober W, Hanson LA, Sell KW eds. New York, Raven Press, 1982, p233
72. Takahashi I., Nakane P.K., Brown W.R.: Ultrastructural events in the translocation of polymeric IgA by rat hepatocytes. J Immunol **128**:1181,1982
73. Chandy K.G., Hubscher S.G., Elias E., Berg J., Khan M., Burnett D.: Dual role of the liver in regulating circulating polymeric IgA in man: studies on patients with liver disease. Clin Exp Immunol **52**:207,1983
74. Brown T.A., Russell M.W., Mestecky J.: Hepatobiliary transport of IgA immune complexes: molecular and cellular aspects. J Immunol **128**:2183,1982
75. Peppard J., Orlans E., Payne A.W.R., Andrew E.: The elimination of circulating complexes containing polymeric IgA by excretion in the bile. Immunology **42**:83,1981
76. Kraft S.C.: The liver as an "IgA pump." Gastroenterology **80**:623,1981
77. Hall R.P., Lawley T.J., Heck J.A.: IgA-containing cir-

culating immune complexes in dermatitis herpetiformis, Henoch-Schoenlein purpura, systemic lupus erythematosus and other diseases. Clin Exp Immunol **40**:431,1980

78. Kater L., Jobsis A.C., de la Faille-Kuyper E.H.B., Vogten A.J.M., Grijm R.: Alcoholic hepatic disease. Specificity of IgA deposits in liver. Am J Clin Pathol **71**:51,1979
79. Nagura H., Tsutsumi Y., Watanabe K., Hasegawa H., Kobayashi K.: Studies on the relationships of IgA in human liver. Digestive Organ and Immunology **8**:315,1982
80. Delacroix D.L., Reymaert M., Pauwels S., Geubel A.P., Vaerman J.P.: High serum levels of secretory IgA in liver disease. Possible liver origin of the circulating secretory component. Dig Dis Sci **27**:333,1982
81. Fukuda Y., Imoto M., Hayakawa T.: Serum levels of secretory immunoglobulin A in liver diseases. Am J Gastroenterol **80**:237,1985
82. Fukuda Y., Nagura H., Asai J., Satake T.: Possible mechanisms of elevation of serum immunoglobulin A in liver diseases. Am J Gastroenterol **81**:315,1986
83. Kleinman R.E., Harmatz P.R., Walker W.A.: The liver: an integral part of the enteric mucosal immune system. Hepatology **2**:379,1982
84. Nagura H., Koshikawa T., Fukuda Y., Asai J.: Hepatic vascular endothelial cells heterogeneously express surface antigens associated with monocytes, macrophages and T lymphocytes. Virchows Arch A **409**:407,1985
85. Berzofsky J.A., Richman L.K., Strober W.: Determinant-specific antigen presentation by liver Kupffer cells under control of H-2-linked Ir genes. In Recent Advances in Mucosal Immunity. Strober W., Hanson L.A., Sell K.W. eds, New York, Raven Press, 1982, p215
86. Praaning-van Dalen D.P., Brouwer A., Knook D.L.: Clearance capacity of rat liver Kupffer, endothelial, and parenchymal cells. Gastroenterology **81**:1036,1981
87. Souhami R.L.: The effect of colloidal carbon on the organ distribution of sheep red blood cells and the immune response. Immunology **22**:685,1972
88. Richman L.K., Klingenstein R.J., Richman J.A., Strober W., Berzofsky J.A.: The murine Kupffer cell. I. Characterization of the cell serving accessory function in antigen-specific T cell proliferation. J Immunol **123**:2602,1980
89. Strober W., Richman L.K., Elson C.O.: The regulation of gastrointestinal immune responses. Immunology Today, August:**156**,1981
90. Richman L.K., Graeff A.S., Yarchoan R., Strober W.: Simultaneous induction of antigen-specific IgA helper T cells and IgG suppressor T cells in the murine Peyer's patch after protein feeding. J Immunol **126**:2079,1981
91. Andre C., Lambert R., Bazin H.: Interference of oral immunization with the intestinal absorption of heterologous albumin. Eur J Immunol **4**:701,1974
92. Stokes C.R., Swarbrick E.T., Soothill J.F.: Immune elimination and enhanced antibody responses: functions of circulating IgA. Immunology **40**:455,1980
93. Cunningham-Rundles C., Brandeis W.E., Good R.A., Day N.K.: Bovine antigens and the formation of circulating immune complexes in selective immunoglobulin A deficiency. J Clin Invest **64**:272,1979
94. Thomas H.C., Derilliers D., Potter B.J., Hodgson H., Jain S., Jewell D.P., Sherlock S.: Immune complexes in acute and chronic liver disease. Clin Exp Immunol **31**:150,1978
95. Triger D.R., Alp M.H., Wright R.: Bacterial and dietary antibodies in liver disease. Lancet **1**:60,1972
96. Cantor H.M., Dumont A.H.: Hepatic suppression of sensitization to antigen absorbed into the portal system. Nature (London) **215**:744,1967

# 10

# Crohn's Disease in Japan—A Clinicopathologic Study

Haruki Wakasa, M.D.
Hidemasa Ishikawa, M.D.
Hikaru Watanabe, M.D.

There have been an increasing number of reports[1-10] describing morphologic features of inflammatory bowel disease (IBD), particularly Crohn's disease, in recent years. Previously, there were thought to be two forms of Crohn's disease, acute and chronic; the acute form has been excluded by the finding that it was induced by Yersinia[11-13] or Anisakis.[14] Actually, the term Crohn's disease[15] includes regional granulomatous ulcerative colitis,[16] right-sided (regional) colitis,[17,18] regional colitis[19] and regional segmental colitis.[20]

Crohn's disease has long been considered a rather rare disease in Japan. To clarify the state of Crohn's disease in Japan, a research committee concerned with this disease was organized under the auspices of the Japanese Gastroenterological Society. This committee has consulted on cases on a nationwide scale and selected cases that were unmistakably Crohn's disease. Of course, during the course of this work, the development of endoscopic procedures and X-ray examination yielded much useful information.

Herein, we describe some characteristic clinicopathologic features of Japanese Crohn's disease, which were seen during the course of the study.

## CRITERIA FOR DIAGNOSIS PROPOSED BY THE COMMITTEE

The Japanese Research Committee[23,24] proposed the criteria composed of six key findings as follows: (1) discontinuity of lesions, (2) cobblestone-like appearance and/or longitudinal ulcers, (3) transmural inflammation, (4) noncaseous epithelioid cell granulomas, (5) fissures and/or fistulae, and (6) anal lesions. These diagnostic criteria were based on the descriptions of Evans and Acheson,[23] Lennard-Jones,[24,25] Fahrländer and Baerlocher[26] and Korelitz et al.[27] The committee consulted on cases of Crohn's disease and allied disorders on the basis of these criteria, and diagnosed each case according to the steps shown in Table 10-1, ranging from clinical examination to diagnostic biopsy and surgical specimen.

In diagnosis of Crohn's disease, however, intestinal tuberculosis, ulcerative colitis, ischemic enterocolitis, radiation (entero-) colitis, intestinal Behçet's disease, simple (nonspecific) ulcer of the small or large intestine, "nonspecific multiple ulcers of the small intestine" and acute terminal ileitis, etc., should be excluded beforehand, even when a combi-

**TABLE 10-1**
Diagnostic Criteria for Crohn's Disease (Japanese Research Committee)

| | Examination | X-ray | Endoscopy | Biopsy | Surgical specimen |
|---|---|---|---|---|---|
| Discontinuity of lesion | | + | + | + | + |
| Cobblestone appearance and/or longitudinal ulcer | | + | + | | + |
| Transmural inflammation | + (tumor) | + (stenosis) | + (stenosis) | | + |
| Granuloma | | | | $\oplus$ | $\oplus$ |
| Fissures and/or fistulae | +′ | +′ | +′ | +′ | +′ |
| Anal lesion | +′ | | | | +′ |

Crohn's disease diagnosis requires findings of at least + + $\oplus$ or + + + +′.

nation of all six of the above-mentioned findings is noted.

During the period from 1978 to 1982, the committee was able to select 102 cases consisting of 75 surgically resected cases and 27 biopsied cases of the disease according to the criteria.

## MATERIALS AND METHODS

These findings are based on data from 102 cases in which there was consultation, 11 cases that involved surgical resection, and 10 cases in which biopsy was done.

Clinical observation of 113 cases consisting of the cases in which there was consultation and those that involved resection was carried out. For morphologic study, biopsy and surgical specimens from 10 cases were processed for light microscopic, immunohistochemical, and electronmicroscopic observation as standard procedure.

Sections from paraffin blocks were stained with hematoxylin-eosin, Masson's trichrome, Gram, Ziehl-Neelsen, and Grocott's silver, and for immunohistochemical procedures sections were processed for lysozyme, $\alpha_1$-antitrypsin, $\alpha_1$-antichymotrypsin and S-100 protein according to the peroxidase antiperoxidase method (PAP method). In some cases, monoclonal antibodies for T or B cell aggregates were used to clarify the characterization of lymphoid cell aggregates in the intestinal wall.

For electronmicroscopic observation, fresh specimens were fixed with glutaraldehyde-formalin and then postfixed with osmium. After embedding with Epon, thin sections were made using an LKB ultramicrotome and stained with uranyl-lead.

## CLINICAL FEATURES

Age and sex distributions are shown in Figure 10-1. About 60% of the patients were in their third decade at the time of diagnosis, followed by those in their second decade. Males outnumbered females. Regarding lesion site, 26 patients had lesions in the small intestine only, and 38 patients had them in the large intestine. In 59 cases, lesions were found in both the small and large intestines (Table 10-2). Among these 113 cases, surgery was performed in 86, the rate of surgical procedure for each type of lesion being 88.5% for ileitis, 76.5% for ileocolitis, and 47.5% for colitis. With regard to symptoms, abdominal pain was the most common complaint at the onset, followed by diarrhea, fever, bloody stools, anemia, abdominal discomfort, emaciation, nausea, and vomiting. As to the relation of symptoms to lesion sites, there was a tendency for cases with small intestinal lesions to have fever and anemia, and for those with

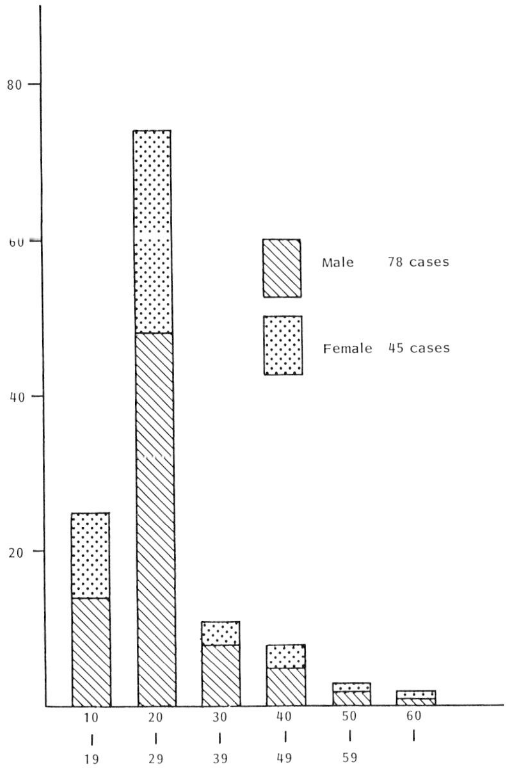


**Fig. 10-1.** Age distribution in patients with Crohn's disease. Abscissa: year range, Ordinate: number of cases.

large intestinal lesions to have bloody stools in addition to abdominal pain and diarrhea.

Symptoms at diagnosis were also similar to those at onset. Cases with small intestinal lesions seem to show more symptoms of obstruction in comparison to those with large intestinal lesions.

With regard to laboratory data, an increased erythrocyte sedimentation rate was found in 86% of the males and 94% of the females. Anemia, characteristically hypochromic anemia, was more frequently observed in the females than in the males. Decreased serum iron and leukocytosis were also observed in connection with hypoproteinemia with decreased A/G ratio. An increased serum $\alpha_2$-globulin was found in 70% of the cases.

The most frequently observed complication was protein-losing enteropathy, followed by malabsorption syndrome, fistulae, massive hemorrhage, disturbance of growth, and arthralgia.

**TABLE 10-2**
Site of Lesion

| | |
|---|---|
| Small intestine | 26 cases |
| Small and large intestines | 59 |
| Large intestine | 38 |
| Total | 123 |

## PATHOLOGIC FEATURES

Macroscopic findings: It is very important to observe the endoscopical finding and/or gross appearance of resected intestine when diagnosing Crohn's disease. In typical Crohn's disease, macroscopic findings are usually characteristic, and therefore, a definite diagnosis of Crohn's disease should not be made when the gross appearance is atypical. It is well known that the terminal ileum and the right-sided colon are more frequently involved than the left-sided colon in Crohn's disease. Resected small intestine is usually covered with mesenteric fibroadipose tissue throughout its entire length. Fibroadipose tissue becomes irregularly nodular, a condition induced by granulomatous infiltration characteristic of the disease. The segmental and/or discontinuous lesions characterized by intestinal wall thickening accompanying consequent obstructive symptoms, cobblestone-like appearance, and ulceration are often compared to the lesions of ulcerative colitis in which the rectum and the left colon are diffusely affected, which then spread throughout the entire colon.[28] Cobblestone-like appearance is characterized by edematous swelling of mucosa, which is surrounded by intercommunicating and fissuring ulceration.

In surgically resected specimens of the small intestine in cases of Crohn's disease, intestinal wall thickening was the most frequent feature, followed by longitudinal ulcers and

**TABLE 10-3**
Macroscopic Findings of Resected Samples

| | Small Intestinal Lesion | Large Intestinal Lesion |
|---|---|---|
| Longitudinal ulcer | 51 (82)* | 28 (52) |
| Cobblestone appearance | 29 (47) | 44 (81) |
| Thickening of intestinal wall | 55 (89) | 46 (85) |
| Stenosis | 23 (37) | 12 (22) |
| Fistulae | 11 (18) | 13 (24) |
| Aphthoid ulcer | 18 (29) | 9 (17) |
| Total | 62 | 54 |

* Percent in parenthesis.

cobblestone-like appearance (Table 10-3). On the other hand, in cases with large intestinal lesions intestinal wall thickening and cobblestone-like appearance were almost equally observed (Table 10-3). Gross observation shows cobblestone-like mucosal appearance with intestinal wall thickening to be the most common morphologic feature of Crohn's disease in Western countries,[29] but such cases are rather less prominent in Japan.

Among Japanese cases, the most characteristic feature of resected intestine is the existence of longitudinal ulcers located on the side of mesenteric attachment. Such ulcers were observed in 82.3% of the cases with small intestinal lesions (Table 10-3; Figs. 10-2, 10-3). This observation was also supported by other studies of cases in Japan.[5] It is not infrequent that the length of longitudinal ulcers in the terminal ileum is as great as 50 cm accompanied by edematous swelling in the surrounding mucosa. The mesenteric attachment opposite the longitudinal ulcer site, that is, the side with Peyer's patches, is usually intact, covered with normal appearing mucosa. A mild to moderate inflammatory cell infiltration, however, is usually present in the mucosa proper and the submucosal layer. In cases with short ulcers, sequential cobblestone-like swelling is found in the mucosa surrounding the ulcer in the terminal ileum, and short stick-like inflammatory polyps are also observed in the lesion.

Aphthoid ulcers, considered to be early lesions of Crohn's disease and probable extensions of longitudinal ulcers, were found in one-third of the cases with small intestinal lesions and one-fifth of those with large intestinal lesions.

The occurrence of longitudinal ulcers in

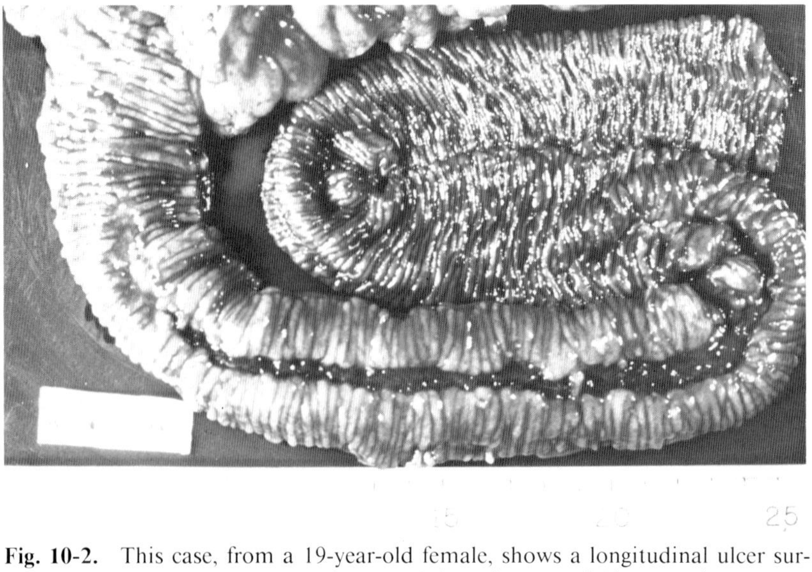

**Fig. 10-2.** This case, from a 19-year-old female, shows a longitudinal ulcer surrounded by edematous mucosa of the small intestine (Iwaki City Hospital case).

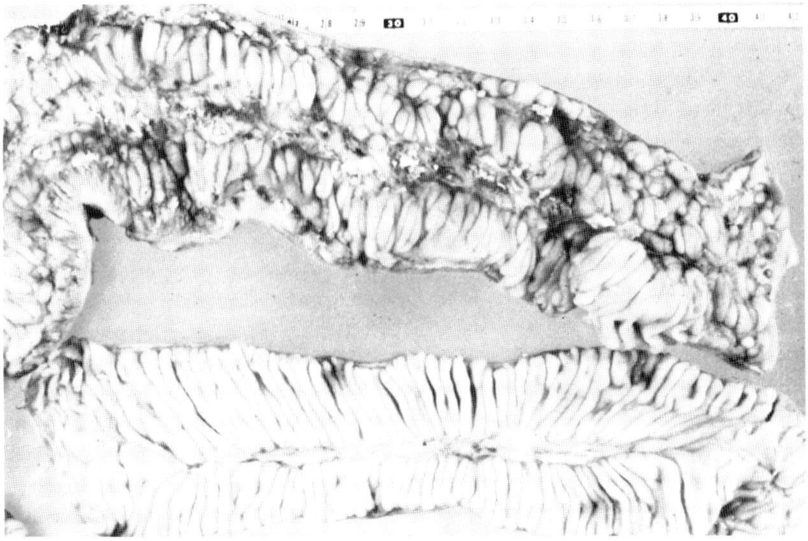

**Fig. 10-3.** In this case, from a 27-year-old male, longitudinal ulcer and serpiginous and irregularly shaped long ulcers are observed in the small intestine (Ōgaki Municipal Hospital case).

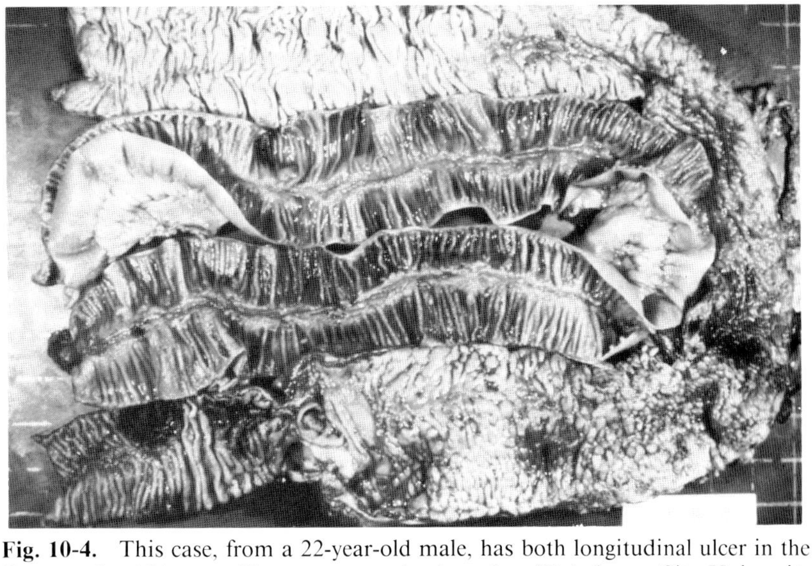

**Fig. 10-4.** This case, from a 22-year-old male, has both longitudinal ulcer in the ileum and cobblestone-like appearance in the colon (Yokohama City University case).

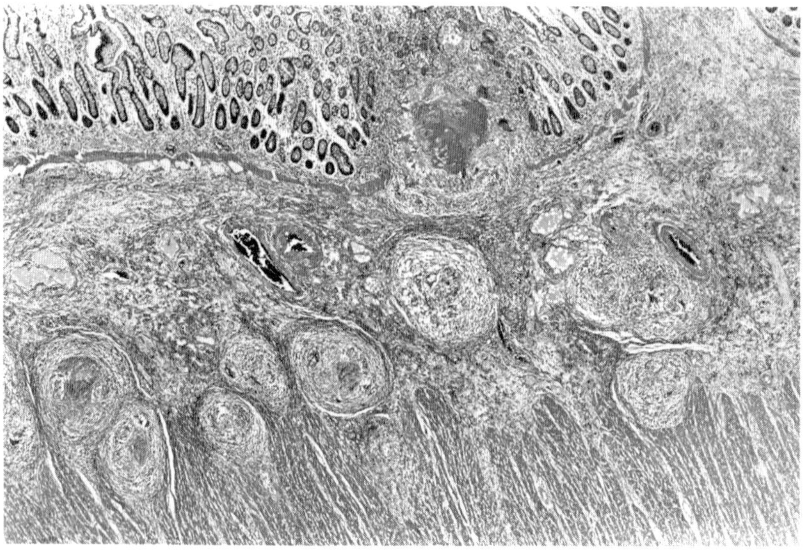

**Fig. 10-5.** Caseous tubercle in mucosa proper and several tubercles are formed in the submucosal and muscular layers. H&E × 20

cases with large intestinal lesions was observed in 57% of the cases, which is markedly lower than the rate of occurrence in the terminal ileum (Table 10-3). Regarding these ulcers observed in the large intestine, there were usually 2 or 3 in line, and they were short and irregular in shape and mainly observed at the site of colonic teniae.

In very rare cases, longitudinal ulcers in the ileum and a prominent cobblestone-like appearance in the large intestine with several fissures were both seen (Fig. 10-4). Such a finding suggests that both longitudinal ulcers and a cobblestone-like appearance are recognized as morphologic characteristics of Crohn's disease. Fissures and/or fistulae, having a reddish inflammatory mucosal appearance with necrotic tissue, were often present in resected intestines.

## GENERAL HISTOLOGICAL FEATURES

It is rather difficult to make a definite diagnosis of Crohn's disease when only histologic slides are used in the absence of information on gross appearance. In addition, it is also necessary to obtain clinical information such as that provided by X-ray, endoscopical findings and clinical history for proper diagnosis of the disease.

The diagnostic criteria used in Japan are very strict compared to those of Western countries, because of the need to differentiate this disease from other diseases, particularly intestinal tuberculosis (Fig. 10-5).[30,31] With routine endoscopic biopsy specimens of the intestine, diagnosis has to be based on microscopic observation of the mucosal and upper portion of submucosal layers. In addition to gross appearance, disproportionate findings, for example, a more intense inflammatory process in the submucosal layer than in the mucosal layer, are very helpful for diagnosing Crohn's disease.

The following findings are histological features of resected specimens of Crohn's disease: (1) transmural inflammatory process, (2) sarcoidlike noncaseous granuloma formation, (3) lymphoid aggregates in the intestinal wall, (4) ulceration, fissures and/or fistula formation, (5) fibrosis in the submucosal layer, (6) lymphangiectasia of the intestinal wall, and

**TABLE 10-4**
Microscopic Findings of Resected Samples

| | Small Intestinal Lesion | Large Intestinal Lesion |
|---|---|---|
| Transmural inflammation | 62 (100)* | 51 (96) |
| Granuloma | 56 (90) | 44 (83) |
| Fissures | 48 (77) | 42 (98) |
| Lymphangiectasia | 41 (66) | 32 (60) |
| Total | 62 | 53 |

* Percent in parenthesis.

(7) longitudinal ulcers with formation of subsequent amputation neuroma at the ulcer base.

There were also some differences in histological features between cases with small intestinal lesions and with large intestinal lesions. Thickening of intestinal wall and ulceration with subsequent formation of amputation neuroma at the ulcer base were more prominent in the small intestine than in the large intestine (Table 10-4).

As described above, longitudinal ulcers are characteristically found in the ileum in 80–90% of the cases of Crohn's disease (Table 10-4). These ulcers usually extend to the submucosal layer (Fig. 10-6), but in rare instances, the muscle layers are involved (Fig. 10-7). Aphthoid ulcers usually develop over lymphoid aggregates and contain a small number of granulocytes. In rare cases it is also observed that aphthoid ulcers detected by endoscopy extend to the longitudinal ulcers after some time. It is also possible that longitudinal ulcers may arise from aphthoid ulcers in some instances. It is difficult, however, to explain why ulcers of the small intestine with Crohn's disease are always formed on the mesenteric side. There is no direct correlation between granuloma formation and longitudinal ulceration based on our observations. At the ulcer base, extensive fibrosis and formation of so-called traumatic or amputation neuromas are usually present indicating that the ulcer is old.

As inflammatory cells, plasma cells, lymphocytes, eosinophils, and some mast cells are observed in the lesion. Granulocytes usually appear in the central portion of fissures and/or fistulae. Lymphocytic infiltration showing some aggregation is not so prominent in the mucosal layer, but it is rather prominent in the submucosal and subserosal layers.[32] These lymphocytes are mainly helper

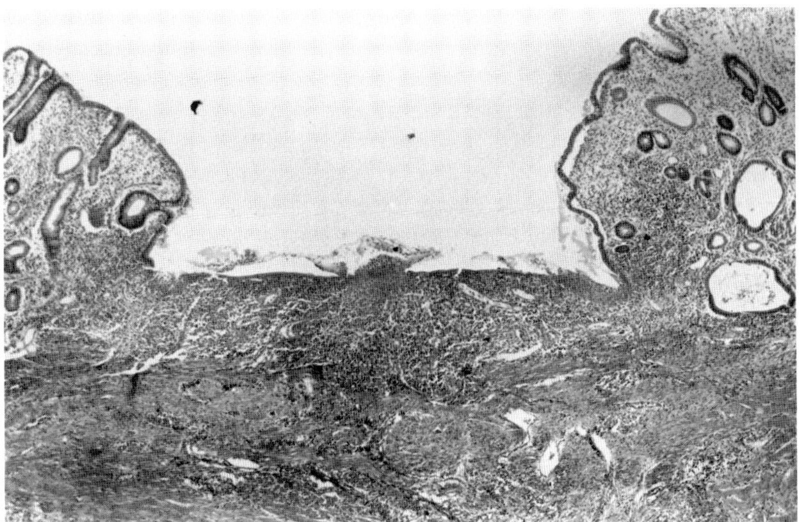

**Fig. 10-6.** Histologic low power view of longitudinal ulcer. H&E × 40

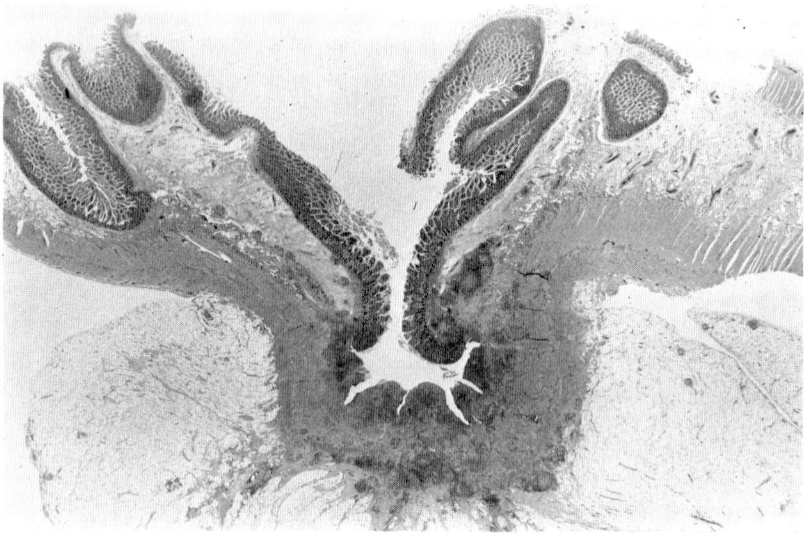

**Fig. 10-7.** Deep longitudinal ulcer and several fissures are distinctly formed on the side of mesenteric attachment. H&E × 5

T-lymphocytes as analyzed by monoclonal antibodies of Leu-series using frozen sections of fresh biopsy specimens. In the mucosa proper, small lymphocytes surround periglandular tissue, and they are also mainly helper T-lymphocytes (Fig. 10-8).[33] In regenerating mucosa, pseudopyloric glands are often observed.

Fibrosis is histologically more extensive than expected from macroscopic appearances. Peyer's patches usually contain an active hyperplastic germinal center in which nu-

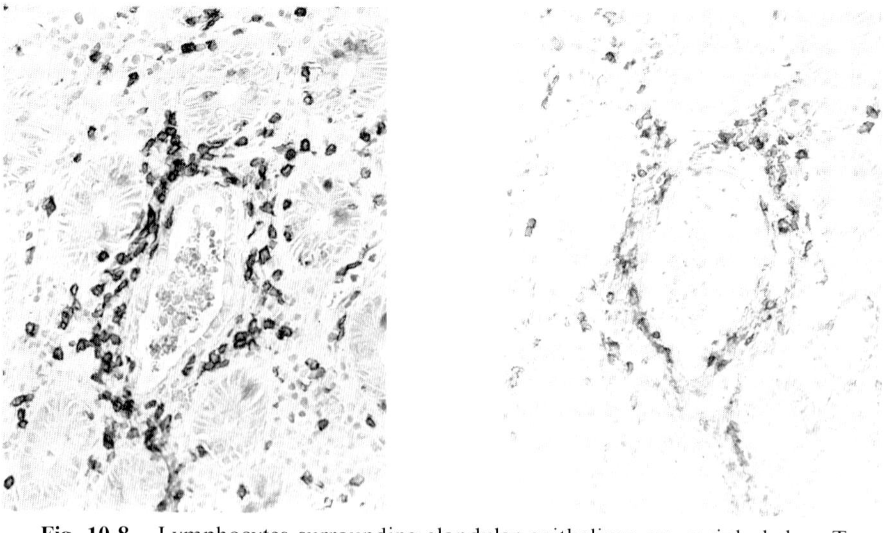

**Fig. 10-8.** Lymphocytes surrounding glandular epithelium are mainly helper T lymphocytes, analyzed by a) Leu 4 (Pan T) and b) Leu 3a (helper) monoclonal antibodies. PAP, × 250

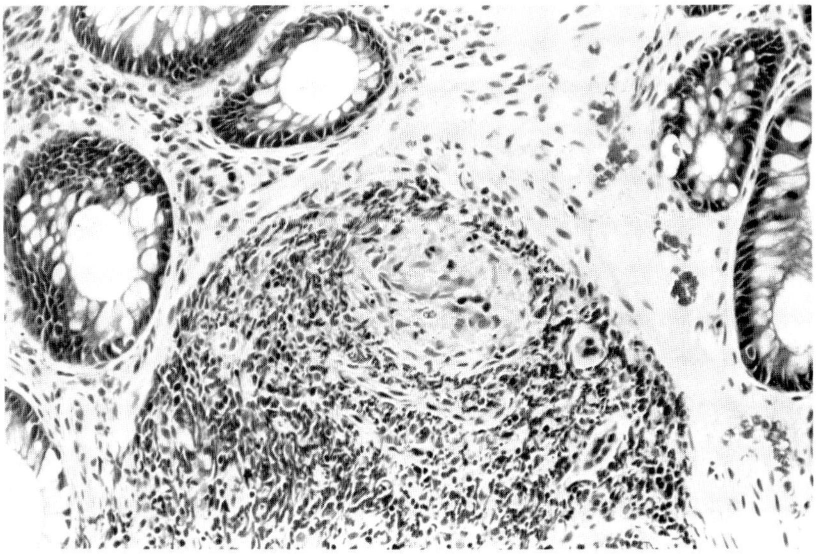

**Fig. 10-9.** Granuloma observed in rectal biopsy from normal appearing mucosa of the patient with active Crohn's disease in the small intestine. H&E × 200

merous tingible body macrophages appear. It is very useful to examine mesenteric lymph nodes in order to differentiate Crohn's disease from tuberculosis and Yersinia enterocolitica. In tuberculous infection, epithelioid granulomas in the lymph nodes are usually characterized by caseous necrosis, and tend to fuse with each other, usually resulting in large tubercles. Yersinia enterocolitica is characterized by the occurrence of granulocytes in the granuloma centers. On the other hand, granulomas in Crohn's disease are similar in size and have no tendency to fuse with each other.

## MORPHOLOGIC FEATURES OF EPITHELIOID CELL GRANULOMA—HISTOLOGIC AND ELECTRONMICROSCOPIC OBSERVATION

Although it is well recognized that epithelioid granulomas, which are considered to be a diagnostic clue, are found in the intestinal wall with varying incidence, their occurrence varies. Especially in biopsy specimens, the existence of granulomas is very helpful in correctly diagnosing the disease. In our study, granulomas were found in 90% of the cases in which there were small intestinal lesions and in over 80% of the cases in which there were large intestinal lesions. The occurrence of granulomas in Crohn's disease in Western countries, however, is usually encountered in 50–70% of the cases.[34] Even in cases without evidence of granulomas in one histologic slide only, granulomas are almost always found if serial sections are made, and it is sometimes necessary to make over 300 sections.

It is possible to find granulomas in rectal biopsy specimens even when the rectal mucosa appears to be normal in cases that are in the active phase of Crohn's disease. Watanabe[35] examined up to 2040 serial sections in an attempt to find granulomas and found such granulomas in 3 cases out of 4 with ileocolonic lesion and 3 out of 3 with large intestinal lesion (Fig. 10-9). The rate of occurrence of granuloma detected by serial sections is markedly higher than in those studies performed in Western countries.[36–40] The difference in frequency of granulomas in cases of Crohn's disease between Japan and Western countries is probably based on some difference in diagnostic clues. In our study granulomas were found to form not only in lymphatic tissue of

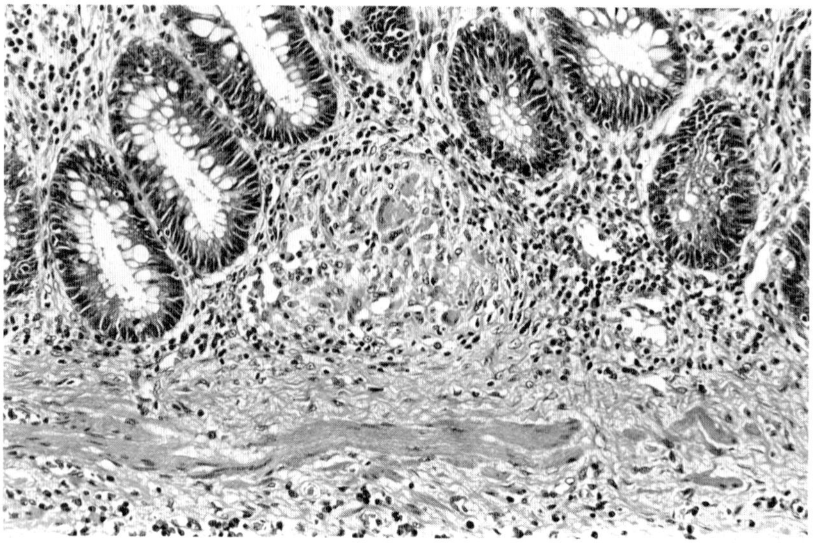

**Fig. 10-10.** Granuloma in mucosa proper. Epithelioid cells with formation of Langhans type giant cells are observed. H&E × 150

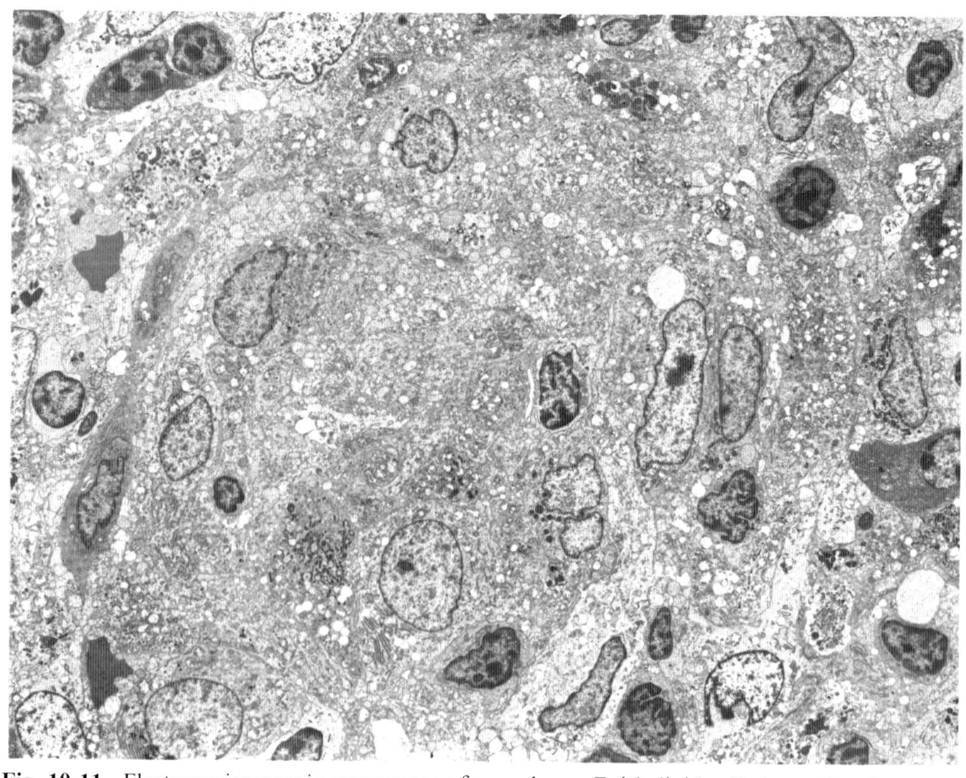

**Fig. 10-11** Electronmicroscopic appearance of granuloma. Epithelioid cells have abundant cytoplasm with or without lysosomes. ×1,800

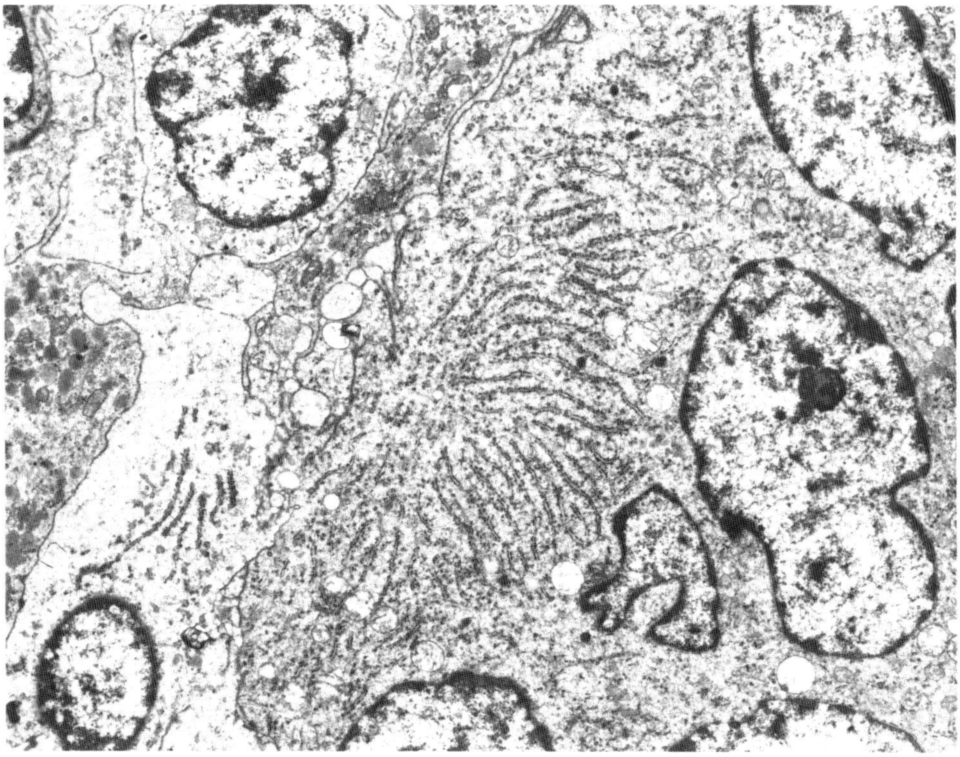

**Fig. 10-12.** Well developed rough endoplasmic reticulum arranged parallel in peripheral portion of Langhans type giant cell. ×2,700

the mucosal layer, but in all layers of the intestine. This observation was previously described by Rappaport.[41]

*Cellular component of granuloma:* Granulomas observed in mucosal and submucosal layers are composed of numerous epithelioid cells characterized by abundant cytoplasm and oval nuclei (Fig. 10-10). Epithelioid cells in granulomas of the mucosal and submucosal layers are rather compactly arranged in comparison to those found in other layers. Epithelioid cell granulomas often contain Langhans-type giant cells that are smaller in size and have fewer nuclei in comparison to those of tuberculous granulomas. Foreign body type giant cells phagocytizing calcified material are sometimes found in the subserosal layer, but they are not specific for the disease and might be formed as a reaction of macrophages to necrotic tissue caused by ulceration. With PAP method, lysozyme, $\alpha_1$-antitrypsin, and $\alpha_1$-antichymotrypsin are always positively stained in epithelioid cells,[42] and are especially intensely positive in Langhans-type giant cells. Electronmicroscopic observation reveals that epithelioid cells have abundant cytoplasm containing many organelles and lysosomes (Fig. 10-11). Cell nuclei are usually round to oval with distinct small nucleoli. Langhans-type giant cells usually contain numerous mitochondria and parallel arrangement of the endoplasmic reticulum is observed in the peripheral portion of the cytoplasm (Fig. 10-12).

*Size and frequency of granulomas in each layer:* The size of granulomas and the frequency of occurrence in each layer of the intestinal wall were calculated to differentiate epithelioid granulomas of Crohn's disease

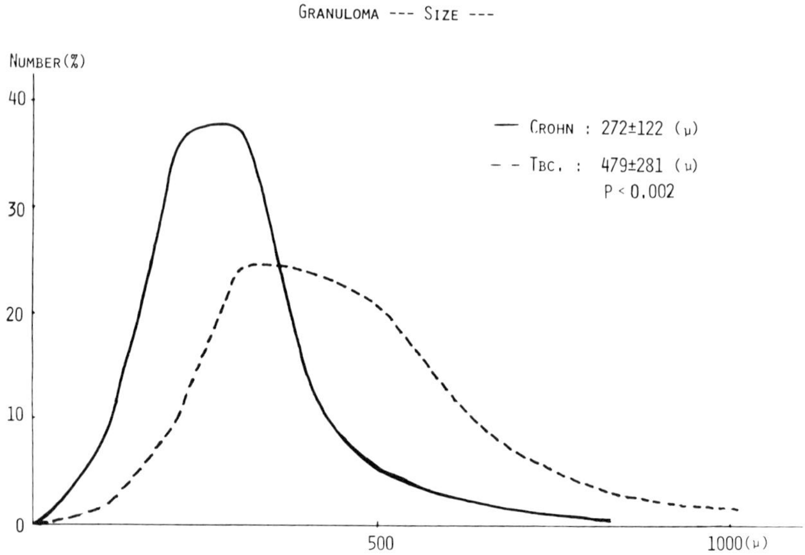


**Fig. 10-13.** Size of granulomas in each layer.

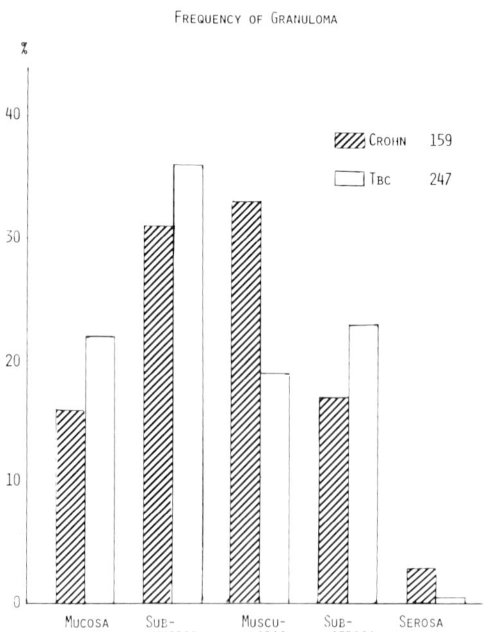


**Fig. 10-14.** Frequency of granulomas.

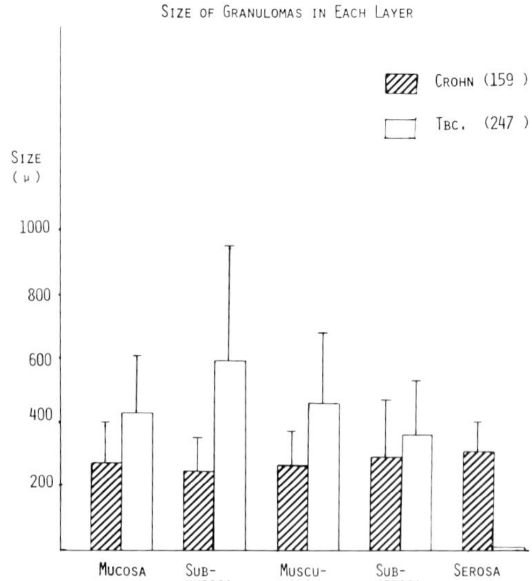


**Fig. 10-15.** Size of granulomas: TBC vs Crohn's disease.

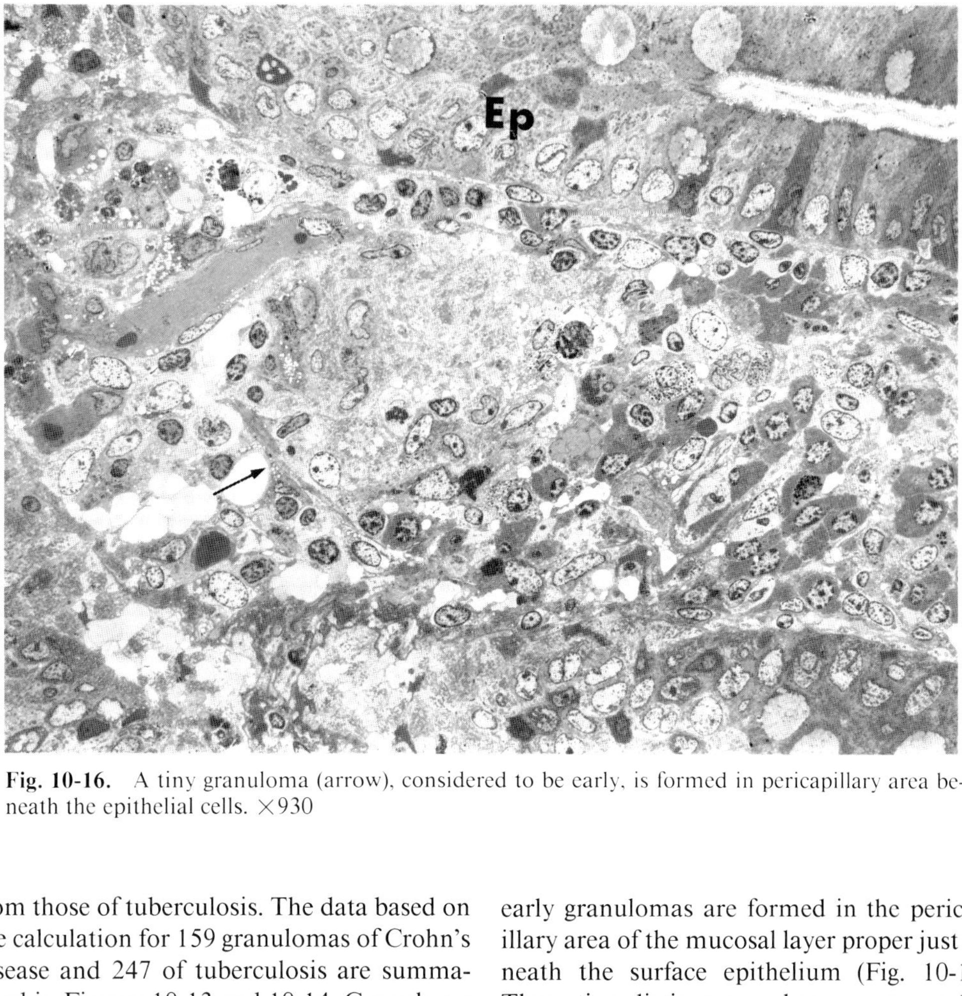


**Fig. 10-16.** A tiny granuloma (arrow), considered to be early, is formed in pericapillary area beneath the epithelial cells. ×930

from those of tuberculosis. The data based on the calculation for 159 granulomas of Crohn's disease and 247 of tuberculosis are summarized in Figures 10-13 and 10-14. Granuloma size as calculated by diameter is similar in all layers in Crohn's disease, but different in different layers in the case of tuberculosis. The size of tuberculous granulomas in the submucosal layer is larger than those of other layers because of the confluent tendency of granulomas. The relation between the size of granulomas and frequency in two diseases is shown in Fig. 10-15, and the mean size in Crohn's disease is $272 \pm 122\ \mu$ and that in tuberculosis is $479 \pm 281\ \mu$.

With regard to the frequency of granulomas in each layer, it is not so different between the two diseases, except that it was slightly higher in the muscular layer in Crohn's disease. Electronmicroscopic observation indicates that early granulomas are formed in the pericapillary area of the mucosal layer proper just beneath the surface epithelium (Fig. 10-16). These tiny distinct granulomas composed of a small number of epithelioid cells are observed to be sharply demarcated from surrounding cells. On the basis of electronmicroscopic observation, it is difficult to determine whether granuloma formation in the mucosal layer is closely related to lymphatics, because lymphatics are not distinct in this area. Electronmicroscopic observation using a wide hole mesh was performed to define the relation of granulomas to lymphatics,and it was found that granulomas were distinctly formed in perilymphatic tissue and/or intralymphatic spaces. Epithelioid granulomas intermingled with small lymphocytes are clearly formed in the lumina of lymphatics (Fig. 10-17). Even in histologic slides, granulomas are often found

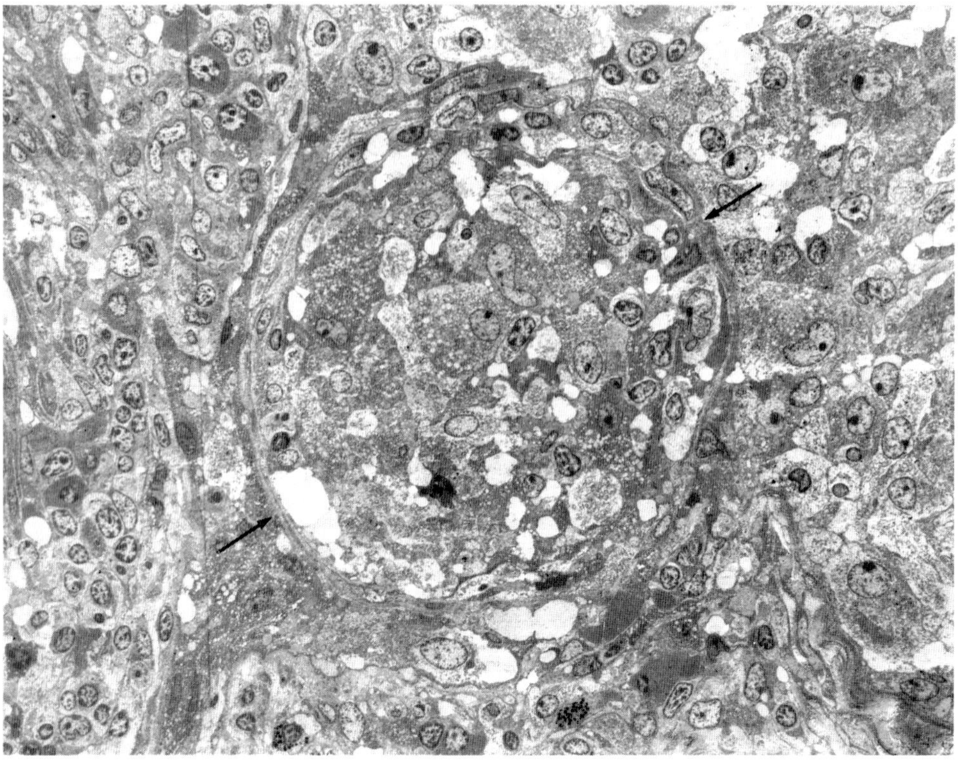

**Fig. 10-17.** Cluster of epithelioid cells intermingled with small lymphocytes are clearly present in lymphatic lumen (arrows). ×830

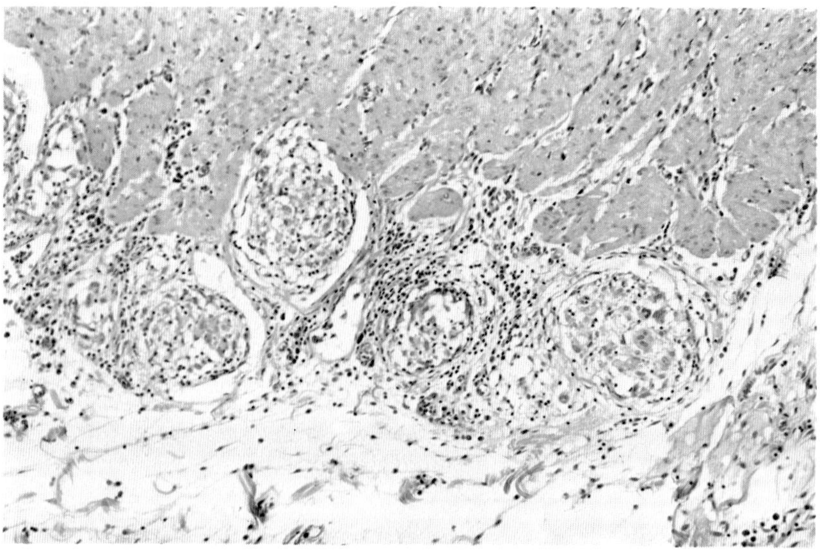

**Fig. 10-18.** Granulomas in the subserosal layer are present in the lymphatics showing luminal obstruction. H&E × 100

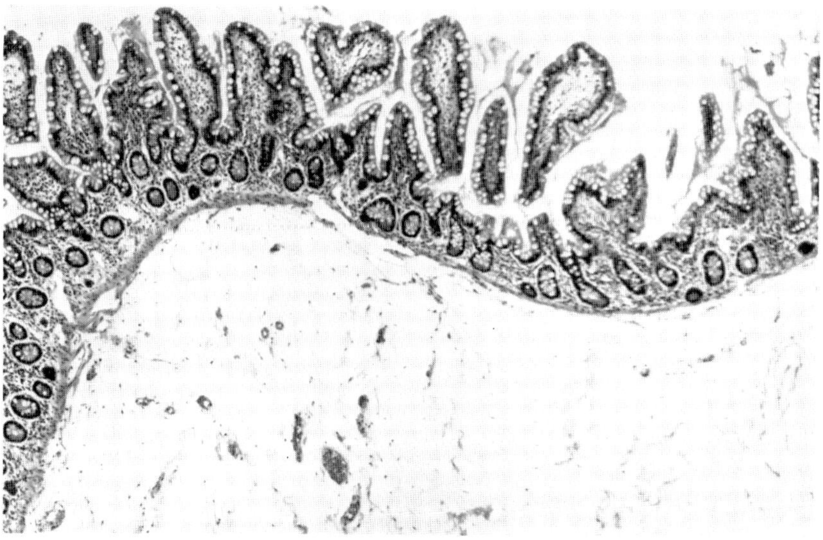

**Fig. 10-19.** Marked submucosal edema, probably in accord with cobblestone-like swelling, is formed by the obstruction of the lymphatics by granuloma. H&E × 40

in dilated lymphatics and in the perineural space of Auerbach's plexus of muscular layers.

Similar findings show that granulomas are even more intimately related to lymphatics in the subserosal layer (Fig. 10-18) and outside the serosa where lymphangitis or perilymphangitis might obstructively induce lymphangiectasia with consequent lymphedema in the submucosal layer (Fig 10-19). Such edematous swelling of mucosal and submucosal layers might be correlated with the cobblestone-like gross appearance. It is reasonably recognized that in case of longstanding cob-

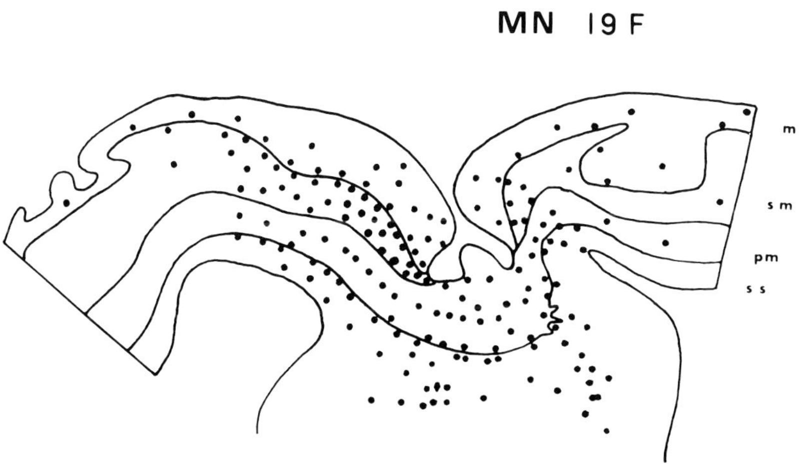


**Fig. 10-20.** This schema shows the distribution of granulomas revealed by serial sections from a 19 year old female. m = mucosa, sm = submucosa, pm = pars muscularis, ss = subserosa.

blestone-like edematous swelling, fibrosis may finally occur mainly in the submucosal layer on the mesenteric side.

*Distribution of granulomas:* Light microscopic observation of serial sections of histologic specimens shows the frequency of granulomas to be quite different from case to case. Granulomas are scattered in the submucosal layer, but were observed in clusters in the area surrounding Peyer's patches and in the deeper mucosal layer close to the lamina muscularis mucosae. The tendency of granulomas to cluster was also observed in the muscular and subserosal layers.

Schematic distribution and extension of granulomas are shown in Figure 10-20. From our morphologic observations, it is concluded that lymphatics have a close relationship to the formation and extension of granulomas in the intestinal wall.

## DISCUSSION

Inflammatory bowel disease is a disorder in which immunological background is necessary for understanding.[43, 44]

Crohn's disease has been considered rare in Japan, because there have been no definite diagnostic criteria. However, cases have been increasing in number since the establishment of clinicopathologic criteria proposed by the Japanese Research Committee for Crohn's Disease. This committee, composed of clinicians and pathologists, consulted on cases of intestinal disorders suspected of being Crohn's disease on a nationwide scale and diagnosed each case. In Japan, it is necessary to differentiate cases of Crohn's disease from tuberculosis, but in recent years cases of tuberculosis have been decreasing markedly.

In Western countries, there are two peaks in age distribution, but in the Japanese cases of the present series, there is no such tendency. The data in the present study were obtained at time of diagnosis, not at onset.

The most prominent feature of Crohn's disease in Japan is the existence of longitudinal ulcers in the small intestine exclusively on the side of the mesenteric attachment. On the other hand, ulcers in the large intestine are usually irregular in shape and are seen in short lines at the sites of colonic teniae.

Cases in Western countries reveal a marked wall thickening with a cobblestone-like appearance, often accompanied by stenosis. It is rather infrequent to observe cases with such classic morphologic features in Japan. The occurrence of both cobblestone-like appearance and longitudinal ulcers in the same case suggests that these two features should be recognized as basic attributes of Crohn's disease.

Regarding longitudinal ulcers, it was confirmed in only one case of our series that aphthoid ulcers definitely extended to the ulcer after some time. In most cases, however, no such clinicopathologic finding was obtained. It is also suggested that the site of longitudinal ulcers in Crohn's disease is similar to that of ischemic enteritis frequently occurring in cases with cardiac disorder or in elderly persons.

Morphometric data on the thickness of intestinal arteries in Crohn's disease show an increase in thickness of the arterial wall outside of the intestine, which may indicate that ischemic change previously existed in the wall.[45] It is also suggested that blood flow is decreased in intestinal arteries of Crohn's disease.[46] In Western countries, the frequency of longitudinal ulcers is low, even sometimes showing railtrack-like appearance in figures. At present, it is speculated that an inflammatory process including granulomatous lesions develops around the lymphatics and involves blood vascularity, and then the occurrence of ischemic change.

Epithelioid cell granulomas, which are noncaseous, rather smaller and more similar in size compared with those of tuberculosis, are formed in all layers of the intestine and lymph nodes. Among Japanese cases, epithelioid cell granulomas are highly useful for diagnostic purposes, because of their frequency, which is high compared with that in Western countries. Examination of 300 serial sections revealed granulomas not only in the overt lesion but also in the biopsy specimens from normal appearing rectal mucosa of cases in the active phase of Crohn's disease. Such a finding showing granulomas and inflammatory process in rectal mucosa apart from any grossly visible lesion confirms that the intestine may be involved extensively,[47, 48] even when it is covered with normal looking mucosa. Therefore, wide surgical resection is sometimes ineffective in preventing recurrence.[8]

As described above, epithelioid cells are formed from macrophages, which are positive for lysozyme, $\alpha_1$-antitrypsin and $\alpha_1$-antichymotrypsin as shown by the PAP method. It is thought that macrophages may appear first and that granulomas are then formed as the result of early reaction in the intestinal wall. With electronmicroscopic observation, early tiny granulomas are seen to be formed in the pericapillary area of the upper mucosal layer just beneath the surface epithelium. They eventually extend to the deeper layers through the lymphatics. Granulomas formed in or around lymphatics in the subserosal layer may induce the obstruction of lymphatics with subsequent submucosal edema of the intestinal wall. Lymphangiectasia and cobblestone-like appearance may ensue in accord with intestinal edema induced by the obstruction of lymphatics in the subserosal layer and outside the intestine. Ultrastructural abnormalities of intestinal lymphatics in Crohn's disease, reported by Kovi,[49] who found no gaps in lymphatic walls, may also play a role in intestinal edema. It is suggested that granulomas formed with relation to lymphatics may be an important factor in the etiopathogenesis of Crohn's disease.

## SUMMARY

Morphological study of cases of Crohn's disease in Japan revealed a high frequency of longitudinal ulcers in the terminal ileum and epithelioid cell granuloma formation in the intestinal wall. The pathogenesis of longitudinal ulcers is still uncertain, but the location of such ulcers is similar to that of ischemic change suggesting that the inflammatory process may induce vascular change.

Epithelioid cell granulomas found in the lesion of the mucosal layer proper may be considered as an early cellular reaction in Crohn's disease, and these granulomas are closely related to lymphatics as shown by electron- and light-microscopic observation. No definitive causative agent was confirmed by our intensive observation.

## ACKNOWLEDGMENTS

We are very grateful to the members of the Japanese Research Committee for Crohn's Disease (Chairman: Prof. S. Yamagata). We express our appreciation to Mr. T. Ito and Mr. Y. Sasaki for their technical assistance and to Mrs. M. Hangai for the preparation of the manuscript.

## REFERENCES

1. Morson B.C., Dawson I.M.P.: Gastrointestinal Pathology, Blackwell, Oxford, London, Edinburgh and Melbourne, 1979
2. Dvorak A.M., Dickersin R.: Crohn's disease: Transmission electron microscopic studies. I. Barrier function. Possible changes related to alterations of cell coat, mucous coat, epithelial cells, and Paneth cells. Human Pathol **11**:561, 1980
3. Dvorak A.M., Monahan R.A., Osage J.E., Dickersin R.: Crohn's disease: Transmission electron microscopic studies. II. Immunologic inflammatory response. Alterations of mast cells, basophils, eosinophils and the microvasculature. Human Pathol **11**:606, 1980
4. Dvorak A.M., Monahan R.A., Osage J.E., Dickersin R.: Crohn's disease: Transmission electron microscopic studies. III. Target tissues. Proliferation of and injury to smooth muscle and the autonomic nervous system. Human Pathol **11**:620, 1980
5. Watanabe H.: Histopathological diagnosis of inflammatory bowel disease of the large intestine. Clinical Radiology **25**:789, 1980 (in Japanese)
6. Wakasa H., Yamazaki T.: Pathology of inflammatory bowel disease. Naika Mook **14**:35, 1980 (in Japanese)
7. Rowland R., Pounder D.J.: Crohn's colitis. Pathol Annu 17 (Pt 1), 267, 1982
8. Hamilton S.R.: Pathologic features of Crohn's disease associated with recrudescence after resection. Pathol Annu 18, 191, 1983
9. Wakasa H., Ishikawa H., Asano S.: Crohn's disease, morphologic features. J Jpn Soc Colo-Proctol **36**:472, 1983 (in Japanese)

10. Saito K.: Crohn's disease; some problems on histopathological diagnosis. Pathology & Clinical Medicine **2**:163, 1984 (in Japanese)
11. Winblad S., Niléhn B., Sternby N.H.: Yersinia enterocolitica (Pasteurella X) in human enteric infections. Brit Med J **2**:1363, 1966
12. Sjöström B.: Acute terminal ileitis and its relation to Crohn's disease. In "Regional Enteritis (Crohn's Disease)" Engel A, Larsson T (eds), Nordiska Bokhandelns Förlag, Stockholm, p 73, 1971
13. Kato Y., Hattori T., Oh-ya H., Suzuki T., Yoshino S., Kato H., Nishikawa H.: A case of acute terminal ileitis by Yersinia enterocolitica. Jap Gastroenterology **73**:56, 1976 (in Japanese)
14. Ishikura H., Hayasaka H., Kikuchi Y.: Acute regional ileitis at Iwanai Kokkaido. With special reference to intestinal Anisakiasis. Sapporo Med J **12**:183, 1967
15. Diseases of the gastrointestinal tract. Vol III, Provisional International Nomenclature. ed. Btesh S, CIOMS, Geneva, 1973
16. Bargen J.A., Weber H.M.: Regional migratory chronic ulcerative colitis. Surg Gynec Obstet **50**:964, 1930
17. Crohn B.B., Ginzburg L., Oppenheimer G.D.: Regional ileitis. A pathologic and clinical entity. JAMA **99**:1323, 1932
18. Crohn B.B., Berg A.A.: Right-sided (regional) colitis. JAMA **110**:32, 1938
19. Dubins J.A.: Regional colitis (with report of two cases). Rev Gastroenterol **6**:293, 1939
20. Castro Barbosa J. de, Bargen J.A., Dixon C.F.: Regional segmental colitis. Proc Staff Meet Mayo Clin **20**:134, 1945
21. The Japanese Research Committee for Crohn's Disease (Chairman: Yamagata S.): Diagnostic criteria for Crohn's disease. Jap Gastroenterology **73**:1467, 1976 (in Japanese)
22. The Japanese Research Committee for Crohn's Disease (Chairman: Yamagata S.): Crohn's disease in Japan. Gastroenterol Jpn **14**:366, 1979
23. Evans J.G., Achsen E.D.: An epidemiological study of ulcerative colitis and regional enteritis in the Oxford area. Gut **6**:311, 1965
24. Lennard-Jones J.E.: Definition and diagnosis. In "Regional Enteritis (Crohn's Disease)", ed. Engel A., Larsson T., Nordiska, Bokhandelns Förlag, Stockholm, p 105, 1971
25. Lennard-Jones J.E.: Etiology and epidemiology of Crohn's disease. Canad J Surg **17**:379, 1974
26. Fahrländer H., Baerlocher C.H.: Clinical features and epidemiological data in the Basle area. In "Regional Enteritis (Crohn's Disease)", ed. Engel A., Larsson T., Nordiska, Bokhandelns Förlag, Stockholm, p 131, 1971
27. Korelitz B.I., Present D.H., Alpert L.I. Marshak R.H., Janowitz, H.D.: Recurrent regional ileitis after ileostomy and colectomy for granulomatous colitis. N Engl J Med **287**:110, 1972
28. Lockhart-Mummery H.E., Morson B.C.: Crohn's disease (regional enteritis) of the large intestine and its distinction from ulcerative colitis. Gut **1**:87, 1960
29. Muto T.: Comparative appearances of Crohn's disease in England and Japan: A preliminary personal experience. Stomach and Intestine **13**:385, 1978 (in Japanese)
30. Watanabe H., Enjoji M., Yao T.: Histopathology of intestinal tuberculosis. Stomach and Intestine **12**:1481, 1977 (in Japanese)
31. Yao T.: Current state of intestinal tuberculosis. Naika Mook **14**:165, 1980 (in Japanese)
32. Meuwissen S.G.M.: Analysis of the lymphoplasmacytic infiltrate in Crohn's disease with special reference to identification of lymphocyte populations. Gut **17**:770, 1976
33. Ishikawa H.: Macroscopical, microscopical and immunohistological studies on intestinal lesion of Crohn's disease. Fukushima J Med Sci **37** (1) [in press] (in Japanese)
34. Schachter H., Kirsner J.B.: Crohn's Disease of the Gastrointestinal Tract. John Wiley & Sons, New York, 1980
35. Watanabe H., Endo K., Sato T., Unoura A., Okata T., Namiki T., Nakamura K., Ōto T., Kobayashi M.: Identification of granulomas by rectal biopsies from patients with active Crohn's disease. Annual Research Committee Report for Inflammatory Bowel Disease p. 269 from Ministry of Health and Welfare, 1983 (in Japanese)
36. Korelitz B.I., Sommers S.C.: Rectal biopsy in patients with Crohn's disease. JAMA **237**:2742, 1977
37. Rotterdam H., Korelitz B.I., Sommers S.C.: Microgranulomas in grossly normal rectal mucosa in Crohn's disease. Amer J Clin Pathol **67**:550, 1977
38. Goodman M.J., Kirsner J.B., Riddell R.H.: Usefulness of rectal biopsy in inflammatory bowel disease. Gastroenterology **72**:952, 1977
39. Hill R.B., Kent T.H., Hansen R.N.: Clinical usefulness of rectal biopsy in Crohn's disease. Gastroenterology **77**:938, 1979
40. Iliffe G.D., Owen D.A.: Rectal biopsy in Crohn's disease. Digest Dis Sci **26**:321, 1981
41. Rappaport H., Burgoyne F.H., Smetana H.F.: The pathology of regional enteritis. Milit Surgeon **109**:463, 1951
42. Wakasa H., Ishikawa H.: Crohn's disease; special reference to granulomas. Annual Research Committee Report on Inflammatory Bowel Disease, p. 369, from Ministry of Health and Welfare, 1984 (in Japanese)
43. Shorter R.G., Huizenga K.A., Spencer R.J.: A working hypothesis for the etiology and pathogenesis of non-specific inflammatory bowel disease. Am J Dig Dis **17**:1024, 1972
44. Kobayashi J.: Crohn's disease. Medicina **20**:220, 1983 (in Japanese)
45. Sasaki I., Funayama Y., Imamura M., Konno Y., Sato T.: Morphometric analysis of intestinal arteries in Crohn's disease. Annual Research Committee Report on Inflammatory Bowel Disease, p. 387, from Ministry of Health and Welfare, 1984 (in Japanese)
46. Hultén L., Lindhagen J., Lundgren O,. Fasth S., Åhrén C.: Regional intestinal blood flow in ulcerative colitis and Crohn's disease. Gastroenterology **72**:388, 1977
47. Goodman M.J., Skinner J.M., Truelove S.C.: Abnormalities in the apparently normal bowel mucosa in Crohn's disease. Lancet I: 275, 1976
48. Dunne W.T., Cooke T.W., Allan R.N.: Enzymatic and morphometric evidence for Crohn's disease as a diffuse lesion of the gastrointestinal tract. Gut **18**:290, 1977
49. Kovi J.: Ultrastructure of intestinal lymphatics in Crohn's disease. Am J Clin Pathol **76**:385, 1981

# Index

Numerals in *italics* indicate a figure, "t" following a page number indicates tabular matter.

# Plant Allelopathy: Mechanisms and Applications in Regenerative Agriculture

Guest Editors

**Margot Schulz**
**Vincenzo Tabaglio**

MDPI

Basel • Beijing • Wuhan • Barcelona • Belgrade • Novi Sad • Cluj • Manchester

*Guest Editors*

Margot Schulz
Institute of Molecular
Physiology and
Biotechnology of Plants
University of Bonn
Bonn
Germany

Vincenzo Tabaglio
Department of Sustainable
Crop Production
Section Agronomy and Plant
Biotechnologies
Università Cattolica del Sacro
Cuore
Piacenza
Italy

*Editorial Office*
MDPI AG
Grosspeteranlage 5
4052 Basel, Switzerland

This is a reprint of the Special Issue, published open access by the journal *Plants* (ISSN 2223-7747), freely accessible at: https://www.mdpi.com/journal/plants/special_issues/Plant_Allelopathy_Mechanisms.

For citation purposes, cite each article independently as indicated on the article page online and as indicated below:

Lastname, A.A.; Lastname, B.B. Article Title. *Journal Name* **Year**, *Volume Number*, Page Range.

**ISBN 978-3-7258-3495-2 (Hbk)**
**ISBN 978-3-7258-3496-9 (PDF)**
**https://doi.org/10.3390/books978-3-7258-3496-9**

Cover image courtesy of Margot Schulz and Vincenzo Tabaglio

# Contents

# About the Editors

**Margot Schulz**

Margot Schulz works since many years in the field of allelopathy, focusing on biochemical responses of target plants, allelochemical detoxification of benzoxazinoids, and glucosinolates by plants and microorganisms, and on molecular effects of terpenoids. She published more than 150 articles, most of them dealing with allelopathy, book chapters and conference abstracts. After studying chemistry and biology and finishing her PhD at the University of Cologne, Germany, she had a postdoc position at the University of Wisconsin, Madison, USA, before starting her habilitation at the University of Bonn. Germany. She got her qualification for a teaching career in higher education in 1993. Presently, she is involved in projects addressing the role of microorganisms in allelopathy and plant-microbe interactions.

**Vincenzo Tabaglio**

Vincenzo Tabaglio, working at the DI.PRO.VE.S., University of Cattolica del Sacro Cuore, Piacenza, Italy, is an established scientist in the field of allelopathic weed control, agroecology, crop residue decomposition, soil fertility and health, conservation tillage systems, carbon farming, nitrogen fertilization and mitigation of greenhouse gasses. He is engaged in projects and research for promoting of the rural development in India, in sustainable crop production for food security in Africa and low-income countries. He has published more than 90 articles, book chapters, and conference abstracts/papers, eleven of them dealing with allelopathy.

# Preface

The use of allelopathic interaction for weed control is a promising component of integrated crop management in sustainable agriculture. Our conviction, that the use of allelopathy can mitigate environmental risks and contribute to maintaining soil fertility and biodiversity, motivated us to design this Special Issue. The functional agents in plant-plant, plant-microbe interactions are allelochemicals/secondary metabolites, which are entirely produced by the organisms and released into the environment. The isolation of the compounds from allelopathic plants and other organisms and the structural identification of the compounds is of outstanding importance to develop efficient application methods and to elucidate the specific mode of action on the physiological, biochemical, and molecular level, including changed protein abundancy and altered gene expression in target plants. This Special Issue contains 15 contributions, 10 research articles and 5 review articles. Altogether, 75 Authors from Brazil, China, Colombia, Egypt, France, Germany, Japan, Iran, Italy, Jordan, Poland, Spain, Tunisia, and USA contribute to the success of the Special Issue, demonstrating a word-wide interest in the field of allelopathy. We think that the theme will find a broad audience at relevant Universities and Research Stations, and we hope that the Special Issue motivates young scholars engaged in science and agriculture to continue research on allelopathy for improving its applications and promotion of Green Technologies development. Finally, we want to thank all Authors for all their work and the Editorial Office, particularly Bobo Wang, for their help and support to complete this Special Issue.

**Margot Schulz and Vincenzo Tabaglio**
*Guest Editors*

*plants*

*Editorial*

# Allelopathy: Mechanisms and Applications in Regenerative Agriculture

**Margot Schulz [1,*] and Vincenzo Tabaglio [2]**

1 IMBIO Institute of Molecular Physiology and Biotechnology of Plants, University of Bonn, Karlrobert-Kreiten Str. 13, 53115 Bonn, Germany
2 Department of Sustainable Crop Production DI.PRO.VE.S., Section Agronomy and Plant Biotechnologies, Università Cattolica del Sacro Cuore, Via Emilia Parmense 84, 29122 Piacenza, Italy; vincenzo.tabaglio@unicatt.it
* Correspondence: ulp509@uni-bonn.de

**Citation:** Schulz, M.; Tabaglio, V. Allelopathy: Mechanisms and Applications in Regenerative Agriculture. *Plants* **2024**, *13*, 3301. https://doi.org/10.3390/plants13233301

Received: 17 November 2024
Accepted: 19 November 2024
Published: 25 November 2024



Allelopathy is an important mechanism in plant communication and interference, involving the release of plant/microorganism self-produced, special featured organic molecules into the environment. These molecules (allelochemicals) inhibit or stimulate the growth of neighbored plants and microorganisms (targets), depending on their type and dosage. They are therefore regarded as natural plant growth modulators, with the effects also influenced by the developmental and other characteristics of the target plants. When used as a form of negative interaction between species, allelopathy in agriculture serves as a proven, sustainable tool for integrated weed control in organic farming, thereby mitigating environmental risks, a key objective of the Green Deal and Farm to Fork Strategy of the EU Agricultural Policy. Allelopathy can reduce the use of synthetic herbicides or of chemically upgraded natural compounds which cannot be no longer considered natural products.

The adoption of allelopathy (plant-plant and plant-microbe interactions) in regenerative agricultural practices still requires thorough multidisciplinary research (encompassing chemistry, genetics, metabolism, and agronomy) to address two complementary areas of focus. First, screening is needed to identify new allelopathic plants and their allelochemicals. Second, it is crucial to investigate the agronomic feasibility of effectively using these plants and their metabolites in conventional agroecosystems through field studies. For the latter, it is important to assess the potential for incorporating these allelopathic plants into crop rotations, often as cover crops, without adversely affecting subsequent crops.

This special issue on allelopathy aims to gather current experimental findings from around the world, covering both basic and applied aspects. It serves as a convenient and accessible resource for researchers working in this field and may contribute to promote future research on allelopathic interactions.

It compiles fourteen articles (nine original research and five original reviews) covering different aspects of allelopathy. The original research articles present recent investigations on allelochemical identification, on tritrophic interaction, on molecular effects in plant growth modulation and on undesired pathogen propagation via allelochemicals.

As can be observed, there is a lack of articles in the more strictly agronomic significance, specifically regarding the application of these results in open-field conditions. This highlights the need for greater research efforts in this important area, which is certainly more costly from an experimental perspective but is absolutely necessary for transitioning from basic knowledge to applied knowledge.

Following, some key points of the research articles are listed.

Vieites-Álvarez et al. [1] characterize the chemical profile of shoots, roots, and root exudates of four buckwheat accessions, emphasizing on polyphenol accumulation and exudation. The buckwheat Gema (accession number 01Z5000112) appeared to be most promising for sustainably control of the two herbicide-resistant target weeds *Lolium rigidum*

Gaud. and *Portulaca oleracea* L. Espinosa-Colín et al. [2] present phytotoxic propiophenone, 4-ethylacetophenone, and 2,4-dimethylacetophenone obtained from *Cistus ladanifer*. Using *Lactuca sativa* and *Allium cepa* as target plants, dosage dependency of inhibitory and hormetic effects of the compounds were investigated.

The study of Amri et al. [3] addresses the chemical composition of essential oils from *Eucalyptus falcata*, *E. sideroxylon* and *E. citriodora*. They determined remarkable antioxidant, antimicrobial and phytotoxic properties of the essential oils. Germination and growth of *Sinapis arvensis*, *Phalaris canariensis*, and *Triticum durum* seedlings were inhibited. Marques et al. [4] contribute with a work on phytotoxic, water-soluble quillaic acid-based triterpene saponins isolated from the leaves of *Quillaja lancifolia*. Kato-Noguchi et al. [5] investigated the hitherto unknown allelopathic properties of *Osmanthus fragrans*, *Osmanthus heterophyllus* and of a hybrid of these two species, *Osmanthus* × *fortunei* Carrière. Main allelopathic substances of *O.* × *fortunei* and *O. fragrans* were identified as (+)-pinoresinol and 10-acetoxyligustroside, which are released into the environment during decomposition.

The contribution of Preusche et al. [6] demonstrated the concentration-dependent influence of the *Mentha x piperita* volatilome, *Mentha* essential oil fraction and limonene on the expression profile of distinct TCP transcription factors that modulate *Arabidopsis thaliana* and cabbage leaf growth under different culture conditions. Staszek et al. [7] investigated the phytotoxic effect of the digestive fluid of *Nepenthes x ventrata* on tomato seed germination and seedlings root growth. Oxidative stress elicited by the digestive fluid is supposed to inhibit tomatoes. A study dealing with the trophic interaction between *Peudosphinx tetrio* L. larvae and the toxic Apocynaceae *Allamanda cathartica* L. is presented by Matignon et al. [8]. The chemical profiles of the leaves of healthy and herbivorous *A. cathartica* and of the excretions of the caterpillars was analyzed. Larval excretion of the bioactive compounds from the host plant is one possibility to escape the harmful effects of these compounds.

Xin et al. [9] present investigations on the interactions of the allelochemicals and pathogens of potato including *A. solani*, *B. cinerea*, *F. solani*, *F. oxysporum*, *C. coccodes*, and *V. dahlia*. 7-Methoxycoumarin had inhibitory effects but, for instance, caffeic acid and chlorogenic acid promoted the pathogens. The results led to the conclusion that autotoxic allelopathy and promotion of pathogens caused by the accumulation of distinct allelochemicals can result in replant problems of potato.

The five original reviews summarize important features of *Cyperus esculentus*, *Solidago species*, *Abutilon theophrasti*, and microalgae allelopathy, whereas the contribution of Lewerenz et al. [10] attends to translocation of allelochemicals between plants, emphasizing on pyrrolizidine alkaloids. Zhang et al. [11] present the current state of *Cyperus esculentus* L. including the allelopathic potential and antibacterial, antioxidant and insecticidal activities of this plant. Kato-Noguchi and Kato [12] give an overview of *Solidago canadensis* L. and *Solidago altissima* L. allelopathy, two species which are aggressive invaders in many parts of the world. Tabaglio et al. [13] thematize properties and microorganisms possibly involved in the resilience of velvetleaf (*Abutilon theophrasti* Medik.) against allelochemicals, such as benzoxazinoids. Casanova et al. [14] reviewed the great variety of allelochemicals found in microalgae. These compounds may be valuable to biocontrol weeds, insects, phytopathogenic fungi and bacteria.

This special issue demonstrates that the sustainable use of allelopathy in agriculture demands in-depth knowledge about the bioactive molecules responsible for influencing the complex interactions between organisms. It is imperative that microorganisms must be considered in allelopathic interactions. This knowledge is the first step in designing smart agroecosystems that ensure both the sustainable intensification of agricultural production, as advocated by the FAO to meet global food demands and combat poverty, and the protection of the environment and species diversity, as outlined in the European Green Deal.

**Author Contributions:** The authors contribute to this article in equal shares. All authors have read and agreed to the published version of the manuscript.

**Funding:** This research received no external funding.

**Conflicts of Interest:** The authors declare no conflict of interest.

## References

1. Vieites-Álvarez, Y.; Otero, P.; López-González, D.; Prieto, M.A.; Simal-Gandara, J.; Reigosa, M.J.; Hussain, M.I.; Sánchez-Moreiras, A.M. Specialized Metabolites Accumulation Pattern in Buckwheat Is Strongly Influenced by Accession Choice and Co-Existing Weeds. *Plants* **2023**, *12*, 2401. [CrossRef] [PubMed]
2. Espinosa-Colín, M.; Hernandez-Caballero, I.; Infante, C.; Gago, I.; García-Muñoz, J.; Sosa, T. Evaluation of Propiophenone, 4-Methylacetophenone and 2′,4′-Dimethylacetophenone as Phytotoxic Compounds of Labdanum Oil from *Cistus ladanifer* L. *Plants* **2023**, *12*, 1187. [CrossRef] [PubMed]
3. Amri, I.; Khammassi, M.; Ben Ayed, R.; Khedhri, S.; Mansour, M.B.; Kochti, O.; Pieracci, Y.; Flamini, G.; Mabrouk, Y.; Gargouri, S.; et al. Essential Oils and Biological Activities of *Eucalyptus falcata*, *E. sideroxylon* and *E. citriodora* growing in Tunisia. *Plants* **2023**, *12*, 816. [CrossRef]
4. Marques, M.E.M.; de Carvalho, A.C.; Yendo, A.C.A.; Magedans, Y.V.S.; Zachert, E.; Fett-Neto, A.G. Phytotoxicity of Quillaja lancifolia Leaf Saponins and Their Bioherbicide Potential. *Plants* **2023**, *12*, 663. [CrossRef]
5. Kato-Noguchi, H.; Hamada, Y.; Kojima, M.; Kumagai, S.; Iwasaki, A.; Suenaga, K. Allelopathic Substances of *Osmanthus* spp. for Developing Sustainable Agriculture. *Plants* **2023**, *12*, 376. [CrossRef] [PubMed]
6. Preusche, M.; Vahl, M.; Riediger, J.; Ulbrich, A.; Schulz, M. Modulating Expression Levels of TCP Transcription Factors by *Mentha x piperita* Volatiles—An Allelopathic Tool to Influence Leaf Growth? *Plants* **2022**, *11*, 3078. [CrossRef] [PubMed]
7. Staszek, P.; Piekarniak, M.; Wal, A.; Krasuska, U.; Gniazdowska, A. Is the Phytotoxic Effect of Digestive Fluid of *Nepenthes x ventrata* on Tomato Related to Reactive Oxygen Species? *Plants* **2023**, *12*, 755. [CrossRef] [PubMed]
8. Matignon, L.; Lo, M.M.; Monpierre, M.; Correia, M.V.; Valencia, D.P.; Palmeira-Mello, M.V.; Sylvestre, M.-N.; Pruneau, L.; Sylvestre, M.; Domenech, A.; et al. Phytochemical and Biological Study of Trophic Interaction between *Pseudosphinx Tetrio* L. Larvae and *Allamanda Cathartica* L. *Plants* **2023**, *12*, 520. [CrossRef]
9. Xin, A.; Jin, H.; Yang, X.; Guan, J.; Hui, H.; Liu, H.; Cui, Z.; Dun, Z.; Qin, B. Allelochemicals from the Rhizosphere Soil of Potato (*Solanum tuberosum* L.) and Their Interactions with the Soilborne Pathogens. *Plants* **2022**, *11*, 1934. [CrossRef]
10. Lewerenz, L.; Abouzeid, S.; Yahyazadeh, M.; Hijazin, T.; Selmar, D. Novel Cognitions in Allelopathy: Implications from the "Horizontal Natural Product Transfer". *Plants* **2022**, *11*, 3264. [CrossRef] [PubMed]
11. Zhang, S.; Li, P.; Wei, Z.; Cheng, Y.; Liu, J.; Yang, Y.; Wang, Y.; Mu, Z. Cyperus (*Cyperus esculentus* L.): A Review of Its Compositions, Medical Efficacy, Antibacterial Activity and Allelopathic Potentials. *Plants* **2022**, *11*, 1127. [CrossRef] [PubMed]
12. Kato-Noguchi, H.; Kato, M. Allelopathy and Allelochemicals of *Solidago canadensis* L. and *S. altissima* L. for Their Naturalization. *Plants* **2022**, *11*, 3235. [CrossRef] [PubMed]
13. Tabaglio, V.; Fiorini, A.; Sterling, T.M.; Schulz, M. Abutilon theophrasti's Resilience against Allelochemical-Based Weed Management in Sustainable Agriculture—Due to Collection of Highly Advantageous Microorganisms? *Plants* **2023**, *12*, 700. [CrossRef] [PubMed]
14. Casanova, L.M.; Macrae, A.; de Souza, J.E.; Neves Junior, A.; Vermelho, A.B. The Potential of Allelochemicals from Microalgae for Biopesticides. *Plants* **2023**, *12*, 1896. [CrossRef] [PubMed]

plants

Article

# Specialized Metabolites Accumulation Pattern in Buckwheat Is Strongly Influenced by Accession Choice and Co-Existing Weeds

Yedra Vieites-Álvarez [1], Paz Otero [2], David López-González [1], Miguel Angel Prieto [2], Jesus Simal-Gandara [2,3], Manuel J. Reigosa [1,3], M. Iftikhar Hussain [1] and Adela M. Sánchez-Moreiras [1,3,*]

1 Departamento de Bioloxía Vexetal e Ciencia do Solo, Facultade de Bioloxía, Campus Lagoas-Marcosende s/n, Universidade de Vigo, 36310 Vigo, Spain; yedra.vieites.alvarez@uvigo.es (Y.V.-Á.); davidlopez@uvigo.es (D.L.-G.); mreigosa@uvigo.es (M.J.R.); iftikhar@uvigo.es (M.I.H.)
2 Nutrition and Bromatology Group, Department of Analytical and Food Chemistry, Faculty of Food Science and Technology, Universidade de Vigo, Ourense Campus, 32004 Ourense, Spain; potero@uvigo.es (P.O.); mprieto@uvigo.es (M.A.P.); jsimal@uvigo.es (J.S.-G.)
3 Instituto de Agroecoloxía e Alimentación (IAA), Universidade de Vigo, Campus Auga, 32004 Ourense, Spain
* Correspondence: adela@uvigo.es; Tel.: +34-6-5059-9150

**Abstract:** Screening suitable allelopathic crops and crop genotypes that are competitive with weeds can be a sustainable weed control strategy to reduce the massive use of herbicides. In this study, three accessions of common buckwheat *Fagopyrum esculentum* Moench. (Gema, Kora, and Eva) and one of Tartary buckwheat *Fagopyrum tataricum* Gaertn. (PI481671) were screened against the germination and growth of the herbicide-resistant weeds *Lolium rigidum* Gaud. and *Portulaca oleracea* L. The chemical profile of the four buckwheat accessions was characterised in their shoots, roots, and root exudates in order to know more about their ability to sustainably manage weeds and the relation of this ability with the polyphenol accumulation and exudation from buckwheat plants. Our results show that different buckwheat genotypes may have different capacities to produce and exude several types of specialized metabolites, which lead to a wide range of allelopathic and defence functions in the agroecosystem to sustainably manage the growing weeds in their vicinity. The ability of the different buckwheat accessions to suppress weeds was accession-dependent without differences between species, as the common (Eva, Gema, and Kora) and Tartary (PI481671) accessions did not show any species-dependent pattern in their ability to control the germination and growth of the target weeds. Finally, Gema appeared to be the most promising accession to be evaluated in organic farming due to its capacity to sustainably control target weeds while stimulating the root growth of buckwheat plants.

**Keywords:** buckwheat; polyphenols; sustainable weed control; allelopathy; competition

**Citation:** Vieites-Álvarez, Y.; Otero, P.; López-González, D.; Prieto, M.A.; Simal-Gandara, J.; Reigosa, M.J.; Hussain, M.I.; Sánchez-Moreiras, A.M. Specialized Metabolites Accumulation Pattern in Buckwheat Is Strongly Influenced by Accession Choice and Co-Existing Weeds. *Plants* **2023**, *12*, 2401. https://doi.org/10.3390/plants12132401

Academic Editor: Ippolito Camele

Received: 27 April 2023
Revised: 17 May 2023
Accepted: 15 June 2023
Published: 21 June 2023



## 1. Introduction

Pests and weeds are probably the primary biotic limitation that farmers face when attempting to increase the yield of their crops. Therefore, research, development, and the use of chemical products exclusively produced for the control of weeds/pests in the field has increasingly grown in the last decades. However, these synthetic chemical products, which have been extensively applied in the field, are dangerous to terrestrial environment and to human health [1], and increase weed resistance [2]. Several synthetic herbicides, including glyphosate, exhibit significant potential for soil adsorption and cannot move around freely in the environment. The effects of herbicides on human health depend on the concentration, length, and frequency of exposure, and often lead to cytotoxic and DNA damage and carcinogenicity [3]. Reducing their use is an increasing necessity in order for more sustainable food production.

There are several recent reports that highlight the development of resistance in different *Lolium* sp., including *Lolium rigidum* Gaudin, the species used in this study, which is likely the cause of the significant loss in cereal crop yield in Mediterranean countries and Australia [4,5]. In the US, populations of Italian ryegrass (*L. perenne* ssp. *multiflorum* (Lam.) Husn.) have also been found to be resistant to glufosinate [6]. As a result of the quick evolution of resistance in *L. rigidum*, comprehensive weed management measures, including crop allelopathic varieties, are required to slow down this rapid evolution and sustainable control. In several European countries, including Spain and Portugal, resistance to acetyl-CoA carboxylase (ACCase), acetolactate synthase (ASL), photosystem II (PSII), 5-enolpyruvylshikimate-3-phosphate synthase (EPSPS), glutamine synthase, very long-chain fatty acid (VLCFA) synthesis, and protoporphyrinogen oxidase (PPO)-inhibiting herbicides has been reported in *L. rigidum*, which is mainly associated with winter cereals, vineyards, and orchards [7,8]. The other species used in this study, *Portulaca oleracea* L., commonly known as purslane, is a weed belonging to the Portulacaceae family that has been ranked ninth out of the world's worst weeds, and has been recorded in 45 crops in 81 countries [9]. According to the International Herbicide-Resistant Weed Database, *P. oleracea* has been already found to develop resistance to Group 5 (Legacy C1 C2) herbicides, which are referred to as PSII inhibitors—Serine 264 Binders. These specific biotypes are resistant to the atrazine and linuron herbicides, and may also be cross-resistant to other members of the Group 5 (Legacy C1 C2) family. Other researchers have also reported *P. oleracea* as a resistant weed to linuron [10]. This is a common phenomenon in many weeds due to the massive use of synthetic herbicides.

Several integrated weed management strategies can be employed to limit herbicide use, such as harrowing or hoeing, flames or hot water, allelopathic cover crops, smother crops, and green mulching, which are crucial for controlling the weed seed population in the soil for green economy, plant biodiversity, and environmental sustainability [11]. The circular economy, promoted by the European Commission, defends the reuse of various types of organic biomass and organic waste, thus transforming waste management into economic opportunities [12,13]. In this context, screening suitable allelopathic crops and crop genotypes that are competitive with weeds can be a secure and environmentally responsible weed control strategy [14]. By releasing specialized metabolites into the surrounding environment that may act as phytotoxins to suppress weeds, they fall in the framework of a process known as allelopathy and provide themselves a competitive edge [15,16]. By encouraging diversification of the agricultural system and reducing the reliance on herbicides, this approach can also reduce the risk of the development of herbicide resistance in monocot and dicot weeds populations. Weed management must protect environmental quality and human health, and allelochemicals released from live crops and crop residues can be used in this way to manage weeds and improve crop performance [17].

The *Fagopyrum* genus is a dicotyledonous pseudo-cereal crop of the family Polygonaceae. It is comprised of both perennial and annual species with diploid (2n = 2x = 16) and tetraploid (2n = 4x = 32) chromosome numbers with a haploid genome size of −1.2 Gb. Out of the 34 reported species to date, this genus is recognized primarily by two cultivated species, common buckwheat (*F. esculentum* Moench.) and Tartary buckwheat (*F. tataricum* (L.) Gaertn.), along with the wild species *F. cymosum* (Trev.) Meisn. [18]. Buckwheat, which is known for its high nutritional value and bioactive components, is cultivated mainly for the production of food and pharmacological products for humans, and is increasingly considered as a promising emergent crop, as it can be an important source of proteins with well-balanced amino acid composition, dietary fibre, and phenolic substances [19]. Buckwheat is rich in phenolic acids and flavonoids, and exhibits antioxidative properties [20–22]. Besides well-known antioxidative effects, it has recently been suggested that buckwheat, as a source of the flavonoid quercetin, may prevent health problems in patients with diabetes [19].

Regarding its allelochemical potential, Kumar et al. [23] demonstrated that buckwheat residues in the soil were able to reduce powell amaranth, shepherd's purse, and corn chamomile growth. There are several research and review manuscripts published advocating that buckwheat tissues possess abundant specialized metabolites, especially phenolic acids and flavonoids, with a significant allelopathic potential [24–26] that could be responsible for the weed-suppressive activity of buckwheat [23,27,28]. In addition, it has been reported that the suppression of some weeds is caused by the light competition of rapidly growing buckwheat plants [29]. However, previous studies have shown that common buckwheat, thanks to allelochemicals, can also significantly reduce the biomass of certain weed species such as *Thlaspi arvense* L., *Cirsium arvense* (L.) Scop., and *Plantago lanceolata* L. [30].

Phenolic compounds, abundant metabolites in buckwheat [31,32], are well known for their allelochemical properties. Phenolic acids such as cinnamic, dihydroxybenzoic, ferulic, *p*-coumaric, phthalic, syringic, *m*-toluic, or protocatechuic have been related to the allelochemical-induced growth inhibition of several weed species [33]. These compounds can be found in different parts of the buckwheat plant, such as the leaves, stems, and roots [34]. When buckwheat residues, such as decomposed plant material or root exudates, are present in the soil, the phenolic acids released can exert inhibitory effects on weed germination, growth, and development [23,29]. The specific mechanism through which phenolic acids inhibit weeds is not fully understood, but it is believed to involve interference with weed seed germination, root elongation, and nutrient uptake. The research has demonstrated the allelopathic effects of buckwheat on various weed species. For example, studies have shown that buckwheat residues can inhibit the germination and growth of weeds such as common lambsquarters (*Chenopodium album*), pigweed (*Amaranthus* spp.), and barnyard grass (*Echinochloa crus-galli*) [23,34]. It is important to note that the allelopathic effects can vary depending on factors such as the buckwheat cultivar and the weed species in question.

Both competition and allelopathy, as mechanisms of plant interference, have been well documented under controlled conditions [35]. The combined effects of allelopathy and crop competition determine the total weed-suppressive potential of a given variety, and research groups worldwide have been working to improve both traits simultaneously in order to achieve maximum gains in weed suppression [36,37], particularly in cereal crops. The root length of ryegrass, mustard, and lettuce was significantly reduced when their seeds co-germinated with buckwheat [30]. Although more recent studies are mostly focused on the allelopathic action of common buckwheat on weeds, Tartary buckwheat has also been studied for years regarding its potential for weed management [38].

However, little is known about the direct relation among allelochemicals exudation or accumulation and weed control by common or Tartary buckwheat. Therefore, the objective of this research was to examine the impact of three accessions of common buckwheat *Fagopyrum esculentum* Moench. (Gema, Kora, and Eva), and one accession of Tartary buckwheat, *Fagopyrum tataricum* (L.) Gaertn. (PI481671), on monocot (*Lolium rigidum* Gaud.) and dicot (*Portulaca oleracea* L.) weeds under laboratory-based germination and seedling growth bioassays. The potential of allelopathic compounds was carried out through identifying and quantifying a broad polyphenols profile (phenolic acids and flavonoids) in the roots, shoots, and root exudates of the different buckwheat accessions to compare the abundance of these allelochemicals with their weed suppressive capacity. The specific objectives of this study include the elucidation of the allelopathic potential of selected buckwheat accessions and their possible use to promote plant-based herbicides and their use in sustainable weed management strategies.

## 2. Results

### 2.1. Germination and Seedling Growth

Our results show that the germination rate of both weed species, *L. rigidum* and *P. oleracea*, was significantly decreased following being co-cultured with the four tested buckwheat accessions (Gema, Kora, Eva, and PI481671), which showed the strong capacity to control weed germination following a 7-day co-culture and it was species-specific

(Table 1). Only *P. oleracea* could maintain its germination unaltered in the presence of the Eva accession. Although different buckwheat accessions behaved differently, they induced significant inhibition of germination when compared with the control, with Gema (19%) and PI481671 (35%) being the most inhibitory accessions for *L. rigidum* followed by Eva (50%) and Kora (54%). On the contrary, Kora (41%) was the most inhibitory accession for *P. oleracea* (41%), followed by PI481671 (55%) and Gema (59%).

**Table 1.** Allelopathic impact of different buckwheat genotypes (Gema, Kora, Eva, and PI481671) on the germination (Germ: number of seeds as % of the control), fresh plant weight (PW; g given as % of the control) (i.e., weed species grown alone), and shoot and root lengths (cm given as % of the control) in monocot (*Lolium rigidum*) and dicot (*Portulaca oleracea*) weeds. Grey cells indicate significant inhibition, while bold numbers indicate significant stimulations compared with the control. The asterisk indicates statistical significant differences compared to the control at $p < 0.05$.

| | *Lolium rigidum* | | | | *Portulaca oleracea* | | | |
|---|---|---|---|---|---|---|---|---|
| *Accession* | Germ | PW | SL | RL | Germ | PW | SL | RL |
| PI481761 | 35 * | 68 * | 106 | 78 | 55 * | **162** * | **186** * | 134 |
| Eva | 50 * | 52 * | **149** * | 122 | 73 | 107 | **146** * | 90 |
| Kora | 54 * | 73 * | 127 | 119 | 41 * | 91 | 100 | 126 |
| Gema | 19 * | 79 | 135 | 29 * | 59 * | 107 | **158** * | **166** * |

Regarding the impact of the presence of buckwheat accessions on weed growth and development, we obtained a species dependent behaviour again, with *L. rigidum* as the most sensitive weed species to buckwheat co-cultivation (Table 1). The most inhibited parameter was the fresh plant weight for *L. rigidum* in the presence of Kora (73%), PI481761 (68%), and Eva (52%), while the most stimulated parameter was the shoot length of *P. oleracea* in the presence of PI481761 (186%), Gema (158%) and Eva (146%). *L. rigidum* was especially sensitive to Eva, as shoot length significantly increased (149%) while reducing fresh plant weight (52%), which resulted in longer but weaker plants. Something similar was found for *P. oleracea* in front of Gema accession, which significantly increased both, shoot (158%) and root (166%) length while maintaining unaltered the total weight of the plant (107%).

Regarding the germination and growth parameters of the different buckwheat accessions in front of the two tested weeds (Table 2), our results show that the shoot and root lengths of Eva were significantly inhibited in front of *P. oleracea*, as well as the root length in front of *L. rigidum*. In fact, Eva was the only accession where the shoot and root length were statistically inhibited in the presence of the weeds, while Gema and PI481671 also showed significant stimulation of root length when co-cultured with *P. oleracea*. PI481671 showed a stimulation of leaf weight in front of *P. oleracea* when compared with the buckwheat plants growing alone. Finally, the root weight was only inhibited in Kora in the presence of the monocot weed *L. rigidum*. From the parameters measured in the different accessions, we could see also that common buckwheat accessions (Eva, Gema, and Kora) grew much more than Tartary buckwheat (PI481671), which showed shoot length values that were two times lower than common buckwheat and root lengths values that were even three times lower than Eva and Kora and two times lower than Gema. These differences were even stronger in the case of leaf weight, where Tartary buckwheat values were ten times under common buckwheat accessions.

**Table 2.** Mean values and standard deviation of growth parameters for different buckwheat accessions (Gema, Kora, Eva, and PI481671) when growing alone or in co-culture with the monocot weed *Lolium rigidum* (LR) or the dicot weed *Portulaca oleracea* (PO). The parameters measured are plant and root weight (g), and shoot and root lengths (cm). Grey cells indicate significant inhibition, while bold numbers indicate significant stimulations compared with the control.

| | | Leaf Weight | Root Weight | Shoot Length | Root Length |
|---|---|---|---|---|---|
| Eva | Alone | 3.12 ± 0.70 | 1.01 ± 0.24 | 13.3 ± 2.09 | 27.2 ± 0.50 |
| | LR | 2.97 ± 0.54 | 0.71 ± 0.10 | 12.8 ± 3.11 | 20.6 ± 4.95 |
| | PO | 2.43 ± 0.21 | 0.87 ± 0.02 | 9.84 ± 0.83 | 17.3 ± 3.19 |
| Gema | Alone | 1.68 ± 0.22 | 0.37 ± 0.15 | 9.81 ± 1.83 | 13.8 ± 1.82 |
| | LR | 1.65 ± 0.17 | 0.53 ± 0.10 | 9.14 ± 3.97 | 14.9 ± 2.73 |
| | PO | 1.76 ± 0.34 | **0.59 ± 0.05** | 11.9 ± 2.9 | **20.3 ± 2.85** |
| Kora | Alone | 2.69 ± 0.25 | 1.20 ± 0.28 | 12.6 ± 1.07 | 21.4 ± 0.62 |
| | LR | 1.99 ± 1.04 | 0.50 ± 0.20 | 10.7 ± 4.33 | 18.7 ± 6.58 |
| | PO | 1.91 ± 0.44 | 0.76 ± 0.19 | 12.5 ± 2.46 | 19.6 ± 1.27 |
| PI481761 | Alone | 0.25 ± 0.07 | 0.56 ± 0.34 | 4.18 ± 1.12 | 6.63 ± 2.36 |
| | LR | 0.33 ± 0.10 | 0.43 ± 0.29 | 4.04 ± 0.04 | 8.07 ± 2.26 |
| | PO | **0.95 ± 0.07** | 0.46 ± 0.17 | 4.43 ± 0.60 | **12.7 ± 4.56** |

### 2.2. *Polyphenols Profile in Different Buckwheat Accessions*

The identification and quantification of different polyphenols (phenolic acids and flavonoids), such as 4-chlorobenzoic acid (4-CBA), vanillic acid (VA), cinnamic acid (CA), dihydroxybenzoic acid (DA), ferulic acid (FA), p-coumaric acid (P-CA), phthalic acid (PA), syringic acid (SA), m-toluic acid (M-TA), luteolin (LU), syringaldehyde (SY), protocatechuic acid (PTA), quercetin (QE), vanillin (VN), salicylic acid (SAA), 4-hydroxyacetophenone (4-HA), catechin (CAT), epicatechin (ECAT), orientin (OR), vitexin (VIT), hypericin (HYP), and rutin (RU) showed different profiles for each of the four tested buckwheat accessions. In fact, while DA, FA, P-CA, SA, LU, QE, VN, 4-HA, ECAT, OR, VIT, and RU were present in the four buckwheat accessions (Gema, PI481671, Kora, and Eva), VA, SY, and SAA were only present in Gema, PI481671, and Eva; 4-CBA and PTA in Gema and Eva; CAT in Gema, Kora, and Eva; PA in Eva and PI481671; and HYP only in Gema, while M-TA was missed in this buckwheat accession (Table 3).

From all of the polyphenols measured, DA, P-CA, LU, 4-HA, OR, and VIT were the most commonly accumulated compounds, especially in the roots, for most of the four buckwheat accessions in the presence of both weeds, *L. rigidum* and *P. oleracea*, while DA, LU, 4-HA, CAT, ECAT, and OR were the most altered compounds in the roots, shoots, and root exudates of the different buckwheat accessions (Table 3). Although in the presence of *L. rigidum* buckwheat tended to accumulate the compounds indistinctly in roots or shoots, depending of the buckwheat accession, there was a clear trend in the four buckwheat accessions to accumulate the compounds in the roots when co-grown with *P. oleracea*, as DA, P-CA, LU, OR, and VIT were significantly accumulated in the roots in three of the four buckwheat accessions tested when *P. oleracea* was present in the medium. On the contrary, *L. rigidum* was the weed that more root exudates induced from the buckwheat accessions tested, especially for Eva (Table 3). Finally, the Tartary buckwheat accession (PI481671) showed a generally reduced root exudation of polyphenols in comparison with the three common buckwheat accessions (Gema, Kora, and Eva), which reacted more to the presence of weeds exuding more or less phenolic acids and flavonoids, but also exuding more polyphenols when growing alone.

**Table 3.** Significant increases and decreases ($p \leq 0.05$) for different polyphenols (PP) in the shoots, roots, or root exudates of the buckwheat accessions Gema (G), Kora (K), Eva (E), and PI481671 (PI) after co-culture with *L. rigidum* (LR) or *P. oleracea* (PO) compared to the control (each accession growing alone). The PP detected were 4-chlorobenzoic acid (4-CBA), vanillic acid (VA), dihydroxybenzoic acid (DA), ferulic acid (FA), *p*-coumaric acid (*P*-CA), syringic acid (SA), luteolin (LU), syringaldehyde (SY), protocatechuic acid (PTA), quercetin (QE), rutin (RU), vanillin (VN), salicylic acid (SAA), 4-hydroxyacetophenone (4-HA), catechin (CAT), epicatechin (ECAT), orientin (OR), vitexin (VIT), phthalic acid (PA), *m*-toluic acid (*M*-TA), and hypericin (HYP).

| **INCREASED** | | **4-CBA** | **VA** | **DA** | **FA** | ***P*-CA** | **SA** | **LU** | **SY** | **PTA** | **QE** | **RU** |
|---|---|---|---|---|---|---|---|---|---|---|---|---|
| Co-cultured with LR | Shoots | | E | G; E | E | E | | E | E | E | E; PI | |
| | Roots | | | | | E | | E | E | E | | G |
| | Root exudates | | E | E; PI | E | E | E; PI | E | E | E | E; PI | E |
| Co-cultured with PO | Shoots | E | E | PI | PI | | | | | G | | |
| | Roots | | E; PI | G; K; PI | G; PI | G; E; PI | PI | G; K; E | E; PI | E | G | G; PI |
| | Root exudates | | | K | K | K | | | | E | G | |
| INCREASED | | VN | SAA | 4-HA | CAT | ECAT | OR | VIT | PA | *M*-TA | HYP | |
| Co-cultured with LR | Shoots | E | | K; E | | | | | | K; PI | | |
| | Roots | | | G; E | E | E | E; PI | E | | | | |
| | Root exudates | E | E | E | G; E | G; E; PI | G; K; E | E | E | | | |
| Co-cultured with PO | Shoots | | G; PI | G; E; PI | | PI | | | | | | |
| | Roots | PI | PI | G; K; PI | E | E; PI | G; K; E | G; K; E | | K | | |
| | Root exudates | | | K; E | E | | K | PI | | K | | |
| DECREASED | | 4-CBA | VA | DA | FA | *P*-CA | SA | LU | SY | PTA | QE | RU |
| Co-cultured with LR | Shoots | | | K | | K | K | | | | K | K |
| | Roots | | | K | K | K | | K | | | K | K |
| | Root exudates | E | | K | K | K | K | K | | | K | K |
| Co-cultured with PO | Shoots | | PI | G; K; E | K; E | K; E | K | G; K; E | G | E | K; E | E; K |
| | Roots | | | | | | K | | | | | K |
| | Root exudates | G; | | G; E | G | ECAT | PI | | G; E | | K | G |
| DECREASED | | VN | SAA | 4-HA | CAT | ECAT | OR | VIT | PA | *M*-TA | HYP | |
| Co-cultured with LR | Shoots | G | | PI | G; K; | G; K; E | | | | | | |
| | Roots | | | PI | | | G; K | G; K | PI | PI | | |
| | Root exudates | PI | | K | K | K | | K | PI | E | | |
| Co-cultured with PO | Shoots | G | E | K | K; E | G; K; E | G; K; E | G; K; E | E; PI | K | | |
| | Roots | G | | | G; K | G; K | PI | | PI | PI | | |
| | Root exudates | K; PI | | | K; G | G | | | PI | | | |

During the comparison of the polyphenol content of shoots, roots, and root exudates of the four buckwheat varieties (Eva, Gema, Kora, and PI481671), the generated score plot of the PCA (Figure 1A) revealed a complex accession distribution pattern that, in the largest distance, was not mainly accession-dependent, but organ-dependent as the root exudates showed strong dissimilarity with shoots and roots, especially for Gema, Eva, and PI491671. The supervised PLS-DA analysis (Figure 1B) confirmed the separation, previously observed with the PCA. The separation was achieved by virtue of the first two principal components, which explained a total variance of 60.2%. Component 2 explained the highest variance (40.5%), while component 1 explained 19.7% of the total variance. The hierarchical cluster showed similarity in the root and shoot polyphenol contents of each accession, being the root and shoot contents of the four accessions grouped together in the same cluster of the dendrogram, but each species constituting and independent subclusters of the tree (Figure 1C). Surprisingly, this division was not species dependent, as there was more distance among the common accessions Eva and Gema with Kora than among the common accessions Gema and Eva with the Tartary accession PI481671.

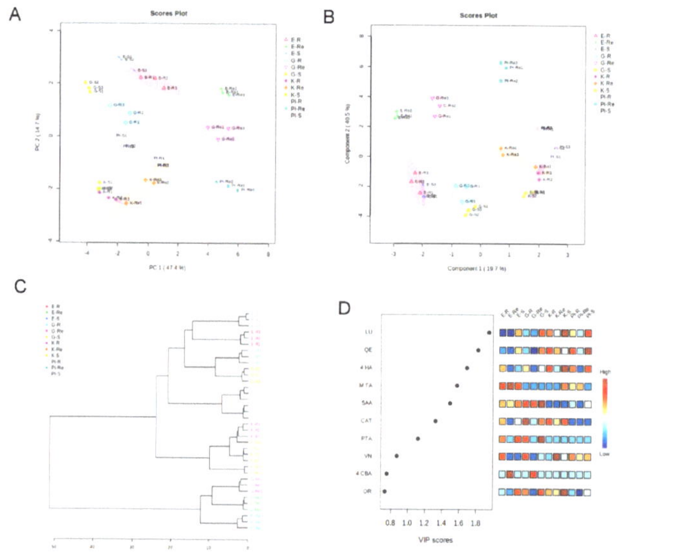


**Figure 1.** Analyses of the polyphenol content in the shoots (S), roots (R), and root exudates (Re) in the three common buckwheat accessions Eva (E), Gema (G), and Kora (K) and the Tartary buckwheat accession PI481671 (PI). (**A**) PCA scores plot between the selected PCs; (**B**) PLS-DA scores plot between the selected PCs, the explained variances of PCA and PLS-DA are shown in brackets; (**C**) clustering result shown as a dendrogram (distance measured using Euclidean, and clustering algorithm using ward). (**D**) Important features identified by PLS-DA. E−S (chemical profile of Eva shoots; dark blue), E-R (chemical profile of Eva roots; red), E-Re (chemical profile of Eva root exudates; dark green), G-S (chemical profile of Gema shoots; yellow), G-R (chemical profile of Gema roots; light blue), G-Re (chemical profile of Gema root exudates; dark pink), K-S (chemical profile of Kora shoots; light green), K-R (chemical profile of Kora roots; violet), K-Re (chemical profile of Kora root exudates; orange), PI-S (chemical profile of PI481671 shoots; malva), PI-R (chemical profile of PI481671 roots; light pink), and PI-Re (chemical profile of PI481671 root exudates; dark green). The coloured boxes on the right indicate the relative concentrations of the corresponding polyphenol in each group under study. N = 3.

In contrast, the root exudates of Gema, Eva, and PI481671 were grouped in a totally independent cluster, showing its dissimilarity from the rest of the samples and indicating a characteristic behaviour of exudation in buckwheat. Moreover, although the content of root exudates of common and Tartary accessions was grouped in the same cluster of the dendrogram, Gema and Eva were grouped in a different subcluster than PI481671, suggesting a species-dependent dissimilarity among accessions at this level of distance. The compounds that had stronger weight in this classification were LU, QE, 4-HA, M-TA, SAA, CAT, and PTA (over 1.0 VIP score). LU, QE, and 4-HA were characterized to be increased in Gema, Kora, and PI481671 shoots, roots, and root exudates in comparison with Eva, while M-TA was increased in Eva shoots, roots, and root exudates in comparison with Gema, Kora, and PI481671 (Figure 1D).

### 2.2.1. Chemical Profile of EVA Polyphenols

When Eva was co-cultured with *L. rigidum*, the concentration of most of the polyphenols was significantly increased in the shoots, roots, and especially root exudates, following a co-culture of 7 days (Table 4).

**Table 4.** Quantification of polyphenols (PP) from shoots, roots, and root exudates from buckwheat accession Eva, alone (control) or in association with *L. rigidum* (LR) or *P. oleracea* (PO). Quantities are expressed in μg $kg^{-1}$ dry weight (shoots and roots) and μg $L^{-1}$ (root exudates). Means followed by different lowercase letters within a column show significant differences among treatments ($p \leq 0.05$). Bold numbers indicate a significant increase when compared with the control, while grey cells indicate a significant decrease.

| Sample | Treatment | 4-CBA | VA | DA | FA | P-CA | PA | SA |
|---|---|---|---|---|---|---|---|---|
| Shoot | Alone | <0.01 b | <0.01 b | 2472 b | 83.41 b | 553.2 b | 350.9 a | 3.187 a |
| | +LR | <0.01 b | **238.8 a** | **3956 a** | **289.1 a** | **998.4 a** | 539.4 a | 28.13 a |
| | +PO | **5.173 a** | **108.5 a** | 131.4 c | 28.69 c | 98.88 c | 31.55 b | 6.337 a |
| Root | Alone | <0.01 a | 471.9 b | 928.9 a | 152.8 a | 49.71 b | 147.4 a | 291.0 a |
| | +LR | <0.01 a | 892.9 ab | 1122 a | 242.9 a | **122.6 a** | 186.2 a | 578.7 a |
| | +PO | <0.01 a | **1067 a** | 1214 a | 326.9 a | **145.0 a** | 218.1 a | 222.5 a |
| Root exudates | Alone | 4.533 a | <0.01 b | 14.47 b | <0.01 b | 123.4 b | 28.02 b | <0.01 b |
| | +LR | <0.01 b | **345.5 a** | **6924 a** | **511.3 a** | **1171 a** | **448.0 a** | **47.23 a** |
| | +PO | 3.980 a | <0.01 b | <0.01 c | <0.01 b | <0.01 c | 10.83 b | <0.01 b |
| Sample | Treatment | M-TA | LU | SY | PTA | QE | VN | RU |
| Shoot | Alone | 418.8 a | 57.66 b | 3.513 b | 366.8 b | 1174 b | <0.01 b | 9011 a |
| | +LR | 553.5 a | **205.5 a** | **14.07 a** | **1384 a** | **3211 a** | **1.948 a** | 9164 a |
| | +PO | 775.9 a | 1.031 c | 2.987 b | 55.64 c | 299.4 c | <0.01 b | 283.2 b |
| Root | Alone | 855.3 a | <0.01 b | 2.658 b | 219.1 b | 122.0 a | 106.1 a | 409.9 a |
| | +LR | 775.1 a | **3.070 a** | **31.83 a** | **2105 a** | 160.6 a | 197.2 a | 899.9 a |
| | +PO | 627.2 a | **1.810 a** | **33.92 a** | **1589 a** | 173.7 a | 116.2 a | 791.9 a |
| Root exudates | Alone | 1089 a | <0.01 b | 2.143 b | <0.01 c | 12.54 b | <0.01 b | 29.08 b |
| | +LR | 323.0 b | **199.9 a** | **10.54 a** | **2837 a** | **3817 a** | **22.61 a** | **13583 a** |
| | +PO | 900.2 a | <0.01 b | <0.01 c | **3.710 b** | 30.44 b | <0.01 b | 23.66 b |
| Sample | Treatment | SAA | 4-HA | CAT | ECAT | OR | VIT | |
| Shoot | Alone | 25.94 a | 0.603 b | 260.5 a | 3143 a | 4220 a | 3078 a | |
| | +LR | 42.41 a | **2.590 a** | 365.4 a | 1573 b | 3547 a | 3504 a | |
| | +PO | 16.16 b | **2.958 a** | 41.35 b | 67.32 c | 314.7 b | 549.9 b | |
| Root | Alone | 23.76 a | 26.59 b | 532.3 b | 33.95 b | 34.92 b | 30.78 b | |
| | +LR | 35.64 a | **137.3 a** | **2616 a** | **414.5 a** | **241.9 a** | **449.0 a** | |
| | +PO | 25.20 a | 59.02 b | **1782 a** | **291.6 a** | **299.3 a** | **430.0 a** | |
| Root exudates | Alone | 18.20 b | <0.01 b | <0.01 c | <0.01 b | 20.36 b | 54.87 b | |
| | +LR | **39.66 a** | **5.327 a** | **346.1 a** | **1034 a** | **4400 a** | **4481 a** | |
| | +PO | 17.34 b | **6.415 a** | **2.110 b** | <0.01 b | 14.40 b | 24.27 b | |

4-chlorobenzoic acid (4-CBA); vanillic acid (VA); dihydroxybenzoic acid (DA); ferulic acid (FA); *p*-coumaric acid (*P*-CA); syringic acid (SA); *m*-toluic acid (*M*-TA); luteolin (LU); syringaldehyde (SY); protocatechuic acid (PTA); quercetin (QE); vanillin (VN); rutin (RU); salicylic acid (SAA); 4-hydroxyacetophenone (4-HA); catechin (CAT); epicatechin (ECAT); orientin (OR); vitexin (VIT).

Different specialized metabolites such as VA, DA, FA, *P*-CA, LU, SY, PTA, QE, VN, and 4-HA were significantly increased in the **shoot tissues** after the co-culture of Eva with *L. rigidum* (Table 4). Even VA and VN were found in high concentrations after co-growth with annual ryegrass, although could not be detected in Eva shoots when growing alone.

In contrast, there was a clear trend to reduce most of the detected polyphenols (DA, FA, *P*-CA, PA, LU, PTA, QE, SAA, CAT, ECAT, OR, VIT, and RU) in Eva shoot tissues when co-cultured with *P. oleracea*, especially LU, ECAT, and RU, which were reduced for more than 57 times, 47 times, and 31 times, respectively, followed by OR and PA, with reductions of more than 12 times. There was also a significant reduction in PTA (6.6 times), and QE (4 times). In contrast, a significant increase was only obtained in 4-CBA, VA, and 4-HA levels in the shoot tissues of Eva when co-cultured with *P. oleracea* (Table 4).

In **root tissues**, the significant increase in the content of phenolic acids and flavonoids, such as *P*-CA, LU, SY, PTA, 4-HA, CAT, ECAT, OR, and VIT when Eva was co-cultured with *L. rigidum* was coherent with the increase observed in the shoots and root exudates of this buckwheat accession in the presence of annual ryegrass. Especially interesting were the results of SY, ECAT, and VIT that increased their contents by more than 12 times, and of LU, which could not be detected in the control, although it appeared in Eva when co-growing with *L. rigidum*. In Eva roots co-cultured with *P. oleracea*, there was also an increase in VA, *P*-CA, LU, SY, PTA, CAT, ECAT, OR, and VIT following the pattern previously described for Gema and Kora. Surprisingly, LU was found to be increased after co-culture with both weeds, but was absent in the root tissues of the control plants of Eva. As a result, Eva root tissues accumulated in general significantly strong levels of polyphenols (Table 4).

In contrast, Eva **root exudates** were strongly increased only in the presence of *L. rigidum*, with 18 significantly increased exuded compounds (VA, DA, FA, *P*-CA, PA, SA, LU, SY, PTA, QE, VN, RU, SAA, 4-HA, CAT, ECAT, OR, and VIT) out of 20 compounds detected (Table 4). In fact, nine of the polyphenols significantly increased after *L. rigidum* co-culture did not practically appear in the control samples (when Eva was growing alone), which could not be detected in the analyses. Especially interesting is the exudation of PTA (2836-times), ECAT (1034-times), FA (511-times), DA (477-times), RU (467-times), CAT (346-times), VA (345-times), QE (304-times), OR (216-times), LU (200-times), VIT (81.6-times), SA (47-times), and VN (22.6-times). In contrast, in general, root exudates significantly decreased following the co-cultivation of Eva with *P. oleracea* and even the polyphenols DA, *P*-CA, and SY practically disappeared from the medium, while the content was only significantly increased for the polyphenols PTA, 4-HA, and CAT, which could not be detected in the root exudates when the Eva buckwheat plants were growing alone (Table 4).

2.2.2. Chemical Profile of GEMA Polyphenols

As shown in Table 5, the distribution of polyphenols in the shoots, roots, and root exudates of Gema was different depending on whether this accession was grown with *L. rigidum* or with *P. oleracea*.

Compared with the control, where Gema plants were growing alone, only the concentration of DA was significantly increased in **shoot tissues** when Gema was co-cultured with *L. rigidum* (Table 5), while the level of PTA, SAA, and 4-HA significantly increased in the shoot tissues when Gema was co-cultured with *P. oleracea*. Although the increases in PTA and SAA were not especially relevant, 4-HA increased by 24 times its concentration in the shoot tissues in the presence of *P. oleracea*. In addition, there were more polyphenols inhibited in the shoots when Gema was co-cultured with *P. oleracea* (DA, LU, SY, VN, ECAT, OR, and VIT) than with *L. rigidum* (VN, CAT, and ECAT). Curiously, the concentration of the polyphenol VN almost disappeared in the shoot tissues when Gema was co-cultured with either weed species. Similar to the shoot analyses, Gema increased significantly more polyphenols in **root tissues** when co-cultured with *P. oleracea* (DA, *P*-CA, LU, 4-HA, RU, OR, and VIT) than with *L. rigidum*, where only 4-HA and RU showed a significantly increased content. In fact, a significantly strong accumulation in the amounts of DA (56-times), LU (98-times), OR (5-times), VIT (4-times), and RU (3-times) was found in the **roots** of Gema when co-cultured with *P. oleracea* (Table 5).

**Table 5.** Quantification of polyphenols (PP) from shoots, roots, and root exudates from buckwheat accession Gema, alone (control) or in association with *L. rigidum* (LR) or *P. oleracea* (PO). Quantities are expressed in μg $kg^{-1}$ dry weight (shoots and roots) and μg $L^{-1}$ (root exudates). Means followed by different lowercase letters within a column show significant differences among treatments ($p \leq 0.05$). Bold numbers indicate a significant increase when compared with the control, while grey cells indicate a significant decrease.

| **Sample** | **Treatm.** | **4-CBA** | **VA** | **DA** | **FA** | ***P*-CA** | **SA** | **PA** |
|---|---|---|---|---|---|---|---|---|
| Shoot | Alone | <0.01 a | 432.7 a | 22123 b | 1004 a | 1317 a | 92.40 a | <0.01 a |
| | +*LR* | <0.01 a | 499.3 a | **33720 a** | 933.7 a | 944.7 a | 131.7 a | <0.01 a |
| | +*PO* | <0.01 a | 395.1 a | 417.3 c | 605.0 a | 2057 a | 132.7 a | <0.01 a |
| Root | Alone | <0.01 a | 232.5 ab | 286.2 b | 125.3 b | 35.47 b | 223.3 a | <0.01 a |
| | +*LR* | <0.01 a | 343.1 a | 352.8 b | 203.7 ab | 53.13 b | 197.0 a | <0.01 a |
| | +*PO* | <0.01 a | 140.4 b | **16210 a** | **297.7 a** | **103.0 a** | 276.3 a | <0.01 a |
| Root exudates | Alone | 2.713 ab | <0.01 a | 3.397 a | 7.573 a | <0.01 a | <0.01 a | 2.710 ab |
| | +*LR* | 1.133 a | <0.01 a | 2.770 a | 3.797 ab | <0.01 a | <0.01 a | 1.130 a |
| | +*PO* | 0.640 b | <0.01 a | <0.01 b | <0.01 b | <0.01 a | <0.01 a | 0.640 b |
| Sample | Treatm. | LU | SY | PTA | QE | VN | SAA | RU |
| Shoot | Alone | 146.8 a | 19.64 a | 593.7 b | 2208 ab | 22.73 a | 183.7 b | 399.8 a |
| | +*LR* | 94.40 a | 17.77 a | 636.3 b | 1447 b | <0.01 b | 113.8 b | 544.9 a |
| | +*PO* | 2.870 b | <0.01 b | **2827 a** | 2720 a | <0.01 b | **265.0 a** | 411.1 a |
| Root | Alone | 2.517 b | 21.00 a | 244.0 a | 293.0 ab | 159.9 a | 37.53 a | 475.0 b |
| | +*LR* | 2.193 b | 34.80 a | 236.3 a | 247.7 b | 47.73ab | 43.73 a | **1275 a** |
| | +*PO* | **245.7 a** | 38.23 a | 490.0 a | 454.3 a | 33.77 b | 48.40 a | **1617 a** |
| Root exudates | Alone | 0.560 ab | 2.331 a | <0.01 a | 12.73 b | <0.01 a | 26.47 a | 16.41 a |
| | +*LR* | 0.420 b | 1.227 a | <0.01 a | 13.77 b | <0.01 a | 29.47 a | 17.64 a |
| | +*PO* | 1.070 a | <0.01 b | <0.01 a | **28.77 a** | <0.01 a | 25.33 a | <0.01 b |
| Sample | Treatm. | 4-HA | CAT | ECAT | OR | VIT | HYP | |
| Shoot | Alone | 9.240 b | 1070 a | 951.8 a | 4642 a | 7825 a | 0.097 a | |
| | +*LR* | 14.15 b | 268.5 b | 61.66 c | 3019 a | 6542 a | 0.120 a | |
| | +*PO* | **224.0 a** | 1842 a | 302.0 b | 259.1 b | 779.9 b | 0.093 a | |
| Root | Alone | 14.14 c | 2442 a | 386.6 a | 697.1 b | 1619 b | 0.033 a | |
| | +*LR* | **44.00 a** | 2134 a | 429.7 a | 97.16 c | 279.1 c | 0.050 a | |
| | +*PO* | **25.96 b** | 209.2 b | 45.44 b | **3610 a** | **6859 a** | 0.073 a | |
| Root exudates | Alone | <0.01 a | 3.910 b | 3.197 a | 5.523 b | 19.05 a | <0.01 a | |
| | +*LR* | 0.167 a | **21.52 a** | 4.213 a | **16.51 a** | 43.40 a | <0.01 a | |
| | +*PO* | <0.01 a | <0.01 c | <0.01 b | 6.490 b | 21.14 a | <0.01 a | |

4-chlorobenzoic acid (4-CBA); vanillic acid (VA); dihydroxybenzoic acid (DA); ferulic acid (FA); *p*-coumaric acid (*P*-CA); syringic acid (SA); luteolin (LU); syringaldehyde (SY); protocatechuic acid (PTA); quercetin (QE); vanillin (VN); salicylic acid (SAA); rutin (RU); 4-hydroxyacetophenone (4-HA); catechin (CAT); epicatechin (ECAT); orientin (OR); vitexin (VIT); hypericin (HYP).

Regarding the presence of polyphenols in **root exudates**, the levels of many of the specialised metabolites decreased significantly when Gema plants were grown in co-culture with *P. oleracea* (4-CBA, DA, FA, SY, RU, CAT, and ECAT) and some of them (DA, FA, SY, RU, CAT, and ECAT) practically disappeared in Gema root exudates following co-growth with common purslane. In fact, only one polyphenol (QE) was slightly more exuded in front of common purslane than when Gema plants were grown alone. In contrast, none of the polyphenols was decreased in the presence of annual ryegrass while CAT and OR significantly increased their exudation to the medium with increases of more than five times for CAT and more than three times for OR (Table 5).

2.2.3. Chemical Profile of KORA Polyphenols

When Kora was co-cultured with *L. rigidum* (Table 6), there was a general decrease in polyphenols in the roots (DA, FA, *P*-CA, LU, QE, RU, OR, and VIT) and root exudates (DA, FA, *P*-CA, SA, LU, QE, 4-HA, RU, CAT, ECAT, and VIT) that was not found for common purslane, which showed the most inhibited polyphenols in the **shoots**, with DA, FA, *P*-CA, SA, *M*-TA, LU, 4-HA, CAT, and ECAT practically disappearing from the shoot tissues, and QE, OR, RU, and VIT also significantly reduced in the presence of this weed compared with the control. As a result, no polyphenols were found to be accumulated in the shoots of Kora after co-growth with *P. oleracea*.

**Table 6.** Quantification of polyphenols (PP) from shoots, roots, and root exudates from buckwheat accession Kora, alone (control) or in association with *L. rigidum* (LR) or *P. oleracea* (PO). Quantities are expressed in μg kg$^{-1}$ dry weight (shoots and roots) and μg L$^{-1}$ (root exudates). Means followed by different lowercase letters within a column show significant differences among treatments ($p \leq 0.05$). Bold numbers indicate a significant increase when compared with the control, while grey cells indicate a significant decrease.

| Sample | Treatment | DA | FA | *P*-CA | SA | *M*-TA | LU | QE |
|---|---|---|---|---|---|---|---|---|
| Shoot | Alone | 1967 a | 173.2 a | 830.9 a | 180.6 a | 39.94 b | 206.9 a | 1022 a |
| | +*LR* | 490.0 b | 168.5 a | 290.0 b | <0.01 b | **365.5 a** | 458.6 a | 406.8 b |
| | +*PO* | <0.01 c | <0.01 b | <0.01 c | <0.01 b | <0.01 c | <0.01 b | 14.97 c |
| Root | Alone | 476.3 b | 245.3 a | 659.2 a | 342.1 a | <0.01 b | 111.1 b | 4785 a |
| | +*LR* | <0.01 c | 21.86 b | 35.86 b | 147.1 a | <0.01 b | 22.04 c | 476,5 b |
| | +*PO* | **7609 a** | 230.6 a | 674.9 a | <0.01 b | **919.2 a** | **1178 a** | 3124 ab |
| Root exudates | Alone | 239.8 b | 42.34 b | 90.87 b | 41.42 a | <0.01 b | 18.23 a | 2296 a |
| | +*LR* | <0.01 c | <0.01 c | <0.01 c | <0.01 b | <0.01 b | <0.01 b | 13.77 c |
| | +*PO* | **2373 a** | **238.0 a** | **289.9 a** | 24.96 a | **321.1 a** | 13.32 a | 109.5 b |
| Sample | Treatment | VN | 4-HA | CAT | ECAT | OR | VIT | RU |
| Shoot | Alone | 42.96 a | 13,541 b | 2230 a | 516.8 a | 4788 a | 5632 a | 176.5 a |
| | +*LR* | 34.38 a | **33,077 a** | 18.25 b | <0.01 b | 2589 ab | 4121 a | <0.01 b |
| | +*PO* | 57.69 a | <0.01 c | <0.01 c | <0.01 b | 2436 b | 31.52 b | 1.791 b |
| Root | Alone | 23.95 ab | 2214 b | 2440 a | 463.8 a | 472.1 b | 793.9 b | 1041 a |
| | +*LR* | 65.56 a | 2199 b | 2264 a | 513.6 a | 36.16 c | 39.10 c | 64.32 b |
| | +*PO* | 25.70 b | **38,173 a** | 64.30 b | 8.760 b | **2650 a** | **5490 a** | <0.01 b |
| Root exudates | Alone | 134.5 a | 1412 b | 462.6 a | 68.51 a | 283.0 b | 224.2 a | 109.1 a |
| | +*LR* | 106.7 ab | <0.01 c | <0.01 c | <0.01 b | **3362 a** | 19.57 b | <0.01 b |
| | +*PO* | 66.41 b | **205,000 a** | 229.9 b | 32.26 a | **1531 a** | 269.7 a | 132.3 a |

Dihydroxybenzoic acid (DA); ferulic acid (FA); *p*-coumaric acid (*P*-CA); syringic acid (SA); *m*-toluic acid (*M*-TA); luteolin (LU); quercetin (QE); vanillin (VN); 4-hydroxyacetophenone (4-HA); catechin (CAT); epicatechin (ECAT); orientin (OR); vitexin (VIT); rutin (RU).

In contrast, once more, different polyphenols were found to be significantly accumulated in the presence of *P. oleracea* in **root tissues**, as *M*-TA (919-times), 4-HA (17-times), DA (16-times), LU (10-times), VIT (7-times), and OR (5.6-times), while most of the polyphenols, were strongly reduced after co-cultivation with *L. rigidum*, as already explained above.

This reduction in the polyphenols in root tissues of annual ryegrass was consistent with the general reduction of polyphenols found in Kora **root exudates** when co-grown with *L. rigidum*, with many of them, such as DA, FA, *P*-CA, SA, LU, 4-HA, CAT, and ECAT, practically disappearing from the root exudates following co-growth with *L. rigidum*. In contrast, Kora strongly exuded a higher amount of several phenolic acids and flavonoids in the presence of *P. oleracea*, such as *M*-TA (321-times), 4-HA (145-times), DA (10-times), FA (5.6-times), OR (5.4-times), and *P*-CA (3.2-times). Finally, OR was the only polyphenol more exuded when Kora was co-cultivated with *L. rigidum* compared with the control (Table 6).

### 2.2.4. Chemical Profile of PI481671 Polyphenols

In general, the root and shoot tissues of PI481671 were more sensitive to the presence of *P. oleracea* than *L. rigidum* in the medium (Table 7). In fact, while only three polyphenols were altered in **PI481671 shoot tissues** in the presence of annual ryegrass (increases in *M*-TA and QE, and a decrease in PA), the content of seven polyphenols was altered in the presence of common purslane (increases in DA, FA, SAA, 4-HA, and ECAT, and decreases in VA and PA). This pattern was even more obvious in the **root tissues**, where the content of four polyphenols was altered in the presence of annual ryegrass, while the content of up to 14 polyphenols was altered in the presence of common purslane. In fact, after co-growth with *P. oleracea*, the **root tissues** of PI481671 accumulated strong amounts of polyphenols, showing a significant increase in the concentration of different specialized metabolites, such as VA, DA, FA, *P*-CA, SA, VN, SAA, 4-HA, RU, and ECAT. Especially interesting are the strong increases of ECAT (200-times), RU (26-times), and SAA (23-times). In contrast, the results only showed a significant increase in one polyphenol, OR (278-times), in the root tissues after the co-cultivation of PI481671 with *L. rigidum* (Table 7).

**Table 7.** Quantification of polyphenols (PP) from the shoots, roots, and root exudates from buckwheat accession PI481671, alone (control) or in association with *L. rigidum* (LR) or *P. oleracea* (PO). Quantities are expressed in μg $kg^{-1}$ dry weight (shoots and roots) and μg $L^{-1}$ (root exudates). Means followed by different lowercase letters within a column show significant differences among treatments ($p \leq 0.05$). Bold numbers indicate a significant increase when compared with the control while grey cells indicate a significant decrease.

| **Sample** | **Treatment** | **VA** | **DA** | **FA** | ***P*-CA** | **PA** | **SA** |
|---|---|---|---|---|---|---|---|
| Shoot | Alone | 911.4 a | 1703 b | 190.4 b | 355.5 ab | 74.54 a | 112.2 a |
| | +*LR* | 930.7 a | 1597 b | 190.1 b | 293.6 b | 61.38 a | 136.6 a |
| | +*PO* | 540.5 b | **5940 a** | **480.0 a** | 472.6 a | 8.597 b | 79.17 a |
| Root | Alone | 325.9 b | 97.73 b | 27.52 b | 17.08 b | 20.91 a | 78.81 b |
| | +*LR* | 368.4 b | 71.74 b | 71.02 b | 22.65 b | 3.853 b | 84.35 b |
| | +*PO* | **2146 a** | **276.8 a** | **283.2 a** | **148.9 a** | 5.613 b | **360.9 a** |
| Root exudates | Alone | <0.01 a | <0.01 b | <0.01 a | <0.01 a | 26.71 a | <0.01 b |
| | +*LR* | <0.01 a | **18.48 a** | <0.01 a | <0.01 a | 3.300 b | **51.82 a** |
| | +*PO* | <0.01 a | <0.01 b | <0.01 a | <0.01 a | 2.660 b | <0.01 b |
| Sample | **Treatment** | ***M*-TA** | **LU** | **SY** | **QE** | **VN** | **SAA** |
| Shoot | Alone | <0.01 b | 144.9 a | 19.62 a | 16,993 b | 49.77 a | 9.467 b |
| | +*LR* | **3.497 a** | 115.5 a | 11.41 a | **19,610 a** | 37.03 a | 14.95 b |
| | +*PO* | <0.01 b | 85.45 a | 12.37 a | 19,429 ab | 25.56 a | **69.19 a** |
| Root | Alone | 13.28 a | 21.93 a | 7.620 b | 4372 a | 72.55 b | 5.537 b |
| | +*LR* | <0.01 b | 23.68 a | 7.293 b | 3850 a | 37.30 b | 8.903 b |
| | +*PO* | <0.01 b | 32.50 a | **30.95 a** | 5581 a | **417.6 a** | **131.5 a** |
| Root exudates | Alone | 33.09 a | 4.397 a | <0.01 a | 535.7 b | 57.48 a | <0.01 a |
| | +*LR* | 18.50 a | 3.793 a | <0.01 a | **1668 a** | <0.01 b | <0.01 a |
| | +*PO* | 13.27 a | 2.467 a | <0.01 a | 546.5 b | <0.01 b | <0.01 a |
| Sample | Treatment | 4-HA | ECAT | OR | VIT | RU | |
| Shoot | Alone | 1756 b | 330.0 b | 98.37 ab | 1786 ab | 905.3 a | |
| | +*LR* | 1.177 c | 175.0 b | 101.9 a | 2236 a | 105.2 a | |
| | +*PO* | **4260 a** | **6603 a** | 38.71 b | 1311 b | 39.05 a | |
| Root | Alone | 1754 b | 23.50 b | 22.12 b | 193.5 a | 57.65 b | |
| | +*LR* | 0.907 c | 19.83 b | **6157 a** | 229.5 a | 31.10 b | |
| | +*PO* | **4461 a** | **4807 a** | 7.701 c | 167.1 a | **327.5 a** | |
| Root exudates | Alone | <0.01 a | 1.543 b | 0.274 ab | 22.57 b | 15.84 a | |
| | +*LR* | <0.01 a | **401.3 a** | 0.586 a | 25.21 b | 18.83 a | |
| | +*PO* | <0.01 a | 1.247 b | <0.01 b | **4404** a | 6.040 a | |

Vanillic acid (VA); dihydroxybenzoic acid (DA); ferulic acid (FA); *p*-coumaric acid (*P*-CA); phthalic acid (PA); syringic acid (SA); *m*-toluic acid (*M*-TA); luteolin (LU); syringaldehyde (SY); quercetin (QE); vanillin (VN); salicylic acid (SAA); 4-hydroxyacetophenone (4-HA); epicatechin (ECAT); orientin (OR); vitexin (VIT); rutin (RU).

Although there was a general lower **root exudation** in the Tartary buckwheat accession PI481671 when compared with the common buckwheat accessions (Kora, Gema, and Eva), there was a significant increase in the root exudates of DA, SA, QE, and ECAT following the co-cultivation of PI481671 with *L. rigidum*, indicating that the levels of polyphenols in the root exudates had a propensity to rise. In contrast, only VIT increased in the root exudates after co-cultivation with *P. oleracea*.

2.2.5. Multivariate Analyses of Polyphenols' Profile of Shoots, Roots, and Root Exudates of the Four Buckwheat Accessions

When independently comparing the polyphenol profile of the shoots (Figure 2A), roots (Figure 2B) and root exudates (Figure 2C) of Gema, Eva, Kora, and PI481671, the results of the PLS-DA analysis further exacerbated the separation among accessions for both shoots and roots (Figure 2A left, Figure 2B left, respectively), but not for the root exudates. The root exudates of each accession alone or in co-culture with *L. rigidum* or *P. oleracea* were separated and, at the same time, overlapped with the samples of the other accessions (Figure 2C left). PLS-DA explained a total variance of 54.2% for shoots (component 1: 23% and component 2: 31.2%), 46.1% for roots (component 1: 29.4% and component 2: 16.7%), and 60.5% for root exudates (component 1 23.1%: and component 2: 37.4%). In fact, the polyphenol profile of the roots of the accessions Gema (G), Eva (E), Kora (K), and PI481671 (PI) were perfectly separated from each other but perfectly grouped into each accession for all of the plants growing alone (A) or co-cultured with *L. rigidum* (L) or *P. oleracea* (P) (Figure 2B left). The same was found for the shoot polyphenol profile of the accessions Gema, PI481671, and Eva (Figure 2A left). In contrast, no clear groups were found for root exudates, where the polyphenol profile of the plants of the different accessions growing alone or in co-culture with *L. rigidum* or *P. oleracea* were completely overlapped for the four accessions tested in this study (Figure 2C left).

The variable importance in projection (VIP) scores (built on the polyphenols with a VIP score higher than 1.0) revealed that PTA and *M*-TA were the only polyphenols with VIP scores higher than 1.0 that were found in all of the analyses (shoots, roots, and root exudates), while CAT and RU were also common for the shoots and roots. In particular, the compounds with a higher VIP score in the shoots were, in order of importance, CAT, PTA, RU, VN, *M*-TA, 4-HA, and OR, while in the roots they were LU, CAT, PTA, QE, *M*-TA, RU, and PA, and in the root exudates they were OR, 4-CBA, SAA, SY, PTA, PA, and *M*-TA (Figure 2A right, Figure 2B right, Figure 2C right, and Table 8).

**Table 8.** Variable importance of projection (VIP) features for the groups from the PLS-DA analysis for roots, shoots, and root exudates of the three common buckwheat accessions Eva (E), Gema (G), and Kora (K), and the Tartary accession PI481671 (PI) growing alone or in co-culture with *L. rigidum* or *P. oleracea*. The compounds included in the table are those compounds with a VIP score higher than 1.0 for each type of sample (shoots, roots, and root exudates). Bold numbers indicate compounds with important VIP score in the shoots, roots, and root exudates, while italic numbers indicate compounds with significant VIP score in the shoots and roots.

| | Shoots | Roots | Root Exudates |
|---|---|---|---|
| CAT | *1.954* | *1.929* | |
| PTA | **1.868** | **1.632** | **1.279** |
| RU | *1.605* | *1.111* | |
| VN | 1.582 | | |
| *M*-TA | **1.572** | **1.343** | **1.183** |
| 4-HA | 1.321 | | |
| OR | 1.293 | | 1.722 |
| LU | | 1.955 | |
| QE | | 1.626 | |
| PA | | 1.047 | 1.24 |
| 4-CBA | | | 1.607 |

**Table 8.** *Cont.*

| | Shoots | Roots | Root Exudates |
|---|---|---|---|
| SAA | | | 1.521 |
| SY | | | 1.481 |

Catechin (CAT); protocatechuic acid (PTA); rutin (RU); vanillin (VN); *m*-toluic acid (M-TA); 4-hydroxyacetophenone (4-HA); orientin (OR); luteolin (LU); quercetin (QE); phthalic acid (PA); 4-chlorobenzoic acid (4-CBA); salicylic acid (SAA); syringaldehyde (SY).

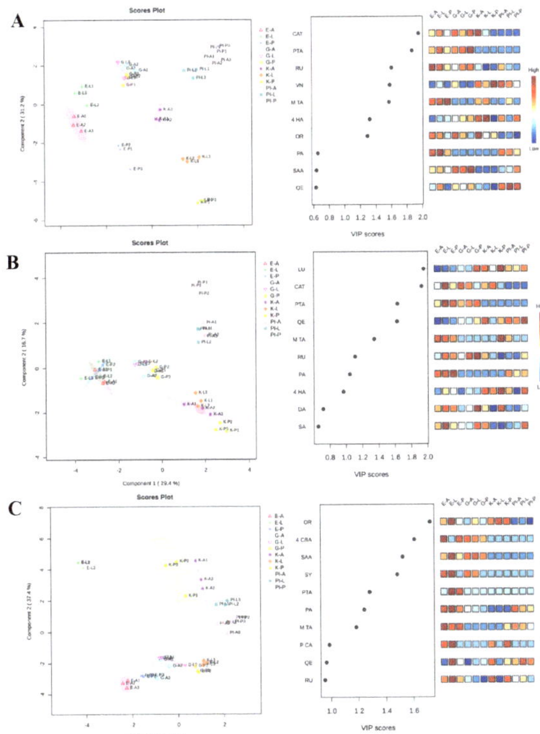

**Figure 2.** Partial least square discriminant analysis—(PLS-DA) multivariate analysis (left, scores plot between the selected PCs, the explained variances of PLS-DA are shown in brackets) and variable importance of projection (VIP) features (right, the coloured boxes on the right indicate the relative concentrations of the corresponding metabolite in each group under study) for the groups from the PLS-DA analysis, of the polyphenols' profile in the (**A**) shoots, (**B**) roots, and (**C**) root exudates of the three common buckwheat accessions Eva (E), Gema (G), and Kora (K) and the Tartary accession PI481671 (PI) growing alone (A) or in co-culture with *L. rigidum* (L) or *P. oleracea* (P). E-A (Eva growing alone; red colour), G-A (Gema growing alone; light blue), K-A (Kora growing alone; violet), PI-A (PI481671 growing alone; light pink), E-L (Eva growing with *Lolium*; dark green), G-L (Gema growing with *Lolium*; dark pink), K-L (Kora growing with *Lolium*; orange), PI-L (PI481671 growing with *Lolium*; blue green), E-P (Eva growing with *Portulaca*; dark blue), G-P (Gema growing with *Portulaca*; yellow), K-P (Kora growing with *Portulaca*; light green), and PI-P (PI481671 growing with *Portulaca*; malva). N = 3.

## 3. Discussion

Crop species with allelopathic activity are known as good options for reducing weed damage in sustainable agroecosystems [39]. Although the allelochemical potential of buckwheat crops to manage weeds in the field has not been deeply studied up until now, different papers suggest the presence of bioactive compounds on their extracts and residues that can control the development of different weeds [23,26]. Moreover, different genotypes may produce specialized metabolites differently, opening a wide variety of allelopathic potentials and, consequently, suppressive effects on weeds [40,41]. For this reason, studies such as those carried out in this work, evaluating different varieties of buckwheat that, by themselves, as a crop (alive plants), can control the presence of weeds in their environment, are highly indispensable.

The current study provides further evidence that phenolic compound synthesis, distribution, and exudation vary among buckwheat accessions, and that these compounds play a role in the interference among plants of crops and weeds. Phenolic compounds are specialized metabolites that can behave as phytotoxic when exuded into the medium, affecting the growth of neighbouring plants, as reported for several phenolic acids [42]. Meanwhile, the identification of allelochemical substances and their particular mode of action and interference in different physiological processes is required to make use of the allelopathic capabilities of crop plants in weed control [43]. Additionally, previous studies revealed that production of phenolic compounds differ greatly between buckwheat accessions in the different tissues [40,44].

Phenolic compounds, and especially flavonoids, have been reported for decades as strong antioxidant compounds, behaving as protectors into the plant metabolism against any external biotic or abiotic damage to which the plant can be exposed [45,46]. In fact, flavonoids are the most reported specialized metabolites in the plant defence system [47], so they may play an important role in plant–plant competition other than allelopathy, by accumulating in the different organs of the plant (leaves, roots, stems, seeds, etc.), and make plants more resistant and resilient against external attacks [48].

Moreover, as reported by Uddin et al. [41], different buckwheat cultivars can show different contents of phenolic compounds, and even the same cultivar can show organ-related differences in the phenolic composition. Studying three common buckwheat cultivars (Suwon1, Suwon 2, and Suwon 12), they found that Suwon 1 had the highest levels of catechin and epicatechin, while the greatest amount of 4-hydroxybenzoic acid, chlorogenic acid, and 4-hydroxy-3-methoxybenzoic acid was present in the cultivar Suwon 2. In this context, the Suwon 2 cultivar dominated over the other two cultivars, with the highest phenolic compound content in the stem, flowers, and roots of common buckwheat. Something similar was found in this study, as when comparing the four accessions, the hierarchical cluster showed more dissimilarities between the samples, grouping shoots, and roots separately from the root exudates, than between species, as common and Tartary accessions were grouped together in the same branch of the dendrogram, although each accession was separated from the others in the sub-branches of the tree.

When analysing the response of the different buckwheat accessions to the weeds, our results showed that the most relevant polyphenolic compounds were DA, LU, 4-HA, CAT, ECAT, and OR, as were the compounds whose chemical profile changed more in the roots or shoots and root exudates of the different buckwheat accessions along the study.

4-HA was discovered in buckwheat root exudates and in soil extracts following buckwheat cultivation, in addition to flavonoids and phenolic acids [26]. On the other hand, CAT was found to be highly phytotoxic against *Arabidopsis thaliana* (L.) Heynh. and *Festuca idahoensis* Elmer [49]. According to previous research, the phytotoxicity of CAT on the root cell tissues of *A. thaliana* is caused by the cytoplasm condensing due to the rapid induction of reactive oxygen species, which is followed by an increase in $Ca^{2+}$ and acidification of the cytoplasm, resulting in cell death [50]. In our results, a strong significant increase in the root exudates (346-fold higher than the control) of CAT was observed in buckwheat variety Eva when co-cultured with *L. rigidum*. Golisz et al. [25] also established the effective concentrations for lettuce to be in this range (0.4 mM). These findings suggest that CAT is highly phytotoxic, but less selective against different weeds. In a similar way, Serniak [51] showed, in a comparative allelochemical study, that ECAT exerted strong phytotoxic effects on radish seedling growth. Moreover, ECAT significantly decreased the growth of *Lepidium sativum* L. [52], and radish root growth was also inhibited in vivo as the result of the phytotoxic activity of ECAT [51].

Because of the quick evolution of resistance in *L. rigidum* and *P. oleracea*, comprehensive weed management measures including crop allelopathic varieties are required to slow down this rapid evolution and promote sustainable control [53]. Determination of the mechanism(s) associated with weed suppression is essential to determine if the use of crop varieties for allelopathic and competitive weed suppression in cereal and pseudo-cereal crops is going to provide sustainable solutions for weed management and to overcome resistance problems in weeds.

In this study, the variety Gema showed the strongest crop competitive ability against mono and dicot weeds compared with the other buckwheat accessions of Eva, Kora, and PI481671. This common buckwheat accession greatly inhibited the germination and root length of the monocot *L. rigidum* in more than 70% when compared with the control (i.e., *L. rigidum* growing alone). Strong effects of Gema were also observed on the dicot weed *P. oleracea*, where shoot and root lengths were stimulated, while no increases in fresh plant weight could be detected, resulting in longer, but much weaker, shoots and roots. Gema accumulated more DA, FA, *P*-CA, LU, 4-HA, OR, RU, and VIT in the roots when co-cultured with *P. oleracea*, while QE was the only polyphenol significantly more exuded to the medium after co-growing with this dicot weed. Previous works have reported that buckwheat varieties can accumulate polyphenols in the roots and shoots as a means of defence or protection [27,54]. Our results indicate that strong competition may be taking place between Gema and *P. oleracea*, and that *P. oleracea* might be trying to colonize more space (via longer roots) at the cost of making its roots weaker. The pressure that Gema has on *P. oleracea* can be related to the significant increase in root length of Gema in the presence of this weed, which would be competing with *P. oleracea* by colonizing the medium. In this context, flavonoid accumulation in the roots might be protecting Gema in front of this dicot weed. Root exudation represents a carbon cost to the plant [55]; therefore, the reduced root exudation of polyphenols could save energy that the buckwheat plant could use for defence or protection against *P. oleracea*. Several researchers have reported the antioxidant properties of flavonoids from different buckwheat varieties [45,56]. In this sense, the significant increase in some polyphenols in the roots and shoots of Gema plants could be protecting them from the damage induced by the presence of this dicot weed.

Allelochemical plants, such as buckwheat, have distinct mechanisms for inducing the phytotoxic effects on monocot and dicot weeds, so that biological action on the target weed differs from one weed to another [24,26]. In this sense, the behaviour of Gema with the monocot weed *L. rigidum* was totally different than with *P. oleracea*. In fact, no alterations in leaf and root weight or shoot and root length were observed in Gema plants when co-growing with *L. rigidum*. On the contrary, the germination and root length of *L. rigidum* were strongly inhibited by Gema, with 80% and 70% inhibitions, respectively. Gema increased the exudation of CAT by more than five times and OR by more than three times in the presence of *L. rigidum*, which could be enough to inhibit the germination and growth of *L. rigidum*, as there is no relevant accumulation of polyphenols on the roots or shoots of buckwheat plants and neither growth parameters of Gema plants are affected in front of this monocot weed, which suggests that *L. rigidum* does not represent a threat to Gema plants. The phytotoxic activity of CAT and OR would be enough for Gema to handle *L. rigidum* development [22].

The next accession with a strong capacity to sustainably control weeds was the Eva variety. This common buckwheat accession greatly inhibited the germination and fresh plant weight of the monocot *L. rigidum*, while it strongly stimulated the shoot length of this weed, which resulted in longer but weaker plants. Something similar was observed on the dicot *P. oleracea*, where Eva stimulated the shoot length but did not increase the plant weight. We revealed that this competitive ability of Eva was related to its robust root exudation of different polyphenols (phenolic acids and flavonoids), such as VA, DA, FA, *P*-CA, PA, SA, LU, SY, PTA, QE, VN, 4-HA, RU, CAT, ECAT, OR, and VIT, when co-cultured with both weeds; this was especially true for *L. rigidum*, which induced a significant increase in the exuded content for 16 polyphenols out of the 19 analysed. This increased the production and exudation of different polyphenols, especially PTA (2836-times), ECAT (1034-times) FA (511-times), DA (477-times), RU (467-times), CAT (346-times), VA (345-times), QE (305-times), OR (215-times), and LU (200-times) by Eva compared with the control, which would ensure the success in the inhibition of the germination and development of *L. rigidum* and in the induction of increased weakness in *P. oleracea*. Our results demonstrated that when buckwheat recognizes the presence of the weeds it subsequently changes its root exudation profile to impede their growth. These results are consistent with those found by Gfeller et al. [57] for buckwheat in the presence of redroot pigweed. Moreover, although previous studies [20,54] have suggested the accumulation and exudation of RU as the responsible allelochemical molecule to inhibit the growth of different weeds, our results showed that there are a plethora of compounds participating in this phenomenon, and that there are other polyphenols, such as PTA, ECAT, or FA, that can playing an even more strong allelochemical role than RU. In this sense, in recent research, Krumsri et al. [58] evaluated the phytotoxic potential of *Dalbergia cochinchinensis* Pierre ex Laness. and found that PTA, the most exuded compound by Eva roots, caused growth inhibition on *Echinochloa crus-galli* (L.) P. Beauv. and *L. sativum* at low concentrations. At concentrations greater than 10 mM, ECAT, the second most exuded compound by Eva, significantly decreased the growth of *L. sativum* [52]. Radish root growth was also inhibited in vivo because of the ECAT phytotoxic activity [51]. In another study, Hussain and Reigosa [43] evaluated the effects of FA and DA on the photosynthesis of *Rumex acetosa* L., and found that both compounds behaved as potent inhibitors of photosynthetic traits, leading to weaker plants. The strong increase in the root exudation by living plants indicates that Eva molecules attacked the herbicide-resistant weeds (*L. rigidum* and *P. oleracea*), inhibiting the germination of *L. rigidum* and hindering the development of both monocot and dicot weeds. The exudation of several flavonoids (QE, VN, 4-HA, CAT, ECAT, OR, RU, and VIT) demonstrates that the defence strategy of Eva is alive and working closely with the attacking phenomena to obtain access to the available resources (space and light) for its growth and development. Moreover, polyphenols can also play a role of defence and protection in the plant, as previously demonstrated by several authors [27,54]. In this context, Eva also significantly increased the production of several polyphenols in the shoots (VA, DA, FA, *P*-CA, LU, SY, PTA, QE, VN, and 4-HA) and roots (*P*-CA, LU, SY, PTA, 4-HA, CAT, ECAT, OR, and VIT) after growing with *L. rigidum*, and in root tissues (VA, *P*-CA, LU, SY, PTA, CAT, ECAT, OR, and VIT) after growing with *P. oleracea*. Especially interesting were the polyphenols *P*-CA, LU, SY, PTA, CAT, ECAT, OR, and VIT, which were found to increase in the root tissues in the presence of both weeds in very high concentrations.

Kora was the common buckwheat accession that affected the development of *L. rigidum* and *P. oleracea* less in the present study, although it showed a strong effect on the germination of both monocot and dicot weeds. Although Kora did not exude phenolic compounds and flavonoids after growth with *L. rigidum*, the accumulation in the roots and shoots of different polyphenols, such as *M*-TA, 4-HA, and OR could improve the antioxidant activity in buckwheat plants, providing an advantage in plant–plant competition [59].

In contrast, Kora exuded significant amounts of DA, FA, *P*-CA, *M*-TA, 4-HA, and OR after growth with *P. oleracea*, which were not only related to the strongest decrease in *P. oleracea* germination for the four tested accessions, but also to the chemical control of *P. oleracea* by Kora, where the weed seedlings could normally grow, without affecting the growth and development of Kora plants.

The Tartary buckwheat accession PI481671 followed a similar chemical profile and buckwheat plant development to the common buckwheat accession Gema, although this accession did not affect the weeds in a similar pattern. PI481671 stimulated the weed total biomass and shoot length of *P. oleracea* while inhibiting the total weight of *L. rigidum*. This could be explained by the results previously found by Sijahović et al. [38], who demonstrated that buckwheat–weed interactions are dependent on the type of weed present in the neighbours, resulting in changes in the exudation behaviour of buckwheat plants. The root tissues of PI481671 indeed accumulated considerable levels of polyphenols after co-growing with *P. oleracea*, displaying a marked rise in the content of many specialized metabolites, including VA, DA, FA, *P*-CA, SA, VN, SAA, RU, 4-HA, and ECAT. The significant increases in ECAT (200 times) and SAA (23 times), a well-known defence compound, are particularly fascinating. Competitive genotypes can better access light, nutrients, and water resources in limited space, thus suppressing the growth and reproduction of nearby weed species [37]. Although the Tartary buckwheat (PI481671) showed generally less root exudation than the common buckwheat accessions, PI481671 increased, as Eva, the exudation of DA, SA, and QE, by several folds after co-culture with *L. rigidum*. In a recent study, Šćepanović et al. [60] showed that strong doses of VA, DHA, and *P*-CA, as well as the phenolic acid mixture, inhibited the early growth of *Ambrosia artemisiifolia* L.

As shown by the multivariate analyses, in this study, no differences were found among species (*F. esculentum* and *F. tataricum*), but among the analysed samples. In fact, the roots and shoots were grouped separately from the root exudates. When having a look at the compounds with a higher VIP score (weight) for the comparison of the different samples, the polyphenols PTA and *M*-TA were common to all of the analyses (shoots, roots, and root exudates), while CAT and RU were also common for the shoots and roots. Most of these compounds (i.e., CAT, RU, and PTA) have been shown to have antioxidant properties [61–63] against different stress factors, which could be one main reason for their accumulation in the roots and shoots of common and Tartary buckwheat accessions, giving an advantage to buckwheat plants in front of the surrounding weeds.

Our findings show that different buckwheat accessions have varying capacities to release or accumulate specific metabolites in the presence of surrounding weeds, as well as varying capacities to manage those weeds sustainably. Additionally, each accession exhibited varied the inhibitory capacities and chemical profiles against monocot or dicot weeds, depending on the type of weed in their vicinity [20,25]. These results are consistent with those of Kalinova [30], who found varietal differences for the inhibition of lettuce by three different buckwheat varieties and related these differences to allelochemical action of buckwheat by measuring the production of the known allelochemical compounds ECAT and RU.

The findings of this study indicate that the buckwheat accessions that most significantly impacted the growth of the tested weeds were those with the highest production of allelopathic compounds and their exudation into the rhizosphere. The inhibitory effect on weed germination and growth could be caused by the allelochemicals that were exuded to the medium, because in the current experiments, there was no direct physical contact between the roots or shoots of the buckwheat and weeds. This was particularly true for the variety Eva, which demonstrated a high potential for controlling monocot weed *L. rigidum* trough root exudates. However, the superior competitive ability that the accumulation of polyphenols in shoots and roots provided buckwheat plants in front of weeds could be driving the negative impact of the tested buckwheat accessions on the two target weeds, even though these weeds showed resistance against different herbicides.

The present results highlight the necessity to screen different buckwheat accessions to find the better ones to be used in organic agriculture, due to the variation in the synthesis, distribution, and exudation of polyphenols, which can provide a different allelopathic or competitive ability to different accessions.

## 4. Materials and Methods

### 4.1. Germination and Growth Bioassays

Four different buckwheat accessions (Gema, Kora, Eva, and PI481671), previously pre-selected for their potential to be used in organic farming (in the frame of the EU project ECOBREED), were screened for their allelopathic potential against germination and seedling growth of common purslane (*Portulaca oleracea* L.) and annual ryegrass (*Lolium rigidum* Gaud.) using perlite as an inert substrate. Eva is a commercial variety from Kmetijski inštitut Slovenije/Agricultural Institute of Slovenia (KIS), Slovenia. Gema, Kora, and PI481671 were provided by the Czech Gene Bank—Crop Research Institute of Prague (Czech Republic).

| Identification Number | Species | Name | Origin |
|---|---|---|---|
| 01Z5000095 | *Fagopyrum esculentum* | Kora | Poland |
| 01Z5000112 | *Fagopyrum esculentum* | Gema | Poland |
| 01Z5100009 | *Fagopyrum tataricum* | PI 481671 | Bhutan |

Seeds of common purslane and annual ryegrass were obtained commercially from "Semillas Cantueso" (Cantueso Natural Seeds, Cordoba, Spain) and Herbiseed (Herbiseed Twyford, Berkshire, UK), respectively. Surface-sterilized seeds of each buckwheat accession were grown alone in individual plastic trays (32 × 20 × 6 cm) filled with a 5 cm deep layer of perlite (500 g/tray), watered with distilled water, and kept in a growth chamber with a day and night temperature of 20 °C and 12/12 h light/dark photoperiod. The light was supplied by cool white fluorescent tubes and irradiance was maintained at 275 $\mu$mol $m^{-2}$ $s^{-1}$. The buckwheat seeds were sown and left to germinate for 5 days before transferring to treatment plastic trays.

Ten buckwheat seedlings per plastic tray and three plastic trays per treatment were used in these experiments for each common and Tartary buckwheat accession. At day 1, similar seedlings for each buckwheat accession were selected and sown in a plastic tray with perlite and were watered each other day. The seedlings were placed in three rows on one half of the tray and placed in a controlled environment growth cabinet with a daily photoperiod of 12L:12D and continuous temperature of 20 °C. After 10 days of growth for the buckwheat accessions, *L. rigidum* or *P. oleracea* seeds were added to the other half of the tray. The arrangement was such that the allelochemicals produced and released by the buckwheat seedlings could diffuse throughout the perlite medium to influence weed germination and growth, but no physical contact was allowed among the roots or shoots of buckwheat seedlings and weeds.

After growing together (buckwheat and weeds) under the same conditions for 7 days, the germination rate, total weight, shoot and root length, and plant height were measured in the two target weeds, *L. rigidum* and *P. oleracea*.

The five treatments established for each buckwheat accession were as follows:

(1) Buckwheat alone (Gema, Kora, Eva, or PI481671);
(2) Buckwheat seedlings (10 days germinated) + *L. rigidum* (10 ungerminated seeds);
(3) Buckwheat seedlings (10 days germinated) + *P. oleracea* (10 ungerminated seeds);
(4) *P. oleracea* alone;
(5) *L. rigidum* alone.

### 4.2. Plant Harvest and Metabolite Extraction

After harvesting the shoots and roots of the buckwheat seedlings and collecting the root exudates from each treatment tray, the samples were stored at −80 °C until extraction. The samples from each buckwheat accession were separately processed for the identification and quantification of phenolic compounds and flavonoids from the shoots, roots, and root exudates. The plant tissues (shoots and roots) were lyophilized, ground into powder with a mortar and pestle after the addition of liquid nitrogen, and macerated with 9 mL of HCl

(1 mM). Afterwards, the whole solution was transferred into a vial, sonicated for 15 min (Branson SINIFIER 250; microTip limit, output 3), and centrifuged at 20,000 rpm at 10 °C for 15 min (SORVALL RC 5B Plus, Du Pont). The supernatant was collected and extracted three times with diethyl ether (DE). The aqueous layers were discarded, and the corresponding organic layers were combined. The organic phases were evaporated in a multivapor (P-12; Buchi, Switzerland) with 12 simultaneous evaporating positions. The multivapor (P-12) comprised of a vacuum pump (V-700), vacuum controller (V-850), rotavapor (R-210), heating bath (B-491), and recirculating chiller (F-105). The temperature of the recirculating chiller was set to −10 °C. The organic layers (DE) were placed in 15 mL plastic tubes and attached to the multivapor to evaporate the organic solvent under reduced pressure (456 mbar for DE) at 35 °C. Because of the chilling temperature (−10 °C) of recirculating chiller, and the temperature of the heating bath (35 °C), the organic solvent was evaporated and condensed in the attached crystal balloon. The final volume of the residual solution was approximately 1 mL and this solution was further dried with $N_2$. Methanol was used to dissolve the residual powder and was injected for the LC-MS analysis.

The perlite-based nutrient-free water-growth medium was collected and adjusted to pH 3.0 with 0.06 M HCl. Then, 25 mL of the root exudated water was extracted three times with 25 mL DE. Further treatment of the root exudated water samples was identical to the preparation of shoots or roots extraction as described above.

### 4.3. *Identification of Phenolic Compounds by LC-MS*

Shoots, roots, and root exudates were extracted from each buckwheat accession using diethyl ether. Specialized metabolites (phenolic acids and flavonoids) were separated on ultra-high performance liquid chromatography coupled to a quadrupole time-of-flight high-definition mass spectrometry detector (UHPLC-qTOF-MS, Thermo Fisher Scientific Inc., Madrid, Spain) according to Wu et al. [64] with small slight amendments according to Hussain et al. [65].

High Performance Liquid Chromatography−Mass Spectrometry (HPLC-MS, 1260 Series, Agilent, Santa Clara, CA, USA) was performed using a system consisted of compact mass detector equipment (TRIPLE QUAD 3500; AB SCIEX INSTRUMENTS, AB Sciex Pte. Ltd., Framingham, MA, USA). Polyphenols were separated with a C18 column (PHENOMENEX LUNA, 150 mm × 2 mm and 3 μm, Phenomenex, Inc., Torrance, CA, USA) using different chromatographic conditions depending of the compounds. Hypericin was separated at a flow rate of 400 μL $min^{-1}$ with a column temperature of 40 °C, an injection volume of 10 μL, and the column was equilibrated for 6 min between runs. The isocratic elution used was a mixture of two solvents: A, consisting of 5 mM ammonium acetate and 0.1% acetic acid in water, and B, consisting of acetonitrile. The isocratic conditions were 25% A and 75% B for 10 min. The other phenolic acids were separated at a flow rate of 300 μL $min^{-1}$, the column temperature was 40 °C, the injection volume was 10 μL, and the column was equilibrated for 6 min between runs. The gradient elution used was a mixture of two solvents: A, consisting of 0.1% formic acid in water, and B, consisting of 0.1% formic acid in acetonitrile. Initial conditions (98% A and 2% B) were held for 4 min before ramping to 20% B at 7 min and 90% B at 14 min. Initial conditions were recovered at 15 min and held until 21 min. The instrument parameters were as follows: curtain gas (CUR), 25 psi; collision gas (CAD), 7 psi: ion spray voltage (IS), −4500 V; temperature (TEM), 400 °C; ion source gas 1 (GS1), 55 psi; ion source gas 2 (GS2), 55 psi; interface heater, on.

The quantification of the concentration of the compounds was obtained from calibration curves that related the detector's response to the pure analyte's concentration of those compounds identified in the chemical analyses.

### 4.4. *Data Analyses*

The experiments were carried out using a completely randomized design with three replications (each replication was a bulk of 10 buckwheat plants and 10 weed plants). IBM SPSS software (SPSS Inc., Chicago, IL, USA, version 22.0) was used to analyse the data. To detect outliers, an exploratory data analysis was performed. The Kolmogorov–Smirnov test was used to check for deviation from normality, and the Levene test was used to check for homogeneity. Depending on the homoscedasticity of the samples, one-way ANOVA or Kruskal–Wallis tests were performed for germination and seedling growth data to establish the significant effect ($p \leq 0.05$) of the treatments (different accessions). The results are presented in the tables as the percentage of increase or decrease when compared with the control. Different letters represent significant differences in treatment. Polyphenol (phenolic compounds and flavonoids) data were analysed through analysis of variance and the Duncan multiple range test was performed to establish the significant effect ($p \leq 0.05$) within the treatments (alone, co-cultured with *L. rigidum*, or co-cultured with *P. oleracea*).

The identified polyphenols were analysed using the Metaboanalyst 5.0 software. The missing values were replaced with half of the minimum value found, and then data were $Log_{10}$ transformed and Pareto scaled. Data were then analysed through unsupervised principal component analysis (PCA), to visualize group discrimination, and through the supervised partial least square discriminant analysis (PLS-DA). Feature selection with the highest discriminatory power was based on their variable importance in projection (VIP) score > 1.0. To avoid overfitting, the PLS-DA model was validated using Q2 as a performance measure, the 10-fold cross-validation and setting in the permutation test a permutation number of 20 (see tables reported in Supplementary Table S1).

## 5. Conclusions

We conclude that the selection, evaluation, and development of buckwheat accessions with an increased competitive ability and strong allelopathic potential will be a good option for sustainable weed management. Our results confirm the ability of different buckwheat accessions to suppress monocot and dicot weeds, and this ability clearly appears to be accession dependent. In this regard, Gema appears to be the accession that should be used for growing in organic agriculture due to its capacity to sustainably regulate the germination and growth of the monocot weed *L. rigidum* and the dicot weed *P. oleracea*, while stimulating the root growth of buckwheat plants. Meanwhile, all four buckwheat accessions showed varying degrees of allelochemical production and release to control weeds through affecting multiple processes, such as germination, growth, and weed biomass. We conclude that different buckwheat genotypes may have different capacities to produce and exude several types of specialized metabolites, which lead to a wide range of allelopathic and defence functions in the agroecosystem to sustainably manage the growing weeds in their vicinity.

**Supplementary Materials:** The following supporting information can be downloaded at: https://www.mdpi.com/article/10.3390/plants12132401/s1. Table S1: Multivariate analyses of the polyphenols quantified in the four buckwheat accessions (Eva, Gema, Kora, and PI481671).

**Author Contributions:** Conceptualization: A.M.S.-M. and M.J.R.; methodology: A.M.S.-M., M.J.R., J.S.-G., M.I.H., Y.V.-Á., P.O. and M.A.P.; data curation: P.O., M.A.P., A.M.S.-M., Y.V.-Á. and M.I.H.; formal analysis: Y.V.-Á., M.I.H. and D.L.-G.; funding acquisition: M.J.R. and J.S.-G.; investigation: Y.V.-Á., M.I.H. and P.O.; project administration: A.M.S.-M.; supervision: A.M.S.-M., M.A.P., J.S.-G. and M.A.P.; visualization: Y.V.-Á., M.I.H., and A.M.S.-M.; writing—review and editing: A.M.S.-M., Y.V.-Á., M.I.H., D.L.-G. and J.S.-G. All authors have read and agreed to the published version of the manuscript.

**Funding:** This work was supported by the European Union's Horizon 2020 research and innovation programme under grant agreement no. 771367, ECOBREED. The seed samples of the buckwheat accessions Gema, Kora and PI481671 were provided by the Gene Bank—Crop Research Institute of Prague (Czech Republic), Eva from the Kmetijski inštitut Slovenije/Agricultural Institute of Slovenia (KIS).

**Data Availability Statement:** The raw data have been deposited at Zenodo webpage (https://zenodo.org/communities/ecobreed/ (accessed on 16 May 2023)), with the following DOI: https://doi.org/10.5281/zenodo.8053668 (accessed on 16 May 2023), as per the rules and regulation.

**Acknowledgments:** The authors want to thank Alberto Acuña Couñago (Centro de Apoio Científico-Tecnolóxico á Investigación, CACTI, Universidade de Vigo) for their help in the performance of the chemical analyses.

**Conflicts of Interest:** The authors declare no conflict of interest.

## References

1. Gandhi, K.; Khan, S.; Patrikar, M.; Markad, A.; Kumar, N.; Choudhari, A.; Sagar, P.; Indurkar, S. Exposure risk and environmental impacts of glyphosate: Highlights on the toxicity of herbicide co-formulants. *Environ. Chall.* **2021**, *4*, 100–149. [CrossRef]
2. Vázquez-García, J.G.; Alcántara-De La Cruz, R.; Palma-Bautista, C.; Rojano-Delgado, A.M.; Cruz-Hipólito, H.E.; Torra, J.; Barro, F.; De Prado, R. Accumulation of target gene mutations confers multiple resistance to ALS, ACCase, and EPSPS inhibitors in *Lolium* species in Chile. *Front. Plant Sci.* **2020**, *11*, 553948. [CrossRef] [PubMed]
3. Koller, V.J.; Fürhacker, M.; Nersesyan, A.; Mišík, M.; Eisenbauer, M.; Knasmueller, S. Cytotoxic and DNA-damaging properties of glyphosate and Roundup in human-derived buccal epithelial cells. *Arch. Toxicol.* **2012**, *86*, 805–813. [CrossRef] [PubMed]
4. Mahmood, K.; Mathiassen, S.K.; Kudsk, P. Multiple herbicide resistance in *Lolium multiflorum* and identification of conserved regulatory elements of herbicide resistance genes. *Front. Plant Sci.* **2016**, *7*, 1160. [CrossRef] [PubMed]
5. Torra, J.; Montull, J.M.; Taberner, A.; Onkokesung, N.; Boonham, N.; Edwards, R. Target-site and non-target-site resistance mechanisms confer multiple and cross-resistance to ALS and ACCase inhibiting herbicides in *Lolium rigidum* from Spain. *Front. Plant Sci.* **2021**, *12*, 625138. [CrossRef]
6. Tehranchian, P.; Nandula, V.K.; Matzrafi, M.; Jasieniuk, M. Multiple herbicide resistance in California Italian ryegrass (*Lolium perenne* ssp. multiflorum): Characterization of ALS-inhibiting herbicide resistance. *Weed Sci.* **2019**, *67*, 273–280. [CrossRef]
7. Fernández-Moreno, P.T.; Travlos, I.; Brants, I.; De Prado, R. Different levels of glyphosate-resistant *Lolium rigidum* L. among major crops in southern Spain and France. *Sci. Rep.* **2017**, *7*, 13116. [CrossRef]
8. Loureiro, I.; Escorial, C.; Plaza, E.H.; Gonzalez-Andujar, J.L.; Chueca, M.C. Current status in herbicide resistance in *Lolium rigidum* in winter cereal fields in Spain: Evolution of resistance 12 years after. *Crop Prot.* **2017**, *102*, 10–18. [CrossRef]
9. Okafor, I.A.; Ayalokunrin, M.B.; Orachu, L.A. A review on *Portulaca oleracea* (purslane) plant—Its nature and biomedical benefits. *Int. J. Biomed. Res.* **2014**, *5*, 75–80. [CrossRef]
10. Masabni, J.G.; Zandstra, B.H. Physiological characteristics of linuron-resistant *Portulaca oleracea* . *Weed Sci.* **1999**, *48*, 420–425. [CrossRef]
11. Liebman, M.; Davis, A.S. Integration of soil, crop and weed management in low-external input farming systems. *Weed Res.* **2000**, *40*, 27–48. [CrossRef]
12. Parisi, M.; Verrillo, M.; Luciano, M.A.; Caiazzo, G.; Quaranta, M.; Scognamiglio, F.; Di Meo, V.; Villani, A.; Cantelli, M.; Gallo, L.; et al. Use of Natural Agents and Agrifood Wastes for the Treatment of Skin Photoaging. *Plants* **2023**, *12*, 840. [CrossRef] [PubMed]
13. Verrillo, M.; Koellensperger, G.; Puehringer, M.; Cozzolino, V.; Spaccini, R.; Rampler, E. Evaluation of Sustainable Recycled Products to Increase the Production of Nutraceutical and Antibacterial Molecules in Basil Plants by a Combined Metabolomic Approach. *Plants* **2023**, *12*, 513. [CrossRef]
14. Mwendwa, J.M.; Jeffrey, D.W.; Weston, L.A. The use of allelopathy and competitive crop cultivars for weed suppression in cereal crops. In *Integrated Weed Management for Sustainable Agriculture*; Zimdhal, R., Ed.; Burleigh Dodds Science Publishing: Cambridge, UK, 2018; pp. 361–388.
15. Hussain, M.I.; Araniti, F.; Schulz, M.; Baerson, S.; Vieites-Álvarez, Y.; Rempelos, L.; Bilsborrow, P.; Chinchilla, N.; Macías, F.A.; Weston, L.A.; et al. Benzoxazinoids in wheat allelopathy-from discovery to application for sustainable weed management. *Environ. Exp. Bot.* **2022**, *202*, 104997. [CrossRef]
16. Mahé, I.; Chauvel, B.B.; Colbach, N.; Cordeau, S.; Gfeller, A.; Reiss, A.; Moreau, D. Deciphering field-based evidences for crop allelopathy in weed regulation. A review. *Agron. Sustain. Dev.* **2022**, *42*, 50. [CrossRef]
17. Liebman, M.; Mohler, C.L. Weeds and the soil environment. In *Ecological Management of Agricultural Weeds*; Liebman, M., Mohler, C.L., Staver, C.P., Eds.; Cambridge University Press: Cambridge, UK, 2001; pp. 210–268.
18. Yasui, Y.; Hirakawa, H.; Ueno, M.; Matsui, K.; Katsube-Tanaka, T.; Yang, S.J.; Aii, J.; Sato, S.; Mori, M. Assembly of the draft genome of buckwheat and its applications in identifying agronomically useful genes. *DNA Res.* **2016**, *23*, 215–224. [CrossRef] [PubMed]
19. Luthar, Z.; Zhou, M.; Golob, A.; Germ, M. Breeding buckwheat for increased levels and improved quality of protein. *Plants* **2021**, *10*, 14. [CrossRef]
20. Kalinova, J.; Triska, J.; Vrchotova, N. Biological activity of phenolic compounds present in buckwheat plants. *Allelopath. J.* **2005**, *16*, 123–129.
21. Golisz, A.; Gawronska, H.; Gawronski, S.W. Influence of buckwheat allelochemicals on crops and weeds. *Allelopath. J.* **2007**, *19*, 337–349.
22. Kalinova, J.; Vrchotova, N. Level of catechin, myricetin, quercetin and isoquercitrin in buckwheat (*Fagopyrum esculentum* Moench), changes of their levels during vegetation and their effect on the growth of selected weeds. *J. Agric. Food Chem.* **2009**, *57*, 2719–2725. [CrossRef]

23. Kumar, V.; Brainard, D.C.; Bellinder, R.R. Suppression of Powell amaranth (*Amaranthus powellii*), shepherd's-purse (*Capsella bursa-pastoris*), and corn chamomile (*Anthemis arvensis*) by buckwheat residues: Role of nitrogen and fungal pathogens. *Weed Sci.* **2008**, *56*, 271–280. [CrossRef]
24. Iqbal, Z.; Hiradate, S.; Noda, A.; Isojima, S.I.; Fujii, Y. Allelopathy of buckwheat: Assessment of allelopathic potential of extract of aerial parts of buckwheat and identification of fagomine and other related alkaloids as allelochemicals. *Weed Biol. Manag.* **2002**, *2*, 110–115. [CrossRef]
25. Golisz, A.; Lata, B.; Gawronski, S.W.; Fujii, Y. Specific and total activities of the allelochemicals identified in buckwheat. *Weed Biol. Manag.* **2007**, *7*, 164–171. [CrossRef]
26. Kalinova, J.; Vrchotova, N.; Triska, J. Exudation of allelopathic substances in buckwheat (*Fagopyrum esculentum* Moench). *J. Agric. Food Chem.* **2007**, *55*, 6453–6459. [CrossRef] [PubMed]
27. Kato-Noguchi, H.; Sugimoto, H.; Yamada, M. Buckwheat seedlings may inhibit other plant growth by allelopathic substances. *Environ. Control Biol.* **2007**, *45*, 27–32. [CrossRef]
28. Kalinova, J. Varietal differences in allelopathic potential of common buckwheat (*Fagopyrum esculentum* Moench). *Cereal Res. Commun.* **2008**, *36*, 397–408. [CrossRef]
29. Björkman, T.; Shail, J.W. Using a buckwheat cover crop for maximum weed suppression after early vegetables. *Hort. Technol.* **2013**, *23*, 575–580. [CrossRef]
30. Kalinova, J. Influence of common buckwheat on growth of other plant species. In Proceedings of the 9th International Symposium on Buckwheat, Prague, Czech Republic, 18–22 August 2004; pp. 529–531.
31. Guo, X.D.; Ma, Y.J.; Parry, J.; Gao, J.M.; Yu, L.L.; Wang, M. Phenolics content and antioxidant activity of tartary buckwheat from different locations. *Molecules* **2011**, *16*, 9850–9867. [CrossRef]
32. Vollmannová, A.; Musilová, J.; Lidiková, J.; Árvay, J.; Šnirc, M.; Tóth, T.; Bojňanská, T.; Čičová, I.; Kreft, I.; Germ, M. Concentrations of Phenolic Acids Are Differently Genetically Determined in Leaves, Flowers, and Grain of Common Buckwheat (*Fagopyrum esculentum* Moench). *Plants* **2021**, *10*, 1142. [CrossRef]
33. John, J.; Sarada, S. Role of phenolics in allelopathic interactions. *Allelopath. J.* **2012**, *29*, 215–230.
34. Mohler, C.L.; Dykeman, C.; Nelson, E.B.; Ditommaso, A. Reduction in weed seedling emergence by pathogens following the incorporation of green crop residue. *Weed Res.* **2012**, *52*, 467–477. [CrossRef]
35. Weston, L.A. History and current trends in the use of allelopathy for weed management. *HortTechnology* **2005**, *15*, 529–534. [CrossRef]
36. Bertholdsson, N.O.; Andersson, S.C.; Merker, A. Allelopathic potential of *Triticum* spp., *Secale* spp. and *Triticosecale* spp. and use of chromosome substitutions and translocations to improve weed suppression ability in winter wheat. *Plant Breed.* **2012**, *131*, 75–80. [CrossRef]
37. Worthington, M.; Reberg-Horton, S.C.; Brown-Guedira, G.; Jordan, D.; Weisz, R.; Murphy, J.P. Relative contributions of allelopathy and competitive traits to the weed suppressive ability of winter wheat lines against Italian ryegrass. *Crop Sci.* **2015**, *55*, 57–64. [CrossRef]
38. Sijahović, E.; Đikić, M.; Gadžo, D.; Terzić, I. Allelopathic potential of common (*Fagopyrum esculentum* Moench) and Tartary (*Fagopyrum tataricum* L.) buckwheat for weed control in cereals. *Ege Üniversitesi Ziraat Fakültesi Dergisi* **2012**, *2*, 529–533.
39. Worthington, M.; Reberg-Horton, C. Breeding cereal crops for enhanced weed suppression: Optimizing allelopathy and competitive ability. *J. Chem. Ecol.* **2013**, *39*, 213–231. [CrossRef]
40. Seo, J.M.; Lee, D.B.; Valan, M.; Arasu; Wu, Q.; Suzuki, T.; Yoon, Y.H.; Lee, S.W.; Park, S.U.; Kim, S.J. Quantitative differentiation of phenolic compounds in different varieties of buckwheat cultivars from China, Japan and Korea. *J. Agric. Chem. Environ.* **2013**, *2*, 109–116. [CrossRef]
41. Uddin, M.R.; Li, X.; Park, W.T.; Kim, Y.B.; Kim, S.J.; Kim, Y.S.; Lee, M.Y.; Park, C.H.; Park, S.U. Phenolic compound content in different organs of Korean common buckwheat cultivars. *Asian J. Chem.* **2013**, *25*, 424. [CrossRef]
42. Falquet, B.; Gfeller, A.; Pourcelot, M.; Tschuy, F.; Wirth, J. Weed suppression by common buckwheat: A review. *Environ. Control Biol.* **2015**, *53*, 1–6. [CrossRef]
43. Hussain, M.I.; Reigosa, M.J. Secondary metabolites, ferulic acid and *p*-hydroxybenzoic acid induced toxic effects on photosynthetic process in *Rumex acetosa* L. *Biomolecules* **2021**, *11*, 233. [CrossRef]
44. Danila, A.M.; Kotani, A.; Hakamata, H.; Kusu, F. Determination of rutin, catechin, epicatechin, and epicatechin gallate in buckwheat *Fagopyrum esculentum* Moench by micro-high-performance liquid chromatography with electrochemical detection. *J. Agric. Food Chem.* **2007**, *55*, 1139–1143. [CrossRef]
45. Liu, C.L.; Chen, Y.S.; Yang, J.H.; Chiang, B.H. Antioxidant activity of tartary (*Fagopyrum tataricum* (L.) Gaertn.) and common (*Fagopyrum esculentum* Moench) buckwheat sprouts. *J. Agric. Food Chem.* **2008**, *56*, 173–178. [CrossRef]
46. Sharma, A.; Shahzad, B.; Rehman, A.; Bhardwaj, R.; Landi, M.; Zheng, B. Response of phenylpropanoid pathway and the role of polyphenols in plants under abiotic stress. *Molecules* **2019**, *24*, 2452. [CrossRef]
47. Sugiyama, A.; Yazaki, K. Flavonoids in plant rhizospheres: Secretion, fate and their effects on biological communication. *Plant Biotechnol.* **2014**, *31*, 431–443. [CrossRef]
48. Brunetti, C.; Fini, A.; Sebastiani, F.; Gori, A.; Tattini, M. Modulation of phytohormones signaling: A primary function of flavonoids in plant-environment interactions. *Front. Plant Sci.* **2018**, *9*, 1042. [CrossRef] [PubMed]

49. Kaushik, S.; Bais, H.P.; Biedrzycki, M.L.; Venkatachalam, L. Catechin is a phytotoxin and a pro-oxidant secreted from the roots of *Centaurea stoebe* . *Plant Signal. Behav.* **2010**, *5*, 1088–1098. [CrossRef]
50. Bais, H.P.; Vepachedu, R.; Gilroy, S.; Callaway, R.M.; Vivanco, J.M. Allelopathy and exotic plant invasion: From molecules and genes to species interactions. *Science* **2003**, *301*, 1377–1380. [CrossRef] [PubMed]
51. Serniak, T.L. Comparison of the allelopathic effects and uptake of *Fallopia japonica* phytochemicals by *Raphanus sativus* . *Weed Res.* **2016**, *56*, 97–101. [CrossRef]
52. Okada, S.; Iwasaki, A.; Kataoka, I.; Suenaga, K.; Kato-Noguchi, H. Phytotoxic activity of kiwifruit leaves and isolation of a phytotoxic substance. *Sci. Hortic.* **2019**, *250*, 243–248. [CrossRef]
53. Khamare, Y.; Chen, J.; Marble, S.C. Allelopathy and its application as a weed management tool: A review. *Front. Plant Sci.* **2022**, *13*, 1034649. [CrossRef]
54. Iqbal, Z.; Hiradate, S.; Noda, A.; Isojima, S.I.; Fujii, Y. Allelopathic activity of buckwheat: Isolation and characterization of phenolics. *Weed Sci.* **2003**, *51*, 657–662. [CrossRef]
55. Wen, Z.; White, P.J.; Shen, J.; Lambers, H. Linking root exudation to belowground economic traits for resource acquisition. *New Phytol.* **2022**, *233*, 1620–1635. [CrossRef]
56. Sedej, I.; Sakač, M.; Mandić, A.; Mišan, A.; Tumbas, V.; Čanadanović-Brunet, J. Buckwheat (*Fagopyrum esculentum* Moench) grain and fractions: Antioxidant compounds and activities. *J. Food Sci.* **2012**, *77*, C954–C959. [CrossRef] [PubMed]
57. Gfeller, A.; Glauser, G.; Etter, C.; Signarbieux, C.C.; Wirth, J. *Fagopyrum esculentum* alters its root exudation after *Amaranthus retroflexus* recognition and suppresses weed growth. *Front. Plant Sci.* **2018**, *9*, 50. [CrossRef]
58. Krumsri, R.; Iwasaki, A.; Suenaga, K.; Kato-Noguchi, H. Assessment of allelopathic potential of *Dalbergia cochinchinensis* Pierre and its growth inhibitory substance. *Emir. J. Food Agric.* **2020**, *32*, 513–521. [CrossRef]
59. Liu, X.; Ji, D.; Cui, X.; Zhang, Z.; Li, B.; Xu, Y.; Chen, T.; Tian, S. *p*-Coumaric acid induces antioxidant capacity and defence responses of sweet cherry fruit to fungal pathogens. *Postharvest Biol. Technol.* **2020**, *169*, 111297. [CrossRef]
60. Šćepanović, M.; Košćak, L.; Šoštarčić, V.; Pismarović, L.; Milanović-Litre, A.; Kljak, K. Selected phenolic acids inhibit the initial growth of *Ambrosia artemisiifolia* L. *Biology* **2022**, *11*, 482. [CrossRef] [PubMed]
61. Ismail, H.; Dragišic Maksimovic, J.; Maksimovic, V.; Shabala, L.; Živanovic, B.D.; Tian, Y.; Jacobsen, S.E.; Shabala, S. Rutin, a flavonoid with antioxidant activity, improves plant salinity tolerance by regulating $K^+$ retention and $Na^+$ exclusion from leaf mesophyll in quinoa and broad beans. *Funct. Plant Biol.* **2015**, *43*, 75–86. [CrossRef] [PubMed]
62. Popović, B.M.; Štajner, D.; Ždero-Pavlović, R.; Tumbas-Šaponjac, V.; Čanadanović-Brunet, J.; Orlović, S. Water stress induces changes in polyphenol profile and antioxidant capacity in poplar plants (*Populus* spp.). *Plant Physiol. Biochem.* **2016**, *105*, 242–250. [CrossRef] [PubMed]
63. Bernatoniene, J.; Kopustinskiene, D.M. The role of catechins in cellular responses to oxidative stress. *Molecules* **2018**, *23*, 965. [CrossRef]
64. Wu, H.; Haig, T.; Pratley, J.; Lemerle, D.; An, M. Distribution and exudation of allelochemicals in wheat (*Triticum aestivum* L.). *J. Chem. Ecol.* **2000**, *26*, 2141–2154. [CrossRef]
65. Hussain, M.I.; Vieites, Y.; Otero, P.; Prieto, M.A.; Simal-Gandara, J.; Reigosa, M.J.; Sánchez-Moreiras, A.M. Weed pressure determines the chemical profile of wheat (*Triticum aestivum* L.) and its allelochemicals potential. *Pest Manag. Sci.* **2022**, *78*, 1605–1619. [CrossRef] [PubMed]

*plants*

MDPI

*Article*

# Evaluation of Propiophenone, 4-Methylacetophenone and 2′,4′-Dimethylacetophenone as Phytotoxic Compounds of Labdanum Oil from *Cistus ladanifer* L.

**María Espinosa-Colín [1], Irene Hernandez-Caballero [2], Celia Infante [3], Irene Gago [1], Javier García-Muñoz [4] and Teresa Sosa [1,*]**

[1] Department of Plant Biology, Ecology and Earth Sciences, Faculty of Science, University of Extremadura, 06006 Badajoz, Spain

[2] Department of Anatomy, Cellular Biology and Zoology, Faculty of Science, University of Extremadura, 06006 Badajoz, Spain

[3] Department of Forest Resources Technology, Center for Scientific and Technological Research of Extremadura (CICYTEX), 06187 Badajoz, Spain

[4] Toxicology Unit, Faculty of Veterinary Medicine, University of Extremadura, 06006 Badajoz, Spain

* Correspondence: tesosa@unex.es

**Abstract:** This is the first study to evaluate the phytotoxic activity of three phenolic compounds present in the essential oil of the labdanum of *Cistus ladanifer*, an allelopathic species of the Mediterranean ecosystem. Propiophenone, 4′-methylacetophenone, and 2′,4′-dimethylacetophenone slightly inhibit total germination and radicle growth of *Lactuca sativa*, and they strongly delay germination and reduce hypocotyl size. On the other hand, the inhibition effect of these compounds on *Allium cepa* was stronger on total germination than on germination rate, and radicle length compared to hypocotyl size. The position and number of methyl groups will affect the efficacy of the derivative. 2′,4′-dimethylacetophenone was the most phytotoxic compound. The activity of the compounds depended on their concentration and presented hormetic effects. In *L. sativa*, on paper, propiophenone presented greater inhibition of hypocotyl size at greater concentrations, with $IC_{50}$ = 0.1 mM, whereas 4′-methylacetophenone obtained $IC_{50}$ = 0.4 mM for germination rate. When the mixture of the three compounds was applied, in *L. sativa*, on paper, the inhibition effect on total germination and the germination rate was significantly greater compared to the effect of the compounds when they were applied separately; moreover, the mixture inhibited radicle growth, whereas propiophenone and 4′-methylacetophenone did not exert such effect when applied separately. The activity of the pure compounds and that of the mixture also changed based on the substrate used. When the trial was conducted in soil, the separate compounds delayed the germination of the *A. cepa* to a greater extent compared to the trial on paper, although they stimulated seedling growth. In soil, *L. sativa* against 4′-methylacetophenone also showed the opposite effect at low concentrations (0.1 mM), with stimulation of germination rate, whereas propiophenone and 4′-methylacetophenone presented a slightly increased effect.

**Keywords:** phytotoxicity; phenolic compounds; allelopathy; *Cistus ladanifer*; bioherbicides

**Citation:** Espinosa-Colín, M.; Hernandez-Caballero, I.; Infante, C.; Gago, I.; García-Muñoz, J.; Sosa, T. Evaluation of Propiophenone, 4-Methylacetophenone and 2′,4′-Dimethylacetophenone as Phytotoxic Compounds of Labdanum Oil from *Cistus ladanifer* L. *Plants* **2023**, *12*, 1187. https://doi.org/10.3390/plants12051187

Academic Editors: Margot Schulz and Vincenzo Tabaglio

Received: 20 January 2023
Revised: 23 February 2023
Accepted: 1 March 2023
Published: 6 March 2023



## 1. Introduction

In recent years, thanks to different technological innovations and advances, agricultural production has been improved, expanding the irrigated area and thus obtaining greater profit; however, this has also brought major problems related to the deterioration of the natural resources, such as deforestation, soil degradation, biodiversity loss, desertification and contamination due to the use of artificial chemical products [1].

The continuous exponential growth of the human population implies the further exploration of new advances that continue to increase agricultural production. Therefore, it is essential to use pesticides; the question is: where can we find safe products that do not compromise the environment and health? One of the emerging strategies to attain a more sustainable future is to search for solutions in nature itself. Nature has already solved all the challenges we face today; its failures have become fossils, and what surrounds us in the present time is the key to survival. Mimicking these measures is known as biomimicry [2].

In ecosystems where resources are scarce, some plants synthesise phytotoxic compounds, with which they manage to inhibit the growth of other species around them, thereby preventing future competition for resources. This phenomenon is called allelopathy, and it has been widely studied [3]. In addition, other studies have also shown the phytotoxic effect of the essential oils of these allelopathic species on different weeds. This negative effect of essential oils on germination is related to the presence of allelochemical compounds [4–6]. Currently, allelopathic compounds may constitute a natural source of bioherbicides [7], but often these molecules are complex and difficult to reproduce. To avoid this problem, we must focus the search on low molecular weight structures such as phenolic compounds. Although the phytotoxic effect of phenolic compounds is well known [8–10], many of them have not been evaluated to date, due to their diversity and the difficulty in isolating or synthesising them. Acetophenone, due to its chemical, biological, pharmacological, and allelochemical properties, can be a good candidate in different fields such as agronomy. Acetophenone is a common secondary metabolite in plant species [11]. Different studies show that its derivatives are involved in defense mechanisms [11]. Some studies on allelopathic plants have found that acetophenone derivatives such as xanthoxylin and acetosyringone can be good herbicides [12–14]. Another example of an allelopathic species where acetophenone is present is *Cistus ladanifer* Linneo (1753). This shrub is a typical species of the Mediterranean ecosystem that can eventually form monospecific communities known as rock rose thickets. When this species is exploited for the extraction of essential oil and/or labdanum, plant richness increases immediately in the area, although, due to the seed bank preserved in the soil and the regenerative capacity of this species, such plant richness decreases progressively after two years [15]. A large number of studies show that this reduction of biodiversity in rock rose thickets may be due to the allelopathic potential of this species [16–19]. In addition, its essential oil also presents phytotoxic activity [20,21]. The labdanum of its leaves and its essential oil contain a concentrated amount of secondary metabolites with different properties [22]. An important group of this labdanum is constituted of phenolic compounds [21,23–28]. Acetophenone is also found in the essential oil of labdanum. Three derivatives of acetophenone (propiophenone, 4′-methylacetophenone, and 2′,4′-dimethylacetophenone) have been identified in the neutral part of labdanum oil [29,30]. Labdanum oil contains more than 300 constituents, with 186 compounds (154 from the neutral part and 32 from the acidic part) representing about 95% of this oil [30,31].

Propiophenone (Figure 1A), 4′-methylacetophenone (Figure 1B), and 2′,4′-dimethylacetophenone (Figure 1C) are simple and very similar phenolic compounds. All three of them present an acetophenone backbone, with a methyl group in different positions. Phenolic compounds present variable phytotoxicity depending on their formula, and small differences may result in different phytotoxic activity [9]. The inhibitory action of a phenolic compound may also change based on the concentration applied [19,22]. In some cases, even hormetic effects can be observed [32–35]. Furthermore, in soil, phenolic compounds can undergo processes of transportation, retention, and transformation, which can also influence the final result of bioactivity [36]. Moreover, it is worth highlighting that the action of allelopathic plants is commonly caused by the mixture of several allelochemicals that are found in the soil at very low concentrations [9].

Nowadays, thanks to their commercial availability, propiophenone, 4′-methylacetophenone, and 2′,4′-dimethylacetophenone can be easily evaluated through a standardised phytotoxicity bioassay. To date, no adverse effects have been reported in humans from these three compounds, and 4′-methylacetophenone is used in disinfectants, pest-control products, perfumes, and cosmetics [37].

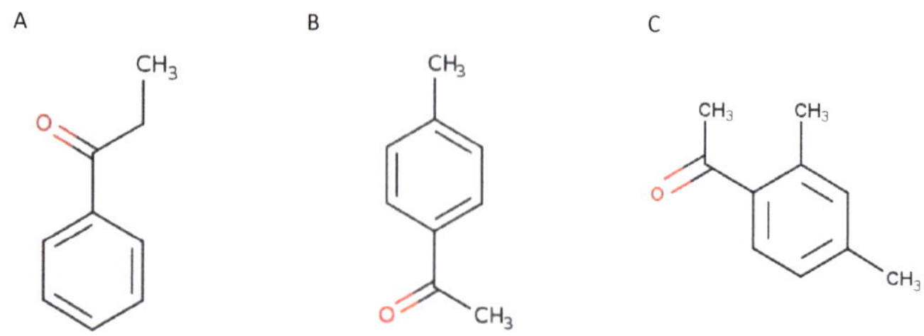


**Figure 1.** Chemical structure of propiophenone (**A**), 4′-methylacetophenone (**B**), and 2′,4′-dimethylacetophenone (**C**). Source: https://echa.europa.eu/ (accessed on 3 January 2023).

A very important aspect that allows the introduction of allelochemicals in the natural management of weeds is the knowledge of target plants and the exact chemicals responsible for the interaction [38]. Therefore, the aim of this study was to evaluate the phytotoxic activity of propiophenone, 4′-methylacetophenone and 2′,4′-dimethylacetophenone through a standard bioassay that contemplates all the possible variables. To this end, seeds of *Lactuca sativa* L., as a representative of monocotyledons, and *Allium cepa* L., as a representative of dicotyledons, were used, due to their sensitivity. In addition, their rapid, complete, and uniform germination grants reliability and duplicity to the assay [39–41]. These seeds were planted on paper and in soil, and they were watered with different concentrations of each of the compounds separately and a mixture of all three. Their phytotoxic activity was assessed by measuring their effect on germination and seedling growth [42]. The results may contribute to finding possible structures that serve as sources of natural bioherbicides that are safer and less contaminant.

## 2. Results

### 2.1. *Effect of Propiophenone, 4′-Methylacetophenone and 2′,4′-Dimethylacetophenone on the Germination of* Lactuca sativa *L.*

The results showed that propiophenone, 4′-methylacetophenone, 2′,4′-dimethylacetop henone and the mixture of the three compounds behaved in a similar manner, the three compounds separately, and their mixture inhibited germination rate (%GR) to a greater extent than total germination (%GT), and, lastly, the greater the concentration, the greater the inhibition effect (Figure 2). Both in soil and on paper, the three compounds separately and their mixture at 1 mM slightly inhibited total germination, except when the mixture was applied on paper, which showed full inhibition of total germination. The results for germination rate showed that propiophenone, 2′,4′-dimethylacetophenone and the mixture strongly inhibited %GR on paper and in soil, whereas 4′-methylacetophenone produced a lower effect; moreover, when the soil was watered with 0.1 mM of 4′-methylacetophenone, the opposite effect was obtained, showing significant stimulation of this parameter.

At the three analysed concentrations, propiophenone strongly inhibited germination rate (over 80%) both on paper and in soil, and it also significantly inhibited total germination (over 10%) in soil.

On paper and in soil, 4′-methylacetophenone significantly inhibited total germination at 0.5 mM and 1 mM. On paper, this compound also significantly inhibited germination rate with all analysed concentrations, showing a significant positive correlation ($R^2$ = 0.99), i.e., the greater the concentration, the greater the inhibition. The effective concentration required to induce half-maximal inhibition ($IC_{50}$) was 0.4 mM. It is worth highlighting that, when the soil was watered with 1 mM of 4′-methylacetophenone, the germination rate was significantly inhibited, whereas the concentration of 0.1 mM stimulated this parameter.

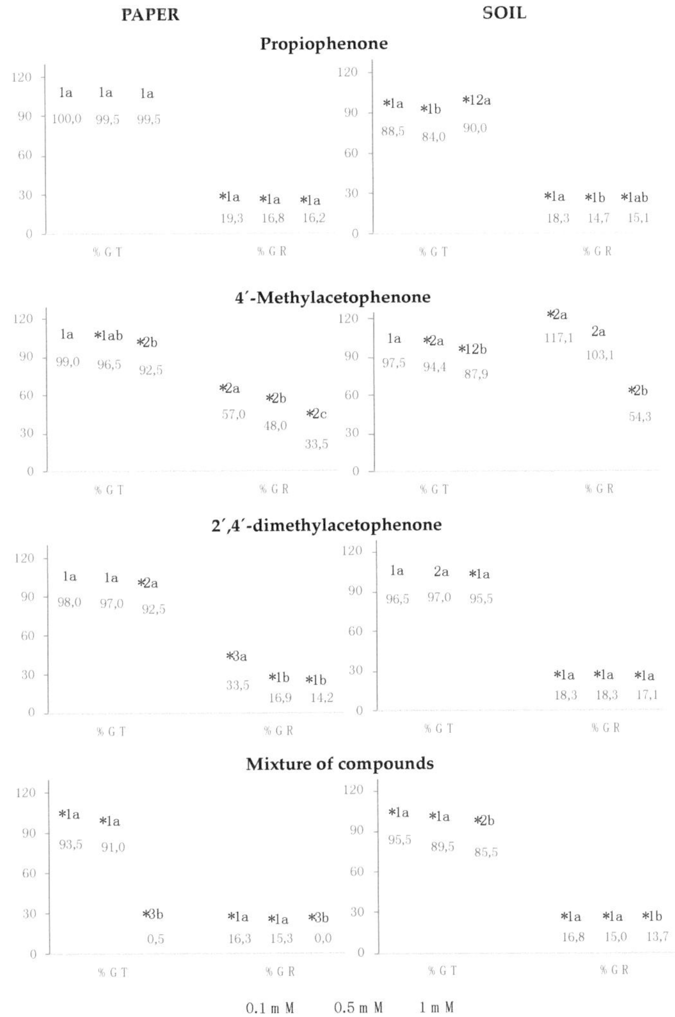


**Figure 2.** The effect of different concentrations of propiophenone, 4′-methylacetophenone, 2′,4′-dimethylacetophenone, and the mixture of the three compounds on the total germination (%GT) and germination rate (%GR) of *Lactuca sativa*, expressed as the percentage relative to the control. Four replicates of each treatment were performed (n = 4 × 50 = 200 seeds in total for each solution). * Significantly different from the controls; 1, 2, 3: differences numbers indicate significant differences between treatments of the same index and for each concentration. a, b, c: differences in small letters indicate significant differences between concentrations of the same index and for each treatment. $p < 0.05$ (Mann–Whitney U test).

In the assays with 2′,4′-dimethylacetophenone at 1 mM, %GT was significantly inhibited both on paper and in soil. This inhibition was only 7.5% and 4.5% on paper and in soil, respectively; however, as in the case of propiophenone, the germination rate was strongly inhibited at all three concentrations analysed, both on paper and in soil, showing no significant differences between the three concentrations.

The mixture inhibited total germination and germination rate at all analysed concentrations both on paper and in soil. When the mixture of the three compounds was applied on paper at 1 mM, %GT, and %GR were inhibited to a significantly greater extent compared to the inhibition obtained with the compounds separately. However, in soil, the inhibition of %GT produced by the mixture at 1 mM was only significantly greater than that obtained with 2′,4′-dimethylacetophenone separately, whereas %GR was inhibited to a significantly greater extent with the mixture than with 4′-methylacetophenone and 2′,4′-dimethylacetophenone separately.

### 2.2. *Effect of Propiophenone, 4′-Methylacetophenone and 2′,4′-Dimethylacetophenone on the Seedling Growth of Lactuca sativa L.*

The results for radicle and hypocotyl growth indicate that propiophenone, 4′-methylac etophenone, 2′,4′-dimethylacetophenone, and the mixture played a similar role on paper, the three compounds separately and the mixture inhibited hypocotyl length (%Hypocotyl length) to a greater extent than radicle length (%Radicle length), and greater inhibition was obtained at greater concentrations (Figure 3). Both in soil and on paper, the three compounds separately and their mixture slightly inhibited radicle growth, except for the soil assay with 2′,4′-dimethylacetophenone, which produced an inhibition of over 42%. The three compounds separately and their mixture strongly inhibited hypocotyl growth on paper; on the other hand, in soil, although the effect was greater with 2′,4′-dimethylacetophenone, it decreased with propiophenone and the mixture, obtaining the opposite effect when 4′-methylacetophenone was applied, with significant stimulation of this index at all three concentrations analysed.

When the assay was carried out in soil, propiophenone significantly inhibited radicle and hypocotyl growth at the three analysed concentrations. When the assay was performed on paper, radicle length was not significantly affected, whereas hypocotyl size decreased by over 52%. This inhibition was greater at higher concentrations, being significantly dependent on concentration ($R^2 = 0.98$) and obtaining an $IC_{50}$ of 0.1 mM.

Both on paper and in soil, 4′-methylacetophenone significantly inhibited radicle length at 1 mM, but not at lower concentrations. When the assay was conducted in paper, hypocotyl size was strongly inhibited at all three concentrations. This inhibition showed a positive correlation with concentration ($R^2 = 0.99$), obtaining an $IC_{50}$ lower than 0.1 mM. Nevertheless, when the assay was carried out in soil, hypocotyl growth was stimulated at all three concentrations.

At all concentrations, both on paper and in soil, 2′,4′-dimethylacetophenone significantly inhibited radicle and hypocotyl growth, observing a greater effect for the assays in soil.

The mixture of propiophenone, 4′-methylacetophenone and 2′,4′-dimethylacetophenone inhibited radicle and hypocotyl length at all three concentrations on paper and in soil, except when the paper was watered with 0.1 mM, where radicle length was significantly greater than in the control. On paper, at 1 mM, radicle and hypocotyl length % was cero, since, at that concentration of the mixture, the seeds did not germinate; at 0.5 mM, the mixture inhibited radicle growth to the same extent as 2′,4′-dimethylacetophenone, whereas propiophenone and 4′-methylacetophenone separately did not show such inhibition; at 0.1 mM, the mixture stimulated radicle growth to the same extent as propiophenone alone. On paper, the mixture inhibited %Hypocotyl length to a lesser extent than the isolated compounds. In soil, the inhibitory effect of the mixture on radicle and hypocotyl length was significantly greater than that of the compounds separately, except for 2′,4′-dimethylacetophenone.

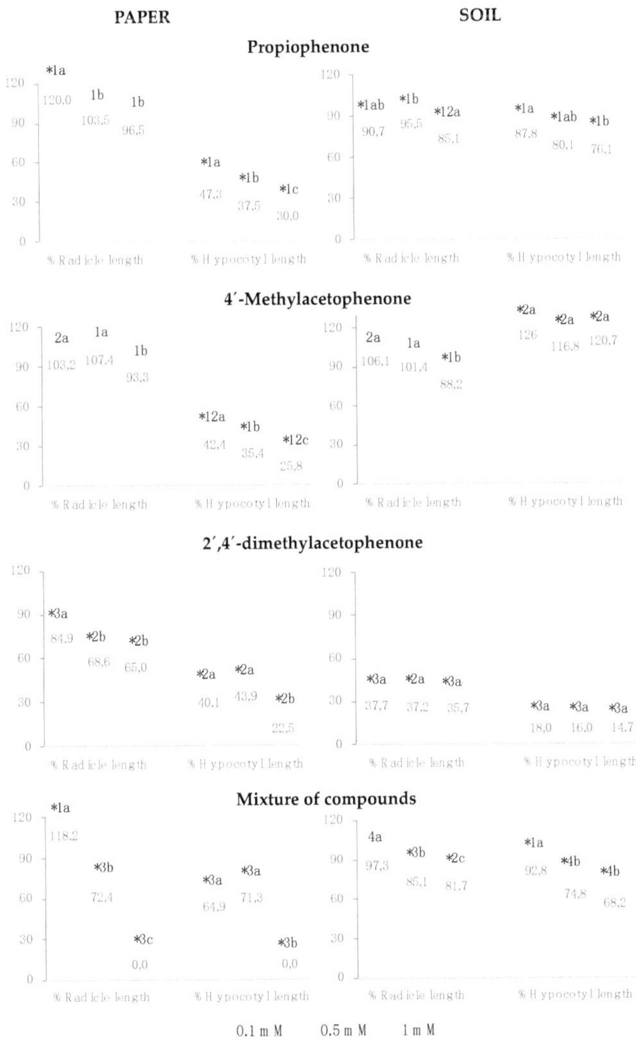


**Figure 3.** The effect of different concentrations of propiophenone, 4′-methylacetophenone, 2′,4′-dimethylacetophenone, and the mixture of the three compounds on the radicle and hypocotyl length of *Lactuca sativa*, expressed as the percentage relative to the control. Four replicates of each treatment were performed (n = 4 × 50 = 200 seeds in total for each solution). * Significantly different from the controls; 1, 2, 3, and 4: differences numbers indicate significant differences between treatments of the same index and for each concentration. The a, b, c: differences in small letters indicate significant differences between concentrations of the same index and for each treatment. $p < 0.05$ (Mann–Whitney U test).

### 2.3. *Effect of Propiophenone, 4′-Methylacetophenone and 2′,4′-Dimethylacetophenone on the Germination of Allium cepa L.*

When the assay was carried out with *Allium cepa*, it was also observed that the inhibition effects of the separate compounds were greater at higher concentrations, although the behaviour was slightly different (Figure 4). Unlike in the case of *Lactuca sativa*, propiophenone, 4′-methylacetophenone, and 2′,4′-dimethylacetophenone inhibited total germination (%GT) to a greater extent than germination rate (%GR). In this case, both in soil and on paper, the three compounds separately at 1 mM strongly inhibited total germination and germination rate, and, in contrast to the results obtained with *Lactuca sativa*, 4′-methylacetophenone did not present hormetic effects, but propiophenone did.

At all three analysed concentrations, propiophenone inhibited %GT more strongly than %GR in soil with respect to the paper assay. Moreover, when the paper was watered with a concentration of 1 mM, the germination rate was significantly inhibited, whereas, at 0.1 mM, it was stimulated by over 20%.

In both paper and soil, 4′-methylacetophenone significantly inhibited total germination and germination rate at all three analysed concentrations. At 1 mM, the inhibition was very strong: over 90% on paper and over 45% in soil. Furthermore, in soil, this inhibition depended on the concentration, presenting a positive correlation ($R^2$ = 0.99 for %GT, $R^2$ = 0.98 for %GR). The effective concentration required to induce the half-maximal inhibition of %GT and %GR ($IC_{50}$) was 0.1 mM.

When the assay was performed with 2′,4′-dimethylacetophenone, a similar behaviour was observed with respect to propiophenone: the inhibition effects of %GT and %GR are greater in soil than on paper, and %GR stimulation was observed when the paper was watered with 0.1 mM. In soil, 2′,4′-dimethylacetophenone strongly inhibited %GT and %GR at the three analysed concentrations. This effect depended on the concentration, presenting a significant positive correlation ($R^2$ = 0.98 for %GT, $R^2$ = 0.99 for %GR). The effective concentration required to induce the half-maximal inhibition of %GT ($IC_{50}$) was 1 mM, and 0.1 mM for %GR.

On its part, the mixture of compounds also presented a different behaviour with respect to that observed in *Lactuca sativa*. On paper, the mixture inhibited total germination and germination rate at the highest concentration; however, in soil, the effect was the opposite. In soil, at the highest and lowest concentrations, %GT and %GR were significantly stimulated by over 26%. When the mixture of the three compounds was applied on paper at 0.5 mM, %GR was inhibited, which was not observed with the separate compounds, and, at 0.1 mM, %GR was inhibited significantly more strongly with the mixture than with propiophenone and 2′,4′-dimethylacetophenone separately.

### 2.4. *Effect of Propiophenone, 4′-Methylacetophenone and 2′,4′-Dimethylacetophenone on the Seedling Growth of Allium cepa L.*

The effect on the seedling growth of *Allium cepa*, when watered with propiophenone, 4′-methylacetophenone, 2′,4′-dimethylacetophenone or the mixture, was different from that observed in *Lactuca sativa*. On paper, the three separate compounds and the mixture inhibited radicle length more strongly (%Radicle length) than hypocotyl length (%Cotyledon length), being greater at higher concentrations (Figure 5). However, in soil, the tendency observed was the opposite. The three compounds separately and the mixture stimulated seedling growth at the three analysed concentrations; only at 0.1 mM of propiophenone and 1 mM of 4′-methylacetophenone, hypocotyl length was significantly inhibited.

On paper, radicle and hypocotyl growth were strongly inhibited when watered with concentrations above 0.5 mM, although it was significantly stimulated when watered with a concentration of 0.1 mM. In soil, radicle size was not significantly affected, unlike hypocotyl size, which decreased by over 25% at 0.1 mM and increased by over 20% at higher concentrations.

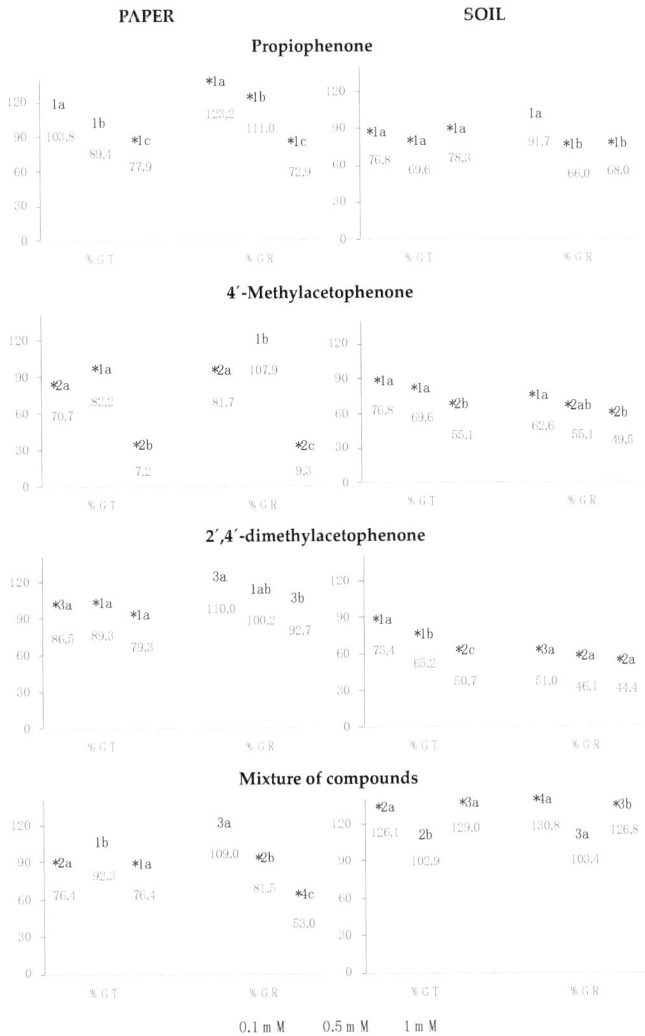


**Figure 4.** The effect of different concentrations of propiophenone, 4′-methylacetophenone, 2′,4′-dimethylacetophenone, and the mixture of the three compounds on the total germination (%GT) and germination rate (%GR) of *Allium cepa*, expressed as the percentage relative to the control. Four replicates of each treatment were performed (n = 4 × 50 = 200 seeds in total for each solution). * Significantly different from the controls; 1, 2, 3, and 4: differences numbers indicate significant differences between treatments of the same index and for each concentration. The a, b, c: differences in small letters indicate significant differences between concentrations of the same index and for each treatment. $p < 0.05$ (Mann–Whitney U test).

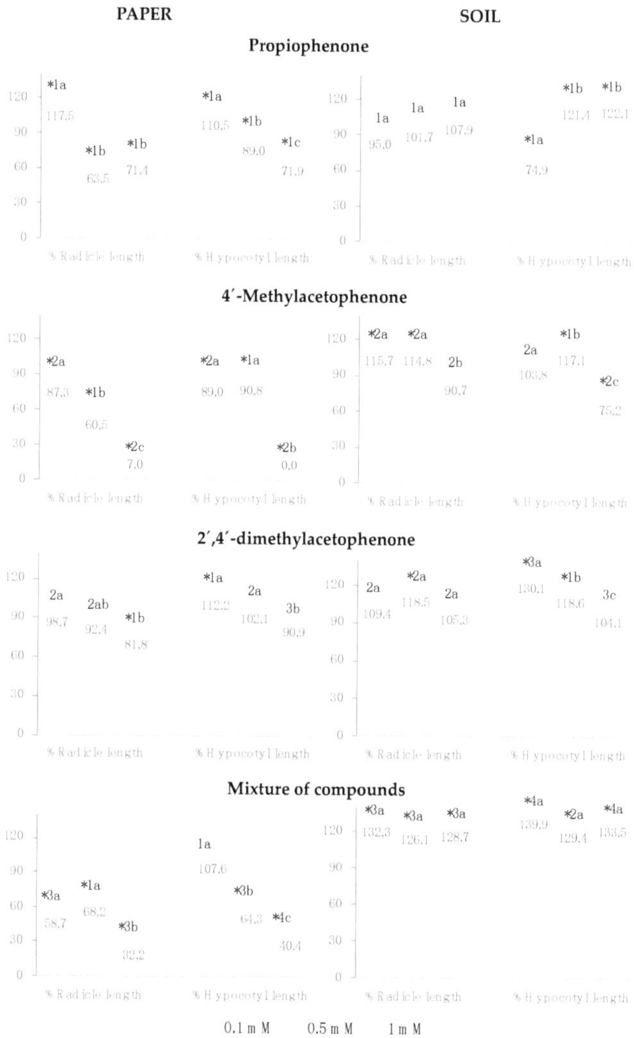


**Figure 5.** The effect of different concentrations of propiophenone, 4′-methylacetophenone, 2′,4′-dimethylacetophenone, and the mixture of the three compounds on the radicle and hypocotyl length of *Allium cepa*, expressed as the percentage relative to the control. Four replicates of each treatment were performed (n = 4 × 50 = 200 seeds in total for each solution). * Significantly different from the controls; 1, 2, 3, and 4: differences numbers indicate significant differences between treatments of the same index and for each concentration. The a, b, c: differences in small letters indicate significant differences between concentrations of the same index and for each treatment. $p < 0.05$ (Mann–Whitney U test).

The same was observed with 4′-methylacetophenone. When the assays were carried out on paper, radicle, and cotyledon length were significantly inhibited at the three analysed concentrations, whereas the opposite effect was observed in soil.

On paper, 2′,4′-dimethylacetophenone significantly inhibited radicle growth at 1 mM, although at 0.1 mM it significantly stimulated hypocotyl length. In soil, this compound stimulated the seedling growth of *Allium cepa* at all concentrations analysed.

On paper, the mixture of propiophenone, 4′-methylacetophenone and 2′,4′-dimethylacetophenone strongly inhibited radicle and hypocotyl length at all three concentrations; however, at 0.1 mM, hypocotyl length was slightly greater than in the control. The effect of the mixture on radicle and hypocotyl length was significantly greater than that of propiophenone or 2′,4′-dimethylacetophenone separately. On the other hand, in soil, the mixture of compounds significantly stimulated seedling growth at the three concentrations analysed, with this stimulation being greater than that observed when each of the compounds were applied separately.

## 3. Discussion

The appearance of resistance in weeds and the contamination of natural areas are currently the main problems derived from the massive use of herbicides. To prevent health problems and a decrease in the productivity of crops, it is necessary to find safer and more innovative products with new target sites [43,44]. This study proposes searching for phytotoxic compounds in essential oils of allelopathic species, such as *Cistus ladanifer*. The process of natural selection has given rise to allelochemicals with great structural diversity and adapted to interact with specific target sites. Therefore, through the study of these natural products, it may be possible to develop new tools for the development of new herbicides. However, in many cases, these compounds are complex and difficult to synthesise at an industrial scale. Distillation is the most common method for the extraction of plant essential oils. This method is a process of physical separation, not a chemical reaction. It consists in heating the plant until its most volatile components reach the vapour phase; then, the vapour is cooled down until these components are recovered in liquid form through a condensation process. In this process, complex molecules are hydrolysed into simpler molecules. This may pose a source of simpler derivatives of allelochemicals. If these derivatives preserve their reaction site, their activity may be the same or even greater. Evaluating the phytotoxic activity of simple and low-molecular-weight molecules may help to find a structure that can be used as a backbone for new bioherbicides. An important group of natural phytotoxic compounds is constituted of phenolic compounds [10,12,45]. In the essential oil of *Cistus ladanifer* labdanum, this group of compounds is very abundant and diverse in the exudate of its leaves and photosynthetic stems, although the impossibility of isolating some of them in sufficient amounts has prevented their evaluation. Currently, the commercial availability of three phenolic compounds present in this labdanum oil of *C. ladanifer*, i.e., propiophenone, 4′-methylacetophenone, and 2′,4′-dimethylacetophenone, allows measuring their phytotoxic activity through a germination bioassay in Petri dishes. The results of the present study showed that propiophenone, 4′-methylacetophenone, and 2′,4′-dimethylacetophenone may act as regulators of germination and growth in *Lactuca sativa* L. and *Allium cepa* L.

Although the assay on paper and in soil showed that 4′-methylacetophenone and 2′,4′-dimethylacetophenone slightly inhibited the germination of *L. sativa* at the highest concentration, on paper, all three analysed compounds strongly delayed germination and hypocotyl length; moreover, 2′,4′-dimethylacetophenone also inhibited radicle growth at concentrations of over 0.5 mM. These effects on the germination rate and seedling growth of *L. sativa* could compromise the survival of the seedling and thus be as harmful as the inhibition of germination [46]. This behaviour is similar to that shown by other phenolic compounds analysed in previous studies [10,12,45], which can be attributed to the multiple effects that this group of compounds may have on the processes of photosynthesis, respiration, and transpiration, as well as on the cell cycle [47–50]. Another characteristic of phenols is that their inhibitory action depends on concentration [9,35,51]. In the case of *L. sativa*, the concentration of 4′-methylacetophenone was positively correlated with %GR and %Hypocotyl length, showing that, the greater the concentration, the greater the inhibition of germination rate and hypocotyl growth. The inhibitory effect of propiophenone on hypocotyl size was also positively correlated with concentration. Furthermore, it is known that some phenolic compounds act as regulators of plant growth, presenting hormesis; that is, their effects are either stimulating or inhibitory depending on their concentration [35,52,53]. This behaviour was shown by 4′-methylacetophenone on %GR of *L. sativa*, when the assay was conducted in soil, obtaining inhibitory and stimulating effects at 1 mM and 0.1 mM, respectively.

When the assay was performed with seeds of *Allium cepa*, the results were somewhat different. Unlike in the case of *Lactuca sativa*, propiophenone, 4′-methylacetophenone, and 2′,4′-dimethylacetophenone showed stronger inhibition of total germination (%GT) than of germination rate (%GR), and radicle length (%Radicle length) compared to hypocotyl length (%Cotyledon length). In this case, propiophenone and 2′,4′-dimethylacetophenone presented hormetic effects when the trial was conducted on paper. This species-dependent activity has been observed with other phenolic compounds present in *C. ladanifer* [35,51]. Monocotyledons are usually more resistant to allelochemicals than dicotyledons [54]. Both in soil and on paper, the most phytotoxic compound against *Lactuca sativa* was 2′,4′-dimethylacetophenone. In paper, 1 mM of 4′-methylacetophenone presented a strong inhibition of %GT and %GR of *Allium cepa*; in soil, this compound also strongly inhibited these parameters at the three concentrations analysed, although, in soil, 2′,4′-dimethylacetophenone was the compound that presented the greatest phytotoxic effect on *A. cepa*. The analysed compounds, as in the case of any phenolic compound, have a hydroxyl group bound to a benzene molecule, and they only differ from each other in the binding of methyl groups. Their effects are different due to these small structural differences. In the analysed parameters, 2′,4′-dimethylacetophenone produced the greatest inhibition, which suggests that having two methyl groups may increase the activity of the molecule. Studies with 3,4-dihydroxyacetophenone isolated from *Picea schrenkiana* Fisch. et Mey. have shown that this compound significantly inhibits the germination of lettuce seeds at concentrations of 1 mM and 0.5 mM. In this case, the inhibitory effect of this compound was greater on radicle growth than on hypocotyl growth. Similarly, 3,4-dihydroxyacetophenone also exerted hormesis on the growth of rice radicles and radish hypocotyls [55]. Other studies on acaricide activity with compounds derived from 2′-hydroxy-4′-methylacetophenone identified in *Angelica koreana* Maxim. radicles have shown that, in terms of structure-activity relationships, the activity changed after the introduction of hydroxyl and methyl groups in the acetophenone backbone. In a contact toxicity bioassay, 3′-methylacetophenone was more effective as an acaricide against *Dermatophagoides farinae* than 2′-methylacetophenone and 4′-methylacetophenone [56]. Several studies have shown that 4-hydroxy-(2H)-1,4-benzoxazin-3(4H)-one, or DDIBOA, stands out for its phytotoxic action [57–59], and it may be used as the basis for the development of new herbicides since it is considered to be the most promising structure for the search of new compounds based on the backbones of benzoxazinones [60]. Its structure also presents a benzene ring, and the studies that have been conducted with some of its derivatives, such as 6-Cl-4-hydroxy-(2H)-1,4-benzoxazin-3(4H)-one and 8-Cl-4-hydroxy-(2H)-1,4-benzoxazine-3(4H)-one, show greater activity and selectivity, respectively, exhibiting greater phytotoxicity than the compounds that do not have substituents in their aromatic ring [61,62]. Other studies show that other derivatives such as o-nitroacetophenone inhibit the germination of *Amaranthus tricolor* L. [63]. The herbicide mechanism of benzoxazinoids is still unclear, although it is known that these compounds interfere with electron transport and ATPase activity in mitochondria, as well as with the functions of $H^+$-ATPase in the plasma membrane [64]. On their part, phenolic compounds increase the production of reactive oxygen species and, consequently, produce oxidative stress [65,66]. Moreover, it has been recently known that carbonyl, aromatic compounds, and azaindole are key interactions of the inhibitors of the enzyme 4-hydroxyphenylpyruvate dioxygenase [63].

In most cases, allelopathy by phenolic compounds is probably never due to a single substance. These compounds are not synthesised separately in plants, and they appear as a mixture. Their individual concentrations in the soil are usually very low, and their phytotoxicity seems to depend on the additive effects of each compound in the mixture [33]. Thus, in order to evaluate the possible interactions among the analysed compounds, they were applied as a mixture, and their effects were analysed. The results showed that, when the mixture of the three compounds was applied to *L. sativa* on paper at 1 mM, the inhibition of %GT and %GR was significantly greater than when the compounds were applied separately. At 0.5 mM, the mixture inhibited radicle growth to the same extent as 2′,4′-dimethylacetophenone, whereas propiophenone and 4′-methylacetophenone separately did not show such inhibition; however, the mixture inhibited % Hypocotyl length to a lesser extent than the isolated compounds. When applied to *Alium cepa* on paper, the mixture showed a greater inhibition effect 2′,4′-dimethylacetophenone, and propiophenone separately, whereas 4′-methylacetophenone showed a greater inhibition effect than the mixture. This behaviour is in line with other studies on volatile compounds that showed a considerable increase in phytotoxicity when applied jointly [67].

Another factor to be considered is the substrate on which the bioassay was carried out. In the soil, phenolic compounds can undergo processes of transportation, retention, and transformation, which, in turn, may influence their availability and action [36].

When the bioassay was conducted on a commercial substrate, in the two species analysed, propiophenone, which did not inhibit germination on paper, did inhibit germination in this substrate at all three analysed concentrations. In *Lactuca sativa*, the inhibition effect of 2′,4′-dimethylacetophenone was greater on all the parameters studied when the assay was carried out in soil; however, in *A. cepa*, although this compound in soil also inhibits %GT and %GR to a greater extent, %radicle length and %Cotyledon length are stimulated. On its part, 4′-methylacetophenone also changed its activity when the assay was performed on paper with *L. sativa*, delaying germination and inhibiting hypocotyl growth at the three analysed concentrations; on the other hand, in soil, this compound stimulated these parameters at the three concentrations, except at 1 mM on %GR. When the assay was conducted with *A. cepa*, 4′-methylacetophenone increased the inhibition of %GT and %GR, although the effect on seedling growth was attenuated and even stimulated at low concentrations. The mixture also seemed to change its action in soil, observing, in the case of *L. sativa*, inhibition of %radicle length at 0.1 mM, whereas, on paper, stimulation was obtained, and, in the case of *A. cepa*, inhibition was observed on paper, while stimulation was observed in soil. These activity changes based on the substrate have also been observed in other phenolic compounds [35,51]. Recent studies show that complex synergistic interactions between volatile and phenolic compounds underlie the efficacy of the allelopathic residues aggregated to the soil for weed control [68]. Propiophenone has moderate mobility in the soil, but also high volatilisation, and, in the vapour phase, it is degraded in the atmosphere by reacting with photochemically-produced hydroxyl radicals with an estimated half-life of approximately 5 days [69]. It is also known that acetophenone can be oxidised to phenol by *Aspergillus* species [70]. This possible, simple, and rapid degradation in the soil of the analysed compounds will influence their availability and concentration, which will affect their activity; however, this also implies that the phytotoxic compound is only found in the environment during the period of time that is adequate for its application, reducing or eliminating the risk of contamination. Therefore, phytotoxicity bioassays must be carried out in the substrates to which they will be applied.

Natural products with high phytotoxic activity and new mechanisms of action could be good options to constitute the basis of new herbicides, although, in most cases, their formulae are too complex to be produced, and the simplification of their structures often reduces their activity [71]. Thus, it is interesting to focus on simple, low-molecular-weight compounds of rapid degradation and low accumulation in the soil, in order to prevent their possible influence on non-target organisms. These characteristics are found in simple phenolic compounds [8–10]. If we search for these types of allelochemicals in essential oils of allelopathic plants, we will find natural products that, due to natural selection, have already been optimised for this activity. It is necessary to evaluate their activity in order to determine the concentration that must be applied in the soil to obtain the desired effect on the target weeds. It is important to highlight that the phytotoxic effects of the allelochemicals observed on paper do not allow extending the results to the field conditions, due to the simultaneous appearance of biotic and abiotic factors that may influence the activity of the mixtures or pure allelopathic compounds [72,73]. Moreover, it is also important to study the effect of formulations of mixtures that allow finding the way of enhancing their activity and attacking several mechanisms of action simultaneously, with the aim of addressing weed resistance.

This is the first study to report that propiophenone, 4′-methylacetophenone, and 2′,4′-dimethylacetophenone have phytotoxic activity and may regulate plant growth depending on the concentration applied and the substrate used. These compounds identified in the essential oil of labdanum from *Cistus ladanifer* may provide relatively simple structures, which allows them to be used as bioagents in weed control. The position and number of methyl groups affected the efficacy of the compound. This finding is consistent with other studies considering the molecular design of new acetophenones that are active against weeds [11,63]. Research on the structure-activity relationship of these types of allelochemicals and their derivatives based on the presence of methyl groups and other functional groups could lead to the development of less polluting and more specific bioherbicides. Furthermore, if their structure is simple, their synthesis and production will be easier.

## 4. Materials and Methods

### 4.1. Plant and Substrate Sources

To carry out the bioassay, seeds of *Lactuca sativa* variety romaine verte maraîchère (Vilmorin jardin—CS70110—38291 St Quentin Fallavier Cedex—France) were used as representatives of dicotyledons. This species is ideal for adequately showing the allelochemical effects on the germination processes [40,74]. Moreover, *Lactuca sativa* is recommended by the US EPA (United States Environmental Protection Agency) for phytotoxicity tests, being among the most sensitive species [75]. *Allium cepa* variety Bianca di Maggio (Vilmorin Jardin—CS70110—38291 St Quentin Fallavier Cedex— France) were used as monocotyledons. *Allium cepa* has proved to be the most useful and has repeatedly been suggested as a standard test material in the list of species historically used in plant testing by the International Organization for Standardization [76] and by the Organisation of Economic Cooperation and Development [77]. The total germination of these seeds was over 98%.

The activity of the allelochemicals can vary according to the planting substrate; for this reason, the experiment was carried out on Whatman No. 118 paper and a commercial substrate. The commercial substrate was of universal type, based on 95% peat, 5% green compost, and 1.3 $Kg/m^3$ fertilizer: 12N + 12P + 17K (Geolia, Aki Bricolage España S.L. B-839857—Spain). The commercial universal soil presented the following characteristics: organic matter per dry matter (60%), electrical conductivity (40 mS/m), apparent dry density (320 g/L), grain size (0–20 mm), and pH 5.5–6.5.

None of the materials (seeds and substrate) was sterilised before the experiment.

### 4.2. Phytotoxic Activity Test

Chemically pure reagents (propiophenone, 4′-methylacetophenone and 2′,4′-dimethyla cetophenone of >99% purity) were obtained from Sigma-Aldrich (Merck KGaA, Darmstadt, Germany). Different solutions were prepared with Milli-Q water from each component separately. The highest concentration was 1 mM, which is the maximum recommended concentration in allelopathic bioassays [78]. The minimum concentration was 0.1 mM, which was the lowest concentration to show the dissipation of the effect of these compounds. In addition, solutions of 0.5 mM were also prepared. For the mixture of the three phenols, three solutions were prepared with equimolar concentrations of each of the compounds at 1 mM, 0.5 mM, and 0.1 mM. To eliminate the effects of pH, we measured these parameters for each solution. The pH varied between 6 and 6.3 from one solution to another. There were no significant differences in pH among solutions.

The study was carried out in Petri dishes with Whatman paper or 25 g of commercial substrate. Four replicates were conducted for each assay, with 50 seeds of *Lactuca sativa* in each repetition (200 in total). They were watered with 5 mL and 16 mL of the different solutions for the paper and soil plates, respectively. The same amount of Milli-Q water was applied to the control. To prevent evaporation, the plates were sealed with Parafilm and were kept in a germination chamber for 5 days at 22 °C and a photoperiod of 15 h of light and 9 h of darkness.

### 4.3. Measured Indices to Quantify the Phytotoxic Effect

Germinated seeds were counted daily and total germination (%TG) [35,51] and germination rate (%GR) [69,75] were calculated according to Equations (1) and (2).

$$\%TG = \frac{N_T \cdot 100}{N}, \quad (1)$$

where $N_T$ is the average number of germinated seeds in each treatment and N is the average number of seeds in the control.

$$GR = (N_1 \cdot 1) + (N_2 - N_1) \cdot \frac{1}{2} + (N_3 - N_2) \cdot \frac{1}{3} + \ldots (N_n - N_{n-1}) \cdot \frac{1}{n}, \quad (2)$$

where $N_1, N_2, N_3, \ldots N_{n-1}, N_n$ are the proportions of germinated seeds obtained in the first (1), second (2), third (3), …, (n − 1), (n) days (for lettuce it was n = 5 and for onion n = 6). All results are expressed as a percentage relative to the control (%GR).

On the last day of the experiment, 10 seedlings per Petri dish were randomly selected. Their radicle and hypocotyl length were measured [79] and the median was expressed as a percentage relative to the control, thus:

$$\%Radicle\ length = \frac{treatment\ root\ length}{control\ root\ length} \cdot 100 \quad (3)$$

$$\%Hypocotyl\ length = \frac{treatment\ cotyledon\ length}{control\ cotyledon\ length} \cdot 100 \quad (4)$$

### 4.4. Statistical Analysis

The significance level of the comparisons among treatments was estimated using the Mann-Whitney U test. The differences were considered significant when $p < 0.05$. The interrelationships between germination and seed growth with the concentration of phenolic compounds were determined by Pearson's determination coefficient. The effective concentrations required to induce half-maximal inhibition of growth ($IC_{50}$) were calculated according to the linear relationship between concentration and percent inhibition or stimulation of plant growth. All statistical analyses were conducted using the statistical software IBM SPSS Statistics version 26.

**Author Contributions:** Conceptualization, T.S.; methodology, J.G.-M.; validation, T.S.; formal analysis, C.I., I.H.-C., I.G., J.G.-M. and M.E.-C.; investigation, C.I., I.H.-C., I.G., J.G.-M. and M.E.-C.; resources, T.S.; data curation, C.I.; writing—original draft preparation, M.E.-C.; writing—review and editing, T.S.; visualization, I.H.-C. and I.G.; supervision, T.S.; project administration, T.S.; funding acquisition, T.S. All authors have read and agreed to the published version of the manuscript.

**Funding:** This research was funded by the Regional Government of Extremadura and the European Regional Development Fund, grant number GR21086.

**Data Availability Statement:** The data presented in this study are available on request from the corresponding author.

**Conflicts of Interest:** The authors declare no conflict of interest.

## References

1. Singh, H.P.; Batish, D.R.; Kohli, R.K. Allelopathic Interactions and Allelochemicals: New Possibilities for Sustainable Weed Management. *Crit. Rev. Plant Sci.* **2003**, *22*, 239–311. [CrossRef]
2. Benyus, J.M. *Biomímesis: Innovaciones Inspiradas Por La Naturaleza*; García, L.A., Ed.; Tusquets Editores: Barcelona, Spain, 2012.
3. Rice, E.L. *Allelopathy*; Academic Press: Orlando, FL, USA, 1984; p. 422.
4. Jouini, A.; Verdeguer, M.; Pinton, S.; Araniti, F.; Palazzolo, E.; Badalucco, L.; Laudicina, V.A. Potential effects of essential oils extracted from mediterranean aromatic plants on target weeds and soil microorganisms. *Plants* **2020**, *9*, 1289. [CrossRef] [PubMed]
5. Mahdavikia, F.; Saharkhiz, M.J. Phytotoxic activity of essential oil and water extract of peppermint (Mentha × piperita L. CV. Mitcham). *J. Appl. Res. Med. Aromat. Plants* **2015**, *2*, 146–153. [CrossRef]
6. Uremis, I.; Arslan, M.; Sangun, M.K. Herbicidal activity of essential oils on the germination of some problem weeds. *Asian J. Chem.* **2009**, *21*, 3199–3210.
7. Blanco, Y. La utilización de la alelopatía y sus efectos en diferentes cultivos agrícolas. *Cultiv. Trop.* **2006**, *27*, 5–16.
8. Kuiters, A.T. Effects of phenolic acids on germination and early growth of herbaceous woodland plants. *J. Chem. Ecol.* **1989**, *15*, 467–479. [CrossRef]
9. Einhellig, F.A. Mode of Allelochemical Action of Phenolic Compounds. In *Allelopathy: Chemistry and Mode of Action of Allelochemicals*; Macías, F.A., Galindo, J.C.G., Molinillo, J.M.G.V., Cutler, H.G., Eds.; CRC Press: Boca Raton, FL, USA, 2003; pp. 217–238. [CrossRef]
10. Inderjit. Plant Phenolics in Allelopathy. *Bot. Rev.* **1996**, *62*, 186–202. [CrossRef]
11. Zubkov, F.I.; Kouznetsov, V.V. Traveling across Life Sciences with Acetophenone—A Simple Ketone That Has Special Multipurpose Missions. *Molecules* **2023**, *28*, 370. [CrossRef]
12. Charoenying, P.; Teerarak, M.; Laosinwattana, C. An allelopathic substance isolated from *Zanthoxylum limonella* Alston fruit. *Sci. Hortic.* **2010**, *125*, 411–416. [CrossRef]
13. Chotsaeng, N.; Laosinwattana, C.; Charoenying, P. Herbicidal Activities of Some Allelochemicals and Their Synergistic Behaviors toward *Amaranthus tricolor* L. *Molecules* **2017**, *22*, 1841. [CrossRef]
14. Zaman, F.; Iwasaki, A.; Suenaga, K.; Kato-Noguchi, H. Allelopathic potential and identification of two allelopathic substances in *Eleocharis atropurpurea*. *Plant Biosyst.-Int. J. Deal. All Asp. Plant Biol.* **2020**, *155*, 510–516. [CrossRef]
15. Márquez-García, F.; García-Alonso, D.; Vázquez, F.M. Notes of Changes in Biodiversity in the Exploited Populations of Cistus Ladanifer, L., (Cistaceae) from SW Iberian Peninsula. *J. Fungi.* **2022**, *2*, 1–7.
16. Agra-Coelho, C.; Rosa, M.L.; Moreira, I. Allelopathic effects of *Cistus ladanifer* L. *III Natl. Symp. Herbol.* **1980**, *1*, 165–178.
17. Pereira, I.P. Allelopathic potential of *Cistus ladanifer* L. and *Cistus salvifolius* L. Master's Thesis, Instituto Superior de Agronomia, Lisboa, Portugal, 1992.
18. Dias, A.S.; Costa, C.T.; Dias, L.S. Allelopathic Plants. XVII. *Cistus ladanifer L. Allelopathy. J.* **2005**, *16*, 1–30.
19. Chaves, N.; Alías, J.C.; Sosa, T. Phytotoxicity of *Cistus ladanifer* L.: Role of allelopathy. *Allelopathy. J.* **2016**, *38*, 113–132.
20. Pérez-Izquierdo, C.; Serrano-Pérez, P.; Rodríguez-Molina, M.C. Chemical composition, antifungal and phytotoxic activities of Cistus ladanifer L. essential oil and hydrolate. *Biocatal. Agric. Biotechnol.* **2022**, *45*, 102527. [CrossRef]
21. Verdeguer, M.; Blázquez, M.A.; Boira, H. Chemical composition and herbicidal activity of the essential oil from a *Cistus ladanifer* L. population from Spain. *Nat. Prod. Res. Former. Nat. Prod. Lett.* **2012**, *26*, 1602–1609. [CrossRef]
22. Frazão, D.F.; Martins-Gomes, C.; Steck, J.L.; Keller, J.; Delgado, F.; Gonçalves, J.C.; Bunzel, M.; Pintado, C.M.B.S.; Díaz, T.S.; Silva, A.M. Labdanum Resin from *Cistus ladanifer* L.: A Natural and Sustainable Ingredient for Skin Care Cosmetics with Relevant Cosmeceutical Bioactivities. *Plants* **2022**, *11*, 1477. [CrossRef]
23. Chaves, N.; Sosa, T.; Alías, J.C.; Escudero, J.C. Identification and effects of interaction phytotoxic compounds from exudate of *Cistus ladanifer* leaves. *J. Chem. Ecol.* **2001**, *27*, 611–621. [CrossRef]
24. Chaves, N.; Sosa, T.; Escudero, J.C. Plant growth inhibiting flavonoids in exudate of *Cistus ladanifer* and in associated soils. *J. Chem. Ecol.* **2001**, *27*, 623–631. [CrossRef]
25. Chaves, N.; Sosa, T.; Alías, J.C.; Escudero, J.C. Germination inhibition of herbs in *Cistus ladanifer* L. soil: Possible involvement of allelochemicals. *Allelopathy. J.* **2003**, *11*, 31–42.
26. Días, A.S.; Dias, L.S.; Pereira, I.P. Activity of water extracts of *Cistus ladanifer* and *Lavandula stoechas* in soil on germination and early growth of wheat and *Phalaris minor*. *Allelopathy. J.* **2004**, *14*, 59–64.
27. Herranz, J.M.; Farrandis, P.; Copete, M.A.; Duro, E.M.; Zalacaín, A. Effect of allelopathic compounds produced by *Cistus ladanifer* on germination of 20 Mediterranean taxa. *Plant Ecol.* **2006**, *184*, 259–272. [CrossRef]
28. Sosa, T.; Valares, C.; Alías, J.C.; Chaves, N. Persistence of flavonoids in *Cistus ladanifer* soils. *Plant Soil.* **2010**, *377*, 51–63. [CrossRef]
29. Ramalho, P.S.; de Freitas, V.A.P.; Macedo, A.; Silva, G.; Silva, A.M.S. Volatile components of *Cistus ladanifer* leaves. *Flavour Fragr. J.* **1999**, *14*, 300–302. [CrossRef]

30. Morales-Soto, A.; Oruna-Concha, M.J.; Stephen Elmore, J.; Barrajón Catalán, E.; Micol, V.; Roldán, C.; Segura-Carretero, A. Volatile profile of Spanish Cistus plants as sources of antimicrobials for industrial applications. *Ind. Crops Prod.* **2015**, *74*, 425–433. [CrossRef]
31. Weyerstahl, P.; Marschall, H.; Weirauch, M.; Thefeld, K.; Surburg, H. Constituents of comercial labdanum oil. *Flavour Fragance J.* **1998**, *13*, 295–318. [CrossRef]
32. Kato-Noguchi, H.; Seki, T.; Shigemori, H. Allelopathy and allelopathic substance in the moss *Rhynchostegium pallidifolium*. *J. Plant Phys.* **2010**, *167*, 468–471. [CrossRef]
33. Einhellig, F.A.; Schon, M.K.; Rasmussen, J.A. Synergistic effects of four cinnamic acid compounds on grain sorghom. *Plant Growth Regul.* **1983**, *1*, 251–258.
34. Batish, D.R.; Singh, H.P.; Kaur, S.; Kohli, R.K.; Yadav, S.S. Caffeic acid affects early growth, and morphogenetic response of hypocotyl cuttings of mung bean *(Phaseolus aureus)*. *J. Plant Phys.* **2008**, *165*, 297–305. [CrossRef]
35. Requesón, E.; Osuna, D.; del Rosario Santiago, A.; Sosa, T. Evaluation of the Activity of Estragole and 2-Isopropylphenol, Phenolic Compounds Present in *Cistus ladanifer*. *Agronomy* **2022**, *12*, 1139. [CrossRef]
36. Cheng, H.H. Characterization of the mechanisms of allelopathy: Modeling and experimental approaches. In *Allelopathy: Organisms, Processes, and Applications*; Inderjit, Dakshini, K.M.M., Einhellig, F.A., Eds.; American Chemical Society: Washington, WA, USA, 1995; pp. 132–141.
37. National Center for Biotechnology Information. PubChem Compound Summary for CID 8500, 4′-Methylacetophenone. Available online: https://pubchem.ncbi.nlm.nih.gov/compound/8500 (accessed on 8 January 2023).
38. Macías, F.A.; Molinillo, J.M.; Varela, R.M.; Galindo, J.C. Allelopathy a natural alternative for weed control. Pest Management. *Science* **2007**, *63*, 327–348.
39. Einhellig, F.A.; Leather, G.R.; Hobbs, L.L. Use of *Lemna minor L.* as a bioassay in allelopathy. *J. Chem. Ecol.* **1985**, *11*, 65–72. [CrossRef] [PubMed]
40. Li, H.H.; Inoue, M.; Nishimura, H.; Mizutani, J.; Tsuzuki, E. Interactions of trans-cinnamic acid, its related phenolic allelochemicals, and abscisic acid in seedling growth and seed germination of lettuce. *J. Chem. Ecol.* **1993**, *19*, 1775–1787. [CrossRef] [PubMed]
41. Waller, G.R. *Allelochemicals: Role in Agriculture and Forestry. ACS Symposium Series 330*; American Chemical Society: Washington, WA, USA, 1987. [CrossRef]
42. Haugland, E.; Brandsaeter, L.O. Experiments on bioassay sensitivity in the study of allelopathy. *J. Chem. Ecol.* **1996**, *22*, 1845–1859. [CrossRef]
43. Tudi, M.; Daniel Ruan, H.; Wang, L.; Lyu, J.; Sadler, R.; Connell, D.; Chu, C.; Phung, D.T. Agriculture Development, Pesticide Application and Its Impact on the Environment. *Int. J. Environ. Res. Public Health* **2021**, *18*, 1112. [CrossRef]
44. Baucom, R.S. Evolutionary and ecological insights from herbicide-resistant weeds: What have we learned about plant adaptation, and what is left to uncover? *New Phytol.* **2019**, *223*, 68–82. [CrossRef]
45. Chung, I.M.; Miller, D.A. Effect of alfalfa plant and soil extracts on germination and seedling growth. *Agronomy J.* **1995**, *87*, 762–767. [CrossRef]
46. Muller, C.H.; Hanawalt, R.B.; McPherson, J.K. Allelopathic control of herb growth in the fire cycle of Californian chaparral. *Bull. Torrey Bot. Club.* **1968**, *95*, 225–231. [CrossRef]
47. Martínez-Otero, A.; González, L.; Reigosa, M.J. Oxygen electrode for seedling metabolism measurement in allelopathy. *Allelopathy J.* **2005**, *16*, 95–104.
48. Zhou, Y.H.; Yu, J.Q. Allelochemicals and photosynthesis. In *Allelopathy: A Physiological Process with Ecological Implications*; Reigosa, M.J., Pedrol, N., González, L., Eds.; Kluwer Academic Publishers: Amsterdam, The Netherlands, 2006; pp. 127–139. [CrossRef]
49. Lorenzo, P.; Pazos-Malvido, E.; González, L.; Reigosa, M.J. Allelopathic interference of invasive *Acacia dealbata*: Physiological effects. *Allelopath. J.* **2008**, *22*, 64–76.
50. Ishii-Iwamoto, E.L.; Abrahim, D.; Sert, M.A.; Bontato, C.M.; Kelmer-Brancht, A.M.; Bracht, A. Mitochondria as a site of allelochemicals action. In *Allelopathy: A Physiological Process with Ecological Implications*; Reigosa, M.J., Pedrol, N., González, L., Eds.; Kluwer Academic Publishers: Amsterdam, The Netherlands, 2006; Volume 12, pp. 267–284.
51. Tena, C.; del Rosario Santiago, A.; Osuna, D.; Sosa, T. Phytotoxic Activity of p-Cresol, 2-Phenylethanol and 3-Phenyl-1-Propanol, Phenolic Compounds Present in *Cistus ladanifer* L. *Plants* **2021**, *10*, 1136. [CrossRef] [PubMed]
52. Belz, R.G.; Cedergreen, N.; Duke, S.O. Herbicide hormesis—Can it be useful in crop production? *Weed Res.* **2011**, *51*, 321–332. [CrossRef]
53. Kaya, C.; Tuna, A.L.; Yokas, I. The role of plant hormones in plants under salinity stress. In *Salinity and Water Stress: Improving Crop Efficiency*; Ashraf, M., Ozturk, M., Athar, H.R., Eds.; Springer: Berlin/Heidelberg, Germany, 2009; pp. 45–50.
54. Soltys, D.; Krasuska, U.; Bogatek, R.; Gniazdowsk, A. Allelochemicals as Bioherbicides-Present and Perspectives. In *Herbicides-Current Research and Case Studies in Use*; Price, A.J., Kelton, J.A., Eds.; IntechOpen: London, UK, 2013; pp. 517–542. Available online: https://www.intechopen.com/chapters/44466 (accessed on 15 February 2023).
55. Yang, L.; Ruan, X.; Jiang, D.; Zhang, J.; Pan, C.; Wang, Q. Physiological effects of autotoxicity due to DHAP stress on *Picea schrenkiana* regeneration. *PLoS ONE* **2017**, *12*, e0177047. [CrossRef] [PubMed]
56. Oh, M.S.; Yang, J.-Y.; Lee, H.S. Acaricidal Toxicity of 2′-Hydroxy-4′-methylacetophenone Isolated from *Angelicae koreana* Roots and Structure–Activity Relationships of Its Derivatives. *J. Agric. Food Chem.* **2012**, *60*, 3606–3611. [CrossRef]

57. Macías, F.A.; Marín, D.; Oliveros-Bastidas, A.; Molinillo, J.M.G. Optimization of benzoxazinones as natural herbicide models by lipophilicity enhancement. *J. Agric. Food Chem.* **2006**, *54*, 9357–9365. [CrossRef]
58. Macías, F.A.; Marín, D.; Oliveros-Bastidas, A.; Molinillo, J.M.G. Rediscovering the bioactivity and ecological role of 1,4- benzoxazinones. *Nat. Prod. Rep.* **2009**, *26*, 478–489. [CrossRef]
59. Macías, F.A.; Molinillo, J.M.; Galindo, J.C.; Varela, R.M.; Simonet, A.M.; Castellano, D. The use of allelopathic studies in the search for natural herbicides. *J. Crop Prod.* **2001**, *4*, 237–255. [CrossRef]
60. Chinchilla, N.; Marín, D.; Oliveros-Bastidas, A.; Molinillo, J.M.G.; Macías, F.A. Soil biodegradation of a benzoxazinone analog proposed as a natural products-based herbicide. *Plant Soil* **2015**, *393*, 207–214. [CrossRef]
61. Macías, F.A.; De Siqueira, J.M.; Chinchilla, N.; Marín, D.; Varela, R.M.; Molinillo, J.M.G. New herbicide models from benzoxazinones: Aromatic ring functionalization effects. *J. Agric. Food Chem.* **2006**, *54*, 9843–9851. [CrossRef]
62. Macías, F.A.; Chinchilla, N.; Varela, R.M.; Molinillo, J.M.G.; Marín, D.; de Siqueira, J.M. Aromatic-ring-functionalised benzoxazinones in the system *Oryza sativa-Echinochloa crusgalli* as biorational herbicide models. *Pest Manag. Sci.* **2009**, *65*, 1104–1113. [CrossRef] [PubMed]
63. Chotpatiwetchkul, W.; Chotsaeng, N.; Laosinwattana, C.; Charoenying, P. Structure–Activity Relationship Study of Xanthoxyline and Related Small Methyl Ketone Herbicides. *ACS Omega* **2022**, *7*, 29002–29012. [CrossRef] [PubMed]
64. Dayan, F.E.; Duke, S.O. Biological activity of allelochemicals. In *Plant Derived Natural Products: Synthesis, Function, and Application*; Osbourn, A., Lanzotti, V., Eds.; Springer: New York, NY, USA, 2009; pp. 361–384.
65. Bais, H.P.; Vepachedu, R.; Gilroy, S.; Callaway, R.M.; Vivanco, J.M. Allelopathy and Exotic Plant Invasion: From Molecules and Genes to Species Interactions. *Science* **2003**, *301*, 1377–1380. [CrossRef] [PubMed]
66. Cruz-Ortega, A.; Lara-Núñez, A.; Anaya, A.L. Allelochemical stress can trigger oxidative damage in receptor plants mode of action of phytotoxicity. *Plant Signal. Behav.* **2007**, *2*, 269–270. [CrossRef]
67. Pardo-Muras, M.; Puig, C.G.; Pedrol, N. *Cytisus scoparius* and *Ulex europaeus* produce volatile organic compounds with powerful synergistic herbicidal effects. *Molecules* **2019**, *24*, 4539. [CrossRef]
68. Pardo-Muras, M.; Puig, C.G.; Pedrol, N. Complex Synergistic Interactions among Volatile and Phenolic Compounds Underlie the Effectiveness of Allelopathic Residues Added to the Soil for Weed Control. *Plants* **2022**, *11*, 1114. [CrossRef]
69. National Center for Biotechnology Information. PubChem Compound Summary for CID 7148, Propiophenone. Available online: https://pubchem.ncbi.nlm.nih.gov/#query=propiophenone (accessed on 8 January 2023).
70. Doi, M.; Shuto, Y. Oxidation of acetophenone by *Aspergillus* species and their possible contribution to Katsuobushi flavor. *Biosci. Biotechnol. Biochem.* **1996**, *59*, 2324–2325. [CrossRef]
71. Dayan, F.E.; Owens, D.K.; Duke, S.O. Rationale for a natural products approach to herbicide discovery. *Pest Manag. Sci.* **2012**, *68*, 519–528. [CrossRef]
72. Anaya, A.L. Alelopatía. In *Ecología Química*; Anaya, A.L., Ed.; Plaza y Valdés: Mexico, Mexico, 2003; pp. 255–298.
73. Prichoa, F.C.; Leyser, G.; Vladimir-Oliveira, J.; Cansian, R.L. Comparative allelopathic effects of *Cryptocarya moschata* and *Ocotea odorifera* aqueous extracts on *Lactuca sativa*. *Acta Sci.* **2013**, *35*, 197–202. [CrossRef]
74. Chiapusio, G.; Sánchez, M.A.; Reigosa, J.M.; González, L.; Pellissier, F. Do germination indices adequately reflect allelochemical effects on the germination process? *J. Chem. Ecol.* **1997**, *23*, 2445–2454. [CrossRef]
75. Wang, W. Literature review on higher plants for toxicity testing. *Water Air Soil Poll.* **1991**, *59*, 381–400. [CrossRef]
76. International Organization for Standarization (ISO). *Soil Quality-Determination of the Effects of Pollutants on Soil Flora. Part 1. Method for the Measurement of Inhibition of Root Growth*; ISO: Geneva, Switzerland, 1993; p. 9.
77. Organization of Economical Cooperation and Development (OECD). *Terrestrial Plants, Growth Test*; Guideline for Testing of Chemicals 208; OECD: Paris, France, 1984; p. 15.
78. Kuuluvaine, T. Gap disturbance, ground microtopography, and the regeneration dynamics of boreal coniferous forest in Finland: A review. *Ann. Zool. Fenn.* **1994**, *31*, 35–51.
79. Arango, M.C.; Ringuelet, J.; Viña, S. Intervención de los Compuestos Secundarios en las Interacciones Biológicas. In *Productos Naturales Vegetales*; Edulp integra la Red de Editoriales Universitarias Nacionales (REUN): Buenos Aires, Argentina, 2013.

*plants*

MDPI

*Article*

# Essential Oils and Biological Activities of *Eucalyptus falcata*, *E. sideroxylon* and *E. citriodora* Growing in Tunisia

**Ismail Amri [1,2,*], Marwa Khammassi [2], Rayda Ben Ayed [3,4], Sana Khedhri [2], Manel Ben Mansour [5], Oumayma Kochti [1], Ylenia Pieracci [6], Guido Flamini [6], Yassine Mabrouk [1], Samia Gargouri [5], Mohsen Hanana [3] and Lamia Hamrouni [1]**

1 Laboratory of Biotechnology and Nuclear Technology, National Center of Nuclear Science and Technology, Sidi Thabet, B.P. 72, Ariana 2020, Tunisia
2 Laboratory of Management and Valorization of Forest Resources, National Institute of Researches on Rural Engineering, Water and Forests, P.B. 10, Ariana 2080, Tunisia
3 Laboratory of Extremophile Plants, Centre of Biotechnology of Borj-Cédria, B.P. 901, Hammam-lif 2050, Tunisia
4 Department of Agronomy and Plant Biotechnology, National Institute of Agronomy of Tunisia (INAT), University of Carthage-Tunis, 43 Avenue Charles Nicolle, El Mahrajène 1082, Tunisia
5 Laboratory of Plant Protection, National Institut of Agronomic Research of Tunisia, P.B. 10, Ariana 2080, Tunisia
6 Dipartimento di Farmacia, via Bonanno 6, University of Pisa, 56126 Pisa, Italy
* Correspondence: amri_amri@live.fr

**Citation:** Amri, I.; Khammassi, M.; Ben Ayed, R.; Khedhri, S.; Mansour, M.B.; Kochti, O.; Pieracci, Y.; Flamini, G.; Mabrouk, Y.; Gargouri, S.; et al. Essential Oils and Biological Activities of *Eucalyptus falcata, E. sideroxylon* and *E. citriodora* Growing in Tunisia. *Plants* **2023**, *12*, 816. https://doi.org/10.3390/plants12040816

Academic Editors: Margot Schulz and Vincenzo Tabaglio

Received: 28 December 2022
Revised: 31 January 2023
Accepted: 2 February 2023
Published: 11 February 2023



**Abstract:** Many plants are able to synthesize essential oils (EOs), which play key roles in defense against weeds, fungi and pests. This study aims to analyze the chemical composition and to highlight the antioxidant, antimicrobial and phytotoxic properties of the EOs from *Eucalyptus falcata*, *E. sideroxylon* and *E. citriodora* growing in Tunisia. EOs were analyzed by gas chromatography coupled to mass spectrometry (GC/MS) and their antioxidant properties were determined by total antioxidant capacity (TAC), DPPH and ABTS assays. The phytotoxic potential was assessed against weeds (*Sinapis arvensis, Phalaris canariensis*) and durum wheat crop (*Triticum durum*) and compared to chemical herbicide glyphosate. The antifungal activity was investigated in vitro against eight target fungal strains. All EOs displayed a specific richness in oxygenated monoterpenes (51.3–90%) and oxygenated sesquiterpenes (4.8–29.4%), and 1,8-cineole, citronellal, citronellol, *trans*-pinocarveol, globulol, spathulenol and citronellyl acetate were the main constituents. *Eucalyptus* EOs exhibited remarkable antioxidant activity and *E. citriodora* oil exhibited significant activity when compared with *E. falcata* and *E. sideroxylon* EOs. The phytotoxic potential of the tested oils had different efficacy on seed germination and the growth of seedlings and varied among tested herbs and their chemical composition variability. Their effectiveness was better than that of glyphosate. At the post-emergence stage, symptoms of chlorosis and necrosis were observed. Furthermore, a decrease in chlorophyll and relative water content, electrolyte leakage and high levels of MDA and proline were indicators of the oxidative effects of EOs and their effectiveness as bioherbicides. Moreover, all the EOs exhibited moderate fungitoxic properties against all the tested fungal strains. Therefore, according to the obtained results, *Eucalyptus* EOs could have potential application as natural pesticides.

**Keywords:** allelochemicals; biopesticides; weeds; fungi; plant interactions

## 1. Introduction

Chemical pesticides are among the most applied agrochemicals for pest control. However, their repeated application has resulted in an increased risk of emergence of pest resistance and soil degradation, making the overuse of these synthetic pesticides a new problem for global environment preservation [1,2]. The potential hazardous effect on the environment and on human and animal health associated with the abuse of chemicals has encouraged scientists to search for eco-friendly alternatives for pest control [3,4]. The search for alternatives to these chemical pesticides with natural-based products and biological molecules would provide a sustainable solution to protect both crops and the environment [5]. In this context, allelochemicals are molecules synthesized by plants and known to have several biological activities. These molecules are particularly involved in the defense systems of plants against pests and are also synthesized as part of the allelopathy process [6–8]. It has been reported that several allelochemical molecules have different biological activities. They can act as phytotoxic molecules and thus inhibit the germination and growth of several plant species [8,9]. They can exert different types of effects against insects, both attractive and repellent, and even insecticidal and larvicidal effects [3]. They are also known to inhibit the growth of various microorganisms, such as bacteria, fungi and yeasts [10–12].

In this way, allelochemicals could be of great interest for the development of new eco-friendly bio-pesticides [11,13]. In fact, these molecules have a short half-life and therefore problems regarding the persistence of residues in the environment can be solved and they can be considered safe and eco-friendly for the environment [13].

EOs plays a crucial role in the allelopathic interactions between plants and species of their biotopes, such as weeds, fungi, bacteria and insects [3,5,10]. Terpenes are known as potent allelochemicals with herbicidal and antifungal activity [6]. These molecules can be a good source for the discovery of natural fungicides and herbicides and can limit the harmful environmental effects caused by chemical pesticides [11]. According to the literature, the EOs of various plants have been reported to possess a significant phytotoxic effect against weeds [5,8,11]. Hence, exploiting the allelopathic potential of molecules with herbicidal properties could be a promising approach for weed control [4,7,11,14].

The *Eucalyptus* genus is part of the *Myrtaceae* family, comprising forest trees native to Australia; the *Eucalyptus* genus includes 13 subgenera and more than 700 species [15]. More than 100 species of *Eucalyptus* have been introduced in Tunisia since the 1950s. These species have been used for reforestation programs. They are mainly exploited for wood production, erosion control and the production of EOs. *Eucalyptus* species EOs are a mixture of volatile terpenes, such as 1,8-cineole, globulol, citronellol, spathunelol, limonene and pinenes [5,8,9].

Various molecules extracted from *Eucalyptus* species have been reported to have toxic effects against weeds, insects and microorganisms [5,8,9,15]. Plants' secondary metabolites, known to possess several activities, and their applications in the field make them good alternatives for chemical pesticides without side effects—in particular, the persistence linked to the non-biodegradability of pesticides and resulting in toxicity to the environment, cultivated plants, wild animals, beneficial microorganisms and several insects [13,16].

The essential oils of *E. falcata*, *E. sideroxylon* and *E. citriodora*, which grow in Tunisia, have been the subject of recent studies [15,17–19]; however, studies of their herbicidal potential have not been performed. Likewise, the majority of studies on their antifungal potential are focused on clinical fungi, and few are studies of phyto-pathogenic fungi [17]. The herbicidal activity of *Eucalyptus citriodora* has been reported in India [20], but their mode of action was not described. On the other hand, knowing that chemical ecology is a very important strategy, it is widely exploited for the discovery of metabolites because plants are able to synthesize various molecules with the aim of adaptation and acclimatization to environmental pressure. The synthesis of these molecules continues to evolve according to the pedoclimatic conditions of their biotopes in order to act in a physiological or ecological way on the maintenance of the plant in its ecological environment [13]. This may explain the variability in the production of essential oils depending on the origin of the plant and the usefulness of testing plant material from different origins.

In this sense, the present work aims to determine the chemical compositions of the EOs of *E. falcata*, *E. sideroxylon* and *E. citriodora* growing in Tunisia, to evaluate their antioxidant potential and to test their antifungal effects against eight strains of phyto-pathogenic fungi, as well as to study their herbicidal activity against the germination and seedling growth of weeds and cultivated crops at the germination stage. Moreover, at the post-emergence stage, our objective is to test the effect of EOs applied by spraying on the physiological effects of plants: the relative water content, the relative leakage of electrolytes, the synthesis of chlorophyll, the rate of malondialdehyde resulting from lipid peroxidation and also the proline content, always referring to the activity of a reference synthetic herbicide: glyphosate.

## 2. Materials and Methods

### 2.1. Plant Material

*Eucalyptus* species used for essential oil extraction and weed species tested for herbicide trials, sampling origin, climatic conditions and dates of collection are listed in Table 1. For each *Eucalyptus* species, five samples were harvested from different trees at least 20 m away. *Eucalyptus* samples were then stored in a greenhouse for drying until constant weight.

**Table 1.** Species, date and site of harvest of the plant material.

| Species | Part Collected | Date of Harvest | Harvest Site | Preserved Specimen | Bioclimatic Stage |
|---|---|---|---|---|---|
| *E. citriodora* | Leaves | December 2020 | Rimel arboreta, Bizerte | EC2026 | Humid inferior with mild winter |
| *Eucalyptus sideroxylon* | Leaves | October 2020 | Henchir En Naâm arboreta, Siliana | ES2027 | Upper semi-arid |
| *E. falcata* | Leaves | October 2020 | Mjez Elbab arboreta, Beja | EF2028 | Upper semi-arid with mild winter |
| *S. arvensis* | Seeds | July 2019 | Sidi Ismail, Beja | SA1948 | Subhumid with mild winter |
| *P. canariensis* | Seeds | | | SA1949 | |
| *T. durum* | Seeds | | | SA1952 | |

Plants were identified by Professor Lamia Hamrouni, and the voucher specimens were deposited in the herbarium section of the Institute (INRGREF).

### 2.2. Extraction of Essential Oils

EOs were obtained by hydrodistillation of dried leaves in a Clevenger-type apparatus. The extraction lasted 4 h for each sample. EOs were collected and dried over anhydrous sodium sulfate and stored in a brown glass bottle at 4 °C until use. Yield was calculated based on dried weight ($w/w$ %).

### 2.3. Gas Chromatography and Mass Spectrometry Analysis

Gas chromatography/electron ionization–mass spectrometry (GC/EI–MS) was performed using an Agilent 7890B gas chromatograph (Agilent Technologies Inc., Santa Clara, CA, USA) equipped with an Agilent HP-5MS capillary column (30 m × 0.25 mm; coating thickness 0.25 μm) and an Agilent 5977B single quadrupole mass detector. The analytical conditions were as follows: oven temperature programmed from 60 °C to 240 °C at 3 °C/min; injector temperature 220 °C; transfer-line temperature 240 °C; carrier gas helium at 1 mL/min. The acquisition parameters were as follows: full scan; scan range: 35–300 $m/z$; scan time: 1.0 s; threshold: 1 count. The identification of the constituents was based on the comparison of their retention times with the retention times of pure reference samples and comparing their linear retention indices (LRIs) relative to the series of n-alkanes. The mass spectra were compared with those listed in the commercial libraries NIST 14 [21] and Adams (2007) [22] and in a home-made mass-spectral library, built using MS literature combined with data experimentally obtained from pure substances.

### 2.4. Antioxidant Activity of EOs

#### 2.4.1. Total Antioxidant Capacity

The total antioxidant capacity (TAC) was estimated by an assay based on the reduction of Mo (VI) to Mo (V) by EOs and on the formation of a green phosphate/Mo (V) complex at acidic pH [23]. One hundred μL of each oil was added to 1 mL of reagent solution containing sodium phosphate (28 mM), $H_2SO_4$ (0.6 M) and ammonium molybdate (4 mM). Then, the mixtures were heated for 90 min at 95 °C, followed by cooling, and the absorbance was read at 695 nm. The antioxidant capacity was expressed as mg gallic acid equivalents per gram of EOs (mg GAE/g EOs). All tested oils were analyzed in triplicate.

#### 2.4.2. DPPH Assay

The free radical scavenging activity of *Eucalyptus* oils was assessed by the DPPH (1,1-diphenyl-2-picrylhydrazyl) radical scavenging method, according to Hanato et al. (1988) [24]. For this, 400 μL of each oil diluted with methanol at different concentrations or pure methanol (control) was mixed with 4 mL of methanolic solution of DPPH (0.1 mM). Then, the samples were vortexed and incubated for 30 min at room temperature in the dark, and the absorbance was measured at 517 nm. The percentage of DPPH scavenging activity was calculated according to the following equation:

$$\% \text{ inhibition} = (\text{A control} - \text{A sample}/\text{A control}) * 100$$

where A sample is the absorbance value of the tested oil and A control is the absorbance value of the control.

The $IC_{50}$ is defined as the concentration of EOs required to scavenge 50% of the free radicals. All tested oils were analyzed in triplicate. Butylated hydroxytoluene (BHT) was used as a positive control.

#### 2.4.3. ABTS Free Radical Scavenging Activity

The ABTS+ assay was assessed following the methods described by Re et al. (1999), with slight modifications [25]. A solution containing ABTS radical cations was prepared by mixing an equal volume of potassium persulfate (2.45 mM) and ABTS (7 mM). The mixture was incubated for 16 h in the dark at room temperature. The absorbance of the ABTS solution was adjusted to 0.70 ± 0.02 at 734 nm. A 400 μL aliquot of various concentrations of *Eucalyptus* EOs or pure methanol for the control was mixed with 4 mL of the ABTS radical solution and allowed to stand at room temperature for 5 min in the dark. Absorbance was then measured at 734 nm. Trolox was used as the standard.

The percentage inhibition of the radical cation $ABTS^+$ was determined using the following formula:

$$\text{Inhibition of ABTS } (\%) = ((\text{Ac} - \text{As})/\text{Ac}) \times 100$$

where Ac is the absorbance of the control and As is the absorbance of the tested oil.

ABTS scavenging activity is expressed as the $IC_{50}$ value (μg/mL). All tested oils were analyzed in triplicate.

### 2.5. Seed Germination and Seedling Growth Experiments

Seeds of two weeds, *P. canariensis* L. and *S. arvensis* L., and a cultivated species, *T. durum* L., were used in herbicidal activity assays. Before germination tests, seeds were disinfected with 5% sodium hypochlorite, and then rinsed with water. Twenty seeds were placed in Petri dishes lined with a double layer of Whatman No. 1 filter paper. They were then treated with different doses (0, 0.5, 1, 1.5, and 2 μL/mL) of *Eucalyptus* oils in a solution of Tween 20 (0.1%) and incubated for 12 days at 25 °C; glyphosate was used as a positive control and the choice of glyphosate was based on the fact that it is the active molecule of several commercial herbicides used for the control of annual and perennial grasses and broad-leaved weeds in the post-planting/pre-emergence of many crops [7,16].

The tests were carried out in a completely randomized manner with three replicates for each dose. After 12 days, germination percentages and measured root and shoot growth (cm) were calculated.

### 2.6. Post-Emergence Assays

The post-emergence application of *Eucalyptus* EOs was performed to study its herbicidal effects on 21-day-old plants under controlled conditions in a glass greenhouse. Twenty seeds of the tested plant species were sown in polypropylene pots containing 500 g of mixture of peat, sand and perlite (1/3 of each). Fifteen days after seedling emergence, only five equal-sized plants per pot were kept.

When plants were 21 days old, they were sprayed with the following different solutions at 100 mL/m$^2$:

- Solution of water/Tween 20 (0.1%) as negative control;
- Solution of 10 μL/mL of *Eucalyptus* EOs dissolved in water/Tween 20 (0.1%);
- Solution of 10 mg/mL of glyphosate dissolved in water/Tween 20 (0.1%) as positive control.

A total of 15 pots were used for each plant test: five treatments and three replicates per treatment. Five days after spraying, the treated plants were used for various tests.

#### 2.6.1. Relative Water Content (RWC)

Relative water content was calculated according to the following equation [26]:

$$RWC = (FW - DW)/FW) \times 100$$

where FW is the fresh weight and DW is the dry weight of treated plants (dried to constant weight at 75 °C).

#### 2.6.2. Determination of Total Chlorophyll Content

Chlorophyll content was determined on fresh leaves five days after plant spraying. Here, 100 mg of leaves were ground in 5 mL acetone and kept for 72 h at 4 °C in the dark. The content of chlorophyll was determined according to the method of Lichtenthaler (1987), by measuring the absorbance at 663 and 646 nm [27].

#### 2.6.3. Relative Electrolyte Leakage

Relative electrolyte leakage was assessed in leaves of treated herbs to study the effect of *Eucalyptus* oils on solute leakage. Leaves were immersed in glass boxes containing distilled water for 60 min, and then the conductivity of the water solution was measured (C1). At this point, the aqueous solution was boiled for 30 min and its conductivity was measured (C2) [28]. The relative electrolyte leakage (REL) was calculated according to the following formula:

$$\% REL = (C1/C2) \times 100$$

#### 2.6.4. Determination of Free Proline Content

Proline levels were assessed according to the method adopted by (Bates et al., 1973) [29]. The fresh leaves of tested plants were digested with 6 mL of sulfosalicylic acid (3%) at 100 °C for 30 min, and then centrifuged at 25 °C at 2000× *g* for 5 min.

A volume of 0.5 mL of the obtained extract was mixed with 0.5 mL of distilled water and 2 mL of a mixture containing 0.5 g of ninhydrin, 30 mL of glacial acetic acid, and 20 mL of distilled water. The mixtures were boiled for 1 h. Then, the different samples were cooled and extracted with 6 mL of toluene. The toluene phase was used for absorbance measurements at 520 nm. The proline content was calculated from a standard curve. Proline content was expressed as mg/g fresh weight. All samples were analyzed in triplicate.

### 2.7. Antifungal Activity

Eight fungal strains (*Bipolaris sorokiniana*, *Fusarium verticillioides*, *F. pseudograminearum*, *F. proliferatum*, *F. nygamai*, *F. graminarium*, *F. avenaceum*, and *F. culmorum*) were obtained from the Laboratory of Plant Protection, Tunisian National Institute of Agronomic Research (INRAT). The antifungal potential of the *Eucalyptus* oils on the mycelial growth of tested fungi was assessed in vitro using the agar dilution method [16]. EOs tested were diluted in a solution (0.1%) of Tween 20 and then mixed in PDA medium to obtain a final concentration of 4 μL/mL. A disk of 5 mm, cut from the periphery of each fungal culture, was placed in the center of the PDA plate and then incubated for 7 days in optimal conditions. The experiments were carried out as three replicates per treatment. Growth inhibition was calculated as the growth percentage of inhibition relative to the control according to the formula:

$$\% \text{ Inhibition } ((C - T)/C) \times 100$$

where C: mean of growth of three replicates (mm) of control plates. T: mean of growth of three replicates (mm) of plates containing *Eucalyptus* oils.

### 2.8. Statistical Analysis

All of the experiments were carried out in three replicates, with the results represented as mean ± standard deviation. Data were subjected to one-way analysis of variance (ANOVA) using the SPSS 18.0 software package. Differences between means were tested through Student–Newman–Keuls and values with $p \leq 0.05$ were considered significantly different.

## 3. Results

### 3.1. Eucalyptus EOs' Yield and Chemical Composition

The hydrodistillation of dried leaves yielded 0.7 ± 0.1%, 1.3 ± 0.1%, and 2.9 ± 0.2% of yellow oils for *E. falcata*, *E. sideroxylon*, and *E. citriodora*, respectively. Oils' components, area percentages, retention indices, formulae, and the chemical classes of components for each oil are reported in Table 2.

**Table 2.** Chemical compositions of essential oils of *Eucalyptus* species.

| Peak | Component | Formula | LRI (Lit.) | LRI | % | | |
|---|---|---|---|---|---|---|---|
| | | | | | *E. falcata* | *E. sideroxylon* | *E. citriodora* |
| 1 | α-pinene | $C_{10}H_{16}$ | 939 | 941 | 6 | 1 | |
| 2 | *p*-cymene | $C_{10}H_{14}$ | 1026 | 1028 | 2.5 | 0.9 | |
| 3 | limonene | $C_{10}H_{16}$ | 1031 | 1032 | 0.7 | 0.9 | 0.1 |
| 4 | 1,8-cineole | $C_{10}H_{18}O$ | 1033 | 1034 | 28.4 | 65.4 | 0.3 |
| 5 | bergamal | $C_{11}H_{18}O$ | 1053 | 1053 | | | 0.3 |
| 6 | isopentyl isovalerate | $C_{10}H_{20}O$ | 1103 | 1104 | | 0.1 | |
| 7 | *cis*-rose oxide | $C_{11}H_{18}O$ | 1111 | 1111 | | | 0.1 |
| 8 | fenchol | $C_{10}H_{18}O$ | 1110 | 1112 | 0.7 | | |
| 9 | α-campholenal | $C_{10}H_{16}O$ | 1124 | 1126 | 0.2 | | |
| 10 | *trans*-rose oxide | $C_{11}H_{18}O$ | 1126 | 1127 | | | 0.2 |
| 11 | *trans*-pinocarveol | $C_{10}H_{16}O$ | 1139 | 1141 | 14.2 | 1.8 | |
| 12 | *iso*pulegol | $C_{10}H_{18}O$ | 1146 | 1146 | | | 8.1 |
| 13 | citronellal | $C_{10}H_{18}O$ | 1153 | 1155 | | | 48.7 |
| 14 | *trans*-β-terpineol | $C_{10}H_{18}O$ | 1162 | 1160 | | | 4.1 |
| 15 | pinocarvone | $C_{10}H_{14}O$ | 1162 | 1164 | 2.2 | 0.2 | |
| 16 | borneol | $C_{10}H_{18}O$ | 1165 | 1166 | 1.1 | 0.2 | |
| 17 | *trans*-ocimenol | $C_{10}H_{16}O$ | 1168 | 1169 | | 0.2 | |
| 18 | 4-terpineol | $C_{10}H_{18}O$ | 1177 | 1179 | 0.6 | 0.4 | |
| 19 | *p*-cymen-8-ol | $C_{10}H_{14}O$ | 1183 | 1184 | 0.4 | 0.3 | |
| 20 | *p*-mentha-1(7),8-dien-2-ol | $C_{10}H_{16}O$ | 1186 | 1186 | 0.7 | 1.5 | |
| 21 | α-terpineol | $C_{10}H_{18}O$ | 1189 | 1191 | 1.5 | 1.4 | |
| 22 | myrtenol | $C_{10}H_{16}O$ | 1191 | 1193 | 0.4 | | |
| 23 | *trans*-carveol | $C_{10}H_{16}O$ | 1217 | 1220 | 0.3 | 0.3 | |
| 24 | *cis*-carveol | $C_{10}H_{16}O$ | 1229 | 1228 | | 1.6 | |

Table 2. *Cont.*

| Peak | Component | Formula | LRI (Lit.) | LRI | % | | |
|---|---|---|---|---|---|---|---|
| | | | | | *E. falcata* | *E. sideroxylon* | *E. citriodora* |
| 25 | citronellol | $C_{10}H_{20}O$ | 1228 | 1230 | | | 20.2 |
| 26 | (*Z*)-tagetone | $C_{10}H_{16}O$ | 1234 | 1231 | | 0.9 | |
| 27 | carvone | $C_{10}H_{14}O$ | 1242 | 1244 | | 0.2 | |
| 28 | geraniol | $C_{10}H_{18}O$ | 1255 | 1256 | | | 0.1 |
| 29 | citronellyl formate | $C_{11}H_{20}O_2$ | 1275 | 1276 | | | 0.1 |
| 30 | carvacrol | $C_{10}H_{14}O$ | 1298 | 1298 | 0.4 | | |
| 31 | *p*-vinylguaiacol | $C_9H_{10}O_2$ | 1312 | 1314 | | | 0.4 |
| 32 | 3,7-dimethyl-6-octenoic acid | $C_{10}H_{18}O_2$ | 1314 | 1315 | | | 1.2 |
| 33 | 2-acetoxy-1,8-cineole | $C_{12}H_{20}O_3$ | 1345 | 1345 | 0.2 | 0.2 | |
| 34 | α-terpinyl acetate | $C_{12}H_{20}O_2$ | 1350 | 1352 | | 0.9 | |
| 35 | citronellyl acetate | $C_{12}H_{22}O_2$ | 1354 | 1354 | | | 8.1 |
| 36 | 2-phenylethyl isobutyrate | $C_{12}H_{16}O_2$ | 1395 | 1394 | | | 0.1 |
| 37 | (*Z*)-jasmone | $C_{11}H_{16}O$ | 1394 | 1395 | | | 0.4 |
| 38 | β-caryophyllene | $C_{15}H_{24}$ | 1418 | 1419 | 0.6 | 0.3 | 1 |
| 39 | isoamyl benzoate | $C_{12}H_{16}O_2$ | 1439 | 1439 | | | |
| 40 | aromadendrene | $C_{15}H_{24}$ | 1440 | 1440 | 3.2 | 2.1 | |
| 41 | α-humulene | $C_{15}H_{24}$ | 1454 | 1455 | | | 0.2 |
| 42 | alloaromadendrene | $C_{15}H_{24}$ | 1460 | 1462 | 0.8 | 0.6 | |
| 43 | β-selinene | $C_{15}H_{24}$ | 1486 | 1487 | 0.4 | | |
| 44 | α-vetispirene | $C_{15}H_{22}$ | 1483 | 1488 | 0.5 | | |
| 45 | β-phenylethyl isovalerate | $C_{13}H_{18}O_2$ | 1489 | 1490 | | 0.3 | |
| 46 | α-selinene | $C_{15}H_{24}$ | 1497 | 1495 | | 0.2 | |
| 47 | bicyclogermacrene | $C_{15}H_{24}$ | 1496 | 1496 | 1.1 | 0.2 | |
| 48 | germacrene B | $C_{15}H_{24}$ | 1556 | 1557 | | 1 | |
| 49 | ledol | $C_{15}H_{26}O$ | 1565 | 1566 | 1 | 0.7 | |
| 50 | spathulenol | $C_{15}H_{24}O$ | 1576 | 1576 | 7.2 | 3.3 | 1.4 |
| 51 | caryophyllene oxide | $C_{15}H_{24}O$ | 1582 | 1582 | | | 2.5 |
| 52 | globulol | $C_{15}H_{26}O$ | 1584 | 1583 | 9.1 | 7.4 | |
| 53 | viridiflorol | $C_{15}H_{26}O$ | 1590 | 1591 | 3.6 | 1.6 | |
| 54 | rosifoliol | $C_{15}H_{26}O$ | 1599 | 1601 | 1.5 | 0.6 | |
| 55 | 10-*epi*-α-eudesmol | $C_{15}H_{26}O$ | 1617 | 1620 | 1.9 | 0.6 | 0.5 |
| 56 | *iso* spathulenol | $C_{15}H_{24}O$ | 1640 | 1640 | 0.7 | | |
| 57 | β-eudesmol | $C_{15}H_{26}O$ | 1649 | 1650 | 4.4 | 2 | |
| 58 | α-cadinol | $C_{15}H_{26}O$ | 1653 | 1652 | | | 0.4 |
| | Monoterpene hydrocarbons % | | | | 9.2 | 2.8 | 0.1 |
| | Oxygenated monoterpenes % | | | | 51.3 | 75.5 | 90 |
| | Sesquiterpene hydrocarbons % | | | | 6.6 | 4.4 | 1.2 |
| | Oxygenated sesquiterpenes % | | | | 29.4 | 16.2 | 4.8 |
| | Non-terpene derivatives % | | | | 0 | 0.4 | 2.4 |
| | Total identified % | | | | 96.5 | 99.3 | 98.5 |

Analysis of the three oils allowed the identification of 58 compounds distributed across five classes of terpene and non-terpene derivatives. All oils showed a specific richness in oxygenated monoterpenes (51.3–90%) and oxygenated sesquiterpenes (4.8–29.4%). In *E. falcata*, 31 components were identified, representing 96.5% of the total EOs. Oxygenated monoterpenes and oxygenated sesquiterpenes were the two main subclasses in this oil (51.3% and 29.4%, respectively). EOs' main constituents were 1,8-cineole (28.4%) and trans-pinocarveol (14.2%) as oxygenated monoterpenes, and globulol (9.1%) and spathulenol (7.2%) as oxygenated sesquiterpenes. Furthermore, appreciable percentages of the monoterpene hydrocarbon α-pinene (6.0%) were also present. The major and characteristic compounds of the essential oils of *E. falcata* are presented in Figure 1.

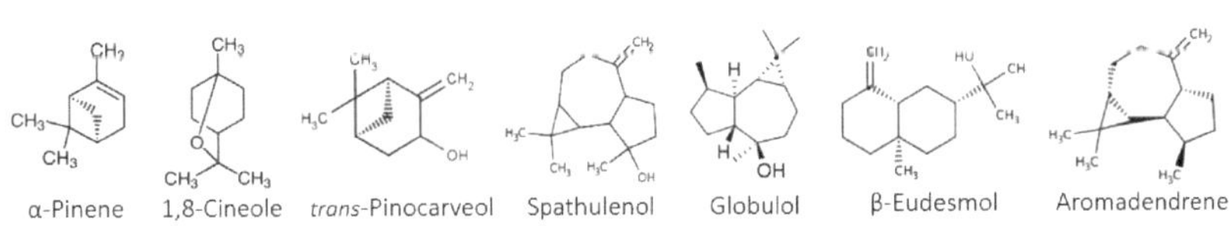


**Figure 1.** Major compounds of essential oils of *E. falcata*.

In *E. sideroxylon* EOs, 33 components were identified, accounting for 99.3% of the oil. Oxygenated monoterpenes and oxygenated sesquiterpenes were the two main subclasses in this oil (75.5% and 16.2%, respectively). The EOs of this species were characterized by a high level of 1,8-cineole (65.4%) as the major oxygenated monoterpene and globulol (7.4%) as an oxygenated sesquiterpene. The major and characteristic compounds of the essential oils of this species are presented in Figure 2.

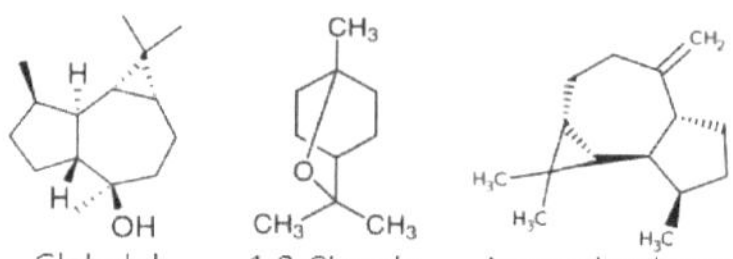

Globulol 1,8-Cineole Aromadendrene

**Figure 2.** Major compounds of essential oils of *E. sideroxylon*.

In *E. citriodora* EOs, 22 different chemical constituents were identified, accounting for 98.5% of the oil. Globally, *E. citriodora* EOs were characterized by the dominance of oxygenated monoterpenes (90%). The major components were citronellal (48.7%), citronellol (20.2%), aitronellyl acetate (8.1%), and isopulegol (8.1%).

Great diversity in the structure and nature of the compounds of *E. citriodora* EOs has been described. The chemical structure of the major compounds is shown in Figure 3.

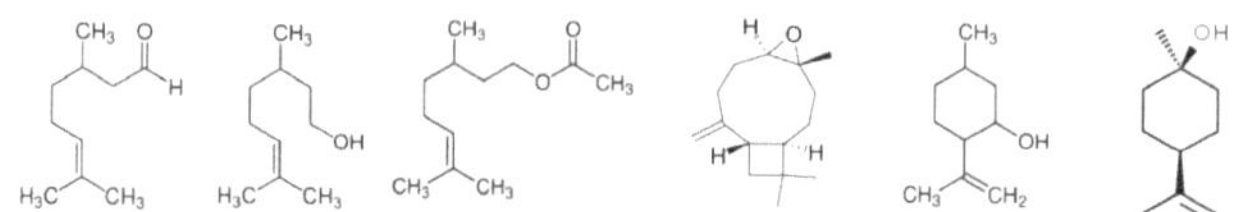

Citronellal Citronellol Citronellyl acetate Caryophyllene oxide <*iso*>Pulegol *trans*-β-Terpineol

**Figure 3.** Major compounds of essential oils of *E. citriodora*.

## 3.2. *Antioxidant Activity*

To establish a better assessment of the antioxidant potential of the EOs, they were evaluated using three different methods. Table 3 details the results obtained in this study.

**Table 3.** Antioxidant activity of the essential oils of the three *Eucalyptus* species.

| Essential Oils | TAC (mg GAE/g) | DPPH ($IC_{50}$ µg/mL) | ABTS ($IC_{50}$ µg/mL) |
|---|---|---|---|
| *E. citriodora* | 80.21 ± 5.72 a | 71.37 ± 3.89 b | 53.26 ± 5.57 b |
| *E. sideroxylon* | 26.68 ± 6.25 b | 96.29 ± 5.58 c | 84.84 ± 1.52 c |
| *E. falcata* | 32.59 ± 3.83 b | 112.61 ± 3.86 d | 90.35 ± 3.27 c |
| BHT | - | 20.53 ± 2.79 a | - |
| Trolox | - | - | 15.75 ± 1.11 a |

TAC: total antioxidant capacity; DPPH: 2,2-diphenyl-1-picrylhydrazyl; ABTS: 2,2′-Azino-bis(3-ethylbenzthiazoline-6-sulfonic acid; GAE: gallic acid equivalent; BHT: butylated hydroxytoluene. Results are expressed as mean ± standard deviation of 3 repetitions. Different letters in the same column indicate significant differences ($p \leq 0.05$) through Student–Newman–Keuls.

According to the statistical analysis, significant differences were noted in the TAC of the three tested EOs. The highest TAC value was observed for *E. citriodora* oil (80.21 mg GAE/g), followed by *E. falcata* oil (32.59 mg GAE/g) and *E. sideroxylon* (26.68 mg GAE/g) oils.

*E. citriodora* EOs showed also the highest antiradical activity with both the DPPH and ABTS assay ($IC_{50}$ = 71.37 and 53.26 µg/mL, respectively).

Hence, the EOs of *E. citriodora* exhibited the highest antioxidant activity in all methods, while the lowest activity was obtained with the EOs of *E. falcata* and *E. sideroxylon*. The observed results could be related to the different compositions of the three oils.

### 3.3. *Phytotoxic Effects of Eucalyptus EOs*

#### 3.3.1. Anti-Germinative Activity

The phytotoxic effect of the *Eucalyptus* EOs was evaluated against two well-known weeds, *S. arvensis* and *P. canariensis*, and on one cultivated crop, *T. durum*. Germination and growth of all tested herbs decreased in a dose-dependent manner, as shown in Table 4.

**Table 4.** Inhibitory effect of *Eucalyptus* species EOs on seed germination.

| Tested Plant | Dose (µL/mL) | Germination % | | | |
|---|---|---|---|---|---|
| | | *E. falcata* | *E. sideroxylon* | *E. citriodora* | Glyphosate |
| *S. arvensis* | 0 | 100 ± 0.0 a | 100 ± 0.0 a | 100 ± 0.0 a | 100 ± 0.0 a |
| | 0.5 | 46.6 ± 11.54 bC | 76.6 ± 5.7 bB | 33.3 ± 5.8 bC | 96.66 ± 3.33 aA |
| | 1 | 23.3 ± 5.8 cB | 40 ± 10 cA | 6.7 ± 5.8 cC | 90 ± 5.77 aA |
| | 1.5 | 16.7 ± 5.8 cB | 23.3 ± 5.7 dB | 0 ± 0 cC | 86.66 ± 3.33 aA |
| | 2 | 0 ± 0 dC | 16.6 ± 5.7 dB | 0 ± 0 cC | 73.33 ± 3.33 bA |
| *P. canariensis* | 0 | 90 ± 10 a | 90 ± 10 a | 90 ± 10 a | 90 ± 10 a |
| | 0.5 | 76.7 ± 5.8 aB | 90 ± 10 aA | 66.7 ± 5.8 bB | 93.33 ± 3.33 aA |
| | 1 | 46.7 ± 11.5 bC | 100 ± 00 aA | 43.3 ± 5.8 cC | 80 ± 0.0 aB |
| | 1.5 | 23.3 ± 5.8 cB | 80 ± 10 aA | 16.7 ± 5.8 dB | 80 ± 0.0 aA |
| | 2 | 26.7 ± 5.8 cB | 30 ± 10 bB | 3.3 ± 5.8 eC | 66.66 ± 3.33 bA |
| *T. durum* | 0 | 96.7 ± 5.7 a | 96.7 ± 5.7 a | 96.7 ± 5.7 a | 96.7 ± 5.7 a |
| | 0.5 | 86.7 ± 5.8 aB | 83.3 ± 5.7 aB | 76.7 ± 5.8 bB | 100 ± 0.0 aA |
| | 1 | 63.3 ± 5.8 bB | 96.6 ± 5.7 aA | 40 ± 10 cC | 93.33 ± 3.33 aA |
| | 1.5 | 30 ± 10 cB | 90 ± 10 aA | 13.3 ± 5.8 dC | 80 ± 0.0 bA |
| | 2 | 36.7 ± 5.8 cC | 63.3 ± 10 bB | 0 ± 0 eD | 76.66 ± 3.33 bA |

Values are means ± standard errors ($n$ = 3). The lowercase letters compare, in the columns, the dose effect for each herb vis-à-vis each oil. The capital letters compare, in the rows, the sensitivity of each herb at the same dose vis-à-vis the samples tested. Means followed by the same letter are not significantly different by the Student–Newman–Keuls test ($p \leq 0.05$).

Data showed that all oils significantly inhibited the seed germination of all tested herbs. The inhibition depended on both the tested species and dose. In fact, the inhibition of seed germination increased with increasing oil concentration.

A significant reduction in the seed germination of all tested herbs was observed at all doses. *E. falcata* oil caused complete germination inhibition in *S. arvensis* at 2 µL/mL. However, at the same dose, seed germination was only reduced for *P. canariensis* and *T. durum* (26.7 and 36.7%), respectively.

The volatile oil of *E. sideroxylon* reduced the germination of *S. arvensis* at the dose of 2.0 µL/mL to 16.6% and that of *P. canariensis* to 30%. On the contrary, *T. durum* appeared to be more resistant at the same dose, observing a higher percentage of germination (63.3%).

The high phytotoxicity of *E. citriodora* oil was remarkable, with a significant inhibitory effect against the germination of all tested herbs at all oil concentrations (0.5, 1.0, 1.5, and 2.0 µL/mL). Indeed, it was also remarkable that the complete inhibition of germination for *S. arvensis* by *E. citriodora* oil was obtained at the dose of 1 µL/mL. However, a partial reduction at the same dose (1.0 µL/mL) was observed in the germination of both *P. canariensis* and *T. durum*, although, at the highest dose (2.0 µL/mL), the seed germination of all tested herbs was totally inhibited.

Similarly, a high herbicidal effect was found with *Eucalyptus* oils against the seedling growth (roots and shoots) of all tested herbs at all doses; see Tables 5 and 6.

**Table 5.** Inhibitory effect of *Eucalyptus* species essential oils on aerial parts growth of germinated seeds.

| Tested Plant | Dose (µL/mL) | Shoots (cm) | | | |
|---|---|---|---|---|---|
| | | *E. falcata* | *E. sideroxylon* | *E. citriodora* | Glyphosate |
| *S. arvensis* | 0 | 7.7 ± 0.68 a | 7.7 ± 0.68 a | 7.7 ± 0.68 a | 7.7 ± 0.68 a |
| | 0.5 | 6.36 ± 1.32 aA | 6.3 ± 0.58 bA | 1.83 ± 0.74 bB | 5.66 ± 0.28 bA |
| | 1 | 4.1 ± 0.96 bA | 4.7 ± 0.37 cA | 1.13 ± 1.06 bcB | 5.96 ± 0.38 bA |
| | 1.5 | 2.93 ± 0.49 bA | 2.73 ± 0.5 dA | 0 ± 0 cB | 3.06 ± 0.58 cA |
| | 2 | 0 ± 0 cC | 2.43 ± 0.49 dA | 0 ± 0 cC | 1.33 ± 0.17 dB |
| *P. canariensis* | 0 | 9.76 ± 0.5 a | 9.76 ± 0.5 a | 9.76 ± 0.5 a | 9.76 ± 0.5 a |
| | 0.5 | 8.4 ± 2.16 abA | 11.8 ± 1.58 aA | 10.53 ± 0.61 aA | 8.46 ± 0.41 bA |
| | 1 | 9.13 ± 0.3 aA | 8.8 ± 0.96 aA | 7.5 ± 1.04 bA | 4.56 ± 0.34 cB |
| | 1.5 | 6.06 ± 0.9 bA | 6.5 ± 2.02 abA | 6.1 ± 0.75 cA | 2.23 ± 0.33 dB |
| | 2 | 3.3 ± 1.6 cA | 3.4 ± 4.2 bA | 0.4 ± 0.7 dA | 0.66 ± 0.16 eA |
| *T. durum* | 0 | 9.16 ± 1.2 a | 9.16 ± 1.2 b | 9.16 ± 1.2 a | 9.16 ± 1.2 a |
| | 0.5 | 8.73 ± 1.27 aB | 11.53 ± 0.98 aA | 8.56 ± 0.45 aB | 5.36 ± 1.12 bC |
| | 1 | 7.73 ± 0.76 aB | 10.1 ± 1.4 abA | 6.1 ± 0.2 bB | 3.63 ± 0.18 bcC |
| | 1.5 | 5.56 ± 0.81 bB | 8.2 ± 0.36 bcA | 4.56 ± 1.15 cB | 2.2 ± 0.17 cdC |
| | 2 | 3.6 ± 1.04 cB | 6.5 ± 0.45 cA | 0 ± 0 dC | 0.9 ± 0.15 dC |

Values are means ± standard errors ($n$ = 3). The lowercase letters compare, in the columns, the dose effect for each herb vis-à-vis each oil. The capital letters compare, in the rows, the sensitivity of each herb at the same dose vis-à-vis the samples tested. Means followed by the same letter are not significantly different by the Student–Newman–Keuls test ($p \leq 0.05$).

**Table 6.** Inhibitory effect of *Eucalyptus* species essential oils on roots growth of germinated seeds.

| Tested Plant | Dose (µL/mL) | Roots (cm) | | | |
|---|---|---|---|---|---|
| | | *E. falcata* | *E. sideroxylon* | *E. citriodora* | Glyphosate |
| *S. arvensis* | 0 | 11.73 ± 0.7 a | 11.73 ± 0.7 a | 11.73 ± 0.7 a | 11.73 ± 0.7 a |
| | 0.5 | 10.07 ± 1.4 bA | 7.8 ± 0.45 bB | 3.77 ± 0.76 bD | 5.86 ± 0.24 bC |
| | 1 | 8.2 ± 0.5 cA | 7.03 ± 1.4 bA | 1.5 ± 1.32 cB | 5.8 ± 0.55 bA |
| | 1.5 | 5.7 ± 0.6 dA | 4.6 ± 0.7 cB | 0 ± 0 cD | 2.36 ± 0.31 cC |
| | 2 | 0 ± 0 eC | 3.87 ± 0.55 cA | 0 ± 0 cC | 1.73 ± 0.21 cB |
| *P. canariensis* | 0 | 10.3 ± 1.18 a | 10.3 ± 1.18 a | 10.3 ± 1.18 a | 10.3 ± 1.18 a |
| | 0.5 | 7.8 ± 0.4 abC | 9.93 ± 1.33 aBC | 11.2 ± 1.31 aA | 9.66 ± 0.43 aBC |
| | 1 | 8.7 ± 1.5 abB | 9.46 ± 0.75 aA | 7.5 ± 0.47 bBC | 6.2 ± 0.25 bC |
| | 1.5 | 6.5 ± 1.3 bcA | 4.5 ± 1.23 bA | 6.06 ± 1.0 bA | 2.36 ± 0.32 cB |
| | 2 | 4.8 ± 1.2 cA | 2.33 ± 0.85 cB | 0.4 ± 0.7 cC | 0.63 ± 0.18 dC |
| *T. durum* | 0 | 10.2 ± 1.09 a | 10.2 ± 1.09 a | 10.2 ± 1.09 a | 10.2 ± 1.1 a |
| | 0.5 | 10.4 ± 0.6 aA | 7.4 ± 1.11 bB | 9.06 ± 1.55 aAB | 8.2 ± 0.5 bAB |
| | 1 | 8.43 ± 0.45 aA | 6.5 ± 0.7 bB | 5.87 ± 0.76 bB | 3.0 ± 0.15 cC |
| | 1.5 | 5.83 ± 1.51 bA | 5.7 ± 0.76 bA | 5.73 ± 0.38 bA | 2.23 ± 0.14 cdB |
| | 2 | 3.9 ± 1.02 cB | 7.36 ± 0.7 bA | 0 ± 0 cD | 1.2 ± 0.15 dC |

Values are means ± standard errors ($n$ = 3). The lowercase letters compare, in the columns, the dose effect for each herb vis-à-vis each oil. The capital letters compare, in the rows, the sensitivity of each herb at the same dose vis-à-vis the samples tested. Means followed by the same letter are not significantly different by the Student–Newman–Keuls test ($p \leq 0.05$).

The growth of *S. arvensis* seedlings was the most affected by *Eucalyptus* oil application, with high inhibition in both aerial parts and root growth when compared to the control at a low dose (0.5 μL/mL). Conversely, no significant effect at the same dose was observed for *P. canariensis* and *T. durum* (monocot species), which are more resistant to oil application.

3.3.2. Post-Emergence Assays

The post-emergent spray treatment with *Eucalyptus* EOs and glyphosate caused chlorosis and necrosis of the leaves, breaking of the stem, and complete wilting of all the tested weeds (*P. canariensis* and *S. arvensis*) and the cultivated species (*T. durum*) when compared to the negative control. Five days after the application of the EOs, significant effects on chlorophyll synthesis were seen. In fact, a significant decrease in the chlorophyll rate was noted for all the tested herbs. This effect varied according to the applied EOs and the tested species (Figure 4).

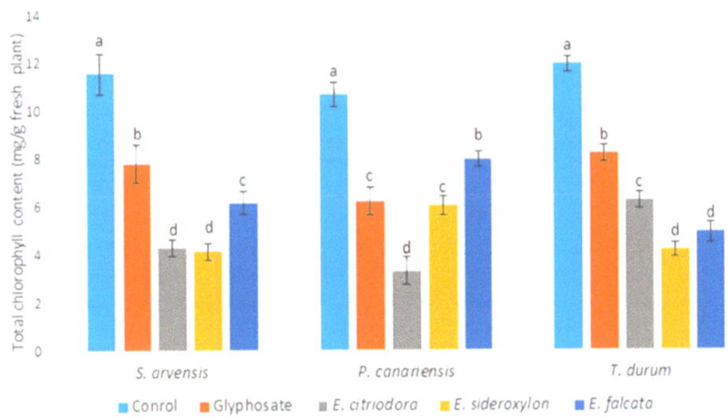


**Figure 4.** Effects of *Eucalyptus* species essential oils and glyphosate on total chlorophyll content as mg/g fresh tested plants measured five days after application. Error bars and letters on graphs represent standard error means and significant differences at $p \leq 0.05$ through Student–Newman–Keuls.

Generally, all the oils showed similar and even better effects than glyphosate. For *S. arvensis* (dicot weed), a significant decrease in the synthesis of chlorophyll was noted in the order of 48.28, 61.74, and 63.37% for *E. falcata*, *E. citriodora*, and *E. sideroxylon*, respectively. On the contrary, glyphosate showed the lowest rate of inhibition (33.96%).

In the case of *P. canariensis* (monocot weed), all oils showed the significant inhibition of chlorophyll synthesis; *E. citriodora* showed the highest rate of inhibition (67.45%), followed by *E. falcata* (24.24%) and *E. sideroxylon* (44.87%), which had effects similar to glyphosate (42.61%).

For *T. durum*, significant inhibition was noted with all *Eucalyptus* oils and its effects outweighed the chemical herbicide used as a positive control. The inhibition of chlorophyll synthesis may explain the herbicidal potential of the *Eucalyptus* EOs and may explain the effects of chlorosis, necrosis, and stunted growth observed after their application.

In the second phase and in relation to the drying effect observed following the application of *Eucalyptus* oils, the relative water content of the treated herbs was determined. The obtained results are presented in Figure 5.

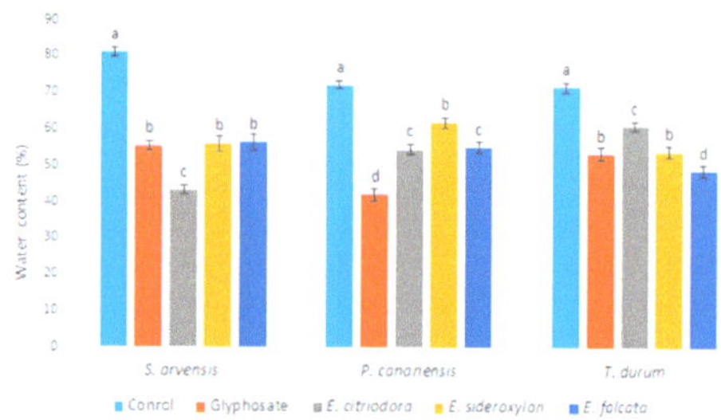


**Figure 5.** Effects of *Eucalyptus* essential oils and glyphosate on water content % of test plants measured five days after application. Error bars and letters on graphs represent standard error means and significant differences at $p \leq 0.05$ through Student–Newman–Keuls.

According to the statistical analysis, a significant and important decrease in the water content of the different tested herbs can be confirmed. This reduction varied according to the applied oil and the tested herb (mono- or dicotyledons and weeds or cultivated species). The effects observed are similar to those obtained with glyphosate. In fact, the water content was reduced for *S. arvensis* by 28.00, 29.26, and 46.4% by *E. falcata*, *E. sideroxylon*, and *E. citriodora*, respectively. For *P. canariensis*, the observed reductions were in the order of 24.6, 15.16, and 27.36%, respectively. In the case of *T. durum*, a smaller decrease in water content was observed with *E. citriodora* and *E. sideroxylon* (10.47 and 25.49%, respectively), while *E. falcata* caused the most significant decrease (49.57%), which outweighed the effects caused by glyphosate (27.5%).

The obtained results reflect the phytotoxic potential of *Eucalyptus* oils and can explain their mechanism of action, which consists in altering the water balance of the plant.

In light of these observations, the effect of *Eucalyptus* oils on the membrane integrity of the tested herbs was evaluated by measuring the relative electrolyte leakage. It has been observed that exposure to *Eucalyptus* EOs induces significant electrolyte leakage from the leaves of the tested herbs, as assessed by the increase in the conductivity of the bathing medium. Hence, these volatile oils disrupt the membrane integrity and cause solute leakage (Figure 6).

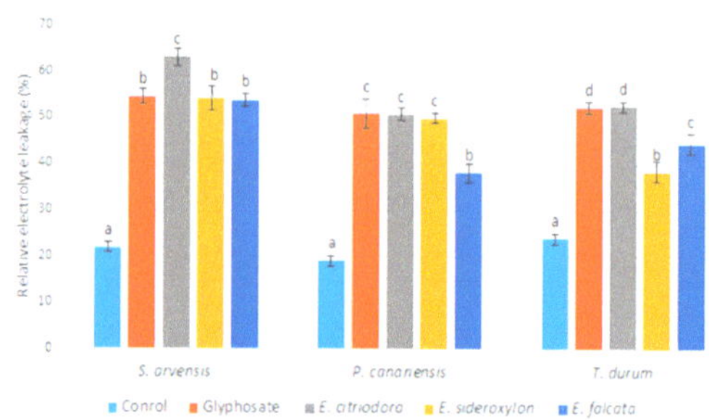


**Figure 6.** Effects of *Eucalyptus* essential oils and glyphosate on relative electrolyte leakage percentage of tested plants measured five days after spray. The errors bars and letters on graphs represent standard errors means and significant differences at $p \leq 0.05$ through Student–Newman–Keuls.

According to the statistical analysis, very pronounced relative electrolyte leakage was noted following the application of EOs and glyphosate compared to the control.

Electrolyte leakage explains the loss of plants' membrane integrity and therefore the observed phytotoxic effects.

The effect of the three oils on electrolyte leakage varied according to the species of *Eucalyptus* and that of the tested plants. Volatile oils of *E. citriodora* induced the most pronounced effects on all herbs: 54.06, 55.23, and 66.93% for *T. durum*, *P. canariensis*, and *S. arvensis*, respectively.

Again, the dicot weed *S. arvensis* was the most sensitive to the action of all applied oils.

The lipid peroxidation of polyunsaturated fatty acids, of which malondialdehyde is a product, could also provide an explanation for the relative leakage of electrolytes and the loss of membrane integrity. For this reason, we measured the level of MDA in the aerial parts of tested species after the application of the oils and the positive and negative controls. The main results are shown in Figure 7.

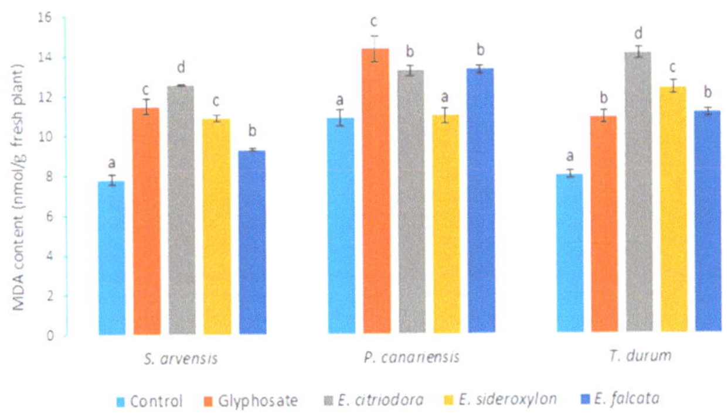


**Figure 7.** Effects of *Eucalyptus* species essential oils and glyphosate on MDA content as nmol/g fresh tested plants measured five days after application. Error bars and letters on graphs represent standard error means and significant differences at $p \leq 0.05$ through Student–Newman–Keuls.

Based on the statistical analysis of the obtained data, an increase in the MDA level was noted for all oils and for glyphosate compared to the control. The highest MDA levels for all the tested herbs were obtained with *E. citrioodora* oil and glyphosate. These results confirm and can be correlated with the loss of membrane integrity and confirm the phytotoxicity of EO application.

It is also known that allelopathic substances generate oxidative stress in plants. This stress is particularly reflected in the accumulation of proline. In this context, the proline level in the aerial parts of the plants sprayed with the three *Eucalyptus* oils was measured.

The results obtained are summarized in Figure 8, which shows an increase in proline levels in the aerial parts of sprayed weeds and crops.

This accumulation varied according to the oils tested and the herbs used for phytotoxicity tests. Generally, EOs showed similar effects to the commercial herbicide. The effect of *E. citriodora* oil was most pronounced for *P. canariensis* (22.36 mg/g f.w.), three times greater than the control (6.39 mg/g f.w.), and *S. arvensis* (12.41 mg/g f.w.), more than two times greater than the control (5.36 mg/g f.w.). In the case of *T. durum*, all the oils showed a similar effect on the accumulation of proline.

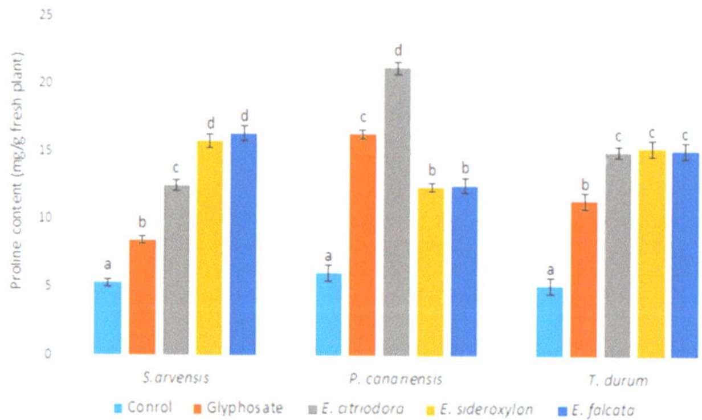


**Figure 8.** Effects of *Eucalyptus* essential oils and glyphosate on proline content as mg/g fresh tested plants measured five days after application. Error bars and letters on graphs represent standard error means and significant differences at $p \leq 0.05$ through Student–Newman–Keuls.

To evaluate the possible antifungal activity, the three *Eucalyptus* EOs were tested against eight phytopathogenic fungi that attack cereals and fruits; the main results are presented in Table 7.

**Table 7.** Antifungal activity of *E. citriodora*, *E. sideroxylon*, and *E. falcata* essential oils.

| Fungal Strain | Essential Oil Inhibition % at the Dose of 4 µL/mL | | |
|---|---|---|---|
| | ***E. citriodora*** | ***E. sideroxylon*** | ***E. falcata*** |
| *F. culmorum* | 100 ± 0.0 a | 80.01 ± 7.51 b | 100 ± 0.0 a |
| *F. pseudograminearum* | 100 ± 0.0 a | 70.49 ± 4.73 b | 100 ± 0.0 a |
| *F. graminearum* | 100 ± 0.0 a | 80 ± 6.65 b | 81.59 ± 4.27 b |
| *F. proliferatum* | 100 ± 0.0 a | 51.07 ± 6.96 b | 87.06 ± 7.41 a |
| *F. avenaceum* | 100 ± 0.0 a | 62.55 ± 5.01 c | 74.77 ± 2.39 b |
| *F.nygamai* | 100 ± 0.0 a | 74.55 ± 1.11 c | 90.00 ± 4.71 b |
| *F. verticillioides* | 100 ± 0.0 a | 78.11 ± 5.23 b | 73.52 ± 4.15 b |
| *B. sorokiniana* | 77.64 ± 6.65 a | 48.70 ± 8.26 a | 66.66 ± 11.78 a |

Results are expressed as mean ± standard errors. Different letters in the same row indicate significant differences ($p \leq 0.05$).

The data in Table 7 show that the oils, at the dose of 4 µL/mL, significantly inhibited the growth of all tested fungi. According to the statistical analysis, the oils exhibited varying degrees of inhibition. *B. sorokiniana* was the most resistant to all the oils, while *Fusarium* species were the most sensitive. *E. citriodora* EOs showed the best antifungal properties, causing total inhibition for all strains, except for *B. sorokiniana*. The other two EOs caused partial inhibition on nearly all tested strains.

## 4. Discussion

The study of the chemical composition of the essential oils of the three species of *Eucalyptus* revealed the great importance and richness of various compounds. According to the literature, among the few studies on *E. falcata* EOs, three studies were performed on plant material from Tunisia [17–19]. The chemical composition of the EOs of *E. falcata* is in agreement with that reported in the present study. In fact, the authors stated that the major components were 1,8-cineole (30.7%), trans-pinocarveol (26%), globulol (7%), and α-pinene (6%) [17]. However, the main differences with the previous studies consist in the absence of spathunelol, the presence of globulol, and the high levels of trans-pinocarveol [17,18].

Similar results were obtained in previous reports for *E. sideroxylon* [15,19]. According to these studies, the EOs of *E. sideroxylon* were characterized by their high content of 1,8-cineole (69–81%), which is in agreement with the present study.

Several investigations on *E. citriodora* EOs have been reported worldwide. In fact, in Colombian *E. citriodora* oils [30,31], in India [20], in Taiwan [32], and in the Congo [33], the major components were citronellal (40–72%), citronellol (6–22%), and iso-pulegol (3–13%), which is in agreement with our obtained data. However, citronellyl acetate was detected for the first time in this study. On the other hand, our study is in contrast with the results of a Tunisian report [2,34] wherein the authors evidenced a different chemotype characterized by a specific richness in 1,8-cineole (54%) and α-pinene (23%) and the total absence of citronellal, citronellol, and iso-pulegone. Apart from this, the data of the current study are in good agreement with the literature. The small differences in the percentages may be due to several factors, such as the genetic background, biotic and abiotic factors, season of collection, and extraction methods [35].

The evaluation of the antioxidant potential of the three oils showed interesting activities that can contribute to the valorization of essential oils of forest species, particularly of the *Eucalyptus* genus. These results are in agreement with the literature.

Indeed, several studies have investigated the antioxidant properties of different *Eucalyptus* species, such as *E. oleosa*, *E. grandis* × *E. urophylla*, *E. gracilis*, *E. citriodora*, *E. salubris*, and *E. salmonophloia* [36–39].

Furthermore, the EOs of *E. citriodora* exhibited higher antioxidant potential than those of *E. falcata* and *E. sideroxylon*. This appears to be related to the high level of oxygenated terpenes in *E. citriodora* oil [36,37].

Similarly, the EOs of *E. citriodora*, collected in India, contain oxygenated monoterpenes such as citronellal (60.66%), exhibiting strong antioxidant activity, in agreement with the current study [38]. In the same report, the authors evaluated and showed the good antioxidant activity of α-citronellal, β-citronellol, and isopulegol, the major compounds of the oil. Furthermore, the synergism between oil components could be related to the remarkable antioxidant capacity of the tested oils [40].

The study of the allelopathic properties of the EOs obtained from the three species of *Eucalyptus* revealed remarkable herbicidal potential, which even exceeds the activity of the synthetic herbicide glyphosate.

The germination- and growth-inhibiting effects of the *Eucalyptus* oils tested in the present study appear to be linked to the presence of several chemical components, particularly monoterpenes and sesquiterpenes, which are the main constituents and are known for their herbicidal potential [41]. Indeed, EOs of species belonging to the *Myrtaceae* family are known for their richness in allelochemicals [5,8,9,16,42]. In particular, in previous studies, we showed the phytotoxic potential of volatile oils and crude extracts of *Eucalyptus erythrocorys* against weeds [16,42].

Recently, the herbicidal potential of 22 *Eucalyptus* species growing in Tunisia has been reported. These studies reveal enormous allelopathic potential linked to the EOs of *Eucalyptus* species; this could be in agreement with the present study [5,8,9,16].

Observing the chemical composition of the *Eucalyptus* oils tested in the present work (Table 2), we can assume that the activity is due to different components, such as 1,8-cineole (0.3–65.4% in *Eucalyptus* oils), citronellal (48.7% in *E. citriodora* oil), citronellol (20.2% in *E. citriodora* oil), and α-pinene (ranging between 0 and 6% in *Eucalyptus* oils), already known for their significant phytotoxic effects [20,43,44].

Several studies report that terpenes, both hydrocarbons and oxygenated, are phytotoxic molecules. Additionally, oxygenated monoterpenes (51.3, 75.5, and 90%, respectively, in *E. falcata*, *E. sideroxylon*, and *E. citriodora*) have been reported to have stronger herbicidal properties than the corresponding hydrocarbon derivatives [20,43,44]; this can explain the high herbicidal activity of *E. citriodora* compared to *E. falcata* and *E. sideroxylon*.

To explain the mode of action of terpenes on the inhibition of germination, various physiological and biochemical mechanisms have been reported.

In fact, such monoterpenes can affect physiological functions, such as cell division, viability, and growth inhibition by the alteration of membrane integrity [45,46].

Other studies have reported that EOs reduce germination and growth by inhibiting the incorporation of nitrogen into amino acid synthesis, leading to the accumulation of ammonia, and by impairing photosynthesis and photorespiration [47].

In the same way, Abrahim et al., 2003 demonstrated that the monoterpene hydrocarbon α-pinene reduces the growth of maize by inhibiting electron transfer and uncoupling oxidative phosphorylation, resulting in the alteration of energy metabolism and the blocking of ATP synthesis in the mitochondria [48]. Similarly, some sesquiterpenes have been reported to have phytotoxic effects by causing oxidative stress, the inhibition of photosynthesis, and the induction of microtubular alterations [47]. Previous reports have shown that EOs induce oxidative stress to weeds and increase peroxidase and superoxide dismutase activities [49–51]. Other studies have shown that EOs and their constituents have remarkable herbicidal potential, the effects of which result in anatomical and physiological effects, such as the formation of lipid globules in the cytoplasm, inhibition of mitochondrial development, and alteration of the integrity of the membrane of the nucleus and mitochondria [52,53].

For post-emergence trials and the application of EOs by spraying, few studies have been undertaken and the exact modes of action still remain poorly known. On the other hand, data obtained in this study are in agreement with those reported in the literature. Several studies have reported that various constituents of EOs, when applied at the post-emergence stage, are able to inhibit the growth of weeds [54], hypothesizing oxidative stress and alteration of the water content [47]. The evidence that emerged in the present study showed a correlation between the decrease in the water content and the arrest of the growth of the plants treated with *Eucalyptus* EOs.

Following the application of *Eucalyptus* EOs, a marked decrease in chlorophyll synthesis was noted, suggesting a correlation between the visible effects on weeds (i.e., chlorosis, necrosis, and photosynthetic functions) and their growth. According to previous studies, several EOs and their pure components have been described to inhibit photosynthesis and chlorophyll synthesis [55]. Indeed, some oxygenated monoterpenes have been reported to induce a photosynthetic decrease by reducing the chlorophyll content in various weeds [56].

In addition, citronellol and 1,8-cineole, major compounds of the *Eucalyptus* species in the current study, reduced the chlorophyll content of *Ageratum conyzoides* by 60 and 66%, respectively [57,58]. Earlier studies concluded that the decrease in chlorophyll content appeared to be related to the inhibition of chlorophyll synthesis and degradation of photosynthetic pigments [59,60].

Among the physiological effects of *Eucalyptus* EOs on membrane integrity, the excessive leakage of electrolytes was noted, which can be explained by the loss of integrity of membrane cells. On the other hand, membrane integrity is essential for vital functions and plays several roles, including that of a barrier, selective permeability to nutrients, and, indeed, control of the electrolyte balance [61]. Various secondary metabolites have been reported to alter the integrity of the cell membrane in plants, particularly EOs and their pure constituents. A previous study has shown that linalool caused increased membrane permeability, further demonstrating that EOs can cause important damage to membrane permeability [62]. According to the data obtained, the application of *Eucalyptus* EOs induced, in the tested herbs, an increase in the rate of MDA and proline compared to the control, in agreement with the previous observations. Indeed, it has been reported that the application of EOs during the post-emergence stage increases the permeability of the membrane by disrupting its integrity because of lipid peroxidation [47,63–65]. Additionally, some EOs and monoterpenes have been reported to induce oxidative stress. α-pinene caused lipid peroxidation when applied to *Cassia occidentalis*, resulting in increased solute leakage [25]. Furthermore, the increase in MDA levels was related to the lipid peroxidation of the membrane and alteration of its permeability.

Finally, the current study has shown that *Eucalyptus* oils have significant in vitro antifungal potential against the growth of phytopathogenic fungi.

The differences in the resistance of different fungal strains to *Eucalyptus* volatile oil seem to be related to the different capacities of the oil components to disrupt the cell membrane [66].

*Eucalyptus* oils are known to have remarkable antimicrobial activity that is related to their richness in oxygenated compounds [67].

Indeed, we have previously reported the antifungal potential of *Eucalyptus erhytrocorys* EOs and its crude extracts against phytopathogenic fungi [16,42], which is in agreement with the current study. Similarly, the inhibitory activity of the volatile oil obtained from *Eucalyptus camaldulensis* against the growth of fungi such as *Thanatephorus cucumeris*, *Aspergillus niger*, *F. oxysporum*, and *Rhizopus oryzae* is also known [67].

In agreement with the current study, Ivanov et al. (2021) demonstrated the fungicidal activity of 1,8-cineole and camphor (major compounds in *Eucalyptus* volatile oils) against the growth of different *Candida* species [68]. In another research work, it was reported that terpinen-4-ol and α-terpineol, terpinolene, and 1,8-cineole, constituents of *Eucalyptus* oils, are fungitoxic against *Botrytis cinerea* [69]. However, with regard to the antimicrobial mechanism, it has been reported that the apolar nature of terpenes may favor their penetration into the lipid bilayer of the fungal membrane, inducing its disruption. Many terpenes have been reported to exert their antifungal activity by increasing the permeability of fungal cells and membrane fluidity [70].

## 5. Conclusions

To conclude, our data showed that *Eucalyptus* EOs are a complex mixture of various compounds. The chemical profile of the tested EOs was characterized by the high content of oxygenated monoterpenes. Great diversity was noted between the three species with the identification of different major compounds; however, the three species belong to the same genus. This is an interspecific diversity, with the identification of 58 compounds. Similarly, the variability of the results obtained in this present study with those in the literature could be considered within the context of ecological variability, which makes this work necessary to appreciate the results obtained with these three species of *Eucalyptus* growing in Tunisia. The essential oils tested for their biological activities have shown efficacy for the control of weeds and phyto-pathogenic fungi, and their antioxidant potential has also been described. These biological activities offer several areas of application for these oils, whether in agronomy or in the chemical and pharmaceutical industries. These molecules are of natural identity; they are biodegradable molecules and are compatible with the environment. Their applications could solve several problems, including the problem of resistance and the undesirable environmental effects. Plants synthesize these substances as allelochemicals; their exploitation can provide an enhancement in forest species and also allow the exploitation of the allelopathic potential of aromatic and medicinal plants. Consequently, the adoption of such bio-molecules as novel compounds in herbicidal formulations could facilitate not only sustainable weed control but also sustainable agriculture. Further studies are required to evaluate their application under field conditions. Such results encourage the use of *Eucalyptus* EOs as natural products in agriculture and for their agro-industrial potential.

**Author Contributions:** Conceptualization, I.A., M.H. and L.H.; Data curation, R.B.A., S.K., O.K. and Y.P.; Formal analysis, M.K. and M.B.M.; Funding acquisition, L.H.; Investigation, I.A. and M.K.; Methodology, R.B.A., G.F. and L.H.; Project administration, L.H.; Resources, I.A.; Supervision, S.G.; Validation, I.A., M.H. and L.H.; Writing—original draft, I.A., M.K., G.F. and Y.M.; Writing—review and editing, I.A. All authors have read and agreed to the published version of the manuscript.

**Funding:** This research received no external funding.

**Data Availability Statement:** All data are available in the manuscript file.

**Conflicts of Interest:** The authors declare no conflict of interest.

## References

1. Oyekunle, J.A.O.; Adekunle, A.S.; Adewole, A.M. Determination of Organochlorine Pesticide Residues in Some Evaporated Milk Samples in Nigeria Using Gas Chromatography-Mass Spectrometry. *Chem. Afr.* **2021**, *4*, 349–366. [CrossRef]
2. Fahed, C.; Hayar, S. Conventional vs. Organic Cucumber Production in Lebanon: Risk Assessment of the Recommended Agrochemicals on Consumer Health and the Environment. *Chem. Afr.* **2021**, *4*, 463–476. [CrossRef]
3. Amri, I.; Lamia, H.; Mohsen, H.; Bassem, J.; Kaouthar, L. Essential oils as biological alternatives to protect date palm (*Phoenix dactylifera* L.) against *Ectomyelois ceratoniae* Zeller (*Lepidoptera*: *Pyralidae*). *Chil. J. Agric. Res.* **2014**, *74*, 273–279. [CrossRef]
4. Oliveira, A.F.; Costa Junior, L.M.; Lima, A.S.; Silva, C.R.; Ribeiro, M.N.S.; Mesquista, J.W.C.; Rocha, C.Q.; Tangerina, M.M.P.; Vilegas, W. Anthelmintic Activity of Plant Extracts from Brazilian Savanna. *Vet. Parasitol.* **2017**, *236*, 121–127. [CrossRef] [PubMed]
5. Khammassi, M.; Polito, F.; Amri, I.; Khedhri, S.; Hamrouni, L.; Nazzaro, F.; Fratianni, F.; De Feo, V. Chemical Composition and Phytotoxic, Antibacterial and Antibiofilm Activity of the Essential Oils of *Eucalyptus occidentalis*, *E. striaticalyx* and *E. stricklandii*. *Molecules* **2022**, *27*, 5820. [CrossRef]
6. Malaspina, P.; Papaianni, M.; Ranesi, M.; Polito, F.; Danna, C.; Aicardi, P.; Cornara, L.; Woo, S.L.; De Feo, V. Eucalyptus cinerea and E. nicholii by-Products as Source of Bioactive Compounds for Agricultural Applications. *Plants* **2022**, *11*, 2777. [CrossRef]
7. Ismail, A.; Mancini, E.; De Martino, L.; Hamrouni, L.; Hanana, M.; Jamoussi, B.; Gargouri, S.; Scognamiglio, M.; De Feo, V. Chemical Composition and Biological Activities of Tunisian *Cupressus arizonica* Greene Essential Oils. *Chem. Biodivers.* **2014**, *11*, 150–160. [CrossRef]
8. Kouki, H.; Polito, F.; De Martino, L.; Mabrouk, Y.; Hamrouni, L.; Amri, I.; Fratianni, F.; De Feo, V.; Nazzaro, F. Chemistry and bioactivities of six Tunisian Eucalyptus species. *Pharmaceuticals* **2022**, *15*, 1265. [CrossRef]
9. Polito, F.; Kouki, H.; Khedhri, S.; Hamrouni, L.; Mabrouk, Y.; Amri, I.; Nazzaro, F.; Fratianni, F.; De Feo, V. Chemical Composition and Phytotoxic and Antibiofilm Activity of the Essential Oils of *Eucalyptus bicostata*, *E. gigantea*, *E. intertexta*, *E. obliqua*, *E. pauciflora* and *E. tereticornis*. *Plants* **2022**, *11*, 3017. [CrossRef]
10. Ullah, N.; Haq, I.U.; Safdar, N.; Mirza, B. Physiological and biochemical mechanisms of allelopathy mediated by the allelochemical extracts of *Phytolacca latbenia* (Moq.) H. Walter. *Toxicol. Ind. Health* **2015**, *31*, 931–937. [CrossRef]
11. Werrie, P.Y.; Durenne, B.; Delaplace, P.; Fauconnier, M.L. Phytotoxicity of Essential Oils: Opportunities and Constraints for the Development of Biopesticides. A Review. *Foods* **2020**, *9*, 1291. [CrossRef]
12. Najar, B.; Mecacci, G.; Nardi, V.; Cervelli, C.; Nardoni, S.; Mancianti, F.; Ebani, V.V.; Giannecchini, S.; Pistelli, L. Volatiles and Antifungal-Antibacterial-Antiviral Activity of South African Salvia Spp. Essential Oils Cul-tivated in Uniform Conditions. *Molecules* **2021**, *26*, 2826. [CrossRef]
13. Shen, S.; Xu, G.; Roy Clemen, D.; Jin, G.; Liu, S.; Zhang, F.; Yang, Y.; Chen, A.; Kato-Noguc, H. Effects of Invasive Plant *Mikania micrantha* on Plant Community and Diversity in Farming Systems. *Asian J. Plant Sci.* **2014**, *14*, 27–33. [CrossRef]
14. Alves-Silva, J.M.; Cocco, E.; Piras, A.; Gonçalves, M.J.; Silva, A.; Falconieri, D.; Porcedda, S.; Cruz, M.T.; Maxia, A.; Salgueiro, L. Unveiling the Chemical Composition and Biological Properties of Salvia cacaliifolia Benth. Essential Oil. *Plants* **2023**, *12*, 359. [CrossRef]
15. Elaissi, A.; Marzouki, H.; Medini, H.; Larbi Khouja, M.; Farhat, F.; Lynene, F.; Harzallah-Skhiri, F.; Chemli, R. Variation in volatile leaf oils of 13 *Eucalyptus* species harvested from Souinet Arboreta (Tunisia). *Chem. Biodivers.* **2010**, *7*, 909–921. [CrossRef]
16. Khedhri, S.; Polito, F.; Caputo, L.; Manna, F.; Khammassi, M.; Hamrouni, L.; Amri, I.; Nazzaro, F.; De Feo, V.; Fratianni, F. Chemical Composition, Phytotoxic and Antibiofilm Activity of Seven *Eucalyptus* Species from Tunisia. *Molecules* **2022**, *27*, 8227. [CrossRef]
17. Elaissi, A.; Rouis, Z.; Salem, N.A.B.; Mabrouk, S.; ben Salem, Y.; Salah, K.B.H.; Aouni, M.; Farhat, F.; Chemli, R.; Harzallah-Skhiri, F.; et al. Chemical composition of 8 *eucalyptus* species' essential oils and the evaluation of their antibacterial, antifungal and antiviral activities. *BMC Complement. Altern. Med.* **2012**, *12*, 81. [CrossRef]
18. Elaissi, A.; Medini, H.; Khouja, M.L.; Monique, S.; Lyenne, F.; Farhat, F.; Chemli, R.; Harzallah-Skhiri, F. Variation in volatile leaf oils of eleven *Eucalyptus* species harvested from Korbous arboreta (Tunisia). *Chem. Biodivers.* **2010**, *7*, 1841–1854. [CrossRef]
19. Elaissi, A.; Medini, H.; Simmonds, M.; Lynen, F.; Farhat, F.; Chemli, R.; Harzallah-Skhiri, F.; Khouja, M.L. Variation in Volatile Leaf Oils of Seven *Eucalyptus* Species Harvested from Zerniza Arboreta (Tunisia). *Chem. Biodivers.* **2011**, *8*, 362–372. [CrossRef]
20. Batish, D.R.; Singh, H.P.; Setia, N.; Kaur, S.; Kohli, R.K. Chemical Composition and Phytotoxicity of Volatile Essential Oil from Intact and Fallen Leaves of *Eucalyptus citriodora*. *Z. Für Nat. C* **2006**, *61*, 465–471. [CrossRef]
21. National Institute of Standards and Technology. *NIST/EPA/NIH Mass Spectral Library*; The NIST Mass Spectrometry Data Center: Gaithersburg, MD, USA, 2014.
22. Adams, R.P. *Identification of Essential Oil Components by Gas Chromatography/Mass Spectrometry*; Allured Publishing Co.: Carol Stream, IL, USA, 2007.
23. Prieto, P.; Pineda, M.; Aguilar, M. Spectrophotometric quantitation of antioxidant capacity through the formation of a phospho-molybdenum complex: Specific application to the determination of vitamin E1. *Anal. Biochem.* **1999**, *269*, 337–341. [CrossRef]

24. Hanato, T.; Kagawa, H.; Yasuhara, T.; Okuda, T. Two new flavonoids and other constituents in licorice root: Their relative astringency and radical scavenging effect. *Chem. Pharm. Bull.* **1988**, *36*, 1090–1097.
25. Re, R.; Pellegrini, N.; Proteggente, A.; Pannala, A.; Yang, M.; Rice-Evans, C. Antioxidant activity applying an improved ABTS radical cation decolorization assay. *Free. Radic. Biol. Med.* **1999**, *26*, 1231–1237. [CrossRef]
26. Downey, L.A.; Miller, J.W. Rapid measurements of relative turgidity in maize (*Zea mays* L.). *New Phytol.* **1971**, *70*, 555–560. [CrossRef]
27. Lichtenthaler, K.H. Chlorophylls and carotenoids: Pigments of photosynthetic biomembranes. *Methods Enzymol.* **1987**, *148*, 350–382. [CrossRef]
28. Singh, H.P.; Batish, D.R.; Kaur, S.; Arora, K.; Kohli, R.K. α-pinene inhibits growth and induces oxidative stress in roots. *Ann. Bot.* **2006**, *98*, 1261–1269. [CrossRef]
29. Bates, L.S.; Waldren, R.P.; Teare, I.D. Rapid determination of free proline for water-stress studies. *Plant Soil* **1973**, *39*, 205–207. [CrossRef]
30. Olivero-Verbel, J.; Nerio, L.S.; Stashenko, E.E. Bioactivity against *Tribolium castaneum* Herbst (*Coleoptera: Tenebrionidae*) of *Cymbopogon citratus* and *Eucalyptus citriodora* essential oils grown in Colombia. *Pest Manag. Sci. Former. Pestic. Sci.* **2010**, *66*, 664–668. [CrossRef]
31. Olivero-Verbel, J.; Tirado-Ballestas, I.; Caballero-Gallardo, K.; Stashenko, E.E. Essential oils applied to the food act as repellents toward *Tribolium castaneum*. *J. Stored Prod. Res.* **2013**, *55*, 145–147. [CrossRef]
32. Su, Y.C.; Ho, C.L.; Eugene, I.C.; Chang, T. Antifungal activities and chemical compositions of essential oils from leaves of four *Eucalypts*. *Taiwan J. For. Sci.* **2006**, *21*, 49–61.
33. Cimanga, K.; Kambu, K.; Tona, L.; Apers, S.; De Bruyne, T.; Hermans, N.; Totté, J.; Pieters, L.; Vlietinck, A.J. Correlation between chemical composition and antibacterial activity of essential oils of some aromatic medicinal plants growing in the Democratic Republic of Congo. *J. Ethnopharmacol.* **2002**, *79*, 213–220. [CrossRef]
34. Elaissi, A.; Salah, K.H.; Mabrouk, S.; Larbi, K.M.; Chemli, R.; Harzallah-Skhiri, F. Antibacterial activity and chemical composition of 20 *Eucalyptus* species' essential oils. *Food Chem.* **2011**, *129*, 1427–1434. [CrossRef]
35. Abd-ElGawad, A.M.; Bonanomi, G.; Al-Rashed, S.A.; Elshamy, A.I. Persicaria lapathifolia Essential Oil: Chemical Constituents, Antioxidant Activity, and Allelopathic Effect on the Weed *Echinochloa colona*. *Plants* **2021**, *10*, 1798. [CrossRef]
36. Gatto, L.J.; Fabri, N.T.; Souza, A.M.; Fonseca, N.S.T.; Furusho, A.; Miguel, O.G.; Dias, J.F.G.; Zanin, S.M.W.; Miguel, M.D. Chemical composition, phytotoxic potential, biological activities and antioxidant properties of *Myrcia hatschbachii* D. Legrand essential oil. *Braz. J. Pharm. Sci.* **2020**, *56*, 18402. [CrossRef]
37. Ben Marzoug, H.N.; Bouajila, J.; Ennajar, M.; Lebrihi, A.; Mathieu, F.; Couderc, F.; Abderraba, M.; Romdhane, M. *Eucalyptus* (*gracilis, oleosa, salubris*, and *salmonophloia*) Essential Oils: Their Chemical Composition and Antioxidant and Antimicrobial Activities. *J. Med. Food* **2010**, *13*, 1005–1012. [CrossRef]
38. Singh, H.P.; Kaur, S.; Negi, K.; Kumari, S.; Saini, V.; Batish, D.R.; Kohli, R.K. Assessment of in vitro antioxidant activity of essential oil of *Eucalyptus citriodora* (lemon-scented Eucalypt; *Myrtaceae*) and its major constituents. *LWT Food Sci. Technol.* **2012**, *48*, 237–241. [CrossRef]
39. Zhou, L.; Li, J.; Kong, Q.; Luo, S.; Wang, J.; Feng, S.; Yuan, M.; Chen, T.; Yuan, S.; Ding, C. Chemical composition, antioxidant, antimicrobial, and phytotoxic potential of *Eucalyptus grandis* × *E. urophylla* leaves essential oils. *Molecules* **2021**, *26*, 1450. [CrossRef]
40. Nafis, A.; Kasrati, A.; Jamali, C.A.; Mezrioui, N.; Setzer, W.; Abbad, A.; Hassani, L. Antioxidant activity and evidence for synergism of *Cannabis sativa* (L.) essential oil with antimicrobial standards. *Ind. Crops Prod.* **2019**, *137*, 396–400. [CrossRef]
41. Amri, I.; Hanana, M.; Jamoussi, B.; Hamrouni, L. Chemical composition of *Thuja orientalis* L. essential oils and study of their allelopathic potential on germination and seedling growth of weeds. *Arch. Phytopathol. Plant Prot.* **2015**, *48*, 18–27. [CrossRef]
42. Ben Ghnaya, A.; Hamrouni, L.; Amri, I.; Ahoues, H.; Hanana, M.; Romane, A. Study of allelopathic effects of *Eucalyptus erythrocorys* L. crude extracts against germination and seedling growth of weeds and wheat. *Nat. Prod. Res.* **2016**, *30*, 2058–2064. [CrossRef]
43. De Martino, L.; Mancini, E.; Rolim de Almeida, L.F.; De Feo, V. The antigerminative activity of twenty-seven monoterpenes. *Molecules* **2010**, *15*, 6630–6637. [CrossRef]
44. Chowhan, N.; Singh, H.P.; Kohl, R.K. Phytotoxic effects of β-pinene on early growth and associated biochemical changes in rice. *Acta Physiol. Plant.* **2011**, *33*, 2369–2376. [CrossRef]
45. Mahdavikia, F.; Saharkhiz, M.J.; Karami, A. Defensive response of radish seedlings to the oxidative stress arising from phenolic compounds in the extract of peppermint (*Mentha* × *piperita* L.). *Sci. Hortic.* **2017**, *214*, 133–140. [CrossRef]
46. Fagodia, S.K.; Singh, H.P.; Batish, D.R.; Kohli, R.K. Phytotoxicity and cytotoxicity of *Citrus aurantiifolia* essential oil and its major constituents: Limonene and citral. *Ind. Crops Prod.* **2017**, *108*, 708–715. [CrossRef]
47. Araniti, F.; Costas-Gil, A.; Cabeiras-Freijanes, L.; Lupini, A.; Sunseri, F.; Reigosa, M.J.; Abenavoli, M.R.; Sánchez-Moreiras, A.M. Rosmarinic acid induces programmed cell death in *Arabidopsis* seedlings through reactive oxygen species and mitochondrial dysfunction. *PLoS ONE* **2018**, *13*, e0208802. [CrossRef]
48. Abrahim, D.; Francischini, A.C.; Pergo, E.M.; Kelmer-Bracht, A.M.; Ishii-Iwamoto, E.L. Effects of α-pinene on the mitochondrial respiration of maize seedlings. *Plant Physiol. Biochem.* **2003**, *41*, 985–991. [CrossRef]

49. Bogatek, R.; Gniazdowska, A.; Stępień, J.; Kupidłowska, E. Sunflower allelochemicals mode of action in germinating mustard seeds. In Proceedings of the 4th World Congress on Allelopathy, "Establishing the Scientific Base", Wagga Wagga, NSW, Australia, 21–26 August 2005; pp. 365–369. Available online: https://www.cabdirect.org/cabdirect/abstract/20073229801 (accessed on 11 July 2022).
50. Hayat, S.; Ahmad, H.; Ali, M.; Ren, K.; Cheng, Z. Aqueous garlic extract stimulates growth and antioxidant enzymes activity of tomato (*Solanum lycopersicum*). *Sci. Hortic.* **2018**, *240*, 139–146. [CrossRef]
51. Ji, X.; Li, J.; Meng, Z.; Dong, S.; Zhang, S.; Qiao, K. Inhibitory effect of allicin against *Meloidogyne incognita* and *Botrytis cinerea* in tomato. *Sci. Hortic.* **2019**, *253*, 203–208. [CrossRef]
52. Koitabashi, R.; Suzuki, T.; Kawazu, T.; Sakai, A.; Kuroiwa, H.; Kuroiwa, T. 1,8-Cineole inhibits root growth and DNA synthesis in the root apical meristem of *Brassica campestris* L. *J. Plant Res.* **1997**, *110*, 1–6. [CrossRef]
53. Zunino, M.P.; Zygadlo, J.A. Effect of monoterpenes on lipid oxidation in maize. *Planta* **2004**, *219*, 303–309. [CrossRef]
54. Sánchez-Muñoz, B.A.; Aguilar, M.I.; King-Díaz, B.; Rivero, J.F.; Lotina-Hennsen, B. The Sesquiterpenes β-Caryophyllene and Caryophyllene Oxide Isolated from *Senecio salignus* Act as Phytogrowth and Photosynthesis Inhibitors. *Molecules* **2012**, *17*, 1437–1447. [CrossRef] [PubMed]
55. Pouresmaeil, M.; Nojadeh, M.S.; Movafeghi, A.; Maggi, F. Exploring the bio-control efficacy of *Artemisia fragrans* essential oil on the perennial weed *Convolvulus arvensis*: Inhibitory effects on the photosynthetic machinery and induction of oxidative stress. *Ind. Crops Prod.* **2020**, *155*, 112785. [CrossRef]
56. Vaid, S.; Batish, D.; Singh, H.; Kohli, R.; Phytotoxic effect of eugenol towards two weedy species. Bioscan 2010, 5: 339–341. Available online: https://www.semanticscholar.org/paper/PHYTOTOXIC-EFFECT-OF-EUGENOL-TOWARDS-TWO-WEEDY-Vaid-Batish/541b664b28a6e3e90cf08e467328286f91bd4024 (accessed on 25 September 2022).
57. Singh, H.P.; Batish, D.R.; Kohli, R.K. Allelopathic effect of two volatile monoterpenes against bill goat weed (*Ageratum conyzoides* L.). *Crop Prot.* **2002**, *21*, 347–350. [CrossRef]
58. Grana, E.; Daaaz-Tielas, C.M.; Sanchez-Moreiras, A.; Reigosa, M. Mode of Action of Monoterpenes in Plant-Plant Interactions. *Curr. Bioact. Compd.* **2012**, *8*, 80–89. [CrossRef]
59. Romagni, J.G.; Allen, S.N.; Dayan, F.E. Allelopathic effects of volatile cineoles on two weedy plant species. *J. Chem. Ecol.* **2000**, *26*, 303–313. [CrossRef]
60. Poonpaiboonpipat, T.; Pangnakorn, U.; Suvunnamek, U.; Teerarak, M.; Charoenying, P.; Laosinwattana, C. Phytotoxic effects of essential oil from *Cymbopogon citratus* and its physiological mechanisms on barnyardgrass (*Echinochloa crus-galli*). *Ind. Crops Prod.* **2013**, *41*, 403–407. [CrossRef]
61. McNeil, P.L.; Steinhardt, R.A. Loss, Restoration, and Maintenance of Plasma Membrane Integrity. *J. Cell Biol.* **1997**, *137*, 1–4. [CrossRef]
62. Varona, S.; Martín, Á.; Cocero, M.J. Formulation of a natural biocide based on lavandin essential oil by emulsification using modified starches. *Chem. Eng. Process* **2009**, *48*, 1121–1128. [CrossRef]
63. Dmitrović, S.; Perišić, M.; Stojić, A.; Živković, S.; Boljević, J.; Nestorović, Ž.J.; Aničić, N.; Ristić, M.; Mišić, D. Essential oils of two *Nepeta* species inhibit growth and induce oxidative stress in ragweed (*Ambrosia artemisiifolia* L.) shoots in vitro. *Acta Physiol. Plant.* **2015**, *37*, 64. [CrossRef]
64. Mahdavikia, F.; Saharkhiz, M.J. Secondary metabolites of peppermint change the morphophysiological and biochemical characteristics of tomato. *Biocatal. Agric. Biotechnol.* **2016**, *7*, 127–133. [CrossRef]
65. Hazrati, H.; Saharkhiz, M.J.; Niakousari, M.; Moein, M. Natural herbicide activity of *Satureja hortensis* L. essential oil nanoemulsion on the seed germination and morphophysiological features of two important weed species. *Ecotoxicol. Environ. Saf.* **2017**, *142*, 423–430. [CrossRef] [PubMed]
66. Obame, L.C.; Edou, P.; Bassolé, I.H.N.; Koudou, J.; Agnaniet, H.; Eba, F. Chemical composition, antioxidant and antimicrobial properties of the essential oil of *Dacryodes edulis* (G. Don) H. J. Lam from Gabon. *Afr. J. Microbiol. Res.* **2008**, 2, 148–152.
67. Siramon, P.; Ohtani, Y.; Ichiura, H. Chemical Composition and Antifungal Property of *Eucalyptus camaldulensis* Leaf Oils from Thailand. *Rec. Nat. Prod.* **2013**, *7*, 49–53.
68. Ivanov, M.; Kannan, A.; Stojković, D.S.; Glamočlija, J.; Calhelha, R.C.; Ferreira, I.C.F.R.; Sanglard, D.; Soković, M. Camphor and Eucalyptol—Anticandidal Spectrum, Antivirulence Effect, Efflux Pumps Interference and Cytotoxicity. *Int. J. Mol. Sci.* **2021**, *22*, 483. [CrossRef]
69. Yu, D.; Wang, J.; Shao, X.; Xu, F.; Wang, H. Antifungal modes of action of tea tree oil and its two characteristic components against *Botrytis cinerea*. *J. Appl. Microbiol.* **2015**, *119*, 1253–1262. [CrossRef]
70. Cristani, M.; D'Arrigo, M.; Mandalari, G.; Castelli, F.; Sarpietro, M.G.; Micieli, D.; Venuti, V.; Bisignano, G.; Saija, A.; Trombetta, D. Interaction of Four Monoterpenes Contained in Essential Oils with Model Membranes: Implications for Their Antibacterial Activity. *J. Agric. Food Chem.* **2007**, *55*, 6300–6308. [CrossRef]

plants

Article

# Phytotoxicity of *Quillaja lancifolia* Leaf Saponins and Their Bioherbicide Potential

**Maria E. M. Marques [1], Ana C. de Carvalho [1], Anna C. A. Yendo [2], Yve V. S. Magedans [1], Eliane Zachert [1] and Arthur G. Fett-Neto [1,*]**

[1] Plant Physiology Laboratory, Center for Biotechnology and Department of Botany, Federal University of Rio Grande do Sul, Porto Alegre 91501-970, RS, Brazil
[2] Arborea Biotechnology, Center for Biotechnology Start Up Incubator (IECBiot), UFRGS, Porto Alegre 91501-970, RS, Brazil
* Correspondence: fett.neto@ufrgs.br

**Abstract:** Weeds are major threats to the integrity of agricultural and natural environments due to their invasive and competing potential. Bioherbicides are substances based on natural compounds that are biodegradable and often have low residual effects. Plant species able to produce and release phytotoxic compounds may represent effective bioherbicide sources. Leaves of *Quillaja lancifolia* D.Don (formerly *Q. brasiliensis* (A.St.-Hil. & Tul.) Mart.) produce water-soluble specialized metabolites of the saponin class that could be evaluated for phytotoxic activity and potential as natural herbicides. This study was conducted to examine the impacts of *Q. lancifolia* total saponins aqueous extract (AE) at 4 and 10% (*w*/*v*) and of two combined reverse-phase chromatography purified saponin fractions (QB) at 1 and 2% (*w*/*v*) on morpho-physiological parameters of *Lactuca sativa* (lettuce) and *Echinochloa crus-galli* (barnyardgrass) in pre- and post-emergence bioassays. QB was only tested in pre-emergence assays. In pre-emergence bioassays, the germination rate and germination kinetics were determined. Post-emergence evaluations included effects on seedling morphology, root and shoot length, dry mass, and chlorophyll content. Osmotic potential and pH analyses ruled out roles for these factors in the observed responses. AE had a high inhibitory impact on the germination of both lettuce and barnyardgrass. QB at 1% and 2% (*w*/*v*) significantly decreased the growth of lettuce seedlings germinated in its presence by more than 10-fold. Phytotoxic effects on the post-emergence growth of lettuce, especially at the highest concentration tested of AE (10% *w*/*v*), was also observed. The presence of quillaic acid-based triterpene saponins in AE and QB was confirmed using different analytical methods. Therefore, both saponin-enriched fraction and aqueous extracts of *Q. lancifolia* inhibited tested plant growth and development. The water solubility of saponins and the availability of a sustainable source of these molecules from the leaves of cultivated young *Q. lancifolia* plants make them attractive candidates for use as bioherbicides.

**Keywords:** soap tree; triterpene saponin; secondary metabolism; germination; seedling

**Citation:** Marques, M.E.M.; de Carvalho, A.C.; Yendo, A.C.A.; Magedans, Y.V.S.; Zachert, E.; Fett-Neto, A.G. Phytotoxicity of *Quillaja lancifolia* Leaf Saponins and Their Bioherbicide Potential. *Plants* **2023**, *12*, 663. https://doi.org/10.3390/plants12030663

Academic Editors: Margot Schulz and Vincenzo Tabaglio

Received: 15 December 2022
Revised: 27 January 2023
Accepted: 30 January 2023
Published: 2 February 2023



## 1. Introduction

The combination of efficient agricultural land use with biodiversity conservation is a challenge [1]. It is estimated that agriculture will need to provide almost 50% more food by 2050 [2]. To sustain this level of production and knowing that 20–40% of global crop yields are lost each year to pests and diseases, pesticide use in agriculture has increased in recent years. Due to its extensive planting area, Brazil is one of the three largest consumers of pesticides in the world [2,3].

"Pests" are considered invasive organisms or pathogens of crops or forest species [4] and include animal pests (insects, mites, nematodes, rodents, slugs, snails, birds), plant pathogens (viruses, bacteria, fungi, chromists), and weeds (i.e., competitive plants) [5]. It has been estimated that weeds represent the most damaging category of pests in agriculture [5,6]. The Weed Science Society of America defines a weed as a plant that causes economic losses or ecological damage, creates health problems for humans or animals, or is undesirable where it is growing [7]. Weeds negatively affect crop yields due to a number of features, including: (a) capacity to grow in disturbed habitats, (b) high environmental plasticity, (c) ability to physically hinder or smother crop growth, (d) capacity to compete with crops for light, nutrients, moisture, and space, (e) rapid emergence, seedling growth, and quick maturation, (f) production of a large numbers of seeds per plant, (g) ability to release natural substances that inhibit crop growth (allelopathy), and (h) host pests or pathogens that may contaminate crops [8,9].

Although pesticides prevent, destroy, and repel most pests growing on crop plants, their continued use can have a significant impact on the environment and human health by contaminating water bodies, air, soil, and food. Moreover, unintentional negative effects on local biodiversity are often observed [10,11]. Thus, there is an increasing demand for pesticides that are safe for the environment and may replace or complement synthetic management methods [12]. This is an important concern in organic farming, given its expansion and the need for environmentally safe management tools [9,10]. Weed management techniques can vary (manual, mechanical, chemical, and biological control) but depend mostly on the use of synthetic herbicides (pre-emergent and post-emergent) [11,13]. Hence, it is important to search for new and effective alternatives for weed management.

Substances obtained from living organisms, e.g., the natural metabolites produced during growth and development, can be ingredients of bioherbicides. Although the use of these metabolites can be efficient and beneficial, few conventional herbicides are derived from natural compounds [14,15]. Accordingly, the use of plant species able to produce and release phytotoxic compounds may represent an effective tool for use alone or in association with other plant protection methods for weed management [12,16].

Saponins are specialized metabolites with complex chemical structures and high variability that are involved in the environmental adaptation of plants [17,18]. These molecules are widely distributed among plants and have several significant industrial and pharmacological applications [19]. Some studies have reported phytotoxic or allelopathic properties for saponins [20–26], which suggests that untested saponins could be evaluated as potential bioherbicides [14].

*Quillaja lancifolia* D.Don (formerly *Q. brasiliensis* (A.St.-Hil. & Tul.) Mart.) (Quillajaceae), known as the soap tree, is distributed throughout Southern Brazil [27]. The species is well known for the abundant presence of saponins and, therefore, a large spectrum of biological activities, including immunoadjuvant properties [28,29], antifungal, and antiherbivore effects [30]. The structure of *Q. lancifolia* saponins is remarkably similar to that of *Quillaja saponaria* Molina bark saponins [31]. The latter is a related Chilean species that has been widely used as an adjuvant in vaccine formulations and is one of the main sources of industrial saponins present in plants. The commercially used saponin fraction obtained from barks of *Q. saponaria* is known as Quil-A® [19]. Studies have reported that *Q. saponaria* shows strong aphicidal, deterrent, nematocidal, molluscicidal, and antifungal activity, indicating that the plant could potentially be used as a biopesticide [32–36]. Some of these features have also been observed for leaf saponins of *Q. lancifolia* [30]. If *Q. lancifolia* saponins prove to be phytotoxic, there is also potential use of these natural products as bioherbicides. In addition, saponins may be used in combination with other molecules at lower concentrations, thereby preventing resistance development in plant enemies. Regardless of its potential use as a biopesticide or bioherbicide, *Q. lancifolia* leaf saponins are a more sustainable and easily renewable alternative compared to *Q. saponaria* bark saponins since they do not require phloem stripping or the use of adult native forests [37]. Miniclonal gardens of young *Q. lancifolia* provide a readily available year-round source of leaf biomass [19].

Herein, the phytotoxic activities of leaf aqueous extract and purified saponin fractions of *Q. lancifolia* on different morpho-physiological parameters of lettuce and barnyard grass were examined. Parameters included germination, growth, chlorophyll concentration, and the presence of morphological anomalies. Exposure of soil-like substrate to *Q. lancifolia* extracts, followed by washing with water, was used to assess retention on the substrate and potential residual effects of bioactive metabolites. Chemical analyses of aqueous extracts and purified saponin fractions were also carried out.

## 2. Results

### *2.1. Phytotoxicity Assay*

#### 2.1.1. Osmotic Potential, pH of Extracts, and Presence of Saponins

PEG solutions up to 0.02 M did not significantly affect the emergence of lettuce and barnyardgrass seeds. Germination reached between 80 and 100% in both cases, being statistically equivalent to respective water controls. Since the osmotic potential of the 0.02 M solution was equivalent to that of the 10% *Q. lancifolia* extract, it was determined that, up to this concentration, the effects on seeds were not due to any osmotic limitation (Table S1). Similarly, the pH of the extract was in the 4–6 range, which was not capable of inhibiting germination of the test species.

Triterpene saponins' presence in aqueous extracts and purified fraction QB-90 were confirmed unequivocally by the analytical tests carried out. The TLC data indicated the presence of saponins matching the Rf of Quil-A, a commercial fraction obtained from *Q. saponaria* bark. Although, as expected, other compounds (e.g., phenolics) were present in aqueous extracts, a prominent band matching Quil-A was evident (Figure S1). Further analyses by HPLC revealed peaks with saponin spectral features within the elution times expected for these metabolites (Figure S2). GC-MS analysis of QB-90 after acid hydrolysis yielded quillaic acid as the main aglycone (Figure S3), confirming the triterpene saponin core identity.

#### 2.1.2. Pre-Emergence Bioassay

Both AE 4% and 10% caused significant inhibitory effects on seed germination. In lettuce, no germination was recorded after 4 days, while the negative control had 97% germinability (Figure 1A). Barnyardgrass had 16% germination in 4% AE and 75% in the negative control; the 10% extract completely inhibited germination (Figure 2A). Both 4 and 10% AE reduced not only the percentage of germination but also the speed of the process in the two species (Table S2). Purified saponins (QB fraction) did not inhibit lettuce germination significantly (Figure 1B). On the other hand, the growth of seedlings germinated in the presence of QB was severely impaired (Figure 3).

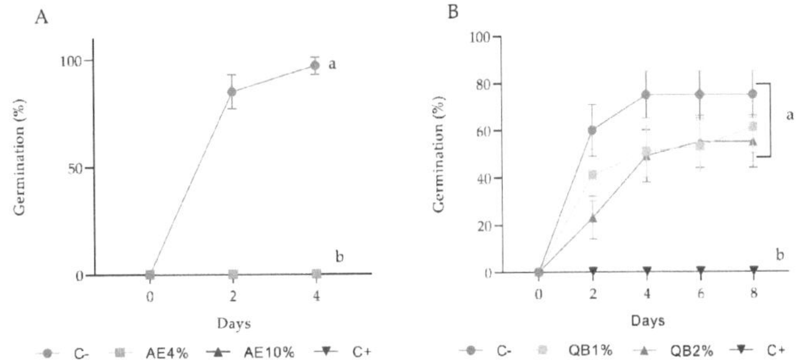


**Figure 1.** Pre-emergence bioassay with lettuce. Effects of (**A**) aqueous extracts (AE) (at 4 and 10%) and (**B**) saponin fraction (QB) (at 1 and 2%) on the number of germinated seeds of *L. sativa* at the end of 4 days and 8 days, respectively. C- represents the negative control (distilled water), and C+ represents the positive control (NaCl). Bars show 95% confidence intervals (Wilson score interval). Treatments not sharing the same letter at the final sampling time differ in germinability ($p \leq 0.05$).

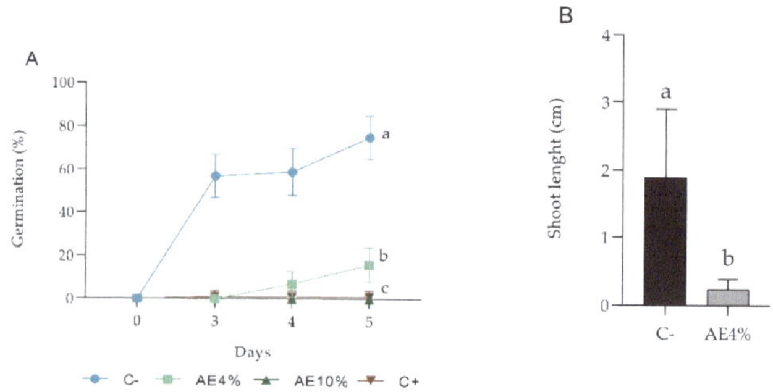


**Figure 2.** Pre-emergence bioassay in barnyardgrass. (**A**) Seed germination in distilled water (C-), aqueous extract (AE) at 4%, AE at 10% and NaCl (C+) and (**B**) seedling growth (shoot length) at the end of 5 days in treatments that showed germination. In (**A**), bars show 95% confidence intervals (Wilson score interval). Treatments not sharing the same letter at the final sampling time differ in germinability ($p \leq 0.05$). In (**B**), bars represent the mean ± SD. Treatments are significantly different by *t*-test ($p \leq 0.05$).

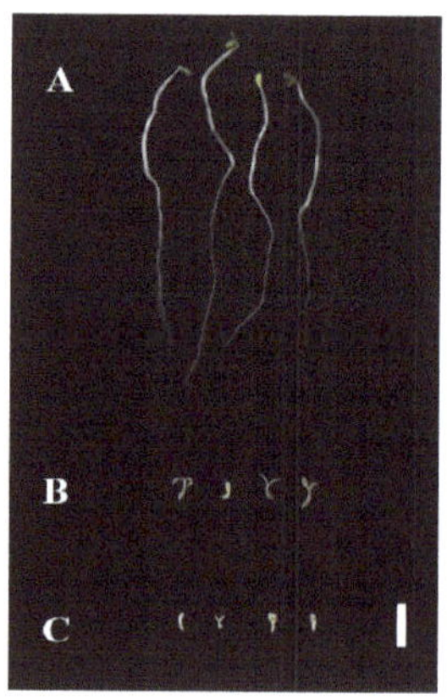


**Figure 3.** Pre-emergence bioassay with lettuce. Seedings at the end of 8 days of application of (**A**) distilled water, (**B**) purified saponin (QB) at 1%, and (**C**) QB 2%. Bar = 1 cm. Statistical data on whole seedling length (cm): distilled water (7.65 ± 0.93 a); QB at 1% (0.60 ± 0.14 b) and QB at 2% (0.38 ± 0.05 b). Numbers in brackets are means ± SD. Means sharing the same letter do not differ by one-way ANOVA and Tukey test ($p \leq 0.05$).

### 2.1.3. Post-Emergence Bioassay

Seven days after the application on lettuce seedlings, exposure to both 4 and 10% AE yielded significant differences from the negative control in every parameter analyzed, except for shoot length and dry weight in the lower concentration (4%) (Figure 4). The chlorophyll content of AE 10% seedlings decreased as much as that of their positive control treatment (NaCl) counterparts (Figure 4C). Plants in AE 4% showed abnormalities and brown spots on the leaves (Figure 5). Moreover, most of the seedlings of the AE 4% were notably fragile. The loss of seedling viability in AE 10% (24%) was comparable to the one recorded in the positive control (16%) (Table S3).

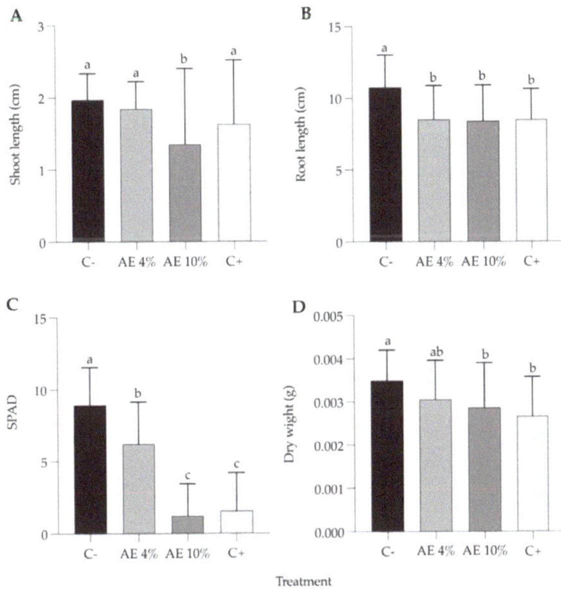


**Figure 4.** Post-emergence bioassay with lettuce. Parameters (7 days after treatment): (**A**) shoot length; (**B**) root length; (**C**) chlorophyll content (SPAD readings); and (**D**) seedling dry weight. Abbreviations: C- (distilled water), AE 4% (aqueous extract at 4%), AE 10% (aqueous extract at 10%), and C+ (NaCl). Bars represent the mean + SD. Different letters indicate significant differences by Kruskal–Wallis test and Dunn's test ($p \leq 0.05$).

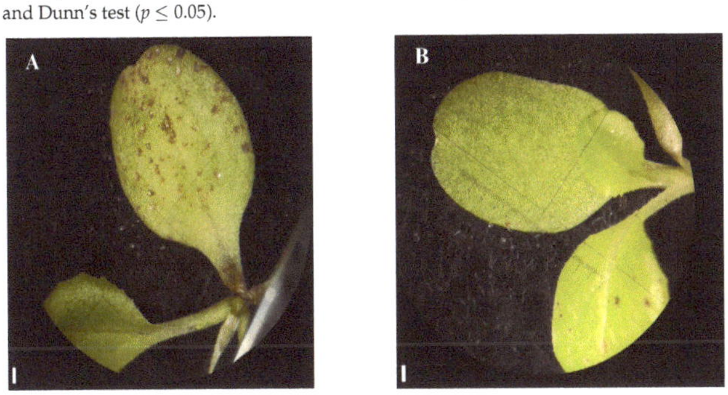


**Figure 5.** *Lactuca sativa* leaves at day 7 in the post-emergence bioassay treated with (**A**) aqueous extract (AE) at 4% and (**B**) negative control (distilled water). Note the brown spots on the leaves of (**A**). Bar = 1 mm.

In barnyardgrass, no significant difference was observed in root length, shoot length, chlorophyll content, and seedling dry weight between the treatments and the controls (Figure S4). However, the plants from the 10% AE appeared wilty (Figure S5).

In the additional post-emergence bioassay growing lettuce in Petri dishes, a significant reduction was observed in root and shoot elongation of seedlings in both AE treatments

(4% and 10%) and the positive control (NaCl) (Figure S6). No significant difference was observed in the seedling dry mass (Figure S6C). The chlorophyll content was not measured in this experiment because the plants were too small.

### 2.1.4. Substrate Leaching Bioassay

The soil-like substrate leaching bioassay carried out with lettuce evaluated germination rates and plant development. Regarding seedling growth, the 10% extract resulted in a significant reduction of shoot length, root length (Figures S7 and 6A,B) and dry mass (Figure 6D). In addition, plants treated with the extracts had a dose–response decrease in chlorophyll content (Figure 6C). Interestingly, the germination rate was higher with AE 10% and AE 4% (56% and 51%, respectively), while the negative control had only 28% seedling emergence (Figure S8). The dry weight was also higher in the 4% extract compared to the control (Figure 6D).

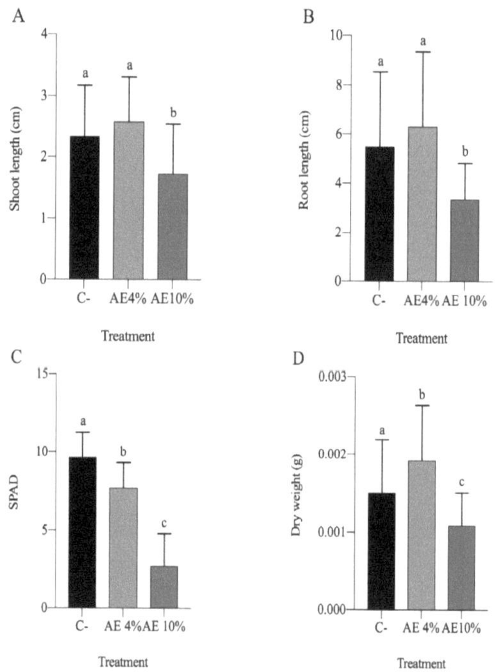


**Figure 6.** Substrate leaching bioassay with lettuce. Parameters (12 days of application of treatments): (**A**) shoot length, (**B**) root length, (**C**) chlorophyll content, and (**D**) seedling dry weight. Abbreviations: C- (distilled water), AE 4% (aqueous extract at 4%), AE 10% (aqueous extract at 10%). Bars represent the mean + SD. Different letters indicate a significant difference by one-way ANOVA and Tukey test ($p \leq 0.05$).

Barnyardgrass plants under extract treatments showed significant growth inhibition, in contrast with those of the negative control (Figure 7). AE 4% and AE 10% revealed a concentration-dependent inhibitory effect on seedlings in terms of shoot length and dry weight (Figure 8A,C).

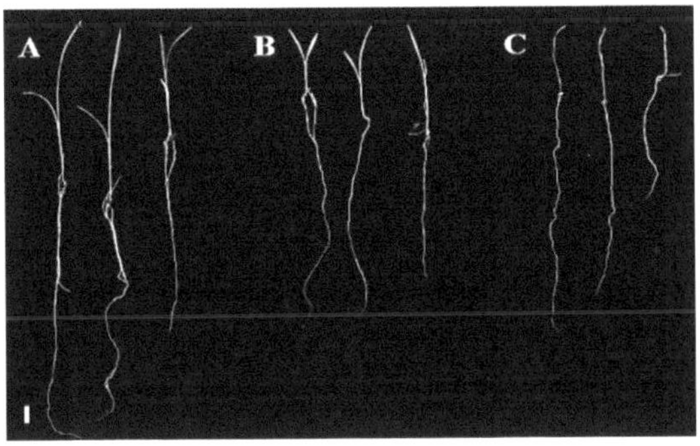


**Figure 7.** Seedlings of barnyardgrass at the end of 8 days in the leaching bioassay. (**A**) Negative control (plants treated with distilled water); (**B**) plants with aqueous extract (AE) at 4% and (**C**) plants with AE at 10%. Bar = 1 cm.

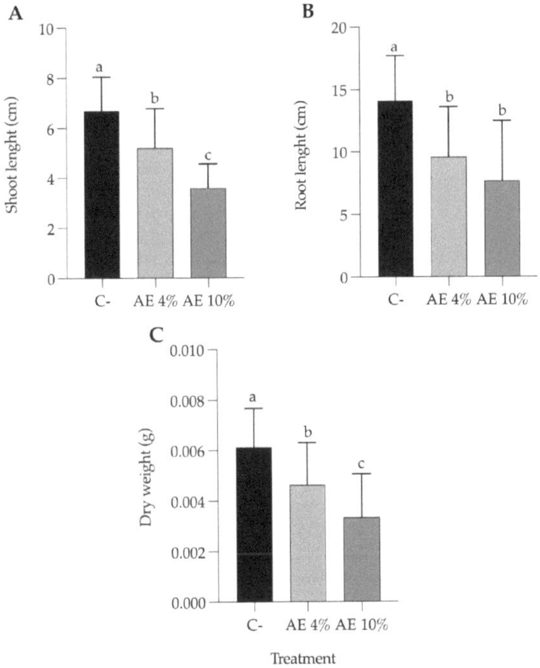


**Figure 8.** Substrate leaching bioassay with barnyardgrass. Parameters after 8 days of leaching (and 4 water applications): (**A**) shoot length, (**B**) root length, and (**C**) seedling dry weight. Abbreviations: distilled water (C-), aqueous extract at 4% (AE 4%), and aqueous extract at 10% (AE 10%). Bars represent the mean + SD. Different letters indicate significant differences by one-way ANOVA and Tukey test ($p \leq 0.05$).

## 3. Discussion

Possible significant impacts of nonspecific factors on the phytotoxic activities of *Q. lancifolia* aqueous extracts and purified saponins at the concentrations used were ruled out. Therefore, the validity of the subsequently recorded data was confirmed. Osmotic and pH values were within non-inhibitory ranges for both tested species [38–40].

Pre-emergence bioassays using 4% and 10% aqueous extracts of *Q. lancifolia* against both lettuce and barnyardgrass revealed a significant reduction of germination rates and root and shoot length of the emerged seedlings. In *L. sativa*, the extracts completely inhibited germination. Extracts and QB fraction significantly inhibited one or more parameters, such as germination percentage and shoot and root length. Considering that even at low concentrations of AE, germination was suppressed, it appears that the extracts showed phytotoxic potential that could be at least partly attributed to the saponins present in the plant. Indeed, analytical methods consistently showed the presence of triterpene saponins with typical quillaic acid aglycone [19,31]. The possible participation of saponins in the phytotoxic effects is also supported by the fact that seeds germinated in the presence of the purified saponin fraction QB-yielded seedlings severely reduced in size. Further studies of these compounds could lead to possible use as an effective pre-emergence bioherbicide.

Phytotoxic effects on the post-emergence growth of lettuce were also observed, especially at AE 10%. Under the AE 4% treatment, numerous leaves exhibited abnormalities that could explain the significantly reduced chlorophyll content recorded. Although the effects on post-emergence were not as intense as those in the germination experiments, *Q. lancifolia* extracts also had phytotoxic effects on seedling growth. In the leaching bioassay, however, there was a significant decrease in the inhibitory effect of the extracts on lettuce, particularly at 4% AE. This could lead to possible use as a post-emergence bioherbicide, alone or in combination, effective at pre- and post-germination with a reduced residual effect.

However, the lack of significant changes shown in the post-emergence bioassays with barnyardgrass can indicate that the extracts are not as effective in repressing the seedling growth of *E. crus-galli* as they are inhibiting its germination. This possibly reflects a higher resistance to biotic stresses in weeds [8]. On the other hand, the leaching bioassay with barnyardgrass showed a significant reduction in the root and shoot length as well as dry weight of plants treated with AE. Perhaps, for this species, longer exposure to the extract residue could affect plants negatively.

Ideally, a bioherbicide residue on the soil surface should be able to undergo leaching and/or degradation, thus avoiding the exposure of subsequent crops to potentially phytotoxic compounds [11]. The leaching assay with lettuce is also considered a pre-emergence experiment since it used seeds grown on substrates exposed to the extracts. Since mixtures of sand and vermiculite are only soil-like substrates, the data obtained with them cannot be directly extrapolated to natural soil conditions. Nonetheless, the use of these substrates provides useful information on the overall behavior of phytotoxic agents in soil. The higher dry biomass of seedlings in AE 4% relative to the water control may indicate a nutritional effect of the extracts caused, for example, by the presence of sugars in saponins [41]. The application of the 10% extract, nonetheless, resulted in lower growth and chlorophyll content, perhaps due to a negative impact on photosynthesis [42].

Antiherbivore and antifungal effects of *Q. lancifolia* saponins were observed in the 1 to 2% concentration range [30]. For saponins to constitute a potential biopesticide, the absence or limited phytotoxic effects at concentrations in which they can inhibit herbivores and pathogens are necessary. Further studies focusing on the compatible use of these molecules in biopesticide and bioherbicide formulations are needed.

In most cases, as has been reported for other saponins, the activity of these triterpenes depends essentially on their effects on membranes [43]. As a result of their amphipathic nature, saponins can interfere with the membrane structure, affecting its integrity and functionality [44]. It seems likely that the growth inhibitory effects recorded in test plants are at least partly caused by saponins present in extracts and their fractions on cell and organelle membranes. However, other compounds, as well as synergistic interactions among metabolites, can also be involved, particularly in AE treatments.

Taken together, the data suggest that AE and QB of *Q. lancifolia* may be considered for use in organic agriculture both as pre- and post-emergence bioherbicide components. In a preliminary assessment, it seems that these agents may be effective for broad leaf and grass weeds. Given the surfactant properties of saponins and based on pilot tests, their application using ordinary sprayers is not difficult. Although it is not possible to estimate more precisely at this point, doses per hectare and the costs of treatment are not likely to be prohibitive. Support for this possibility is based on the renewable and continuous source of saponin supply from the leaves of cultivated plants, as well as on the relatively low active concentrations required. In addition, the combined use of these agents as adjuvants with other products may further contribute to economic feasibility.

## 4. Conclusions

In summary, *Quillaja lancifolia* aqueous extracts and purified saponin fractions showed strong phytotoxic activity against *E. crus-galli* and *L. sativa* (with greater injury levels on the latter) and weed-suppressing abilities. These findings warrant further studies to evaluate the possible uses of these agents in formulations of bioherbicides. Key features of *Q. lancifolia* saponins, such as their water solubility and sustainable supply from leaves obtained in cultivated clonal gardens, are important for potential deployment as bioherbicides. Future work is required to better understand the mechanisms of action of these phytotoxins, notably their interaction with biological membranes and their components.

## 5. Materials and Methods

### *5.1. Plant Material and Extracts*

#### 5.1.1. Plant Source and Extract Preparation

Approximately 5 kg of fresh *Q. lancifolia* leaves were collected from adult plants (about 10 m tall of unknown age) growing in the rural zone of the city of Canguçu, RS, Brazil (31°23′42″ S–52°40′32″ W) in the early fall of 2018 (28 March 2018) (harvest authorization by the Brazilian Board of Management of Genetic Resources—CGEN under number 010540/2011-3). Harvest was done on a sunny day with temperature variations between 17 and 24 °C. Monthly precipitation was typical for the area, around 120 mm. The climate of the site of collection is warm temperate Cfb (Köppen classification).

A voucher specimen was deposited at the ICN Herbarium of the Federal University of Rio Grande do Sul (142,953). Air-dried powdered leaves were extracted in distilled water (1:10, *w*/*v*) for 8 h, filtered, and partitioned with ethyl acetate, followed by lyophilization of the aqueous phase, yielding aqueous extract (AE). AE was submitted to reverse-phase chromatography and gradient of water and methanol to obtain fraction QB-90, as previously described [28]. QB-80 was obtained using the same protocol. QB-80 and QB-90 were also analyzed by thin-layer chromatography (TLC) to further confirm fraction isolation. The two purified saponin fractions were combined for the bioassays constituting QB.

#### 5.1.2. Extract and Saponin Chemical Characterization

Characterization of AE and QB was initially performed by TLC. Silica gel aluminum plates (F254, Supelco, Darmstadt, Germany) were used as the stationary phase. The mobile phase was n-butanol:acetic acid:water (5:1:4, *v*/*v*). Plates were revealed using the anisaldehyde-sulfuric acid protocol [28]. Additional confirmation of saponin presence was obtained by high-performance liquid chromatography (HPLC) analysis using a Shimadzu chromatographer equipped with a PDA-UV detector. Saponins were tracked at 214 nm. The HPLC method was based on Wallace et al. [45] with minor modifications. Finally, Gas Chromatography-Mass Spectrometry (GC-MS) analysis of acid-hydrolyzed saponins was carried out with an oven set to 120 °C for 1 min, then increasing at 6 °C/min to 320 °C. The final hold time was 11.6 min. Spectral data were generated with electron impact ionization at 70 eV (positive mode). Data were acquired in full scans ranging from $m/z$ 50 to 550.

The Agilent MassHunter workstation (version B.07 service pack 2) was used for peak integration of total and extracted ion chromatograms and extraction of mass spectra [46].

### *5.2. Phytotoxicity Assay*

#### 5.2.1. Target Species

The experiments on the phytotoxic effect of the extract were carried out with diaspores (herein referred to as seeds) of *Lactuca sativa* L. (a common model in allelopathy studies), as well as seedlings of the same species; and with seeds and seedlings of *Echinochloa crus-galli* L.P.Beauv (an economically relevant weed species, particularly in rice fields). For these assays, commercially available lettuce seeds were used (Isla®, batch 116377-001, Porto Alegre, Brazil), and barnyardgrass seeds (batches grown at the agronomy campus of UFRGS and harvested in late summer/early fall) were kindly provided by the Department of Crop Plants—Faculty of Agronomy, UFRGS.

#### 5.2.2. Extract Osmotic Potential and pH Measurements

Both the osmotic potential and pH of the extracts were determined in triplicate. The osmotic potential of *Q. lancifolia* extracts was measured in different concentrations (0.1%, 1%, 2%, 4%, 10%, 20%, 40%) with a refractometer-based curve prepared with sucrose. To determine the influence of the osmotic potential of the extracts on both lettuce and barnyardgrass germination bioassays, additional tests were performed with solutions of polyethylene glycol (PEG-6000) [38] at the following concentrations: 0.01 M, 0.02 M, and 0.03 M. This experiment was carried out using the same germination procedure (i.e., pre-emergence) bioassays (Table S1 and Section 5.2.3). The osmotic potential of the different concentrations of PEG was also measured with a refractometer, and it was possible to correlate the solution of PEG at 0.02 M with the 10% *Q. lancifolia* aqueous extract. Extract pH values were determined with a pH meter.

#### 5.2.3. Pre-Emergence Bioassay

The pre-emergence bioassay analyzed the germination of *L. sativa* (lettuce) and *E. crus-galli* (barnyardgrass). Petri dishes (9 cm in diameter) lined with qualitative filter paper were used, and assays were conducted in a growth chamber (25 °C, 12 h/12 h dark/light, 40 μmol photons·$m^{-2}$·$s^{-1}$).

For each one of the species, the Petri dishes were separated into experimental groups and the control, each containing 25 seeds per plate, with 3 plates per experimental group. Seeds were treated with 5 mL in each Petri dish of the AE of *Q. lancifolia* (at 4 and 10% *w*/*v*), distilled water (negative control), and NaCl 0.5 M (positive control). In the case of lettuce, QB at 1% and 2% (*w*/*v*) were also evaluated.

Germination parameters were measured daily (germination time) or on the 5th day of incubation (germination percentage, root and shoot length). The presence of morphological abnormalities was recorded. Germination velocity indexes (GVI) were calculated [47]:

$$GVI = N1/D1 + N2/D2 + \ldots + Nn/Dn$$

where: GVI = germination velocity index; N = number of seeds germinated within the day interval of counting; D = days after sowing until data collection.

An additional experiment using purified saponin fraction QB was performed with lettuce under the same growth conditions described above. Germination and seedling length were analyzed, with treatments consisting of 1 and 2% of QB and controls, in this case ending on the 7th day of incubation.

#### 5.2.4. Bioassay for Post-Emergence

To obtain lettuce seedlings for the effect on initial growth, seeds were put in separate pot trays (each slot with a volume of 15 mL, one plant per slot) containing autoclaved substrate (washed sand: vermiculite—ratio 1:1; *v*/*v*) and kept for 12 days under controlled light and temperature (photoperiod of 16 h per day; 25 ± 2 °C, irradiance 50 μmol·$m^{-2}$·$s^{-1}$).

On the 12th day, plants from germinated seeds were exposed to AE (at 4 and 10% *w*/*v*) and controls (2 mL per slot containing a single plant and sprinkling to dew point). Barnyardgrass seeds were kept for 13 days on the same substrate growth conditions described above, and on the 14th day, seedlings were exposed to the treatments (AE at 4 and 10% *w*/*v*).

Seven days after treatment application, growth parameters were measured (radicle length, shoot length, and whole seedling dry mass). Root and shoot length were recorded with a ruler, and oven dry mass at 60 °C was obtained in an analytical balance. In addition, for lettuce, the chlorophyll content was measured with a SPAD chlorophyllometer (Minolta, Osaka, Japan). With barnyardgrass, due to restrictions of leaf size on the SPAD reading probe, a conventional spectrophotometric evaluation of acetone chlorophyll extracts was carried out [17]. Each individual plant was considered an experimental unit. The number of replicates per treatment and per sampling time was 50 for root length, shoot length, whole seedling dry weight, and SPAD readings. For spectrophotometric chlorophyll measurements, a pooled set of 5 plants was the experimental unit and 4 replicates were used per treatment and sampling time.

In another set of experiments, *Q. lancifolia* extracts and control treatments were applied to post-emergent 12-day-old lettuce seedlings grown in Petri dishes. After 12 days in growth chamber conditions as described above, 5 mL of extracts and controls were applied to each dish containing 25 plants and replicated 3 times. Plants were measured after 7 days of application (root length, shoot length, and whole seedling dry mass).

#### 5.2.5. Substrate Leaching Bioassay

To evaluate whether the extract could be leached from a soil-like substrate, two different bioassays were performed. With *L. sativa*, 50 individual slots of pot trays (each slot with a volume of 15 mL) containing autoclaved soil-like substrate (washed sand: vermiculite—ratio 1:1; *v*/*v*) were inoculated with 2 mL of AE at concentrations of 4 and 10%. In addition, the area comprised of 50 slots was superficially sprayed with 30 mL of the respective extract. Then, each slot was subjected to leaching with 10 mL of distilled water every 2 days until completing 8 days (i.e., 4 washings). In the day of the last water application, 2 lettuce seeds were sown per slot to evaluate germination for 12 days. Root length, shoot length, and seedling dry mass were also recorded at the end of this period. The experiment with barnyardgrass evaluated the leaching potential of seedlings grown on the same untreated substrate previously described for 12 days, with application of the extracts and controls at the end of the 13th day. After 7 days of application, 10 mL of distilled water were applied in each separate slot to leachate the extract away every 2 days until completing 8 days (i.e., 4 washings). The same growth parameters above were measured after the last water application.

#### 5.2.6. Statistical Analyses

Statistical analysis was done with GraphPad Prism 8.1. Results were pre-evaluated for normal distribution by the Shapiro–Wilk or Levene test and then analyzed by one-way ANOVA followed by Tukey test (normal distribution) or Kruskal–Wallis followed by Dunn's test (non-parametric distribution), all at $p \leq 0.05$. For the two treatment comparisons, a *t*-test was applied (after normality verification and at $p \leq 0.05$). Data were expressed as mean ± standard deviation (SD). Germination data were analyzed using 95% confidence intervals (Wilson score interval) [48].

**Supplementary Materials:** The following supporting information can be downloaded at: https://www.mdpi.com/article/10.3390/plants12030663/s1, Figure S1: Thin layer chromatography of *Quillaja* preparations. AE—aqueous extract prepared from *Q. lancifolia* leaves; Quil-A—commercial preparation obtained from *Q. saponaria* barks; QB-90—purified from AE after column chromatography. Triterpenoids stained brown with anisaldehide-sulfuric. Figure S2: HPLC chromatogram (214 nm) of QB-90 (4 mg/mL) from the leaf extract of *Quillaja lancifolia*. The main triterpene saponins elute in the range of 15 to 25 min. The known saponin QS-21 elutes between 20.5 and 20.7 min. Figure S3: GC-MS analysis of QB-90 after acid hydrolysis. Breakdown of saponins produced quillaic acid as the main aglycone (quillaic acid chemical structure shown on the right). The presence of quillaic acid was confirmed with an authentic standard. IS—internal standard (cholestane). Figure S4. Post-emergence bioassay with barnyardgrass. Parameters (7 days after treatment): (A) shoot length, (B) root length, (C) chlorophyll concentration, and (D) seedling dry weight. Abbreviations: C- (distilled water), AE 4% (aqueous extract at 4%), AE 10% (aqueous extract at 10%) and C+ (NaCl). Bars represent the mean + SD. Different letters indicate significant difference by Kruskal-Wallis and Dunn's test (A and D) or one-way ANOVA and Tukey test (B and C) ($p \leq 0.05$). Figure S5. Post-emergence bioassay with barnyardgrass. Seedlings at the end of 7 days treated with (A) distilled water—C- and (B) aqueous extract at 10%—AE 10%. Bar = 1 cm. Figure S6. Post-emergence bioassay with lettuce carried out in petri dishes. Parameters (7 days after treatment): (A) shoot length, (B) root length, and (C) seedling dry weight. Abbreviations: C- (distilled water), AE 4% (aqueous extract at 4%), AE 10% (aqueous extract at 10%) and C+ (NaCl). Bars represent the mean + SD. Different letters indicate significant difference by Kruskal-Wallis and Dunn's test ($p \leq 0.05$). Figure S7. Substrate leaching bioassay with lettuce. Seedlings at the end of 12 days in substrate treated with (A) distilled water—C-, (B) aqueous extract at 4%—AE 4% and (C) aqueous extract at 10%—AE 10%. Bar = 1 cm. Figure S8. Substrate leaching bioassay. Germination rates of lettuce seeds in soil-like substrate with the previous application of the following treatments: distilled water (C-), aqueous extract at 4% (AE 4%) and aqueous extract at 10% (AE 10%), during 12 days of experiment. Bars show 95% confidence intervals (Wilson score interval). Treatments not sharing the same letter at the final sampling time differ in germinability ($p \leq 0.05$). Reference [46] is cited in the supplementary materials.

**Author Contributions:** Conceptualization, M.E.M.M., A.C.A.Y. and A.G.F.-N.; methodology, M.E.M.M., A.C.d.C., A.C.A.Y., Y.V.S.M. and E.Z., investigation, M.E.M.M., A.C.d.C. and A.C.A.Y.; resources, A.G.F.-N.; writing—original draft preparation, M.E.M.M.; writing—review and editing, A.G.F.-N.; supervision, A.G.F.-N.; project administration, A.G.F.-N.; funding acquisition, A.G.F.-N. All authors have read and agreed to the published version of the manuscript.

**Funding:** This research was funded by the Conselho Nacional de Desenvolvimento Científico e Tecnológico (CNPq—Brazil), grant number 310775/2021-3), Rio Grande do Sul State Foundation for Research Support (Fapergs—Brazil), grant number 2019/15477-3, and the Coordenação de Aperfeiçoamento de Pessoal de Nível Superior—(CAPES—Brazil)—Finance Code 001.

**Institutional Review Board Statement:** Not applicable.

**Informed Consent Statement:** Not applicable.

**Data Availability Statement:** The original contributions presented in the study are included in the article/Supplementary Material, and further inquiries can be directed to the corresponding author.

**Conflicts of Interest:** The authors declare no conflict of interest.

## References

1. Rehman, A.; Farooq, M.; Lee, D.J.; Siddique, K.H.M. Sustainable agricultural practices for food security and ecosystem services. *Environ. Sci. Pollut. Res.* **2022**, *29*, 84076–84095. [CrossRef] [PubMed]
2. Food and Agriculture Organization of the United Nations. FAOSTAT-Pesticides Use. 2018. Available online: http://www.fao.org/faostat/en/#data/RP/visualize (accessed on 25 May 2019).
3. Pignati, W.A.; de Lima, F.A.N.S.; de Lara, S.S.; Correa, M.L.M.; Barbosa, J.R.; da Leão, L.H.C.; Pignatti, M.G. Distribuição espacial do uso de agrotóxicos no Brasil: Uma ferramenta para a Vigilância em Saúde (Spacial distribution of agrotoxics use in Brazil: A tool for Health Surveillance). *Cien. Saude Colet.* **2017**, *22*, 3281–3293. [CrossRef]
4. Bebber, D.P.; Holmes, T.; Gurr, S.J. The global spread of crop pests and pathogens. *Glob. Ecol. Biogeogr.* **2014**, *23*, 1398–1407. [CrossRef]
5. Oerke, E.C. Crop losses to pests. *J. Agric. Sci.* **2006**, *144*, 31–43. [CrossRef]
6. Stewart, C.N. Becoming weeds. *Nat. Genet.* **2017**, *49*, 654–655. [CrossRef] [PubMed]
7. Weed Science Society of America. Weeds. 2016. Available online: http://wssa.net/wssa/weed/ (accessed on 25 May 2019).
8. Zimdahl, R.L. *Fundamentals of Weed Science*, 5th ed.; Academic Press: London, UK, 2018; 735p.
9. Schonbeck, M. *Principles of Sustainable Weed Management in Organic Cropping Systems, Workshop for Farmers and Agricultural Professionals on Sustainable Weed Management*, 3rd ed.; Clemson University: Clemson, SC, USA, 2011; 20p.
10. Brühl, C.A.; Zaller, J.G. Biodiversity decline as a consequence of an inappropriate environmental risk assessment of pesticides. *Front. Environ. Sci.* **2019**, *7*, 177. [CrossRef]
11. Abbas, T.; Zahir, Z.A.; Naveed, M.; Kremer, R.J. Limitations of existing weed control practices necessitate development of alternative techniques based on biological approaches. *Adv. Agron.* **2018**, *147*, 239–280. [CrossRef]

12. Cordeau, S.; Triolet, M.; Wayman, S.; Steinberg, C.; Guillemin, J.P. Bioherbicides: Dead in the water? A review of the existing products for integrated weed management. *Crop Prot.* **2016**, *87*, 44–49. [CrossRef]
13. Chauhan, B.S.; Mahajan, G. *Recent Advances in Weed Management*, 1st ed.; Springer: New York, NY, USA, 2014; 411p. [CrossRef]
14. Dayan, F.E.; Duke, S.O. Natural compounds as next-generation herbicides. *Plant Physiol.* **2014**, *166*, 1090–1105. [CrossRef]
15. Duke, S.O.; Pan, Z.; Bajsa-Hirschel, J.; Boyette, C.D. The potential future roles of natural compounds and microbial bioherbicides in weed management in crops. *Adv. Weed Sci.* **2022**, *40*, e020210054. [CrossRef]
16. Puig, C.G.; Reigosa, M.J.; Valentão, P.; Andrade, P.B.; Pedrol, N. Unravelling the bioherbicide potential of *Eucalyptus globulus* Labill: Biochemistry and effects of its aqueous extract. *PLoS ONE* **2018**, *13*, e0192872. [CrossRef] [PubMed]
17. De Costa, F.; Fleck, J.; Yendo, A.C.A.; Gosmann, G.; Fett-Neto, A.G. Accumulation of a bioactive triterpene saponin fraction of *Quillaja brasiliensis* leaves is associated with abiotic and biotic stresses. *Plant Physiol. Biochem.* **2013**, *66*, 56–62. [CrossRef] [PubMed]
18. Yu, B.; Patterson, N.; Zaharia, L.I. Saponin biosynthesis in pulses. *Plants* **2022**, *11*, 3505. [CrossRef] [PubMed]
19. Magedans, Y.V.S.; Phillips, M.A.; Fett-Neto, A.G. Production of plant bioactive triterpenoid saponins: From metabolites to genes and back. *Phytochem. Rev.* **2021**, *20*, 461–482. [CrossRef]
20. Faizal, A.; Geelen, D. Saponins and their role in biological processes in plants. *Phytochem. Rev.* **2013**, *12*, 877–893. [CrossRef]
21. Hoagland, R.E.; Zablotowicz, R.M.; Reddy, K.N. Studies of the phytotoxicity of saponins on weed and crop plants. In *Saponins Used in Food and Agriculture*; Waller, G.R., Yamasaki, K., Eds.; Plenum Press: New York, NY, USA, 1996; pp. 57–73.
22. Jelassi, A.; Ayeb-Zakhama, A.E.; Nejma, A.B.; Chaari, A.; Harzallah-Skhiri, F.; Jannet, H.B. Phytochemical composition and allelopathic potential of three Tunisian *Acacia* species. *Ind. Crops Prod.* **2016**, *83*, 339–345. [CrossRef]
23. Pérez, A.J.; Simonet, A.M.; Pecio, Ł.; Kowalczyk, M.; Calle, J.M.; Macías, F.A.; Oleszec, W.; Stochmal, A. Triterpenoid saponins from the aerial parts of *Trifolium argutum* Sol. and their phytotoxic evaluation. *Phytochem. Lett.* **2015**, *13*, 165–170. [CrossRef]
24. Ribeiro, R.C.; de Carvalho, M.G.; de Moraes, M.L.L.; Rossiello, R.O.P.; de Oliveira, D.R.; de Amorim, R.M.Q.; Barbieri, E., Jr. Chemical screening of *Urochloa humidicola*: Methods for characterizing secondary metabolites and allelopathic activity on forage legumes. *Am. J. Plant Sci.* **2018**, *9*, 1260–1278. [CrossRef]
25. Stavropoulou, M.I.; Angelis, A.; Aligiannis, N.; Kalpoutzakis, E.; Mitakou, S.; Duke, S.O.; Fokialakis, N. Phytotoxic triterpene saponins from *Bellis longifolia*, an endemic plant of Crete. *Phytochemistry* **2017**, *144*, 71–77. [CrossRef]
26. Wyman-Simpson, C.L.; Waller, G.R.; Jurzysta, M.; McPherson, J.K.; Young, C.C. Biological activity and chemical isolation of root saponins of six cultivars of alfalfa (*Medicago sativa* L.). *Plant Soil.* **1991**, *135*, 83–94. [CrossRef]
27. Reitz, R.; Reis, A.; Klein, R.M. *Flora Ilustrada Catarinense—Rosáceas (Illustrated Flora of the State of Santa Catarina—Rosaceae)*; Herbário Barbosa Rodrigues: Itajaí, Brazil, 1996; pp. 113–116.
28. Fleck, J.D.; Kauffmann, C.; Spilki, F.; Lencina, C.L.; Roehe, P.M.; Gosmann, G. Adjuvant activity of *Quillaja brasiliensis* saponins on the immune responses to bovine herpesvirus type 1 in mice. *Vaccine* **2006**, *24*, 7129–7134. [CrossRef] [PubMed]
29. Kumar, A.; Sharma, A.; Tirpude, N.V.; Padwad, Y.; Hallan, V.; Kumar, S. Plant-derived immuno-adjuvants in vaccines formulation: A promising avenue for improving vaccines efficacy against SARS-CoV-2 virus. *Pharmacol. Rep.* **2022**, *74*, 1238–1254. [CrossRef] [PubMed]
30. Yendo, A.C.A. Saponinas de *Quillaja brasiliensis*: Purificação e atividade biológica. (Saponins of *Quillaja brasiliensis*: Purification and biological activity). Ph.D. Thesis, Graduate Program in Botany—Universidade Federal do Rio Grande do Sul (UFRGS), Porto Alegre, Brazil, 2016.
31. Kauffmann, C.; Machado, A.M.; Fleck, J.D.; Provensi, G.; Pires, V.S.; Guillaume, D.; Sonnet, P.; Reginatto, F.H.; Shenkel, E.P.; Gosmann, G. Constituents from leaves of *Quillaja brasiliensis*. *Nat. Prod. Res.* **2004**, *18*, 153–157. [CrossRef]
32. González-Cruz, D.; Martín, R.S. Molluscicidal effects of saponin-rich plant extracts on the grey field slug. *Cien. Investig. Agr.* **2013**, *40*, 341–349. [CrossRef]
33. De Geyter, E.; Smagghe, G.; Rahbe, Y.; Geelen, D. Triterpene saponins of *Quillaja saponaria* show strong aphicidal and deterrent activity against the pea aphid *Acyrthosiphon pisum*. *Pest Manag. Sci.* **2011**, *68*, 164–169. [CrossRef] [PubMed]
34. Moya, E.; San, R.M.; Gamboa, M.; Hidalgo, G.E.A. Evaluation of a *Quillaja saponaria* saponin extract for control of powdery mildew of wheat and squash evaluación de un extracto de saponinas de *Quillaja saponaria* para el control de oídios de trigo y zapallo. *Agro Sur* **2010**, *38*, 87–96. [CrossRef]
35. González-Castillo, J.A.; Quezada-D'Angelo, T.P.; Silva-Aguayo, G.I.; Moya, E.A. Effect of saponins of *Quillaja saponaria* extracts in combination with *Pseudomonas protegens* to control *Gaeumannomyces graminis* var. tritici in wheat. *Chil. J. Agric Res.* **2018**, *78*, 378–390. [CrossRef]
36. Giannakou, I.O. Efficacy of a formulated product containing *Quillaja saponaria* plant extracts for the control of root-knot nematodes. *Eur. J. Plant Pathol.* **2011**, *130*, 587. [CrossRef]
37. Martín, R.; Briones, R. Industrial uses and sustainable supply of *Quillaja saponaria* (Rosaceae) saponins. *Econ. Bot.* **1999**, *53*, 302–311. [CrossRef]
38. Meneses, C.H.S.G.; Lima, L.H.G.M.; Lima, M.M.A.; Pereira, W.E.; Bruno, R.L.A.; Vidal, M.S. Potencial hídrico induzido por Polietilenoglicol-6000 na viabilidade de sementes de algodão (Water potential induced by Polyethylene glycol-6000 on cotton seed viability). *Embrapa Agrobiol.* **2007**, *19*, 1–22.
39. Sadeghloo, A.; Asghari, J.; Ghaderi-Far, F. Seed germination and seedling emergence of velvetleaf (*Abutilon theophrasti*) and Barnyardgrass (*Echinochloa crus-galli*). *Planta Daninha* **2013**, *31*, 259–266. [CrossRef]

40. Rice, E.L. *Allelopathy*, 2nd ed.; Academic Press Inc.: New York, NY, USA, 1984; 422p.
41. Yendo, A.C.A.; De Costa, F.; Da Costa, C.T.; Colling, L.C.; Gosmann, G.; Fett-Neto, A.G. Biosynthesis of plant triterpenoid saponins: Genes, enzymes, and their regulation. *Mini Rev. Org. Chem.* **2014**, *11*, 292–306. [CrossRef]
42. Poonpaiboonpipat, T.; Pangnakorn, U.; Suvunnamek, U.; Teerarak, M.; Charoenying, P.; Laosinwattana, C. Phytotoxic effects of essential oil from *Cymbopogon citratus* and its physiological mechanisms on barnyardgrass (*Echinochloa crus-galli*). *Ind. Crop. Prod.* **2013**, *41*, 403–407. [CrossRef]
43. De Costa, F.; Yendo, A.C.A.; Fleck, J.D.; Gosmann, G.; Fett-Neto, A.G. Immunoadjuvant and anti-inflammatory plant saponins: Characteristics and biotechnological approaches towards sustainable production. *Mini Rev. Med. Chem.* **2011**, *11*, 857–880. [CrossRef]
44. De Groot, C.; Müller-Goymann, C.C. Saponin interactions with model membrane systems—Langmuir monolayer studies, hemolysis and formation of ISCOMs. *Planta Med.* **2016**, *82*, 1496–1512. [CrossRef]
45. Wallace, F.; Bennadji, Z.; Ferreira, F.; Olivaro, C. Analysis of an immunoadjuvant saponin fraction from *Quillaja brasiliensis* leaves by electrospray ionization ion trap multiple-stage mass spectrometry. *Phytochem. Lett.* **2017**, *20*, 228–233. [CrossRef]
46. Magedans, Y.V.S.; Phillips, M.A. Soapbark Triterpenes: *Quillaja brasiliensis* cell culture sapogenin and free sterol analysis by GCMS. *Methods Mol. Biol.* **2022**, *2469*, 119–128. [CrossRef]
47. Popinigis, F. *Fisiologia da Semente (Seed Physiology)*; Brazilian Ministry of Agriculture: Brasíla, Brazil; Inter-American Development Bank (BID): Washington, DC, USA, 1977; pp. 275–277.
48. Newcombe, R.G. Two-sided confidence intervals for the single proportion: Comparison of seven methods. *Statist. Med.* **1998**, *17*, 857–872. [CrossRef]

plants

MDPI

Article

# Allelopathic Substances of *Osmanthus* spp. for Developing Sustainable Agriculture

**Hisashi Kato-Noguchi [1,*], Yuri Hamada [1], Misuzu Kojima [1], Sanae Kumagai [1], Arihiro Iwasaki [2] and Kiyotake Suenaga [2]**

[1] Department of Applied Biological Science, Faculty of Agriculture, Kagawa University, Miki, Kagawa 761-0795, Japan
[2] Department of Chemistry, Faculty of Science and Technology, Keio University, 3-14-1 Hiyoshi, Kohoku, Yokohama 223-8522, Japan
* Correspondence: kato.hisashi@kagawa-u.ac.jp

**Abstract:** *Osmanthus fragrans* Lour. has been cultivated for more than 2500 years because of the fragrance and color of the flowers. The flowers and roots have been used in tea, liquors, foods, and traditional Chinese medicine. The species contains more than 180 compounds including terpenoids, phenylpropanoids, polyphenols, flavonoids, and sterols. However, there has been limited information available on the allelopathic properties and allelopathic substances of *O. fragrans*. We investigated the allelopathy and allelopathic substances of *O. fragrans* and *Osmanthus heterophyllus* (G.Don) P.S. Green, as well as *Osmanthus* × *fortunei* Carrière, which is the hybrid species between *O. fragrans* and *O. heterophyllus*. The leaf extracts of *O. fragrans*, *O. heterophyllus*, and *O.* × *fortunei* suppressed the growth of cress (*Lepidium sativum* L.), alfalfa (*Medicago sativa* L.), *Lolium multiflorum* Lam., and *Vulpia myuros* (L.) C.C.Gmel with the extract concentration dependently. The extract of the hybrid species *O.* × *fortune* was the most active among the extracts. The main allelopathic substances of *O.* × *fortunei* and *O. fragrans* were isolated and identified as (+)-pinoresinol and 10-acetoxyligustroside, respectively. (+)-Pinoresinol was also found in the fallen leaves of *O.* × *fortunei*. Both compounds showed an allelopathic activity on the growth of cress and *L. multiflorum*. On the other hand, several allelopathic substances including (+)-pinoresinol may be involved in the allelopathy of *O. heterophyllus*. *O. fragrans*, *O. heterophyllus*, and *O.* × *fortunei* are evergreen trees. but their senescent leaves fall and cover the soil under the trees. It is possible that those allelopathic substances are liberated through the decomposition process of the leaves into their rhizosphere soil, and that they accumulate in the soil and provide a competitive advantage to the species through the inhibition of the growth of the neighboring competing plants. Therefore, the leaves of these *Osmanthus* species are allelopathic and potentially useful for weed management options in some agriculture settings to reduce commercial herbicide dependency for the developing sustainable agriculture systems.

**Keywords:** allelochemical; 10-acetoxyligustroside; decomposition; fallen leaf; growth inhibition; *Osmanthus*; (+)-pinoresinol

**Citation:** Kato-Noguchi, H.; Hamada, Y.; Kojima, M.; Kumagai, S.; Iwasaki, A.; Suenaga, K. Allelopathic Substances of *Osmanthus* spp. for Developing Sustainable Agriculture. *Plants* **2023**, *12*, 376. https://doi.org/10.3390/plants12020376

Academic Editors: Margot Schulz and Vincenzo Tabaglio

Received: 7 December 2022
Revised: 10 January 2023
Accepted: 10 January 2023
Published: 13 January 2023



## 1. Introduction

*Osmanthus fragrans* Lour., belonging to the Oleaceae family, is an evergreen tree that is 3–5 m high, and has been cultivated for more than 2500 years in China and some other countries because of the fragrance and color of the flowers [1–3]. The flowers are used in traditional tea, liquors, and foods. The essential oil is extracted for perfume. Its roots are used in traditional Chinese medicine such as in treatments for stomach ache, toothache, rheumatism, and muscle pain [4]. Pharmacological and phytochemical investigations of the chemical constituents in the plants and its essential oil suggest that the species contains more than 180 compounds, including terpenoids, phenylpropanoids, polyphenols, flavonoids, and sterols. Some of those compounds, such as ionone, flavonoids, iridoids, and polyphenols, have shown pharmacological functions through an anti-hyperglycemic activity, anti-inflammatory activity, anti-melanogenesis activity, antioxidant activity, and antitumor activity [3,5–10]. There has been limited information available on the allelopathic activity of the leaf extracts of *O. fragrans* in a publication using it as Chinese medicine [11]. However, no information is available on the compounds involved in the allelopathy of *O. fragrans*.

Allelopathy is the interaction between donor plants and receiver plants through certain secondary metabolites defined as allelochemicals, which are synthesized in some plant parts and released into the vicinity of the donner plants, including the rhizosphere soil, through the volatilization and rainfall leachates from the plants, root exudation, and decomposition process of plant residues, including fallen leaves. Allelopathy is able to provide a competitive advantage to the donner plants for resources such as nutrients, water, and light, through the inhibition of the germination and growth of the neighboring competitive plants [12–15]. The plant parts and the extracts of several plant species have shown an excellent weed control ability as mulch and soil additives due to their allelopathic characteristic [16–18]. Therefore, the allelopathy of plants is potentially useful for weed management options in several agriculture settings in order to reduce commercial herbicide dependency for the development of sustainable agriculture [19,20].

The *Osmanthus* genus consists of about 30 species, mostly native to Eastman Asia. *Osmanthus × fortunei* Carrière is a hybrid species between *O. fragrans* and *Osmanthus heterophyllus* (G.Don) P.S.Green. The leaves of *O. heterophyllus* show a serrate leaf margin and *O. fragran* leaves show no serration, and the hybrid species *O. × fortunei* has a combination of both of these characteristics (Figure 1). These plant species are evergreen trees but their senescent leaves fall, and the fallen leaves accumulate on the soil surfaces under the trees (Figure 2). Tree plants are able to release allelopathic substances into their rhizosphere soil over many years through the decomposition process of their fallen leaves. Those liberated compounds from the leaves may accumulate in the soil, and suppress the germination and growth of other plant species [21–23]. Therefore, some allelopathic substances can be released into the rhizosphere soil during the decomposition process of the fallen leaves of *O. fragrans*, *O. heterophyllus*, and *O. × fortune*, and act as allelopathic agents [13–15]. The objective of this study was the investigation of the allelopathic activity of the leaves of *O. fragrans*, *O. heterophyllus*, and *O. × fortune*, and the determination of the main allelopathic substances in their leaves for the development of sustainable agriculture.

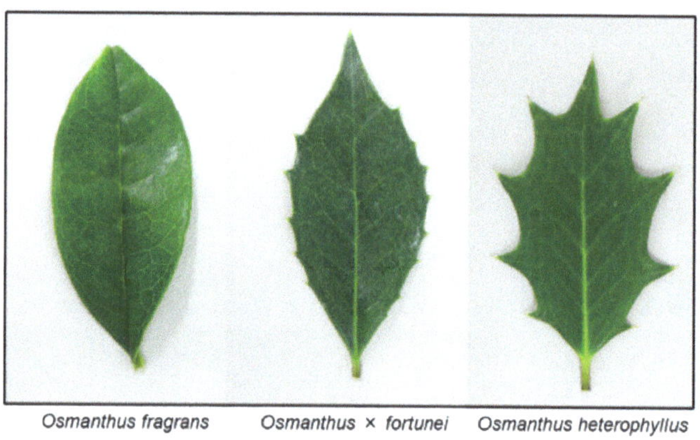


**Figure 1.** The leaves of *O. fragrans*, *O. × fortunei*, and *O. heterophyllus*.

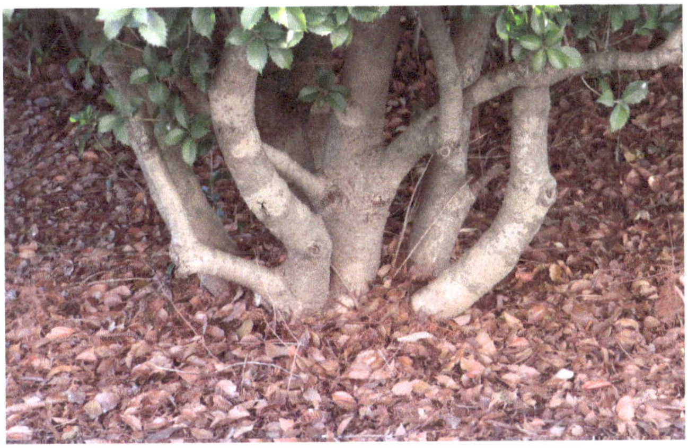

**Figure 2.** The accumulation of the fallen leaves on the soil under the tree of *O.* × *fortune*.

## 2. Results

### 2.1. Allelopathic Activity of the Leaves of O. fragrans, O. heterophyllus and O. × fortunei

The extracts of *O. fragrans* leaves significantly inhibited the hypocotyl and root growth of the dicotyledonous plants, namely cress and alfalfa at concentrations greater than 30–100 mg leaf equivalent extract per mL. The extract also significantly inhibited the coleoptile and root growth of the monocotyledonous weed plants, namely *V. myuros* and *L. multiflorom* at concentrations greater than 10–30 mg leaf equivalent extract per mL (Figure 3). The extracts of *O. heterophyllus* and *O.* × *fortunei* also showed an inhibitory activity on the growth of cress, alfalfa, *V. myuros*, and *L. multiflorom* (Figures 4 and 5). Increasing the extract concentration of *O. fragrans*, *O. heterophyllus*, and *O.* × *fortunei* resulted in an increase in the growth suppression of the hypocotyls/coleoptiles and roots of both dicotyledonous and monocotyledonous plant species (Figures 3–5).

Table 1 shows the $IC_{50}$ values of the extracts of *O. fragrans*, *O.* × *fortune*, and *O. heterophyllus*, which can cause 50% growth inhibition on the hypocotyls/coleoptiles and roots of the test plant species, and indicate that smaller values show a higher growth inhibitory activity than large values. All $IC_{50}$ values of the *O.* × *fortune* extracts, except the $IC_{50}$ value for *V. myuros* roots, were smaller than those of the *O. fragrans* and *O. heterophyllus* extracts.

**Table 1.** $IC_{50}$ values (mg leaf equivalent extract per mL) of the extracts of the leaves of *O. fragrans*, *O.* × *fortunei*, and *O. heterophyllus* on the growth of hypocotyls/coleoptiles and the roots of bioassay plant species. $IC_{50}$ values were determined with GraphPad Prism. Different letters in the same column indicate significant differences (Tukey's HSD test, $p \leq 0.05$).

| | *Osmanthus fragrans* | | *Osmanthus* × *fortunei* | | *Osmanthus heterophyllus* | |
|---|---|---|---|---|---|---|
| | **Hypocotyl/ Coleoptile** | **Root** | **Hypocotyl/ Coleoptile** | **Root** | **Hypocotyl/ Coleoptile** | **Root** |
| Cress | 63.8 ± 4.2 b | 63.7 ± 4.7 b | 24.8 ± 1.9 c | 36.5 ± 1.9 c | 11.7 ± 1.1 bc | 59.1 ± 4.7 b |
| Alfalfa | 107 ± 8.1 a | 153 ± 9.7 a | 53.1 ± 4.2 bc | 68.5 ± 7.4 b | 76.5 ± 6.7 b | 114 ± 9.9 a |
| *Lolium multiflorum* | 82.6 ± 4.9 ab | 30.4 ± 2.5 c | 21.5 ± 1.6 c | 12.4 ± 0.9 d | 29.5 ± 3.1 c | 13.8 ± 0.9 d |
| *Vulpia myuros* | 25.9 ± 2.1 c | 8.8 ± 0.9 d | 21.4 ± 1.7 c | 11.5 ± 0.9 d | 36.8 ± 3.2 c | 13.8 ± 1.1 d |

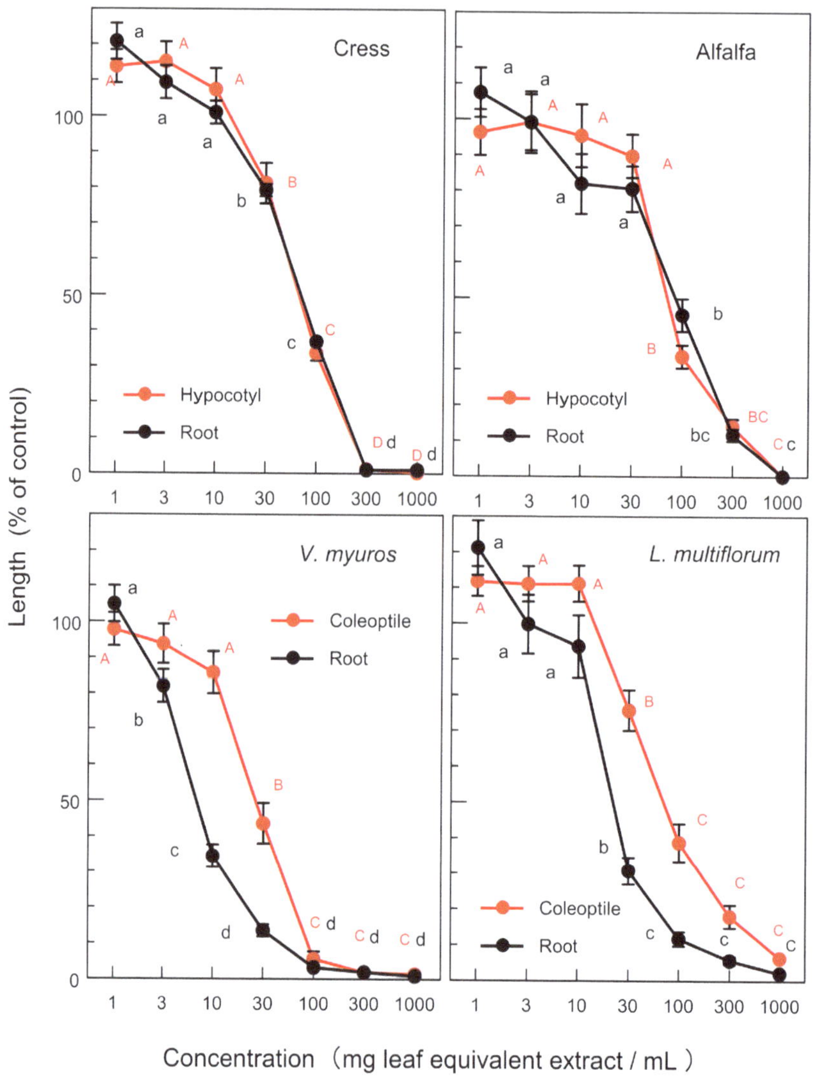


**Figure 3.** Effects of the extracts of *O. fragrans* leaves on the growth of the hypocotyls and roots of cress and alfalfa, and the growth of the coleoptiles and roots of *L. multiflorum* and *V. myuros*. Concentration (mg leaf equivalent extract/mL) indicates the concentration of the tested sample corresponding to the extracts obtained from 1, 3, 10, 30, 100, 300, and 1000 mg leaves per mL. Different letters on the symbols in the same panels indicate significant differences (Tukey's HSD test, $p \leq 0.05$).

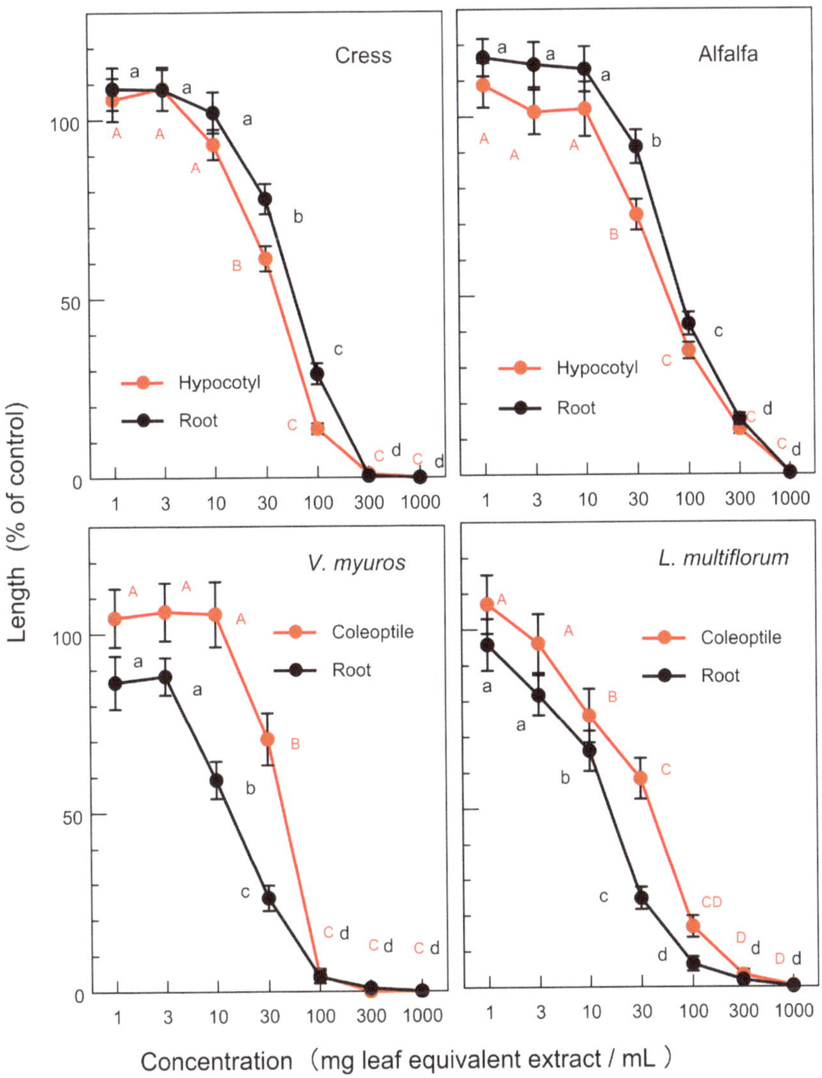


**Figure 4.** Effects of the extracts of *O. heterophyllus* leaves on the growth of the hypocotyls and roots of cress and alfalfa, and the growth of the coleoptiles and roots of *L. multiflorum* and *V. myuros*. Concentration (mg leaf equivalent extract/mL) indicates the concentration of the tested sample corresponding to the extracts obtained from 1, 3, 10, 30, 100, 300, and 1000 mg leaves per mL. Different letters on the symbols in the same panels indicate significant differences (Tukey's HSD test, $p \leq 0.05$).

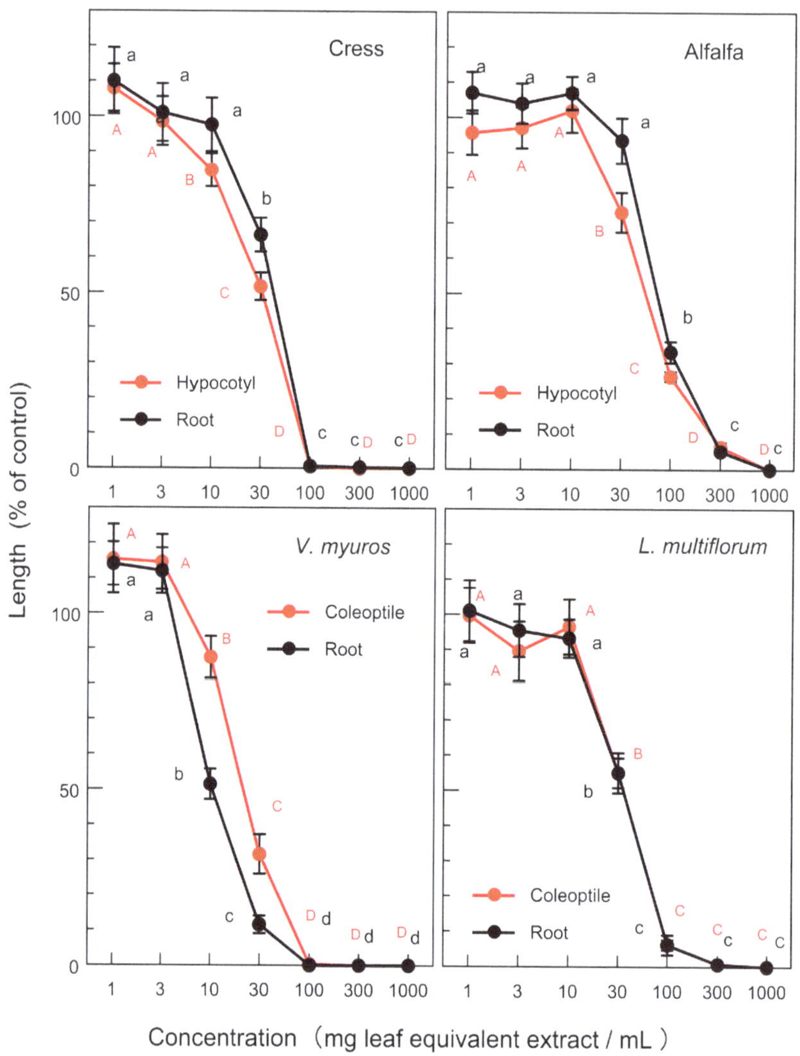


**Figure 5.** Effects of the extracts of *O.* × *fortunei* leaves on the growth of the hypocotyls and roots of cress and alfalfa, and the growth of the coleoptiles and roots of *L. multiflorum* and *V. myuros*. Concentration (mg leaf equivalent extract/mL) indicates the concentration of tested sample corresponding to the extracts obtained from 1, 3, 10, 30, 100, 300, and 1000 mg leaves per mL. Different letters on the symbols in the same panels indicate significant differences (Tukey's HSD test, $p \leq 0.05$).

### 2.2. Identification of Compound 1 and Its Activity

The extract of *O.* × *fortunei* leaves was partitioned with ethyl acetate. The activity of the obtained ethyl acetate phase was much greater than that of the aqueous phase (Table 2). Therefore, the ethyl acetate phase was separated using the chromatography of the silica gel, Sephadex LH-20, and ODS cartridge. The allelopathic activity of all of the separated fractions was determined by a cress bioassay after each chromatographic separation, as described above, and the most active fraction was carried out following chromatographic separation. Finally, active compound **1** was isolated by HPLC.

**Table 2.** Effects of the aqueous and ethyl acetate phase obtained after the partition of the extracts of *O. fragrans*, *O. heterophyllus*, and *O.* × *fortunei* on the growth of the hypocotyl and roots of the cress (% of control). The activity was determined using the test samples obtained from 100 mg of leaf equivalent extract/mL. Different letters in the same column indicate significant differences (Tukey's HSD test, $p \leq 0.05$).

| | *Osmanthus fragrans* | | *Osmanthus* × *fortunei* | | *Osmanthus heterophyllus* | |
|---|---|---|---|---|---|---|
| | **Hypocotyl** | **Root** | **Hypocotyl** | **Root** | **Hypocotyl** | **Root** |
| Aqueous phase | 76.8 ± 7.5 a | 101 ± 9.8 a | 76.2 ± 4.3 a | 62.4 ± 4.8 a | 87.1 ± 4.0 a | 70.9 ± 4.6 b |
| Ethyl acetate phase | 46.8 ± 4.4 b | 27.1 ± 2.7 b | 22.4 ± 3.6 b | 19.9 ± 3.9 b | 31.9 ± 3.7 b | 29.7 ± 2.9 b |

The molecular formula of compound **1** is $C_{20}H_{22}O_6$, as suggested by HRESIMS at $m/z$ 359.1478 $[M + H]^+$ (calcd for $C_{20}H_{23}O_6$ 359.1495). The $^1$H NMR (400 MHz, $CD_3OD$) spectrum of compound **1** showed $\delta_H$ 6.95 (d, $J$ = 1.9 Hz, 2 H, H-2/2′), 6.81 (dd, $J$ = 8.4, 1.9 Hz, 2 H, H-6/6′), 6.77 (d, $J$ = 8.4 Hz, 2 H, H-5/5′), 4.71 (d, $J$ = 4.5 Hz, 2 H, H-7/7′), 4.23 (dd, $J$ = 9.5, 7.0 Hz, 2 H, H-9a/9a′), 3.86 (s, 6 H, H-10/10′), 3.84 (dd, $J$ = 9.5, 3.9 Hz, 2 H, H-9b/9b′), and 3.14 (m, 2 H, H-8/8′). The optical rotation of the compound was $[\alpha]_D^{27}$ = +84.5 ($c$ = 0.215, $CH_3OH$). The chemical structure of compound **1** was determined as (+)-pinoresinol (Figure 6) by the comparison of those spectra data with the published data [24]. (+)-Pinoresinol (1) significantly inhibited the growth of hypocotyls/coleoptiles and the roots of the cress and *L. multiflorum* at concentrations greater than 0.3 mM. The inhibition increased with the increasing concentration of (+)-pinoresinol (Figure 7). The $IC_{50}$ values of (+)-pinoresinol of the growth hypocotyls/coleoptiles and the roots of cress and *L. multiflorum* are shown in Table 3.

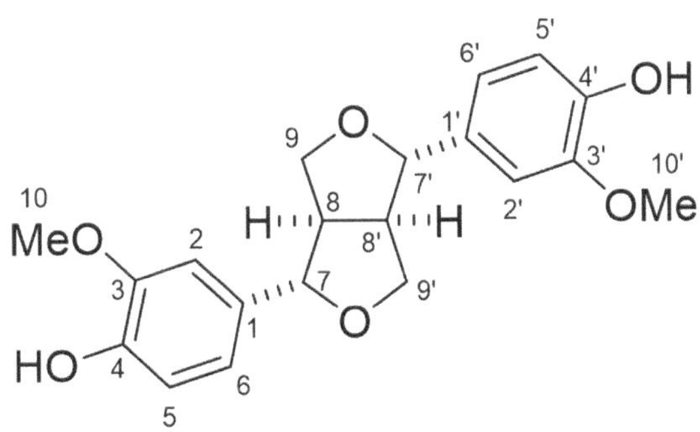


**Figure 6.** Chemical structure of (+)-pinoresinol.

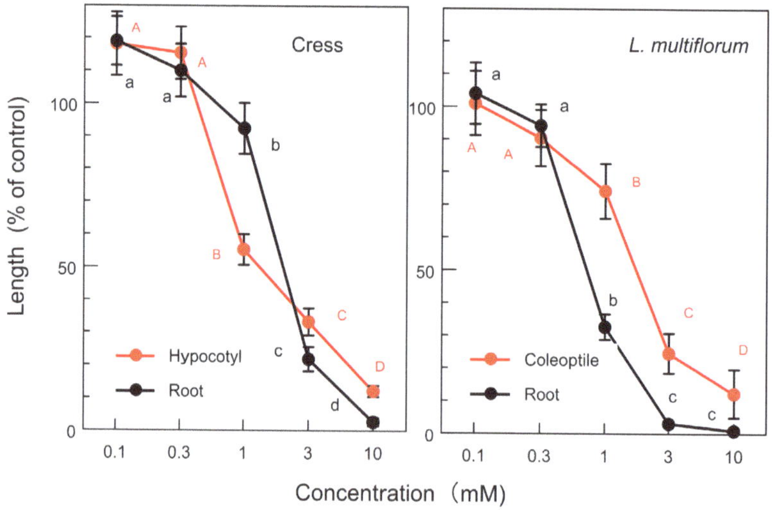


**Figure 7.** Effects of (+)-pinoresinol on the hypocotyl/coleoptile and root growth of cress and *L. multiflorum*. Means ± SE from three independent experiments with 10 seedlings for each determination are shown. Different letters on the symbols in the same panels indicate significant differences (Tukey's HSD test, $p \leq 0.05$).

**Table 3.** $IC_{50}$ values (mM) of (+)-pinoresinol and 10-acetoxyligustroside of the growth of the hypocotyls/coleoptiles and roots of the cress and *L. multiflorum*. $IC_{50}$ values were determined with GraphPad Prism. Different letters in the same column indicate significant differences (Tukey's HSD test, $p \leq 0.05$).

| | **(+)-Pinoresinol** | | **10-Acetoxyligustroside** | |
|---|---|---|---|---|
| | **Hypocotyl/ Coleoptile** | **Root** | **Hypocotyl/ Coleoptile** | **Root** |
| Cress | 1.9 ± 0.2 a | 2.5 ± 0.3 b | 4.7 ± 0.3 b | 4.4 ± 0.3 a |
| *Lolium multiflorum* | 2.1 ± 0.3 a | 0.7 ± 0.1 d | 3.1 ± 0.3 b | 2.2 ± 0.2 b |

### *2.3. Concentration of (+)-Pinoresinol in the Leaves of O. × fortune, O. fragrans, and O. heterophyllus*

The concentration of (+)-pinoresinol (1) in the mature leaves of *O. × fortune* was 4.1 mg/g and the concentration of its fallen leaves was 2.1 mg/g. However, the mature leaves *O. fragrans* and *O. heterophyllus* showed a small amount of (+)-pinoresinol (Table 4).

**Table 4.** The concentration of (+)-pinoresinol in the mature and fallen leaves of *O. × fortunei*, and in the mature leaves of *O. fragrans* and *O. heterophyllus*. Different letters indicate significant differences (Tukey's HSD test, $p \leq 0.05$).

| *Osmanthus × fortunei* | (+)-Pinoresinol (mg/g) |
|---|---|
| Mature leaf | 4.1 ± 0.5 a |
| Fallen leaf | 2.1 ± 0.2 b |
| *Osmanthus fragrans* | 0.22 ± 0.03 c |
| *Osmanthus heterophyllus* | 0.12 ± 0.02 c |

### 2.4. *Identification of Compound 2 and Its Activity*

The extract of *O. fragrans* leaves was partitioned with ethyl acetate. The activity of the obtained ethyl acetate phase was much greater than that of the aqueous phase (Table 2). The ethyl acetate phase was separated using the chromatography of the silica gel, Sephadex LH-20, and $C_{18}$ cartridge. The allelopathic activity of all separated fractions was determined by a cress bioassay after each separation step, and the most active fraction was applied to the next separation, and an active compound **2** was finally isolated by HPLC.

The molecular formula of compound **2** is $C_{27}H_{34}O_{1}$, as suggested by HRESIMS at $m/z$ 605.1836 $[M + Na]^+$ (calculated for $C_{27}H_{34}O_{14}Na$, 605.1846). The $^1$H NMR (400 MHz, $CD_3OD$) spectrum of the compound **2** showed $\delta_H$ 7.53 (s, 1 H, H3), 7.05 (d, $J$ = 8.6 Hz, 2 H, H2′, H6′), 6.71 (d, $J$ = 8.6 Hz, 2 H, H3′, H5′), 6.08 (brdd, $J$ = 7.7, 5.9 Hz, 1 H, H8), 5.98 (brs, 1 H, H1), 4.82 (d, $J$ = 7.7 Hz, 1 H, H1″), 4.76 (dd, $J$ = 13.1, 7.7 Hz, 1 H, H10), 4.56 (ddd, $J$ = 13.3, 5.9, 1.8 Hz, 1 H, H10), 4.24 (ddd, $J$ = 10.8, 7.3, 7.3 Hz, 1 H, H8′), 4.14 (ddd, $J$ = 10.8, 7.3, 7.3 Hz, 1 H, H8′), 4.00 (dd, $J$ = 10.0, 4.1 Hz, 1 H, H5), 3.90 (dd, $J$ = 11.8, 1.4 Hz, 1 H, H6″), 3.72 (s, 3 H, H14), 3.67 (dd, $J$ = 11.8, 5.9 Hz, 1 H, H6″), 3.41 (dd, $J$ = 8.6, 9.2 Hz, H3″), 3.35 (m, 1 H, H5″), 3.34 (m, 1 H, H2″) 3.33 (m, 1 H, H4″), 2.83 (t, $J$ = 7.3 Hz, 1 H, H7′), 2.77 (dd, $J$ = 15.4, 4.1 Hz, 1 H, H6), 2.50 (dd, $J$ = 15.4, 9.5 Hz, 1 H, H6), and 2.02 (s, 3 H, H13). The $^{13}$C NMR (100 MHz, $CD_3OD$) spectrum of the compound showed $\delta_C$ 172.8 (C7), 172.5 (C12), 168.3 (C11), 157.1 (C4′), 154.9 (C3), 133.9 (C9), 131.0 (C2′, C6′), 130.0 (C1′), 124.4 (C8), 116.3 (C3′, C5′), 109.1 (C4), 100.8 (C1″), 94.2 (C1), 78.5 (C3″), 77.9 (C5″), 74.7 (C2″), 71.4 (C4″), 66.9 (C8′), 62.7 (C6″), 61.8 (C10), 52.0 (C14), 41.0 (C6), 35.2 (C7′), 32.4 (C5), and 20.8 (C13). The optical rotation of the compound was $[\alpha]_D^{27}$-163 ($c$ 0.32, $CH_3OH$). Those spectra indicate that the chemical structure of compound **2** is 10-acetoxyligustroside (Figure 8), in comparison with those reported in the literature [25]. The compound significantly inhibited the growth of the hypocotyls/coleoptiles and roots of cress and *L. multiflorum* at concentrations greater than 1 mM (Figure 9). $IC_{50}$ values of 10-acetoxyligustroside of the growth of the hypocotyls/coleoptiles and roots of cress and *L. multiflorum* are shown in Table 3.

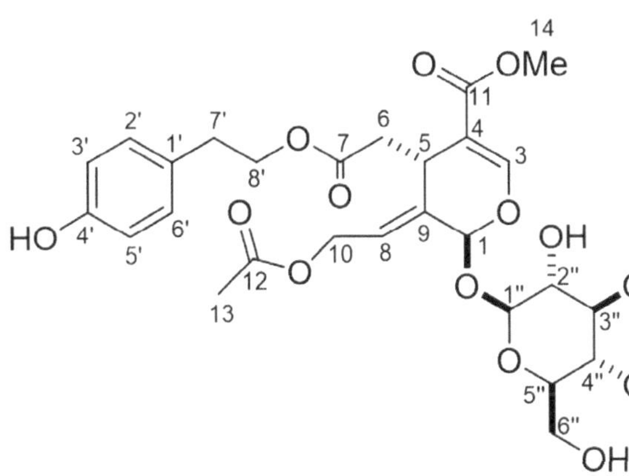


**Figure 8.** Chemical structure of 10-acetoxyligustroside.

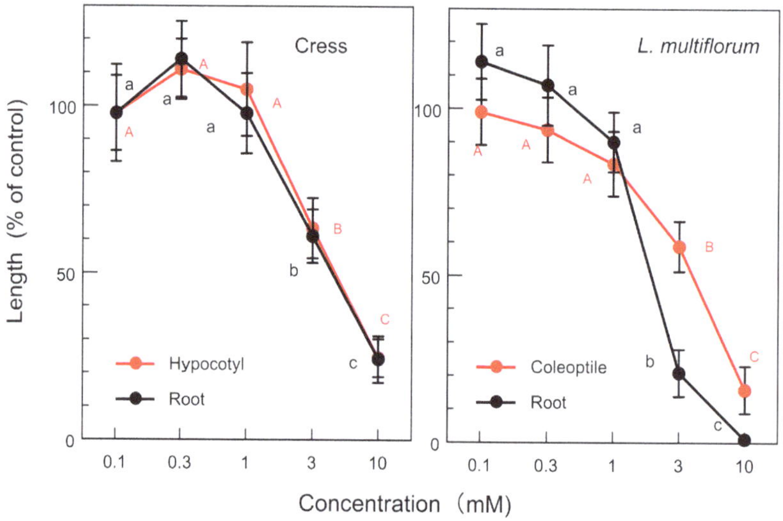


**Figure 9.** Effects of 10-acetoxyligustroside on the hypocotyl/coleoptile and root growth of cress and *L. multiflorum*. Means ± SE from three independent experiments with 10 seedlings for each determination are shown. Different letters on the symbols in the same panels indicate significant differences (Tukey's HSD test, $p \leq 0.05$).

## 3. Discussion

The leaf extracts of *O. fragrans*, *O. heterophyllus*, and *O.* × *fortunei* showed allelopathic activity against the growth of dicotyledonous plants (cress and alfalfa) and monocotyledonous weed plants (*L. multiflorum* and *V. myuros*) (Figures 3–5). As allelopathic substances are synthesized and stored in some plant parts until their release into the environments [12–15], the inhibitory activity of these leaves suggest that these plant species may produce and accumulate the allelopathic substances in their leaves. All of the $IC_{50}$ values of *O.* × *fortunei* on the growth of the hypocotyls/coleoptiles and roots of four test plant species were the smallest compared with those of *O. fragrans* and *O. heterophyllus* except for the $IC_{50}$ value on the root growth of *V. myuros*. $IC_{50}$ values on the root growth of *V. myuros* and *O.* × *fortunei* are not significantly different (Table 1). Thus, the leaf extract of a hybrid species of *O.* × *fortunei* was the most active among the extracts of *O. fragrans*, *O. heterophyllus*, and *O.* × *fortunei*. The accumulation of the allelopathic substances in the leaves of *O.* × *fortunei* could be greater than that of the other two species. *Fallopia japonica* (Houtt.) Ronse Decraene and *Fallopia sachalinensis* (F. Schmidt) Ronse Decraene are highly competitive invasive plant species [26,27]. *F. japonica* and *F. sachalinensis* hybridize unnaturally by asexual reproduction and create a hybrid species, *Fallopia* × *bohemica* (Chrteket Chrtková) J.P. Bailey [28]. Hybridization of the both species gives genetic diversity to *F.* × *bohemica* [29,30], and the invasiveness of the hybrid species *F.* × *bohemica* is high [31,32].

The allelopathic activity is usually evaluated on the basis of the specific activity of the compound such as ppm and $IC_{50}$. However, when we evaluated the contribution of the allelochemicals to the certain plant species, the concentration of the allelochemicals in the plants needs to be considered. For example, allelochemicals, which were contained in large amounts with a moderate activity, contributed more than those that contained a small amount with a very strong activity as the allelopathic agents of the plants. The concept of the total activity included both factors; the specific activity of a compound and its concentration in the plant materials, which indicates the contribution of the compounds to the allelopathy of the plants [33]. When we compare the activity of the extracts and separated fractions obtained from same weight of the plant materials, we could evaluate the total activity of the extracts and fractions, and we chose the most active extracts and fractions as described by Dr. Fujil's group [33]. Therefore, we evaluated the activity of the separated fractions using the concept of total activity, and selected the most active separated fraction.

The most active extract of *O.* × *fortunei* leaves among the extracts of the three species was partitioned with ethyl acetate, and the ethyl acetate phase was separated as described in Section 4.4. After each chromatographic separation, the total activity of all of the separated fractions was determined by a cress bioassay, and the most active fraction was carried out next in chromatographic separation, and an active compound was isolated. The total activity of the fractions was equivalent by the plant material basis (10 and 100 mg plant materials) [33]. During the isolation process of the active compound, the cress seeds were used as the test plant because the sensitivity of the cress to the extracts was not low or high among the four test plant species (Table 1). Based on its spectrum data compared with the published data [24], the chemical structure of the isolated compound 1 was identified as (+)-pinoresinol (Figure 6). (+)-Pinoresinol may be the main contributor to the allelopathic activity of the extract of *O.* × *fortunei* leaves because the compound was isolated from the most active fraction (total activity) of every separation step.

(+)-Pinoresinol is a tetrahydrofuran lignan and is synthesized from two coniferyl alcohol monomers [34–36]. The compound inhibited the growth of cress and *L. multiflorum* (Figure 7), and the $IC_{50}$ values of the compound on the growth of the hypocotyls/coleoptiles and roots of cress and *L. multiflorum* were 0.7–2.5 mM (Table 3). The compound was also reported to show a growth inhibitory activity on the wheat coleoptiles [37], as well as an antifungal activity, antioxidative activity, and hepatoprotective activity in mammalian cells [38–40].

The concentration of (+)-pinoresinol in the fallen leaves of *O.* × *fortune* was less than that in its manure leaves, which indicates that degradation of the compound may occur during the senescence of the leaves or through some other factors. However, the fallen leaves of *O.* × *fortune* still contained 51% (+)-pinoresinol of its mature leaves (Table 4). *O.* × *fortune* is evergreen, but their senescent leaves cover the soil under the trees (Figure 2). The fallen leaves were gradually decomposed and decayed into the soil in the same way as other tree leaves [41–43]. It is possible that (+)-pinoresinol in the fallen leaves may be liberated through the decomposition process of the leaves and accumulate in their rhizosphere soil over many years. The accumulated (+)-pinoresinol may be able to suppress the germination and growth of other plant species as an allelopathic agent.

The concentration of (+)-pinoresinol in the mature leaves *O. fragrans* and *O. heterophyllus* was 0.22 mg/g and 0.12 mg/g, respectively (Table 4). It was also reported that 13 mg of (+)-pinoresinol-β-D-glucopyranoside was isolated from 2.6 kg of *O. heterophyllus* leaves [44], which is equivalent to 0.005 mg/g. The concentration of (+)-pinoresinol in the mature leaves of *O.* × *fortune* was 18.6-fold and 34.2-hfold greater than that of *O. fragrans* and *O. heterophyllus*, respectively. *O. fragrans* and *O. heterophyllus* are the parents of the hybrid species *O.* × *fortune*. Thus, the hybridization of both species may increase the biosynthesis of (+)-pinoresinol.

Based on the $IC_{50}$ values, the allelopathic activity of *O. fragrans* was 38–94% and 40–130% that of *O.* × *fortune* for the growth of the hypocolyls/coleoptiles and roots, respectively, of the four test plant species, and the allelopathic activity of *O. heterophyllus* was 59–72% and 60–89% that of *O.* × *fortune* for their growth of hypocolyls/coleoptiles and roots, respectively (Table 1). However, the concentration of (+)-pinoresinol in the mature leaves of *O. fragrans* and *O. heterophyllus* was only 5% and 3%, respectively, of that in the mature leaves of *O.* × *fortune* (Table 4). Thus, (+)-pinoresinol may not be a main allelopathic substance in the leaves of *O. fragrans* and *O. heterophyllus*.

The extract of *O. fragrans* leaves after being separated is described in Section 4.5, and an allelopathic substance was isolated and identified as 10-acetoxyligustroside (Figure 8) based on its spectrum data compared with the published data [25]. 10-Acetoxyligustroside is an iridoid glycoside and is synthesized from iridodial [45,46]. The compound inhibited the growth of cress and *L. multiflorum* (Figure 9), and the $IC_{50}$ values of the compound on the hypocotyls/coleoptiles and roots of the cress and *L. multiflorum* were 2.2–4.7 mM (Table 3). There is limited information about 10-acetoxyligustroside regarding the biological activity, including the allelopathic activity, in the literature. This paper is the first report showing the allelopathic activity of 10-acetoxyligustroside. In addition, 10-acetoxyligustroside may be the main contributor to the allelopathic activity of *O. fragrans* leaves because the compound was isolated from the most active fraction in every separation step.

The extract of *O. heterophyllus* leaves was also partition with ethyl acetate (Table 2), and the ethyl acetate phase was separated using the chromatography of the silica gel, Sephadex LH-20, and $C_{18}$ cartridge for the isolation of the main allelopathic substances, similar to other leaf extracts of *O. fragrans* and *O.* × *fortunei*. However, many active fractions were identified in every separation step, and we could not isolate the main allelopathic substances from the extracts. Several lignans, neolignan glycosides, and secoiridoid glycosides were isolated from *O. heterophyllus* leaves, but their biological activities have not yet been reported [47–49]. There has also been no information available on the allelopathic substances in *O. heterophyllus* leaves. Considering these investigations, many allelopathic substances including (+)-pinoresinol may be involved in the allelopathy of *O. heterophyllus*. Therefore, the extracts of the leaves of these *Osmanthus* species have allelopathic potential and contain allelopathic substances, which may be species specific. However, it is necessary to determine the concentrations of these compounds in the rhizosphere soil, and to clarify the contribution of these compounds to their allelopathy.

## 4. Materials and Methods

### *4.1. Plant Material*

Mature leaves of *O. fragrans* and *O. heterophyllus*, and mature and fallen leaves of *O.* × *fortunei* were obtained from the campus of Faculty of Agriculture, Kagawa University, and the nearest botanical garden. Collected leaves were weighed and kept at −25 °C. The seeds of cress (*Lepidum sativum* L.) and alfalfa (*Medicago sativa* L.) were used to determine the allelopathic activity because of their stable germination. Weed species of *Vulpia myuros* (L.) C.C. Gmel. and *Lolium multiflorum* Lam. were also used to test the allelopathic activity.

### *4.2. Extraction*

Mature leaves (50 g fresh weight) of *O. fragrans*, *O. heterophyllus* and *O.* × *fortunei* were cut into small pieces and extracted separately with 80% ($v/v$) aqueous methanol (300 mL) for 2 days. The extracts were filtered with a filter paper (No. 2; Toyo Ltd., Tokyo, Japan), and the residue of each extract was extracted again with methanol (300 mL) for 2 days and then filtered. Two filtrates of each species were mixed and concentrated under reduced pressure at 40 °C [50]. The yield of the extracts of *O. fragrans*, *O. heterophyllus*, and *O.* × *fortunei* was 0.62, 0.57 g, and 0.69 g, respectively.

### *4.3. Determination of Allelopathic Activity*

The concentrated extracts of *O. fragrans*, *O. heterophyllus*, and *O.* × *fortunei* were dissolved with methanol, and a given quantity of the methanol solution was applied to a filter paper (No. 2) in a Petri dish (2.8 cm i.d.). After the methanol solution was completely evaporated in a draft chamber, 0.6 mL of Tween 20 solution (0.05%, Nacalai, Kyoto, Japan) was added onto the filter paper. Ten seeds of alfalfa and cress and 10 germinated seeds of *L. multiflorum* and *V. myuros*, which had been germinated for 48 h in the dark at 25 °C, were separately arranged on the filter paper in the Petri dishes. After 48 h of incubation in the dark at 25 °C, the length of the roots and hypocotyls/coleoptiles of these four test plants was measured using a ruler. The percentage length of the hypocotyls/coleoptiles and roots of the test plant species treated with the leaf extracts was determined against that of each of the control seedlings. The control seedlings were treated exactly same process without the extract application [50]. The concentrations of the applied extracts in the Petri dishes were 1, 3, 10, 30, 100, 300, and 1000 mg leaf equivalent extracts per mL. The concentrations of the extract caused for the 50% growth inhibition (defined as $IC_{50}$) of these test plant species were determined with GraphPad Prism 6.0 (GraphPad Software, Inc., La Jolla, CA, USA). The determination of the allelopathic activity was repeated four times using a completely randomized design with 10 plants for each determination.

### 4.4. Separation of O. × fortunei Extract

The leaves (100 g fresh weight) of *O. × fortunei* were extracted with 80% (*v*/*v*) aqueous methanol (600 mL) and methanol (600 mL), and were filtrated. Two filtrates were mixed and evaporated to obtain an aqueous solution, as described above. Then, the aqueous solution was made to pH 7.0 with the buffer of 0.5 M phosphate, and partitioned four times with ethyl acetate. Obtained ethyl acetate phase was concentrated to dryness, and applied to a silica gel (100 g, silica gel 60, 70–230 mesh; Nacarai, Kyoto, Japan) chromatography, which was eluted with 100 mL each of 20, 30, 40, 50, 60, 70, and 80% (*v*/*v*) ethyl acetate in *n*-hexane and ethyl acetate, and 200 mL of methanol. The allelopathic activity of those nine fractions was determined using cress seeds, as described in the Section 4.3. The activity was found in a fraction obtained by an elution of 80% ethyl acetate in *n*-hexane.

After the active fraction was evaporated, the residue was separated by a chromatography of Sephadex LH-20 (50 g, GE Healthcare, Uppsala, Sweden) and eluted with 100 mL each of 20, 30, 40, 50, 60, 70, 80, and 90% (*v*/*v*) aqueous methanol and 200 mL of methanol. An active fraction was obtained with the elution of 60% aqueous methanol, and the active residue was further separated using a reverse-phase ODS cartridge (YMC-Dispo Pack AT ODS-25; YMC Ltd., Kyoto, Japan), which was eluted with 150 mL each of 30, 40, 50, 60, 70, 80, and 90% (*v*/*v*) aqueous methanol. The active fraction was obtained by the elution with 50% aqueous methanol, and the residue was finally subjected to a reverse-phase HPLC (4.6 i.d. × 150 mm, μBondasphere 5μ $C_{18}$-100Å, Waters Co., Ltd. (Milford, MA, USA), detection 220 nm) and eluted with 45% aqueous methanol (flow rate; 1.5 mL/min). The allelopathic activity was found in a peak fraction eluted between 125–130 min, yielding active compound **1**. The chemical structure of compound **1** was characterized by the analyses of the HRESIMS (LCT Premier XE time-of-flight TOF mass spectrometer, Waters, Tokyo) and $^1$H-NMR spectrum (400 MHz, $CD_3OD$; JNM-ECX400, JEOL, Tokyo, Japan), and the optical rotation.

### 4.5. Separation of O. fragrans Extract

The leaves (500 g fresh weight) of *O. fragrans* were extracted with 80% (*v*/*v*) aqueous methanol (3 L) and methanol (3 L), and separated by silica gel chromatography, as described above. An active fraction was obtained with the elution of methanol, and the active residue was applied to the second silica gel chromatography, which was eluted with 100 mL each of ethyl acetate, and 25, 50, and 75% (*v*/*v*) acetone in ethyl acetate, acetone, and methanol. The activity was obtained by the elution of 25% acetone in ethyl acetate, and the residue was applied to a chromatography of Sephadex LH-20, and eluted with 100 mL each of 20, 30, 40, 50, 60, 70, 80, and 90% (*v*/*v*) aqueous methanol. An active fraction obtained with 30% aqueous methanol was further purified using $C_{18}$ cartridges (YMC Ltd.), and eluted with 15 mL each of 30, 40, 50, 60, 70, 80, and 90% (*v*/*v*) aqueous methanol. The active fraction was obtained by the elution of 30% aqueous methanol. The active residue was subjected to a reverse-phase HPLC (10 i.d. × 500 mm, ODS-AQ 5μ YMC-Pack, YMC, detection 220 nm) eluted with 45% aqueous methanol (1.5 mL/min). The allelopathic activity was found in a peak fraction eluted between 104–105 min, yielding active compound **2**. The chemical structure of compound **2** was characterized by the analyses of HRESIMS and $^1$H-NMR (400 MHz, $CD_3OD$), $^{13}$C-NMR (100 MHz, $CD_3OD$) spectra and the optical rotation.

### 4.6. Allelopathic Activity of Isolated Compounds 1 and 2

Each of isolated compounds **1** and **2** was dissolved with methanol, and a given quantity of the methanol solution was added onto a filter paper in the Petri dish. After the evaporation of methanol in the Petri dishes, the filter paper was moistened with 0.6 mL Tween 20. Then, 10 seeds of cress and 10 germinated seeds of *L. multiflorum*, were separately arranged on the filter paper and incubated in the dark at 25 °C for 48 h. The allelopathic activity of the compounds and its $IC_{50}$ values were determined as described in Section 4.3.

### 4.7. Concentration of Compound 1 in the Leaves

Mature and fallen leaves (5 g) of *O.* × *fortune*, and mature leaves (5 g) of *O. fragrans* and *O. heterophyllus* were separately extracted and partitioned with ethyl acetate, as described above. The obtained residue was applied to a silica gel chromatography, and eluted with 100 mL each of 60, 70, and 80% ($v/v$) ethyl acetate in *n*-hexane. After evaporation of the fraction eluted with 80% ethyl acetate in *n*-hexane, the residue was applied to a reverse-phase $C_{18}$ cartridge, and eluted with 15 mL each of 30, 40, and 50% ($v/v$) aqueous methanol. The fraction obtained by the elution of 40% aqueous methanol was subjected to a reverse-phase HPLC (4.6 i.d. × 250 mm, Cosmosil, Nacalai, detection 220 nm) eluted with 40% aqueous methanol (0.8 mL/min). The quantification of compound **1** was performed by the peak area on the HPLC chromatograms of samples. The recovery of compound **1** added to the leave extracts was 95 ± 11% (mean ± SE) as calculated from three replications.

### 4.8. Statistical Analysis

The data were subjected to a one-way analysis of ANOVA and subsequent post hoc analysis with Tukey's HSD test ($p < 0.05$). $IC_{50}$ values were obtained using GraphPad Prism 6.0.

## 5. Conclusions

The leaf extracts of *O. fragrans*, *O. heterophyllus*, and *O.* × *fortunei* showed an allelopathic activity on the four test plant species, including the weed species of *Vulpia myuros* and *Lolium multiflorum*. The allelopathic substances of *O. fragrans* and *O.* × *fortunei* were isolated and identified as 10-acetoxyligustroside and (+)-pinoresinol, respectively, according to the concept of the total activity. Those compounds may be the main contributors to the allelopathy of *O. fragrans* and *O.* × *fortunei*, and provide a competitive advantage to these species through the inhibition of the growth of competing plant species in their vicinity, while several allelopathic substances, including (+)-pinoresinol, may be involved in the allelopathy of *O. heterophyllus*. The present investigation suggests that the extracts of the leaves of these *Osmanthus* species have allelopathic characteristics. Therefore, these extracts and the leaves themselves could potentially be useful for weed management options in some agriculture settings, as mulch, soil additive, and foliar spray, in order to reduce commercial herbicide dependency for the developing sustainable agriculture systems. However, it is necessary to evaluate the weed control activity of these leaves in the field condition.

**Author Contributions:** Conceptualization, H.K.-N.; methodology, Y.H., M.K., S.K., A.I. and H.K.-N.; software Y.H., M.K. and S.K.; validation, K.S. and H.K.-N.; formal analysis, Y.H., M.K. and S.K., investigation, Y.H., M.K., S.K. and A.I.; data curation, H.K.-N.; writing, H.K.-N.; visualization, H.K.-N.; supervision, H.K.-N. All authors have read and agreed to the published version of the manuscript.

**Funding:** This research received no external funding.

**Institutional Review Board Statement:** Not applicable.

**Informed Consent Statement:** Not applicable.

**Data Availability Statement:** No supporting data in this study.

**Conflicts of Interest:** The authors declare no conflict of interest.

## References


1. Ren, Q.J.; Zhu, H.W.; Yu, J.P. The utilization value of *O. fragrans* resources. *Chin. Wild Plant Res.* **1999**, *18*, 34–35.
2. Wu, L.C.; Chang, L.H.; Chen, S.H.; Fan, N.C.; Ho, J.A. Antioxidant activity and melanogenesis inhibitory effect of the acetonic extract of *Osmanthus fragrans*: A potential natural and functional food flavor additive. *Food Sci. Technol.* **2009**, *42*, 1513–1519. [CrossRef]
3. Wang, B.; Luan, F.; Bao, Y.; Peng, X.; Rao, Z.; Tang, Q.; Zeng, N. Traditional uses, phytochemical constituents and pharmacological properties of *Osmanthus fragrans*: A review. *J. Ethnopharmacol.* **2022**, *293*, 115273. [CrossRef]
4. Liao, X.Y.; Hu, F.L.; Chen, Z.L. Identification and quantification of the bioactive components in *Osmanthus fragrans* roots by HPLC-MS/MS. *J. Pharm. Anal.* **2021**, *11*, 299–307. [CrossRef] [PubMed]
5. Casirola, D.M.; Ferraris, R.P. α-Glucosidase inhibitors prevent diet-induced increases in intestinal sugar transport in diabetic mice. *Metabolism* **2006**, *55*, 832–841. [CrossRef] [PubMed]
6. Fang, X.Y.; Zhou, J.L.; Wang, J.Q.; Tang, F.; Zhao, L.G. Preparation of flavonoids from *Osmanthus* dregs and enzymatic modification. *J. For. Eng.* **2020**, *5*, 99–105.
7. Li, G.H.; Wang, M.M.; He, W.; Liu, J.; Zhang, D.; Liu, J.Q.; Tang, W.Z. Iridoid glycoside extraction technology and anti-thrombotic activity of *Osmanthus fragrans* seeds. *Chin. Tradit. Herb. Drugs* **2018**, *49*, 3033–3041.
8. Li, Y.L.; Cai, Q.Y.; Lv, F.; Zhou, L.H.; Tang, X.Y.; Ren, D.X.; Li, Y. Study on immune function of *Osmanthus fragrans* extract Osthin. *Mod. Prev. Med.* **2021**, *48*, 1867–1870.
9. Wang, X.L.; Heraud, S.; Thepot, A.; Santos, M.O.; Luo, Z. The whitening properties of the mixture composed of pomegranate, *Osmanthus* and olive and the protective effects against ultraviolet deleterious effects. *Clin. Cosmet. Invest. Dermatol.* **2021**, *14*, 561–573. [CrossRef]
10. Fu, C.C.; Xu, F.Y.; Qian, Y.C.; Koo, H.L.; Duan, Y.F.; Weng, G.M.; Fan, T.P.; Chen, M.X.; Zhu, F.Y. Secondary metabolites of *Osmanthus fragrans*: Metabolism and medicinal value. *Front. Pharmacol.* **2022**, *13*, 922204. [CrossRef]
11. Li, F.; He, G.; Zhou, Q.; Liang, S. Compare the allelopathic potential of Osmanthus *fragrans* in different habitats. *J. Guangxi Norm. Univ. Nat. Sci.* **2013**, *31*, 88–93.
12. Rice, E.L. *Allelopathy*, 2nd ed.; Academic Press: Orlando, FL, USA, 1984; pp. 1–422.
13. Bais, H.P.; Weir, T.L.; Perry, L.G.; Gilroy, S.; Vivanco, J.M. The role of root exudates in rhizosphere interactions with plants and other organisms. *Annu. Rev. Plant Biol.* **2006**, *57*, 233–266. [CrossRef] [PubMed]
14. Bonanomi, G.; Sicurezza, M.G.; Caporaso, S.; Esposito, A.; Mazzoleni, S. Phytotoxicity dynamics of decaying plant materials. *New Phytol.* **2006**, *169*, 571–578. [CrossRef] [PubMed]
15. Belz, R.G. Allelopathy in crop/weed interactions—An update. *Pest. Manag. Sci.* **2007**, *63*, 308–326. [CrossRef]
16. Kato-Noguchi, H. Involvement of allelopathy in the invasive potential of *Tithonia diversifolia*. *Plants* **2020**, *9*, 766. [CrossRef] [PubMed]
17. Kato-Noguchi, H.; Kurniadie, D. Allelopathy and allelochemicals of *Leucaena leucocephala* as an invasive plant species. *Plants* **2022**, *11*, 1672. [CrossRef]
18. Kato-Noguchi, H. Allelopathy and allelochemicals of *Imperata cylindrica* as an invasive plant species. *Plants* **2022**, *11*, 2551. [CrossRef] [PubMed]
19. Narwal, S.S. Allelopathy in weed management. In *Allelopathy Update Basic and Applied Aspects*; Narwal, S.S., Ed.; Science Publishers Inc.: Enfield, NH, USA, 1999; Volume 2, pp. 203–254.
20. Duke, S.O.; Dayan, F.E.; Romagni, J.G.; Rimando, A.M. Natural products as sources of herbicide, current status and future trends. *Weed Res.* **2000**, *40*, 99–111. [CrossRef]
21. Mallik, A.U. Allelopathy and competition in coniferous forests. *Environ. For. Sci.* **1998**, *54*, 309–315.
22. Kato-Noguchi, H.; Kurniadie, D. Allelopathy of *Lantana camara* as an invasive plant. *Plants* **2021**, *10*, 1028. [CrossRef]
23. Kato-Noguchi, H. Phytotoxic substances involved in teak allelopathy and agroforestry. *Appl. Sci.* **2021**, *11*, 3314. [CrossRef]
24. Xie, L.H.; Akao, T.; Hamasaki, K.; Deyama, T.; Hattori, M. Biotransformation of pinoresinol diglucoside to mammalian lignans by human intestinal microflora, and isolation of *Enterococcus faecalis* strain PDG-1 responsible for the transformation of (+)-pinoresinol to (+)-lariciresinol. *Chem. Pharm. Bull.* **2003**, *51*, 508–515. [CrossRef]
25. Kikuchi, M. Studies on the constituents of *Osmanthus* species. On the components of the leaves of *Osmanthus fragrans* Lour. var. *Aurantiacus makino*. *Yakugaku Zasshi* **1984**, *104*, 535–539. [CrossRef]
26. Global Invasive Species Database, Species Profile: Polygonum cuspidatum. Available online: http://www.iucngisd.org/gisd/speciesname/Polygonum+cuspidatum (accessed on 19 October 2022).
27. Kato-Noguchi, H. Allelopathy of knotweeds as invasive plants. *Plants* **2022**, *11*, 3. [CrossRef]
28. Bailey, J.P.; Bímová, K.; Mandák, B. The potential role of polyploidy and hybridisation in the further evolution of the highly invasive *Fallopia* taxa in Europe. *Ecol. Res.* **2007**, *22*, 920–928. [CrossRef]
29. Parepa, M.; Schaffner, U.; Bossdorf, O. Help from underground soil biota facilitate knotweed invasion. *Ecosphere* **2013**, *4*, 31. [CrossRef]

30. Gaskin, J.F.; Schwarzländer, M.; Grevstad, F.S.; Haverhals, M.A.; Bourchier, R.S.; Miller, T.W. Extreme differences in population structure and genetic diversity for three invasive congeners: Knotweeds in western North America. *Biol. Invasions* **2014**, *16*, 2127–2136. [CrossRef]
31. Mandák, B.; Pyšek, P.; Lysák, M.; Suda, J.; Krahulcová, A.; Bímová, K. Variation in DNA-ploidy levels of *Reynoutria* taxa in the Czech Republic. *Ann. Bot.* **2003**, *92*, 265–272. [CrossRef]
32. Mandák, B.; Pyšek, P.; Bímová, K. History of the invasion and distribution of *Reynoutria* taxa in the Czech Republic: A hybrid spreading faster than its parents. *Preslia* **2004**, *76*, 15–64.
33. Hiradate, S.; Ohse, K.; Furubayashi, A.; Fujii, Y. Quantitative evaluation of allelopathic potentials in soils: Total activity approach. *Weed Sci.* **2010**, *58*, 258–264. [CrossRef]
34. Ward, R.S. Recent advances in the chemistry of lignans. In *Studies in Natural Products Chemistry*; Attaur, R., Ed.; Elsevier: Amsterdam, The Netherlands, 2000; pp. 739–798.
35. Ferrer, J.L.; Austin, M.B.; Stewart, C., Jr.; Noel, J.P. Structure and function of enzymes involved in the biosynthesis of phenylpropanoids. *Plant Physiol. Biochem.* **2008**, *46*, 356–370. [CrossRef]
36. Patyra, A.; Kołtun-Jasion, M.; Jakubiak, O.; Kiss, A.K. Extraction techniques and analytical methods for isolation and characterization of lignans. *Plants* **2022**, *11*, 2323. [CrossRef]
37. Fuentes-Gandara, F.; Torres, A.; Fernández-Ponce, M.T.; Casas, L.; Mantell, C.; Varela, R.; Martínez de la Ossa-Fernández, E.J.; Macías, F.A. Selective fractionation and isolation of allelopathic compounds from *Helianthus annuus* L. leaves by means of high-pressure techniques. *J. Supercrit. Fluids* **2019**, *143*, 32–41. [CrossRef]
38. Jong, T.T.; Chau, S.W. Antioxidative activities of constituents isolated from *Pandanus odoratissimus*. *Phytochemistry* **1998**, *49*, 2145–2148. [CrossRef]
39. Hwang, B.; Lee, J.; Liu, Q.H.; Woo, E.R.; Lee, D.G. Antifungal effect of (+)-pinoresinol isolated from *Sambucus williamsii*. *Molecules* **2010**, *15*, 3507–3516. [CrossRef]
40. Kim, H.Y.; Kim, J.K.; Choi, J.H.; Jung, J.Y.; Oh, W.Y.; Kim, D.C.; Lee, H.S.; Kim, Y.S.; Kang, S.S.; Lee, S.H.; et al. Hepatoprotective effect of pinoresinol on carbon tetrachloride-induced hepatic damage in mice. *J. Pharmacol. Sci.* **2010**, *112*, 105–112. [CrossRef]
41. Kato-Noguchi, H.; Takeshita, S.; Kimura, F.; Ohno, O.; Suenaga, K. A novel allelopathic active substance in *Ginkgo biloba*. *J. Plant Physiol.* **2013**, *170*, 1595–1599. [CrossRef] [PubMed]
42. Kato-Noguchi, H.; Kimura, F.; Ohno, O.; Suenaga, K. Involvement of allelopathy in inhibition of understory growth in red pine forests. *J. Plant Physiol.* **2017**, *218*, 66–73. [CrossRef]
43. Kato-Noguchi, H. Bioactive compounds involved in the formation of the sparse understory vegetation in pine forests. *Curr. Org. Chem.* **2021**, *25*, 1731–1738. [CrossRef]
44. Sakamoto, S.; Machida, K.; Kikuchi, M. Lignan glycosides from the leaves of *Osmanthus heterophyllus*. *J. Nat. Med.* **2008**, *62*, 362–363. [CrossRef]
45. Inouye, H.; Uesato, S. Biosynthesis of iridoids and secoiridoids. In *Progress in the Chemistry of Organic Natural Products*; Herz, W., Grisebach, H., Kirby, G.W., Tamm, C., Eds.; Springer: Wean, Australia, 1986; Volume 50, pp. 169–226.
46. Geu-Flores, F.; Sherden, N.; Courdavault, V.; Glenn, W.S.; Wu, C.; Nims, E.; Cui, Y.; O'Connor, S.E. An alternative route to cyclic terpenes by reductive cyclization in iridoid biosynthesis. *Nature* **2012**, *492*, 138–142. [CrossRef]
47. Kikuchi, M.; Yamauchi, Y. Studies on the constituents of *Osmanthus* species III. On the components of the leaves of *Osmanthus ilicifolius* (Hassk.) Mouillefert. *Yakugaku Zasshi* **1986**, *105*, 442–448. [CrossRef] [PubMed]
48. Machida, K.; Sakamoto, S.; Kikuchi, M. Structure elucidation and NMR spectral assignments of four neolignan glycosides with enantiometric aglycones from *Osmanthus ilicifolius*. *Magn. Reson. Chem.* **2008**, *46*, 990–994. [CrossRef] [PubMed]
49. Sakamoto, S.; Machida, K.; Kikuchi, M. Secoiridoid di-glycosides from *Osmanthus ilicifolius*. *Heterocycles* **2009**, *77*, 557–563.
50. Matuda, Y.; Iwasaki, A.; Suenaga, K.; Kato-Noguchi, H. Allelopathy and allelopathic substances of fossil tree species *Metasequoia glyptostroboides*. *Agronomy* **2022**, *12*, 83. [CrossRef]

*plants*

MDPI

*Article*

# Modulating Expression Levels of TCP Transcription Factors by *Mentha x piperita* Volatiles—An Allelopathic Tool to Influence Leaf Growth?

**Matthias Preusche [1,2], Marvin Vahl [1], Johanna Riediger [1,2], Andreas Ulbrich [1] and Margot Schulz [2,*]**

[1] Department of Horticultural Production, University of Applied Science, 49090 Osnabrück, Germany
[2] Institute of Molecular Physiology and Biotechnology of Plants (IMBIO), University of Bonn, 53127 Bonn, Germany
* Correspondence: ulp509@uni-bonn.de

**Abstract:** Peppermint (*Mentha x piperita*) is a species with inhibitory allelopathic properties due to its high amounts of terpenes. Recent studies have disclosed dosage dependent growth promotion or defense reactions in plants when facing appropriate amounts of *Mentha* bouquet terpenes. These positive effects could be of interest for agricultural applications. To obtain more insights into leaf growth modulations, the expression of *Arabidopsis and Brassica rapa* TCP transcription factors were studied after fumigation with *M. x piperita* bouquets (*Arabidopsis*), with *M. x piperita* essential oil or with limonene (*Arabidopsis* and Chinese cabbage). According to qPCR studies, expression of *TCP3*, *TCP24*, and *TCP20* were downregulated by all treatments in *Arabidopsis*, leading to altered leaf growth. Expressions of *B. rapa TCPs* after fumigation with the essential oil or limonene were less affected. Extensive greenhouse and polytunnel trials with white cabbage and *Mentha* plants showed that the developmental stage of the leaves, the dosage, and the fumigation time are of crucial importance for changed fresh and dry weights. Although further research is needed, the study may contribute to a more intensive utilization of ecologically friendly and species diversity conservation and positive allelopathic interactions in future agricultural systems.

**Keywords:** *Mentha x piperita* volatiles; *Brassica oleracea*; *Arabidopsis thaliana*; TCP transcription factors; leaf growth; fumigation

**Citation:** Preusche, M.; Vahl, M.; Riediger, J.; Ulbrich, A.; Schulz, M. Modulating Expression Levels of TCP Transcription Factors by *Mentha x piperita* Volatiles—An Allelopathic Tool to Influence Leaf Growth? *Plants* **2022**, *11*, 3078. https://doi.org/10.3390/plants11223078

Academic Editor: Lígia R. Salgueiro

Received: 12 October 2022
Accepted: 9 November 2022
Published: 14 November 2022



## 1. Introduction

Terpenoids, one of the largest groups of plant and microbe secondary metabolites, can positively or negatively impact seed germination and plant growth. Depending on the dosage, many terpenoids have phytotoxic properties [1]. For instance, farnesene, a sesquiterpene, influences cell division, abolishes gravitropism in *Arabidopsis*, and downregulates auxin polar transport proteins [2]. Monoterpenes are described as interacting with transcriptional activities, cell division, and cytoskeletal elements in fumigated receiver plants, which results in growth inhibition or even plant death [3–7]. Volatile bouquets emitted from aromatic plants, such as *Mentha x piperita*, affect the transpiration of neighbored *Arabidopsis* plants by inducing stomatal opening [7]. Therefore, terpenes are considered as lead structures for the design of new herbicides. However, the effects of terpenoids are dosage dependent. Consistently, low dosages can have plant growth promoting properties.

*Mentha x piperita* L. belongs to the Lamiaceae, a family with numerous species containing high amounts of essential oil with antifungal, bactericidal, insecticidal, and antifeedant properties. More than 50 constituents have been identified in the essential oil fraction [8], which can quantitatively and qualitatively vary from cultivar to cultivar and from leaf to leaf. The composition is determined by genetic factors, depending on culture methods, plant age and organ, microbial interactions, further interkingdom communication, and other biotic and abiotic parameters such as climate, geographical region, altitude, and irradiation. The most abundant compounds in the essential oil fraction and in the bouquets emitted by *Mentha x piperita* are limonene, linalool, menthone, menthol, and pulegone, while the concentration of single compounds in the emitted bouquets differ from the essential oil fraction of the leaves [9]. Limonene is a precursor of many other monoterpenoids, such as pulegone, menthol, and menthone, and its contents vary over the course of the season [10,11].

In a field study, Sukegawa et al. [9] reported the strong upregulation of *Glycine max* (soybean) defense genes in the leaves when plants are exposed to *Mentha x piperita* volatiles. They found a lower damage of *Brassica rapa* by herbivores when co-cultured with peppermint. We found in a previous study that the volatile bouquet of *Mentha x piperita* (English Mint cv. Mitcham) positively influenced leaf development in young white cabbage (*Brassica oleracea* convar. *capitata* var. *alba*) plants during a 27-day-fumigation, while the influence on leaf growth seemed to depend on responsiveness during early stages of leaf development. A changed leaf shape but no enhanced leaf growth or dry weight was seen when young plants were exposed to menthol or to a combination of menthol and menthone [12]. The observation that the youngest leaves were sensitive to the treatment led to the assumption that fumigation with the *Mentha* volatile bouquet entails modulations of fundamental processes in early leaf development, which results in an enhanced growth of the young leaf. Thus, the responsiveness of transcription factors, in particular of TCPs, to *Mentha x piperita* monoterpenes could be causative for the modulation of leaf growth and development.

The differentiation process in the developing leaf is regulated by a network of hormones and transcription factors, while TCPs (TEOSINTEBRANCHED1/CYCLOIDEA/PROLIFERATING CELL FACTOR) are of particular importance. The roles and interactions of TCPs have been studied intensively during the last few decades [13,14], but many aspects of the complicated, hierarchically organized network with counteracting and redundant functions in controlling plant developmental processes are still elusive [15,16].

The TCP family is composed of two different classes, class I and class II. In *Arabidopsis thaliana*, the class II subfamily is further divided into the subclasses CYC/TB1 and CIN. While being under the control of miRNA 319 (miR319), TCP2, TCP3, TCP4, TCP5, TCP10, TCP13, TCP17, and TCP24 regulate leaf development. The miR319 interaction site is located near the 3′ part of the coding region and not within the *TCP* domain, a characteristic region of the *TCPs* [17]. This TCP domain is necessary for protein–protein interactions [18]. The miR319 interaction site is of importance for class II TCP mRNA abundance, as downregulation of class II TCPs seems to be regulated by miRNA-mediated degradation of their mRNAs [19]. Thus, high levels of miR319 downregulate these TCPs with effects on leaf morphogenesis in *Arabidopsis* [20].

Another group of TCPs have genes lacking the miRNA319 target sequence. The non-miR319-regulated class I TCPs, for instance TCP20 and TCP9, inhibit lipoxygenase 2 gene (*LOX2*) expression, which is crucial for jasmonate biosynthesis. *LOX2* expression is thought to be regulated by the ratios of class I and class II TCP (TCP4) levels [21]. While members of class II TCPs inhibit growth cell division and promote aging, members of class I TCPs have the opposite functions by controlling the expression of specific target genes [22,23]. Non-miR319-regulated TCP20 and TCP9 are also reported to control senescence. TCPs of the same class form homo- or hetero-dimers, which increases the flexibility in interacting with other proteins [19]. The TCP/miRNA interactions, the complex, not yet completely understood regulation processes by TCPs, their known target genes, as well as interaction with plant hormones and jasmonate synthesis, influences of light, temperature, and further factors on TCPs, have recently been reviewed [13].

In this study, the influence of *Mentha* volatiles on the gene expressions of CIN branch TCPs (TCP2, TCP3, TCP4, TCP10, and TCP24), the non-miR319-regulated class 1 TCP 20 and TCP9, and *LOX2* were investigated using the model plant *Arabidopsis thaliana*. These studies were performed to obtain clues concerning the essential interferences of the volatiles with fundamental processes in leaf development after 1, 3, and 7 days of fumigation. The expression of well-known TCP genes of *Brassica rapa* ssp. *Pekinensis*, [24,25] was studied after 7 days of fumigation. The major part of our study deals with the impacts of *Mentha piperita* bouquet volatiles on white cabbage plants in greenhouse and polytunnel trials to reveal conditions that may allow an ecologically acceptable utilization of a positive allelopathic interaction of *Mentha* bouquet terpenoids for the modulation of leaf development in horticulture.

## 2. Results

### 2.1. Effects of Fumigations on the Arabidopsis Phenotype

Fumigation with one *Mentha* plant of 10 shoots and 3 nodes or with larger plants possessing 5 nodes in the growth chamber severely altered the phenotype of *Arabidopsis* plants in comparison to the control plants. In the presence of the smaller *Mentha* plants, *Arabidopsis* developed larger rosettes with longer narrow leaves and longer petioles. A similar result was obtained with *Mentha* essential oil. Limonene led to longer petioles, whereas the leaf shape was not changed. With larger *Mentha* plants, the growth of *Arabidopsis* was heavily reduced (Figure 1), indicating a strong, negative influence of higher volatile concentrations. The negative growth effects are in agreement with the findings that many terpenes have phytotoxic properties when applied in high concentrations [1].

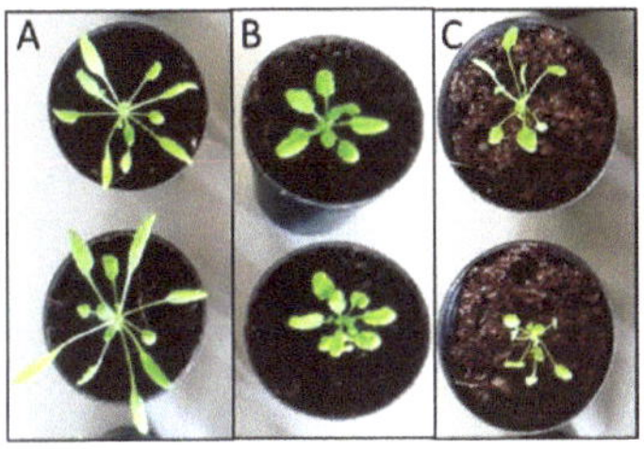


**Figure 1.** Effects of volatile bouquets emitted from different sized *Mentha* plants on the phenotype of *Arabidopsis thaliana* Col-0. (**A**): *Mentha* plant of 10 shoots and 3 nodes; (**B**): control; (**C**): *Mentha* plants of 10 shoots and 5 nodes. Fumigation time was one week.

### 2.2. Determinations of White and Chinese Cabbage Fresh and Dry Weights after Fumigation with Limonene and Mentha Essential Oil

Fresh and dry weights of the above-ground parts of white and Chinese cabbage plants were determined after fumigation with limonene or *Mentha* essential oil for one week to estimate threshold ranges of terpenoid concentrations causing inhibitory effects on cabbage growth. In contrast to *Arabidopsis*, no striking alterations of the phenotypes were observed. Nevertheless, white cabbage developed a significantly higher fresh and dry weight with limonene and a higher dry weight with *Mentha* essential oil, but a slightly reduced fresh weight (Figure 2). Regarding the fresh weight, Chinese cabbage was less responsive than white cabbage to limonene, although dry weight was also significantly enhanced. Here, *Mentha* essential oil increased fresh weight with high significance only with the 16 mL dosage.

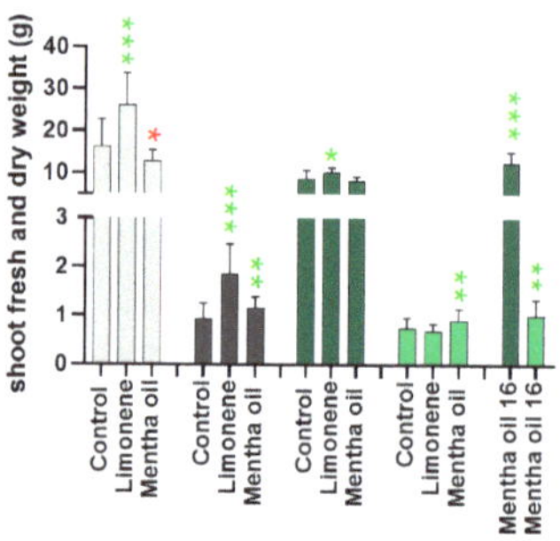


**Figure 2.** Fresh (FW) and dry weight (DW) of above-ground plant material after 1-week-fumigation in the greenhouse with high concentrations of limonene (8 mL/day) and *Mentha* essential oil (14 or 16 mL/day) and controls. White cabbage: light grey (FW), dark grey (DW); Chinese cabbage: dark green (FW), green (DW). *Mentha* oil 16 indicates 16 mL/day, for all other treatments 14 mL/day were used. Significance: * $p < 0.05$; ** $p < 0.005$; *** $p < 0.0005$), green asterisks: increase, red asterisk: reduction.

### 2.3. *TCP Transcription Factors—Targets of Mentha x piperita Emitted Volatiles, Essential Oil Fraction, and Limonene*

Because it was intended to address the growth promotion and phenotype modeling of *Arabidopsis* by *Mentha* volatile bouquets, TCP gene expressions were investigated with plants fumigated with the smaller *Mentha* plants. qPCR analysis with cDNA from growth-promoted *Arabidopsis* plants revealed a strong downregulation of *TCP2* and *TCP3* transcripts, most exhibited after 3 days of fumigation, and a downregulation of *TCP4*, strongest at day 7, while *TCP 9*, *TCP10*, *TCP 20*, and *TCP24* transcript levels showed a much weaker response and were only slightly, if at all, downregulated (Figure 3). The *LOX2* gene expression was ambivalent but tended towards an upregulation at day 7 without significance. Fumigation with the essential oil fraction led to similar results, i.e., a downregulation of *TCP2* transcripts after 1 and 3 day(s) and a slight upregulation at day 7. *TCP3* mRNA was downregulated at all time points. A weaker response of *TCP4* transcripts was stated, with the highest downregulation at day 3. Again, *TCP 9* and *TCP10* transcripts were only slightly affected, with a low upregulation of *TCP9* at day 1 and of *TCP10* at day 7, while *TCP20* and in particular *TCP24* were more strongly downregulated than was found after *Mentha* bouquet fumigation. The *LOX2* transcripts were downregulated. Using limonene for fumigation resulted in similar transcript profiles for *TCP3, TCP9*, and *TCP20; TCP10* was downregulated, but *TCP2* and *TCP4* were almost not affected. The downregulation of *TCP24* was between the one found for the bouquet and essential oil fumigation. Thus, fumigation with limonene had almost no effect on transcripts of *TCP2* and *TCP4*, which were responsive to the complex mixture of the volatiles present in the bouquet and the essential oil. The *LOX2* transcript level was similarly affected, as found after the essential oil fumigation. Most of the expression profiles showed a dependence on the fumigation time, in particular *TCP2*, *TCP3*, *TCP4*, and *LOX2* transcript abundances.

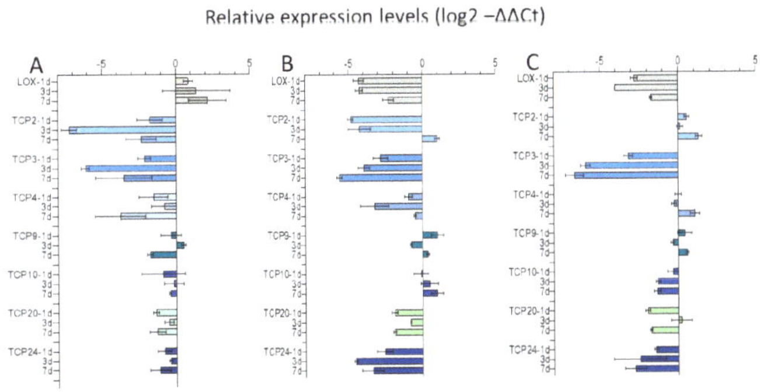


**Figure 3.** TCP gene expression in *Arabidopsis* is modulated by *Mentha* volatiles. Expression of class II *TCP2, TCP3, TCP4, TCP5, TCP10, TCP13, TCP17, TCP24*, and class I *TCP20* and *TCP9* genes, *LOX2* (LOX) after the different types of fumigation. **A**: *Mentha* plant; **B**: *Mentha* essential oil; **C**: limonene. The figure shows mean values and standard error of means (n = 2 samples, each sample prepared from 43–51 plants per time point).

#### 2.3.1. Expression of TCP Transcription Factors in Chinese Cabbage after Exposure to Mentha Essential Oil Fraction and Limonene

In contrast to *Arabidopsis thaliana*, Chinese cabbage has two *BraTCP2*, one *BraTCP3*, three *BraTCP4*, one *BraTCP10*, and two *BraTCP24* genes [24,25]. When fumigated with the *Mentha* essential oil fraction or limonene, expressions of the tested *Brassica rapa* ssp. *Pekinensis* TCP transcription factors were considerably less affected than the *TCPs* of *Arabidopsis*. With limonene, all *TCPs* were downregulated in the rage of −0.5 to −2fold, except for *TCP2a*, which was slightly upregulated, and *TCP24a*, which was not responsive. With the essential oil fraction, the only downregulated TCP was *TCP4a* (−3 fold), while *TCP4b* was 4-fold, but *TCP4c* was only 0.5-fold upregulated (Figure 4). The latter range of upregulation was also found for *TCP2a*, *TCP3*, *TCP9a*, *TCP10*, and *TCP20b*. *TCP24b* was not responsive, and *TCP2b* showed a 2-fold, *TCP9b* and *TCP24a* each showed a 1-fold, and *TCP20a* showed an approximate 2-fold upregulation.

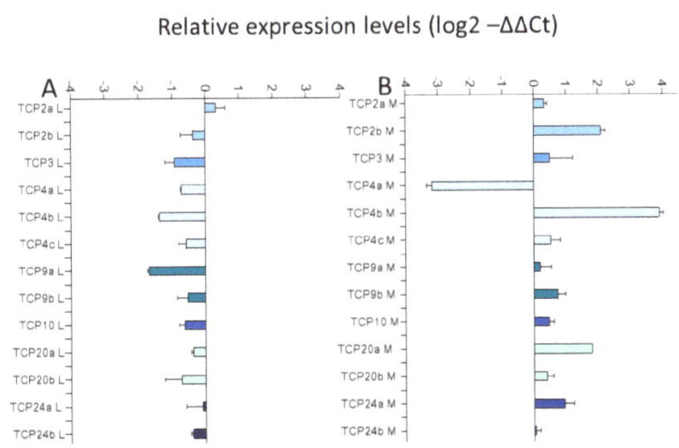


**Figure 4.** Expression of *Brassica rapa* ssp. *Pekinensis* TCP transcription factors in response to *Mentha x piperita* essential oil and limonene. **A**: limonene; **B**: *Mentha* essential oil. The figure shows mean values and standard error of means (n = 2 composed samples).

#### 2.3.2. Choice of White Cabbage for Greenhouse and Polytunnel Trials

In turnips (*Brassica rapa* ssp. *rapa*), *Brr/BraTCP2* is involved in leaf development by regulating cell proliferation [25]. According to Efroni et al. [26], CIN-class TCPs have crucial functions, such as being negative regulators of cell proliferation, therefore causing leaf differentiation [24]. Figures 2 and 4 illustrate that the fumigation with limonene and *Mentha x piperita* essential oil have different impacts on (1) leaf fresh and dry weight and (2) TCP gene expressions. With Chinese cabbage, the study with *Mentha* essential oil disclosed that head shape modulating TCP4a was the only downregulated TCP gene; all others were upregulated or not responsive. Because downregulation of the CIN-class TCP abundance is a prerequisite for cell proliferation, enhanced leaf growth of Chinese cabbage may not occur when the plants were fumigated with *Mentha* plants as the fresh and dry weight determinations after limonene and *Mentha* essential oil fumigation indicated that Chinese cabbage needs higher volatile concentrations than white cabbage to achieve growth responses. Thus, the concentrations of *Mentha* bouquet compounds may not be high enough for modulating Chinese cabbage leaf growth, but could be high enough for white cabbage. Therefore, and by considering the results of the former pilot study [12], fumigation with *Mentha* plants in greenhouse and polytunnel experiments were performed with white cabbage and not with Chinese cabbage. The responsiveness of TCP transcription factors towards *Mentha* volatiles found for *Arabidopsis* was assumed to be similar in white cabbage.

### *2.4. Greenhouse and Polytunnel Trials with* Brassica oleracea convar. capitata var. alba *and* Mentha *plants*

#### Greenhouse Trial—Leaf Length and Width, Growth Increments

Leaf length and width were measured after 1 (T1), 4 (T2), 8 (T3), 11 (T4), and 15 days (T5) after exposure to *Mentha* volatiles emitted by one or four plants (Figure S1). At T1 and T2, where only the first and the emerging (T1) or the further developed (T2) second leaves were present, growth showed no significant differences to the controls. At T3 (8 days), the difference in leaf length of control plants and those exposed to four *Mentha* plants (4M) was significant larger for leaf 2 when the distance to the *Mentha* plants was more than 35 cm. Leaf 1 was not responsive and leaf 3 tended towards an increased length growth but without significance. Leaf width was not affected at T3. The largest differences were seen with leaf 2 and leaf 4, but particularly with leaf 3 after 15 days (T5) when plants were exposed to four *Mentha* plants when the distance to the *Mentha* plants was more than 20 cm. Thus, the number of *Mentha* plants, dependence on the distance, and the dosage are crucial for leaf parameter modulations. The results indicate again that defined developmental stages of a leaf in combination with the dosage of the volatiles are important for the response to the treatments. To summarize, only the second and third leaves at T3, T4, and T5, and also the fourth leaf, clearly responded to the treatment with bouquet volatiles emitted from four *Mentha* plants. The highest increases in leaf length and width were obtained at distances exceeding 35 cm.

Measurements of the leaf increments support the observations (Figure 5). Compared to the controls, leaf growth increments show that the responses of leaves 2, 3, and 4 to the *Mentha* volatiles are significantly higher between 11 and 15 days (T4–T5) of fumigation when the distance to four *Mentha* plants was more than 25 cm. Increments of fumigated leaves at T1–T2, except for leaf 2, and T2–T3 were similar to the control values. The increments of leaf 2 were continuously larger after 8 days of fumigation but not during the early phase of the treatment.

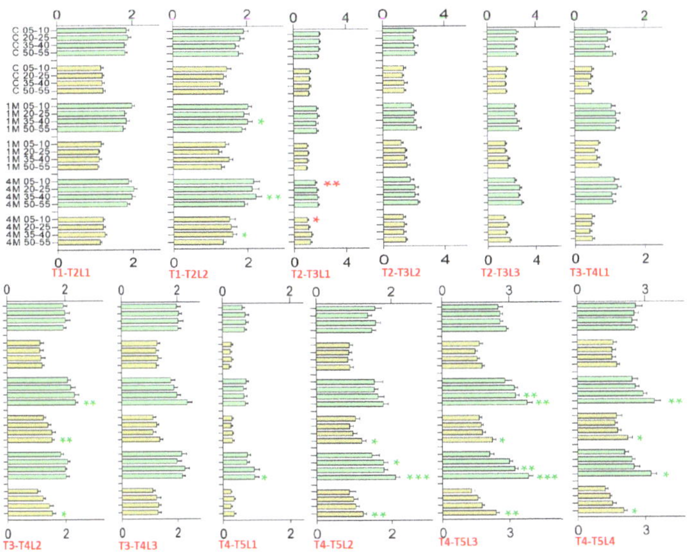


**Figure 5.** Greenhouse Trial: Increments (cm y-axis, consider graph right 90° rotation) in length (green) and width (olive) of the first two to four leaves (T1–T2, T2–T3, T3–T4, and T4–T5) at four difference distances (0.5–10, 20–25, 35–40 and 50–55 cm, x-axis, consider graph right 90° rotation) in control plants (no *Mentha*), plants exposed to one *Mentha* (1 M), and plants exposed to four *Mentha* (4 M) plants. Green asterisks indicate significantly increased growth, red asterisk significant lower growth compared to the controls, bars without asterisk: no significance. Enhanced increments occurred predominantly during the late period of fumigation with leaf 2 (T3–T4) and with leaves 2, 3, and 4 at T4–T5. The figure shows mean values and standard error of means (n = 16). Significance with reference to the appropriate cm control (no fumigation), (*t*-test): * $p < 0.05$; ** $p < 0.005$; *** $p < 0.0005$). Red labels give the increment (T1–T2, T2–T3, T3–T4, and T4–T5) and the leaf number (L1, L2, L3, L4).

### 2.5. *Polytunnel Trial—Leaf Length and Width, Growth Increments*

Leaf length and width were measured after 1 (T1), 4 (T2), 8 (T3), 12 (T4), and 15 days (T5) after exposure of the plants to volatiles emitted by four or nine *Mentha* plants. At all time-points, leaf 1 was comparable to the control, thus without response to the treatment. At T2, T3, and T4, the length growth of leaf 2 and, to a lesser degree, leaf 3 were enhanced by the bouquets of four and nine mint plants at both distances. At T5, the growth promoting effect of the volatiles was almost halted in leaf 2 and leaf 3. Leaf width was enhanced only at T3 with high significance and again only in leaf 2 and leaf 3. Thus, for leaf 2 and leaf 3, length growth was more affected than width growth and overall responsiveness, mainly restricted to leaf 2 and leaf 3, occurred between day 4 and day 12 of the treatment (Figure S2).

The increments of leaf growth, depictured in Figure 6, illustrate the dynamics of leaf growth more distinctly. Increments of leaves 2 and 3 occurred mainly between T1–T2 (leaf 2) and T2–T3 (both leaves), while at T3–T4, only four mints had a positive effect on leaf length at both distances. Leaf width did not increase and was even reduced at the short distance with nine *Mentha* plants. The reduction in increments, compared to control values or even lower values, continued at T4–T5 for all leaves (except for leaf 4) with four mint plants at the larger distance (60–75 cm). The increments demonstrate that the growth promoting effect of *Mentha* bouquet affected leaves in defined developmental stages only temporarily. No growth promotion was found with leaves that were developed during the late period of the treatment (T5, leaves 4, 5, and 6).

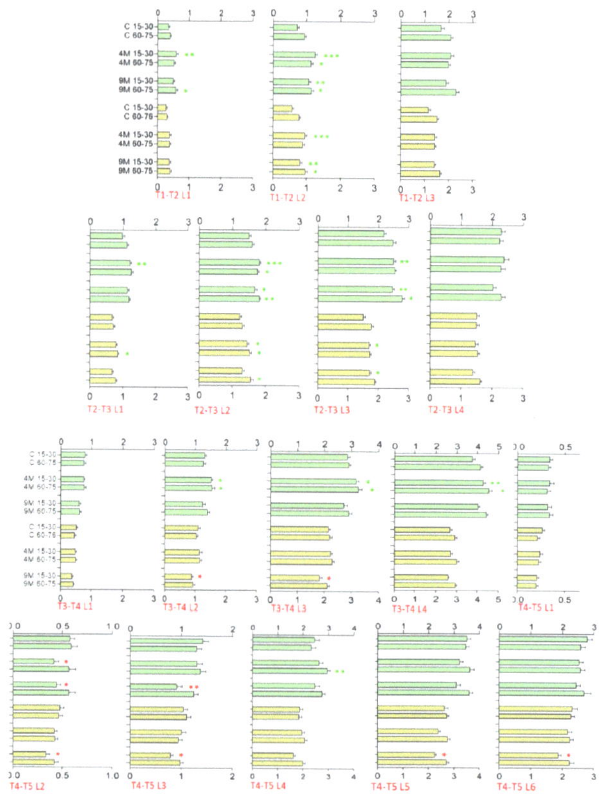

**Figure 6.** Polytunnel Trial: Consider graph right 90° rotation. Increments in length (green) and width (olive) of the first three to four leaves (T1–T2, T2–T3, T3–T4, T4–T5) at two difference distances (15–30 cm and 60–75 cm) in control plants (no *Mentha*), plants exposed to four *Mentha* (4 M), and plants exposed to nine *Mentha* (9 M) plants. Green asterisks indicate significantly increased growth, red asterisks indicates significantly lower growth compared to the controls, bars without asterisk: no significance; n= 24. Enhanced growth is primarily found during the early period of fumigation with leaves 2 and 3, while during the late period, a significantly inhibited or at least a reduced growth of these leaves was predominately seen. Significance with reference to the appropriate cm control (no fumigation), (*t*-test): * $p < 0.05$; ** $p < 0.005$; *** $p < 0.0005$). Red labels give the increment (T1–T2, T2–T3, T3–T4, and T4–T5) and the leaf number (L1, L2, L3, L4, L5, L6).

## 2.6. Greenhous and Polytunnel Trials—Fresh and Dry Weight

The fresh and dry weight of the above-ground plant material was determined after termination of the fumigation at day 21. Fresh and dry weights of the cabbage plants cultured in the greenhouse were enhanced when the distance to one mint was more than 35 cm; with four mint plants, more than 50 cm were necessary to achieve a similar increase

(Figure 7). Four *Mentha* plants led to lower dry masses at the smaller distances. Fresh and dry weights of the entire above-ground plant material mirror the overall growth, while increases must be attributed mainly to the second and third leaves. Nevertheless, the total increase of above-ground biomass fresh weight was in the range of 20% (calculated from mean values) of the above controls for plants growing with a 35–55 cm distance to one *Mentha* plant. The total dry weight was lower than control values, with the exception of the plants growing with a distance of 55 cm to one *Mentha* plant. Here, the increase in dry weight was approximately 10%.

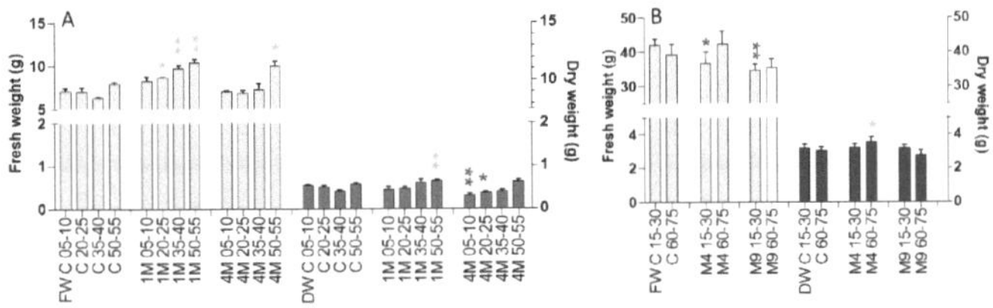


**Figure 7.** (**A**): Greenhouse trial: Fresh and dry weights after termination of the treatment (means + standard error of means). (**B**): Polytunnel Trial: Fresh and dry weights after termination of treatment (means + standard error of means). Light grey bars: fresh weight; dark grey bark dry weight. Green asterisks indicate increase, red asterisk inhibition, significance levels: (*t*-test): * $p < 0.05$; ** $p < 0.005$); bars without asterisk: no significance. Notice that the number of plants used for fresh and dry weight determinations was different compared to the greenhouse trial, due to the different arrangements.

As a consequence of the more or less stagnating leaf growth during the late period of the treatment (T5, 15 days) in the polytunnel trial, no enhanced fresh and dry weights of the above-ground plant material was found after treatment termination (21 days) (Figure 7). The cabbage plants cultured in the polytunnel developed more leaves compared to the plants in the greenhouse, due to the different culture conditions (pre-culture in the greenhouse in pots prior the planting in the polytunnel soil). Leaves 7 and 8 were very small and did not considerably contribute to fresh and dry weights. Because of their small size, these leaves were not evaluated further. Taken together, a higher biomass due to the volatile promoted growth of leaves 2 and 3 at T2, T3, and T4 was not a decisive factor when the fresh and dry weights of the above-ground biomass (Figure 7) was determined after 21 days. In comparison to the greenhouse trial with the strongest effects between 11 and 15 days (T4–T5), growth promoting effects occurred much earlier, namely between 4 and 12 days, when the plants were cultured in the polytunnel with 4 and 9 *Mentha* plants and was characterized by a subsequent decline (Figures 5 and 6).

## 3. Discussion

Presently, approaches to integrate positive allelopathic interactions in agricultural practices are rarely addressed, although the positive effects of many allelochemicals when applied in low concentrations are well known. This study disclosed some of the difficulties associated with the suitable application and maintenance of plant growth promoting concentrations of *Mentha x piperita* emitted volatiles and, on the other side, the dynamics in responses of the receiver plants.

The involvement of TCPs indicates that dosage dependent responsiveness to *Mentha* volatiles starts on superordinated levels that regulate the leaf growth process and is embedded in the entire life cycle of the plant. Causative molecular interactions that lead to modulations of transcriptional activities, resulting perhaps in shifts of the ratios of class I and class II TCP levels, could not be elucidated in this study, nor could the responsiveness of TCP target genes and hormone interactions or levels of miR319. Nevertheless, for a possible interpretation of the results, we would like to address some of the far-reaching downstream events of gene activity cascades that are presumably linked to *Mentha* volatile induced modulations of TCP transcript abundances.

Treatments with limonene, *Mentha* essential oil, and *Mentha* bouquet all downregulated *TCP3*, *TCP24* (both class II CIN branch TCPs), and *TCP20*, a class I non-miR319-regulated TCP in *Arabidopsis*. TCP3 negatively affects auxin responses [27]. Auxin is known to be crucial in leaf development for its functions in leaf initiation and influences on leaf size, shape, and form [28,29]. The effects of TCP3 on the auxin response and on flavonoid biosynthesis have been investigated by Li and Zachgo [30]. Thus, downregulation of TCP3 expression might have reverse effects on auxin triggered processes that are under the control of TCP3. Downregulation of TCP3 by *Mentha* volatiles should therefore influence effects linked with auxin responses. *TCP20* is another partner in the auxin network as it regulates the expression of *GH3.3*. GH3s are known to control the formation of IAA-amino acid conjugates, which are important in maintaining auxin homeostasis [31]. In our study, downregulation of TCP20 gene expression was, however, found to be less severe than that of *TCP3*. *TCP24* suppresses secondary wall thickening [32]; thus, a downregulation of *TCP24* transcription can lead to enhanced secondary cell wall formation, which would be in line with the increased dry weights of white cabbage after fumigation with high amounts of *Mentha* volatiles. Another group of transcription factors (growth-regulating factors (GRFs), which is under the control of miR396 [33], might also be affected, but the study of their expression profiles after *Mentha* fumigation remains to be carried out.

The results indicate that the positive effects of *Mentha* volatiles on leaf development probably proceed first from the interactions of volatile components with TCPs. Growth stimulation may later be due to interactions with the auxin network. Other downstream interactions with hormones and proteins are presumable, but further investigations must prove the assumption. The many antagonistic and synergistic interactions and functional redundancies raise difficulties in unambiguous assignments of the observed effects to defined developmental pathways. In addition, alterations in downstream events, performed as counteracting steps by the plant or its associated microorganisms, for instance monoterpene detoxification, may intercept responses to the volatiles.

Down regulation of the gene expression of other transcription factors, such as MYC-2, ANAC, and SCR-SHR, has been found after the application of the monoterpene citral. A binding of citral to these and further transcription factors (SSBPs WHY1, WHY2, and WHY3) was concluded from in silico molecular docking analyses [3]. Godard et al. [34] reported myrcene or ocimene induced expression of transcription factors, stress, and defense genes in *Arabidopsis*. The gene expression, at least of several plant transcription factors but also of some genes involved in defense, is apparently sensitive to terpenoid volatiles. Thus, it is possible that interactions of terpenoids with transcription factors and perhaps with many other proteins are common features. With MYC-2, ANAC, SCR-SHR, SSBPs WHY1, WHY2, and WHY3, the molecular backgrounds of the modulation are also not yet understood. Sukegawa et al. [11] concluded that there was a fumigation-time dependent epigenetic regulation of the JA- and SA-signaling-dependent defense genes TI and PR1 by *Mentha x piperita* volatiles in soybean. Here, the transient chromatin acetylation levels of the regulatory promoter region of these genes were immediately changed after starting the fumigation [11]. It cannot be discounted that epigenetic regulation of volatile binding is important at certain stages of the plant's life cycle, allowing defined gene responses or hindering them, leading to different gene expression profiles and finally to other protein interactions [35]. Some TCPs also seem to be under circadian clock control [36]; thus, transcriptional responses upon fumigation may succumb to diurnal variations. Transient changes in the gene expressions of the TCPs, in combination with the leaf life cycle and the abundance of miR319, and perhaps also epigenetic regulations, could be one reason for the decrease of the growth promoting effect of *Mentha* volatiles found with the plants grown in the polytunnel during the late phase of fumigation and may explain the failed growth stimulation in oldest leaves.

Further explanations are given by the dosage effects. The greenhouse and the polytunnel trials indicate the possibility of transient TCP-involved interactions. Concentrations of volatiles able to elicit growth effects were reached earlier with a higher number of *Mentha* plants, and thus the threshold concentration necessary for leaf growth induction in the greenhouse is later in place. Leaf surface can be influential, particularly wax layers. Monoterpenoids have been found to precipitate on wax layers and permeate them subsequently [7]; thus, local concentrations on the leaf may be spotted and increase during the course of fumigation. Because wax deposition on cabbage leaves was found to increase with aging [37], inhibitory amounts of terpenoids can finally accumulate in the wax layer, serving as a local source for the release of the molecules that infiltrate leaf cells underneath. We assume that plants with a thinner wax layer than cabbage, such as *Arabidopsis*, are more quickly affected by low monoterpene concentrations, which would explain the rapidly altered expression profiles of sensitive TCPs. More for cabbage than for *Arabidopsis*, the shape of the shoot and the positioning of the leaves are properties that influence the receiving of volatiles by leaves. Nevertheless, with the exception of *TCP24*, the expression profiles of affected TCPs were surprisingly similar in *Arabidopsis* when fumigated with small *Mentha* plants or with *Mentha* essential oil. Are some of the volatiles better trapped in the wax layers than others? In this case, subsequently different TCP gene expression profiles in cabbage would occur, if their expression is compound specific. For volatile trapping, the structure of the wax crystals, the wax composition, and immersed secondary metabolites, for instance flavonoids, may be of importance for species-dependent differences in the responsiveness to *Mentha* volatiles. In addition, many plant species have low quantities of di- and triterpenes, sometimes rare ones, deposited in their wax layers, including *Arabidopsis* and *Brassica oleracea* [38–40], indicating that wax layers are suitable sites for terpenoid deposition. At present, it is speculative to assume an involvement of TCPs, perhaps TCP4, in wax layer modulations and functions.

On the other hand, the amounts of volatiles emitted by the *Mentha* plants can vary as the terpenoid biosynthesis is modulated by many factors such as season, temperature, wind, leaf and whole plant age, growth of the plant, and, as important modulators, by soil and plant microbiomes. The temperature dependency of *Mentha x piperita* essential oil composition is known [41]. Menthol and menthone decrease at high temperature, menthylacetate and pulegone increase, and others, such as limonene, are not affected. Consistently, the maintenance of identical volatile compositions over time is unlikely. Altered volatile compositions can be an additional, important reason for shaping the leaf responsiveness. Alterations should be more presumable in the polytunnel trial, with consequences for the leaf growth, because, in this trial, temperature was not controlled.

In summary, the study disclosed the leaf growth promoting and dosage dependent effect of *Mentha* volatiles in cabbage and *Arabidopsis* at defined developmental stages. Greenhouse cultures may be more suitable for utilizing the positive effects of *Mentha* volatiles on the leaf growth of young cabbage plants, and also on other important vegetables. The maintenance of optimal volatile concentrations over time is, however, an essential problem as the concentration depends on air circulation and temperature as well as alterations in the bouquet composition, and is also due to the different chemical properties, such as the volatility, of the constituents.

Although optimization of culture and fumigation conditions are expected to be species dependent and need further extensive research, the ecologically and environmentally friendly utilization of allelopathic volatiles in suitable concentrations for leaf growth promotion seems to be feasible, when harvest times are adapted. The results presented here are in line with our former pilot study [12]. Moreover, the growth promoting effects of *Mentha* species, when applied in low amounts, have been described by Islam and Kato-Noguchi [42]. Finally, the use of plant volatile bouquets for plant growth promoting effects does not have the potential risk to animal health and the environment as may occur with high amounts of terpenoids [43].

## 4. Material and methods

### 4.1. Plant Material

#### 4.1.1. *Mentha x piperita* Variety English Mint cv. "Mitcham"

For the fumigation of receiver plants, *Mentha x piperita* L. variety English Mint cv. "Mitcham" was used. The young plants were purchased from a local gardener and grown in a greenhouse (20/16 °C day/night) for approximately one and a half month until the start of the experiments. Two weeks after delivery, *Mentha* plants were propagated form cuttings. The uniformly-sized *Mentha* plants were grown for one month under the same conditions as described. The *Mentha* plants were cut again one week before being grown (4 main shoots with 5 nodes each, if not otherwise noted).

#### 4.1.2. *Arabidopsis thaliana* Col-0

Seeds of *A. thaliana* Col-0 were surface sterilized and germinated in petri dishes with standard MS media and 1% sucrose (Murashige & Skoog, without any additives) under sterile conditions. After two days of stratification at 4 °C, the plates were transferred into a growth chamber for germination and growth at 23 °C, 16/8 h day/night. After 10 days, the young seedlings were transferred into small pots (Ø 5 cm) filled with water-saturated soil ("Seedlingsubstrat" from Klaasmann-Deilmann, Germany). Treatments were started one day after pricking.

#### 4.1.3. *Brassica oleracea* cv. *capitata* var. *alba* convar. LENNOX F1 (white cabbage) and *Brassica rapa* (Chinese cabbage)

White cabbages (*Brassica oleracea* cv. *capitata* var. *alba* convar. LENNOX F1, Bejo Germany) were grown as described in [12]. In short, cabbages were sown in pressed peat pots (4.5 × 4 × 5 cm, cf. Figure 1) and germinated under 16/10 °C day/night conditions in a greenhouse and grown for 14–21 days until the second leaf was approximately 1.5–2 cm long. During this period, the plants were watered once a day. The substrate used for germination and growth was "Potground P" (Klaasmann-Deilmann, Germany). Chinese cabbages (*Brassica rapa* ssp. *Pekinensis*, Bilko F1, Bejo, Germany) were similarly cultured.

### 4.2. Fumigation Experiments

#### 4.2.1. Fumigation of *Arabidopsis thaliana* with *Mentha x piperita* Mitcham

For determination of *TCP* gene expression profiles, standardized *Mentha* plants were used. *A. thaliana* seedlings were co-cultured with one *Mentha* plant of 10 shoots and 3 nodes or with larger plants possessing 5 nodes. *A. thaliana* control groups were cultured without *Mentha* plants. These pre-experiments revealed the growth promoting and phenotype modeling properties of smaller *Mentha* plants, while the larger plants led to growth inhibition of the co-cultured *Arabidopsis* plants (Figure 1). The following experiments were therefore performed with the smaller *Mentha* plants. Co-culturing with *A. thaliana* after one day of acclimation was performed for 1, 3, and 7 days in the growth chamber.

#### 4.2.2. Fumigation of *A. thaliana* and *Brassica* plants with Mentha essential oil and limonene for Gene Expression Experiments

*A. thaliana* plants were treated with steam distillates of English mint essential oil, free of organic solvents (Norfolk Essential Oils, Wisbech, UK) or limonene (Merck Chemicals GmbH, Darmstadt, Germany; companies' information regarding the products are given in the Supplementary File). Limonene is one of the known components of the *Mentha* essential oil fractions (in the used essential oil charge: 2.4%) and also of the plant-emitted bouquet. Limonene was also separately applied, because it is the precursor of further monoterpenes. The treatment was performed for one week by injecting the essential oil fraction or limonene into cotton balls swinging approximately 5 cm above the plants (Figures 8 and 9).

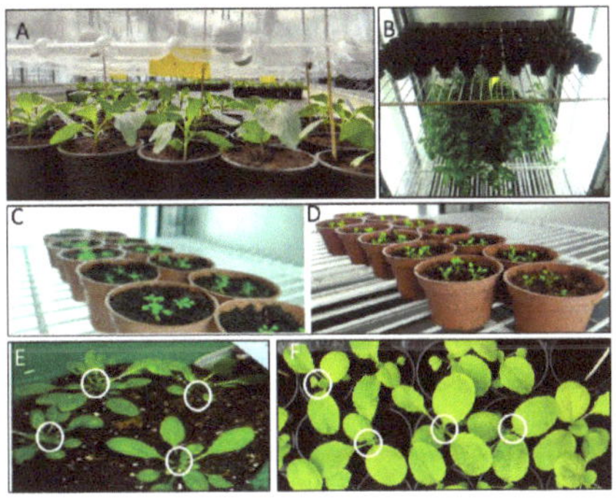

**Figure 8.** One-week-fumigation of cabbage and *Arabidopsis* for gene expression experiments. (**A**): Cabbage plants were fumigated with volatile-loaded cotton balls. Controls were with volatile-free cotton balls. (**B**): Fumigation arrangement of *Arabidopsis* with one *Mentha* plant in the growth chamber. (**C**): Control, (**D**): Limonene-fumigated *Arabidopsis* after 7 days. (**E**,**F**): Harvested shoot material for gene expression studies. The innermost parts of the *Arabidopsis* rosettes and shoot apex containing material of cabbage plants (white rings) were harvested and used for RNA extraction. Pictures (**E**) and (**F**) show control plants. (**E**): *Arabidopsis*; (**F**): Chinese cabbage.

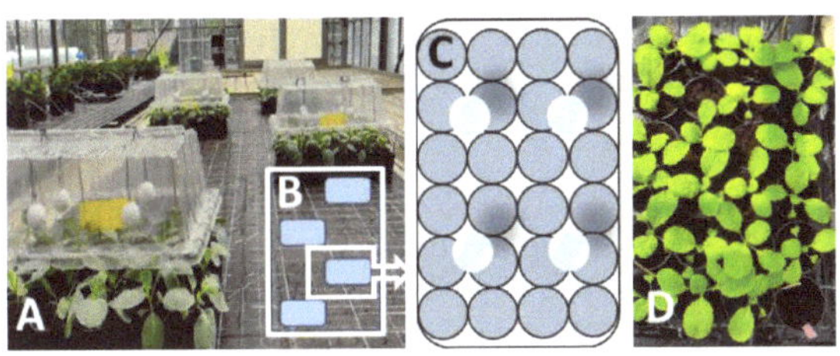

**Figure 9.** Experimental setup of cabbage plants in 4 culture boxes for limonene and *Mentha* essential oil fumigations in the greenhouse. Distances between culture boxes: 60 cm. (**A**,**C**): plants and cotton balls in one box ((**B**): inserted scheme in the picture of culture box arrangements in the greenhouse). (**D**): cabbage plants used for fresh and dry weight determination.

These arrangements allow efficient fumigation of the plants with the terpenoids emitted from the cotton balls. Injection was carried out at the start of the experiment and after 3½ days. In total, 4 mL of the essential oil fraction or limonene were applied to *Arabidopsis* plants per week.

### 4.3. Real Time PCR

Expression studies were performed to reveal the alterations of *TCP* transcript abundances during the first week of fumigation. The material for qPCR were obtained by harvesting the innermost part of the *Arabidopsis* rosettes with the stem apex and emerging leaves. Each sample comprised 43–51 individual plants per time point, i.e., 1, 3, and 7 days after co-cultivation with *Mentha* plants, application of *Mentha* essential oil and limonene, respectively, and the corresponding controls. The plant material was collected in liquid nitrogen and stored at −80 °C, if not immediately used for RNA extraction. Material from *Brassica rapa* (Chinese cabbage) was likewise harvested after 7 days of fumigation with *Mentha* essential oil or with limonene (Figure 8).

Two replicates were obtained at all three dates, resulting in 6 *Arabidopsis* samples for the treated and control groups. For mRNA preparation, 100 mg of plant material was used. RNA was extracted with the NucleoSpin® RNA Plant" extraction kit (Macherey and Nagel, Düren, Germany) according to the manufacturer's instructions. RNA quantity was determined by NanoDrop measurements. For cDNA synthesis, the RevertAid First Strand cDNA Synthesis Kit (Thermo Fisher Scientific) was utilized according to the manufacturer's protocol.

Real time PCR was performed as described in [44], with the qPCR-Mix "my-Budget 5× EvaGreen® QPCR-Mix II (ROX)" (Bio-Budget Technologies GmbH, Krefeld, Germany) and the thermocycler Applied Biosystems 7300 Real Time PCR System (Thermo Fisher Scientific, München, Germany). For all repetition setups with *Arabidopsis* and for all experiments with Chinese cabbage, the thermocycler CFX Connect (Bio-Rad, Feldkirchen, Germany) was used. Quantitative analysis was carried out for *TCP2, TCP3, TCP4, TCP9, TCP10, TCP20, TCP24*, and *LOX2* expression. Actin (*ACT2*) was used as a reference gene. Primers were synthesized by Eurofins Genomics (Ebersberg, Germany) and are listed in Table S1 [24,45]. The qPCR reaction mixtures (20 μL) contained μL 5× EvaGreen® QPCR-Mix II (ROX, Bio-Budget Technologies GmbH, Krefeld, Germany), 5 μL cDNA sample (15.52 ng/μL), 1 μL forward and reverse Primer Mix (1:1, *v*/*v*; 10 μM each), and 10 μL DNase free $H_2O$. For evaluation of RT-qPCR results, the ΔΔCT method was applied.

### *4.4. Determination of Cabbage Dry and Fresh Weights after Fumigation with High Mentha Essential Oil and Limonene Concentrations*

For determinations of fresh and dry weights after applications of high amounts of the volatiles, 18-day-old plants were arranged into groups of 24 plants and set up in rows of 4 × 6 under a transparent hood equipped with four cotton balls, as shown in Figure 9. To ensure that the concentration of chemicals was constantly high throughout the experimental period, the cotton balls were soaked every day with either 8 mL limonene or 14 and 16 mL *Mentha* essential oil. Cotton balls of the control groups had no volatile injections. This experiment was performed to elucidate threshold ranges of inhibitory volatile concentrations.

Watering of the plants was performed automatically by an ebb and flow system, which was adjusted to flood the table once a day for 8 min. The heating temperature in the greenhouse was set to 18/15 °C day/night, and the aeration temperature to 21 °C. Trials were started in May and lasted until the end of July. The duration of the treatments was 7 days; afterwards, the plants were cut above ground and fresh weight (FW) and dry weight (DW) after drying at 60 °C for two days were determined.

### *4.5. Greenhouse Trial with Mentha piperita Plants*

In early May 2018, treatments were started by placing pots with *Mentha* plants next to boxes with 120 ten-day-old white cabbage plants for 21 days (Figure 10). The *Mentha* treatment was run in three plot arrangements with one, four, or no mint plants, the latter as the control. Each plot was placed at a different table with two replicates for each treatment group. The distance between the boxes was 80 cm. The distances of the cabbage plants placed in rows in the boxes to the *Mentha* plants were: 1st row: 5–10 cm; 2nd row: 20–25 cm; 3rd row: 35–40 cm; 4th row: 50–55 cm. Control plants were placed in a neighbored greenhouse and grown under the same conditions (18/15 °C day/night, 16 °C venting temperature, shading when luminous flux was > 60 klx).

Watering was ensured by an automated ebb and flow system (9 min flow, triggered via light integral of 0.6 kWh). Each table (i.e., plot) had its individual immersion pump powering the ebb and flow system. The watering regime was adjusted to 0.4 kWh after four days. The watering conditions for the control plants were correspondingly adjusted. After 11 days, the light integral was changed to 0.9 kWh until the end of the experiment.

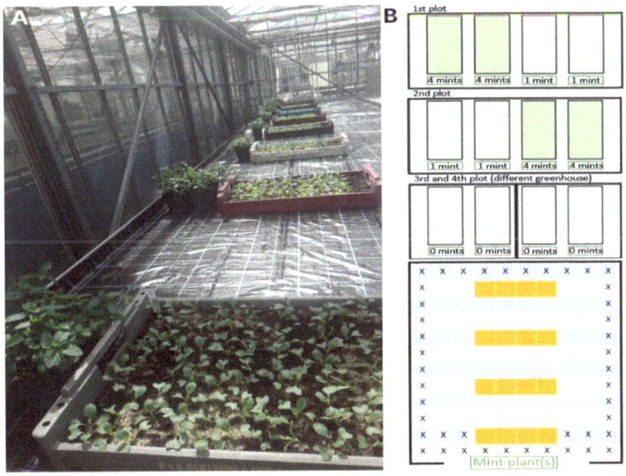


**Figure 10.** Greenhouse trial. Arrangement of plots (**A**,**B** above) and experimental setup of a single box (8 replications) containing 120 plants (**B** below). The setups in two different greenhouses were carried out in a completely randomized design. Orange box = scored plant (repeated measurements); X = unused plant.

### *4.6. Polytunnel Trial*

Three independent sets were conducted in May and July 2018, following the same design as described for the greenhouse experiments. Four blocks were designed, each consisting of three plots: one untreated control and two co-cultivated plots, here with 4 and 9 mint plants, respectively, taking into account that the air exchange was faster than in the greenhouse. The blocks were arranged as shown in Figure 11, and each block was orthogonally aligned towards the prevailing wind direction.

*Mentha* plants were placed in front of their respective plots, allowing the air flow to carry the volatiles into the bulk of the cabbage plants. The squarely designed plots had an edge length of 1.05 m with 8 $\times$ 8 cabbage plants (Figure 11). Each set was conducted in the same polytunnel. Between the sets, weeds were removed and the roots of the *Mentha* plants were cut to prevent growing towards the experimental plots. In addition, *Mentha* plants were cut to maintain equal size and uniformity. The smallest *Mentha* plant served as reference for the mode of cutting.

After sowing, the young cabbage seedlings of each set were grown for 21 days in a greenhouse, as described above, before planting into the soil covered by the polytunnel. Each set of experiments was run for 22 days before cutting the plants for fresh and dry matter determination. Set 2 was started 8 days after set 1, and set 3 was started 6 days after set 2.

Watering in the tunnel was carried out by a sprinkler system; once a day for at least 30 min in the first three days after bedding out, then when necessary but at least two to three times a week.

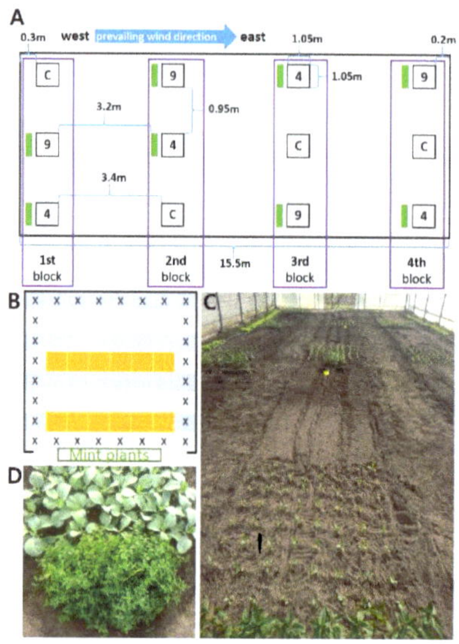


**Figure 11.** Polytunnel trial. Schema of the experimental setup: total experimental design (**A**) and of a single plot (**B**). Dimensions, the prevailing wind direction, and the positions of individual plots and mints are indicated; (**C**): control plants, 9 and 4: plants exposed to 9 and 4 mints (green bars). orange box = scored plant (repeated measurements); X = unused plant. (**C**): Arrangements of cabbage and *Mentha* plants in the Polytunnel soil; (**D**): picture of a single plot.

### *4.7. Measurements of Leaf Parameters*

Leaf parameters were determined with leaves longer than 15 mm. Measurement of leaf length and width was performed after 1, 4, 8, 11, and 15 days after exposure to mint volatiles (T1–T5) with plants at 4 different distances (1st row: 5–10 cm; 2nd: 20–25 cm; 3rd: 35–40 cm; 4th: 50–55 cm), and scored as shown in Figure 10. Regarding the polytunnel trial, the leaf parameters length and width were determined for 12 individual plants/plot and at two different distances (1st row: 15–30 cm; 2nd row: 60–75 cm) once a week, 1 (T1), 8 (T3), and 15 (T5) days after the start of co-cultivation (set 1). In the second set, an additional measurement was taken on day 12 (T4) after treatment, and in the third set additional measurements were conducted after 5 (T2) and 12 (T4) days. The methods were the same as described for the greenhouse trial. Evaluations were performed with data obtained from at least 2 plots of identical conditions. Rates of leaf growth increments were determined for T1–T2, T2–T3, T3–T4, and T4–T5. For calculations, zero growth rates were not considered; the quantity of plants/plots showing no increment are mentioned in the text (or Table S1).

### *4.8. Fresh and Dry Weight*

To determine dry matter percentage, plants used for leaf parameter determinations were cut above ground 21 days after treatment. After fresh weight measurements, the plant material was placed in an oven at 105 °C for five days and then used for dry weight determinations.

### *4.9. Statistics*

All measured variables were subjected to one-way analysis of variance (ANOVA) or to the Kruskal–Wallis test in the case of no Gaussian distribution to verify the differences between the means (GraphPad Software, Inc., La Jolla, CA, USA). Normality was tested according to Anderson–Darling, DÁgostino–Pearson, Shapiro–Wilk, and Kolmogorow–Smirnov. Results are presented in the figures as means + standard error of means. Student's t-tests were performed in addition and *p*-values provided in the results.

**Supplementary Materials:** The following supporting information can be downloaded at: https://www.mdpi.com/article/10.3390/plants11223078/s1, Figure S1: Greenhouse trial leaf growth; Figure S2: Polytunnel trial leaf growth, Table S1: Primer Used for Real Time PCR. Suppliers Volatile Oil Analyses and Certificates.

**Author Contributions:** Conceptualization, M.S. and A.U.; methodology, M.S. and A.U.; investigation, M.P., M.V. and J.R.; writing—original draft preparation, M.S.; writing—review and editing, M.S., M.P. and A.U.; supervision, M.S. and A.U. All authors have read and agreed to the published version of the manuscript.

**Funding:** This research received no external funding.

**Data Availability Statement:** Not applicable.

**Acknowledgments:** The authors thank the technical staff in the greenhouse and polytunnel trials for assistance.

**Conflicts of Interest:** The authors declare no conflict of interest.

## References

1. Verdeguer, M.; Sánchez-Moreiras, A.M.; Araniti, F. Phytotoxic Effects and Mechanism of Action of Essential Oils and Terpenoids. *Plants* **2020**, *9*, 1571. [CrossRef] [PubMed]
2. Araniti, F.; Bruno, L.; Sunseri, F.; Pacenza, M.; Forgione, I.; Bitonti, M.B.; Abenavoli, M.R. The allelochemical farnesene affects *Arabidopsis thaliana* root meristem altering auxin distribution. *Plant Physiol. Biochem.* **2017**, *121*, 14–20. [CrossRef] [PubMed]
3. Graña, E.; Díaz-Tielas, C.; Sánchez-Moreiras, A.M.; Reigosa, M.J.; Celeiro, M.; Abagyan, R.; Teijeira, M.; Duke, M.V.; Clerk, T.; Pan, Z.; et al. Transcriptome and binding data indicate that citral inhibits single strand DNA-binding proteins. *Physiol. Plant.* **2020**, *169*, 99–109. [CrossRef]
4. Sarheed, M.M.; Rajabi, F.; Kunert, M.; Boland, W.; Wetters, S.; Miadowitz, K.; Kazmierczak, A.; Sahi, V.P.; Nick, P. Cellular Base of Mint Allelopathy: Menthone Affects Plant Microtubules. *Front. Plant Sci.* **2020**, *11*, 546345. [CrossRef] [PubMed]
5. Chaimovitsh, D.; Shachter, A.; Abu-Abied, M.; Rubin, B.; Sadot, E.; Dudai, N. Herbicidal activity of monoterpenes is associated with disruption of microtubule functionality and membrane integrity. *Weed Sci.* **2017**, *65*, 19–30. [CrossRef]
6. Kriegs, B.; Jansen, M.; Hahn, K.; Peisker, H.; Samajova, O.; Beck, M.; Braun, M.; Ulbrich, A.; Baluska, F.; Schulz, M. Cyclic monoterpene mediated modulations of *Arabidopsis thaliana* phenotype—Effects on the cytoskeleton and on the expression of selected genes. *Plant Signal. Behav.* **2010**, *5*, 832–838. [CrossRef]
7. Schulz, M.; Kussmann, P.; Knop, M.; Kriegs, B.; Gresens, F.; Eichert, T.; Ulbrich, A.; Marx, F.; Fabricius, H.; Goldbach, H.; et al. Allelopathic monoterpenes interfere with *Arabidopsis thaliana* cuticular waxes and enhance transpiration. *Plant Signal. Behav.* **2007**, *2*, 231–239. [CrossRef]
8. Cappellari, L.D.R.; Santoro, M.V.; Schmidt, A.; Gershenzon, J.; Banchio, E. Improving Phenolic Total Content and Monoterpene in *Mentha x piperita* by Using Salicylic Acid or Methyl Jasmonate Combined with *Rhizobacteria* Inoculation. *Int. J. Mol. Sci.* **2020**, *21*, 50. [CrossRef]
9. Sukegawa, S.; Shiojiri, K.; Higami, T.; Suzuki, S.; Arimura, G.-I. Pest management using mint volatiles to elicit resistance in soy: Mechanism and application potential. *Plant J.* **2018**, *96*, 910–920. [CrossRef]
10. Grulova, D.; De Martino, L.; Mancini, E.; Salamon, I.; De Feo, V. Seasonal variability of the main components in essential oil of *Mentha × piperita* L. *J. Sci. Food Agric.* **2015**, *95*, 621–627. [CrossRef]
11. Kjonaas, R.; Croteau, R. Demonstration that Limonene is the First Cyclic Intermediate in the Biosynthesis of Oxygenated p-Menthane Monoterpenes in *Mentha piperita* and Other *Mentha* Species. *Arch. Biochem. Biophys.* **1983**, *220*, 79–89. [CrossRef]
12. Ulbrich, A.; Kahle, H.; Kramer, P.; Schulz, M. *Mentha x piperita* volatiles promote *Brassica oleracea*—A pilot study for sustainable vegetable production. *Allelopath. J.* **2018**, *43*, 93–104. [CrossRef]
13. Lan, J.; Qin, G. The Regulation of CIN-like TCP Transcription Factors. *Int. J. Mol. Sci.* **2020**, *21*, 4498. [CrossRef]
14. Schommer, C.; Debernardi, J.M.; Bresso, E.G.; Rodriguez, R.E.; Palatnik, J.F. Repression of cell proliferation by miR319-regulated TCP4. *Mol. Plant.* **2014**, *7*, 1533–1544. [CrossRef] [PubMed]
15. Urano, K.; Maruyama, K.; Koyama, T.; Gonzalez, N.; Inzé, D.; Yamaguchi-Shinozaki, K.; Shinozaki, K. CIN-like TCP13 is essential for plant growth regulation under dehydration stress. *Plant Mol. Biol.* **2022**, *108*, 257–275. [CrossRef] [PubMed]
16. Hao, J.; Lou, P.; Han, Y.; Chen, Z.; Chen, J.; Ni, J.; Yang, Y.; Jiang, Z.; Xu, M. GrTCP11, a Cotton TCP Transcription Factor, Inhibits Root Hair Elongation by Down-Regulating Jasmonic Acid Pathway in *Arabidopsis thaliana*. *Front. Plant Sci.* **2021**, *12*, 769675. [CrossRef]

17. Baulies, J.L.; Bresso, E.G.; Goldy, C.; Palatnik, J.F.; Schommer, C. Potent inhibition of TCP transcription factors by miR319 ensures proper root growth in *Arabidopsis*. *Plant Mol. Biol.* **2022**, *108*, 93–103. [CrossRef]
18. Danisman, S. TCP transcription factors at the interface between environmental challenges and the plant's growth responses. *Front. Plant Sci.* **2016**, *7*, 1930. [CrossRef]
19. Palatnik, J.F.; Allen, E.; Wu, X.; Schommer, C.; Schwab, R.; Carrington, J.C.; Weigel, D. Control of leaf morphogenesis by microRNAs. *Nature* **2003**, *425*, 257–263. [CrossRef]
20. Bresso, E.G.; Chorostecki, U.; Rodriguez, R.E.; Palatnik, J.F.; Schommer, C. Spatial Control of Gene Expression by miR319-Regulated TCP Transcription Factors in Leaf Development. *Plant Physiol.* **2018**, *176*, 1694–1708. [CrossRef]
21. Danisman, S.; van der Wal, F.; Dhondt, S.; Waites, R.; de Folter, S.; Bimbo, A.; van Dijk, A.D.; Muino, J.M.; Cutri, L.; Dornelas, M.C.; et al. *Arabidopsis* class I and class II TCP transcription factors regulate jasmonic acid metabolism and leaf development antagonistically. *Plant Physiol.* **2012**, *159*, 1511–1523. [CrossRef] [PubMed]
22. Li, Y.; An, S.; Cheng, Q.; Zong, Y.; Chen, W.; Guo, W.; Zhang, L. Analysis of Evolution, Expression and Genetic Transformation of TCP Transcription Factors in Blueberry Reveal That VcTCP18 Negatively Regulates the Release of Flower Bud Dormancy. *Front. Plant Sci.* **2021**, *12*, 697609. [CrossRef] [PubMed]
23. Li, D.; Zhang, H.; Mou, M.; Chen, Y.; Xiang, S.; Chen, L.; Yu, D. *Arabidopsis* Class II TCP Transcription Factors Integrate with the FT–FD Module to Control Flowering. *Plant Physiol.* **2019**, *181*, 97–111. [CrossRef] [PubMed]
24. Mao, Y.; Wu, F.; Yu, X.; Bai, J.; Zhong, W.; He, Y. microRNA319a-Targeted *Brassica rapa* ssp. *pekinensis* TCP Genes Modulate Head Shape in Chinese Cabbage by Differential Cell Division Arrest in Leaf Regions. *Plant Physiol.* **2014**, *164*, 710–720. [CrossRef]
25. Du, J.; Hu, S.; Yu, Q.; Wang, C.; Yang, Y.; Sun, H.; Yang, Y.; Sun, X. Genome-Wide Identification and Characterization of BrrTCP Transcription Factors in *Brassica rapa* ssp. *rapa*. *Front. Plant Sci.* **2017**, *8*, 1588. [CrossRef]
26. Efroni, I.; Blum, E.; Goldshmidt, A.; Eshed, Y. A Protracted and Dynamic Maturation Schedule Underlies *Arabidopsis* Leaf Development. *Plant Cell* **2008**, *20*, 2293–2306. [CrossRef] [PubMed]
27. Koyama, T.; Mitsuda, N.; Seki, M.; Shinozaki, K.; Ohme-Takagi, M. TCP transcription factors regulate the activities of ASYMMETRIC LEAVES1 and miR164, as well as the auxin response, during differentiation of leaves in *Arabidopsis*. *Plant Cell* **2010**, *22*, 3574–3588. [CrossRef]
28. Xiong, Y.; Jiao, Y. The Diverse Roles of Auxin in Regulating Leaf Development. *Plants* **2019**, *23*, 243. [CrossRef]
29. Saini, K.; Markakis, M.N.; Zdanio, M.; Balcerowicz, D.M.; Beeckman, T.; De Veylder, L.; Prinsen, E.; Beemster, G.T.S.; Vissenberg, K. Alteration in Auxin Homeostasis and Signaling by Overexpression of PINOID Kinase Causes Leaf Growth Defects in *Arabidopsis thaliana*. *Front. Plant Sci.* **2017**, *8*, 1009. [CrossRef]
30. Li, S.; Zachgo, S. TCP3 interacts with R2R3-MYB proteins, promotes flavonoid biosynthesis and negatively regulates the auxin response in *Arabidopsis thaliana*. *Plant J.* **2013**, *76*, 901–913. [CrossRef]
31. Kong, Q.; Low, P.M.; Lim, A.R.Q.; Yang, Y.; Yuan, L.; Ma, W. Functional Antagonism of WRI1 and TCP20 Modulates GH3.3 Expression to Maintain Auxin Homeostasis in Roots. *Plants* **2022**, *11*, 454. [CrossRef] [PubMed]
32. Wang, H.; Mao, Y.; Yang, J.; He, Y. TCP24 modulates secondary cell wall thickening and anther endothecium development. *Front. Plant Sci.* **2015**, *6*, 436. [CrossRef] [PubMed]
33. Omidbakhshfard, M.A.; Proost, S.; Fujikura, U.; Mueller-Roeber, B. Growth-Regulating Factors (GRFs): A Small Transcription Factor Family with Important Functions in Plant Biology. *Mol. Plant* **2015**, *8*, 998–1010. [CrossRef]
34. Godard, K.-A.; White, R.; Bohlmann, J. Monoterpene-induced molecular responses in *Arabidopsis thaliana*. *Phytochemistry* **2008**, *69*, 1838–1849. [CrossRef]
35. Onosato, H.; Fujimoto, G.; Higami, T.; Sakamoto, T.; Yamada, A.; Suzuki, T.; Ozawa, R.; Matsunaga, S.; Seki, M.; Ueda, M.; et al. Sustained defense response via volatile signaling and its epigenetic transcriptional regulation. *Plant Physiol.* **2022**, *189*, 922–933. [CrossRef]
36. Nie, Y.; Han, F.; Ma, J.; Chen, X.; Song, Y.-T.; Niu, S.-H.; Wu, H.X. Genome-wide TCP transcription factors analysis provides insight into their new functions in seasonal and diurnal growth rhythm in *Pinus tabuliformis*. *BMC Plant Biol.* **2022**, *22*, 167. [CrossRef] [PubMed]
37. Laila, R.; Robin, A.H.K.; Yang, K.; Park, J.-I.; Suh, M.C.; Kim, J.; Nou, I.-S. Developmental and Genotypic Variation in Leaf Wax Content and Composition, and in Expression of Wax Biosynthetic Genes in *Brassica oleracea* var. *capitata*. *Front. Plant Sci.* **2017**, *7*, 1972. [CrossRef]
38. Martelanc, M.; Vovk, I.; Simonovska, B. Determination of three major triterpenoids in epicuticular wax of cabbage (*Brassica oleracea* L.) by high-performance liquid chromatography with UV and mass spectrometric detection. *J. Chromatogr. A* **2007**, *1164*, 145–152. [CrossRef]
39. Buschhaus, C.; Jetter, R. Composition and Physiological Function of the Wax Layers Coating *Arabidopsis* Leaves: β-Amyrin Negatively Affects the Intracuticular Water Barrier. *Plant Physiol.* **2012**, *160*, 1120–1129. [CrossRef]
40. Hadacek, F. Cuticular Wax Terpenoids in Plants: Functional Diversity of. In *Encyclopedia of Lipidomics*; Wenk, M., Ed.; Springer: Dordrecht, The Netherlands, 2017. [CrossRef]
41. Heydari, M.; Zanfardino, A.; Taleei, A.; Shahnejat Bushehri, A.A.; Hadian, J.; Maresca, V.; Sorbo, S.; Di Napoli, M.; Varcamonti, M.; Basile, A.; et al. Effect of Heat Stress on Yield, Monoterpene Content and Antibacterial Activity of Essential Oils of *Mentha x piperita* var. Mitcham and *Mentha arvensis* var. piperascens. *Molecules* **2018**, *23*, 1903. [CrossRef]

42. Islam, A.K.M.M.; Kato-Noguchi, H. *Mentha sylvestris*: A Potential Allelopathic Medicinal Plant. *Int. J. Agric. Biol.* **2013**, *15*, 1313–1318.
43. Maes, C.; Meersmans, J.; Lins, L.; Bouquillon, S.; Fauconnier, M.-L. Essential Oil-Based Bioherbicides: Human Health Risks Analysis. *Int. J. Mol. Sci.* **2021**, *22*, 9396. [CrossRef]
44. Girel, S.; Schütz, V.; Bigler, L.; Dörmann, P.; Schulz, M. Bioactive Nitrosylated and Nitrated N-(2-hydroxyphenyl)acetamides and Derived Oligomers: An Alternative Pathway to 2-Amidophenol-Derived Phytotoxic Metabolites. *Molecules* **2022**, *27*, 4786. [CrossRef] [PubMed]
45. Danisman, S.; van Dijk, A.D.J.; Bimbo, A.; van der Wal, F.; Hennig, L.; de Folter, S.; Angenent, G.C.; Immink, R.G.H. Analysis of functional redundancies within the *Arabidopsis* TCP transcription factor family. *J. Exp. Bot.* **2013**, *64*, 5673–5685. [CrossRef] [PubMed]

plants

MDPI

Article

# Is the Phytotoxic Effect of Digestive Fluid of *Nepenthes x ventrata* on Tomato Related to Reactive Oxygen Species?

**Pawel Staszek *, Maciej Piekarniak, Agnieszka Wal, Urszula Krasuska and Agnieszka Gniazdowska ***

Department of Plant Physiology, Institute of Biology, Warsaw University of Life Sciences-SGGW, 02-776 Warsaw, Poland

* Correspondence: pawel_staszek1@sggw.edu.pl (P.S.); agnieszka_gniazdowska@sggw.edu.pl (A.G.)

**Abstract:** The digestive fluid of pitcher plants is a rich source of enzymes and secondary metabolites, but its impact on higher plant growth and development remains unknown. The aim of the study was to determine the phytotoxicity of the digestive fluid of the pitcher plant (*Nepenthes x ventrata*) on the germination of tomato (*Solanum lycopersicum* L.) seeds, elongation growth and cell viability of roots of tomato seedlings. The digestive fluid was collected from pitchers before feeding and four days after feeding; the pH and electrical conductivity of the fluid were determined. Undiluted and 50% fluids were used in the study. An inhibition of germination of tomato seeds, by around 30% and 55%, was respectively observed in 50% and 100% digestive fluids collected before and after feeding. Digestive fluid did not affect the root growth of tomato seedlings; a slight (6%) inhibition was only observed after the application of 100% digestive fluid from an unfed trap. The roots of the tomato seedlings treated with undiluted fluid were characterized by reduced cell viability. Reactive oxygen species ($H_2O_2$ and $O_2^{\bullet-}$) were mainly localized in the root apex regardless of the used phytotoxic cocktail, and did not differ in comparison to control plants.

**Keywords:** carnivorous plant; ROS; root growth; seed germination; allelopathy

**Citation:** Staszek, P.; Piekarniak, M.; Wal, A.; Krasuska, U.; Gniazdowska, A. Is the Phytotoxic Effect of Digestive Fluid of *Nepenthes x ventrata* on Tomato Related to Reactive Oxygen Species? *Plants* **2023**, *12*, 755. https://doi.org/10.3390/plants12040755

Academic Editors: Margot Schulz and Vincenzo Tabaglio

Received: 9 January 2023
Revised: 2 February 2023
Accepted: 6 February 2023
Published: 8 February 2023



## 1. Introduction

*Nepenthes x ventrata* belongs to the Nepenthaceae family and is a natural hybrid of *Nepenthes alata* Blanco and *Nepenthes ventricosa* Blanco. This species is endemic to forests in the Philippines [1]. *N. ventrata* forms jug-shaped containers that function as passive pitcher traps. Pitchers are filled with digestive fluid, being the mixture that enables the release of nutrients from the bodies of the captured prey [2].

Many enzymes have been found in the digestive fluid of pitcher plants: proteases, peptidases, phosphatases, esterases, ribonucleases and chitinases [3–6]. The aspartyl proteinases Nepenthesin-1 and Nepenthesin-2 have also been isolated from the digestive fluid [7]. The digestive fluid also contains a thaumatin-like protein with antibacterial and antifungal properties [8]. In addition, pitcher fluid contains compounds of low molecular weight, e.g., two naphthoquinones: droseron (3,5-dihydroxy-2-methyl-1,4-naphthoquinone) and its derivative 5-O-methyldroserone (2-methyl-3-hydroxy-5-methoxy-1,4- naphthoquinone) [9], of antifungal activity against a wide range of human and plant fungal pathogens [10]. Another low-molecular substance is plumbagin, isolated from *N. alata* [11] and characterized by antimalarial, antibacterial, antifungal and anticancer properties [12–14] and 7-methyl-juglone [11]. The digestive fluid of the Nepenthes species is rich in mineral nutrient composition (boron, calcium, copper, iron and nickel) and anions $Cl^-$, $Br^-$ and $SO_4^{2-}$ [11]. Prey digestion (feeding process) is accompanied by alteration in fluid composition, including reactive oxygen species (ROS) and reactive nitrogen species (RNS) levels [15].

The physicochemical properties of the digestive fluid, such as lower surface tension against water and high viscoelasticity, play an important role in preventing the escape of captured insects [16].

Application of allelopathic cocktails in cultivation can effectively influence weed populations and insect pests. Allelopathy thus offers an attractive environmentally friendly alternative to pesticides in agriculture [17]. Volatile organic compounds belonging to the group of allelochemicals could repel insects or mask the host's odor to confuse them [18,19].

Digestive fluid as a mixture of many compounds with a possible phytotoxic potential may prove to be a key element in research on natural herbicides that would replace artificial and less specific compounds currently used in agriculture. The exact composition of the digestive fluid is unknown, but the digestive fluid of some species is known to contain compounds that have phytotoxic potential.

The aim of our study was to characterize some properties of phytotoxic cocktails and to determine the effect of the digestive fluid from pitchers of *N. ventrata*, collected before and after plant feeding, on tomato (*Solanum lycopersicum* L.) seed germination and root growth.

Based on the mode of action of many allelochemicals and phytotoxins [20], we hypothesized that pitcher plants' digestive fluid impacts the seed germination and root growth of tomato seedlings by the induction of oxidative stress.

## 2. Results

### 2.1. Electrical Conductivity

The electrical conductivity and pH of the phytotoxic cocktail depended on the origin of the fluid (from fed or unfed traps) and the concentration. The highest pH value was found in distilled water used as a control, and the lowest in heat-treated, 100% fluid from fed traps (Table 1). The pH of the fluid from fed pitchers was lower than that from unfed ones, regardless of concentration or heat-treatment (Table 1).

**Table 1.** Electrical conductivity and pH of digestive fluid solutions used in the experiments as phytotoxic cocktails.

| | | pH | Electrical Conductivity [mS cm$^{-1}$] |
|---|---|---|---|
| Control | | 6.29 ± 0.07 c | 0.021 ± 0.017 A |
| | | Crude fluid | |
| Unfed trap | 50% fluid | 5.96 ± 0.17 bc | 0.786 ± 0.078 B |
| | 100% fluid | 5.82 ± 0.03 b | 1.333 ± 0.012 C |
| Fed trap | 50% fluid | 3.78 ± 0.19 a | 0.704 ± 0.042 B |
| | 100% fluid | 3.38 ± 0.08 a | 1.247 ± 0.017 C |
| | | Heat-treated fluid | |
| Unfed trap | 50% fluid | 6.09 ± 0.29 bc | 0.771 ± 0.026 B |
| | 100% fluid | 5.54 ± 0.10 b | 1.364 ± 0.052 C |
| Fed trap | 50% fluid | 3.83 ± 0.31 a | 0.630 ± 0.040 B |
| | 100% fluid | 3.36 ± 0.16 a | 1.127 ± 0.039 C |

Table includes average values ± SD of three replicated experiments. Homogenous groups (a–c or A–C) were evaluated using Fisher's LSD post hoc test with $p < 0.5$.

The highest electrical conductivity (1.364 mS cm$^{-1}$) was recorded for heat-treated undiluted fluid from unfed pitchers, and the lowest (0.0209 mS cm$^{-1}$) for the distilled water (control) (Table 1). Digestive fluids (100%) were characterized by higher electrical conductivity compared to diluted ones, irrespective of the origin of the fluid and heat-treatment.

### 2.2. Germination Tests

Two-way Anova showed that there were no statistically significant differences between the germination of tomato seeds in crude fluid and heat-treated fluid ($p = 0.73$, F = 0.13). Due to the lack of associations, the dataset for crude and heat-treated fluids was not separated in the remaining analyses.

Tomato seeds germinated in 100% fluid after three days of imbibition in water (Figure 1). Undiluted digestion fluids from unfed or fed traps inhibited the germination of tomato seeds by 59% or 53%, respectively. In diluted phytotoxic cocktails of fed and unfed pitchers, tomato seeds germinated in 67% and 75%, respectively (Figure 1).

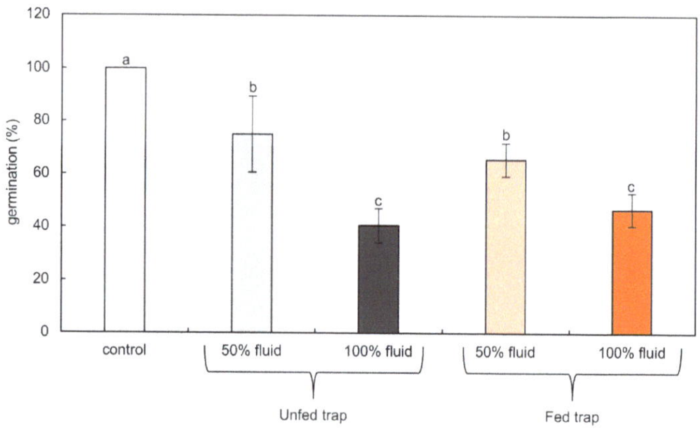


**Figure 1.** Germination of tomato seeds in water (control) or in phytotoxic cocktails of 100% or 50% digestive fluids from fed and unfed traps of pitcher plants. Due to the lack of significant differences, we did not separate data obtained after treatment with crude and heat-treaded fluids. Values are average ± SD of three replications. Homogenous groups (a–c) were evaluated using Fisher's LSD post hoc test with $p < 0.5$.

## 2.3. *Root Growth Biotest*

Two-way Anova showed that there were no statistically significant differences between the growth of tomato seedlings in crude fluid and heat-treated fluid ($p = 0.33$, $F = 0.95$). Due to the lack of associations, the dataset for crude and heat-treated fluids was not separated in the remaining analyses.

Roots of the control tomato seedlings growing in water for 24 h were about 16 mm long. Fluids from traps of pitcher plants repressed the growth of tomato roots in only 6% (Figure 2). The longest roots were observed in seedlings treated with the diluted fluid from unfed traps. The strongest inhibition of root growth was noted for seedlings treated with 100% fluids from unfed traps. Root lengths measured in seedlings treated with diluted and undiluted fluid from fed traps differed by 0.25 mm and 0.5 mm from the control, respectively, but the differences were not statistically significant.

## 2.4. *Test of Root Cell Viability*

The viability of the root cells of seedlings treated for 24 h with crude and heat-treated phytotoxic cocktails slightly differed (Table 2). Excluding the control plants, the highest viability was estimated for roots of seedlings treated with crude, diluted fluid from fed traps, and the lowest viability was noticed for the roots of seedlings grown in 100% crude digestion fluid from unfed pitchers, which was very similar to 100% heat-treated fluid from fed traps (31,8–31,3% of damages, respectively). The roots of seedlings treated with 50% fluid were characterized by a higher viability than the roots of seedlings treated with undiluted fluid, irrespective of heat treatment.

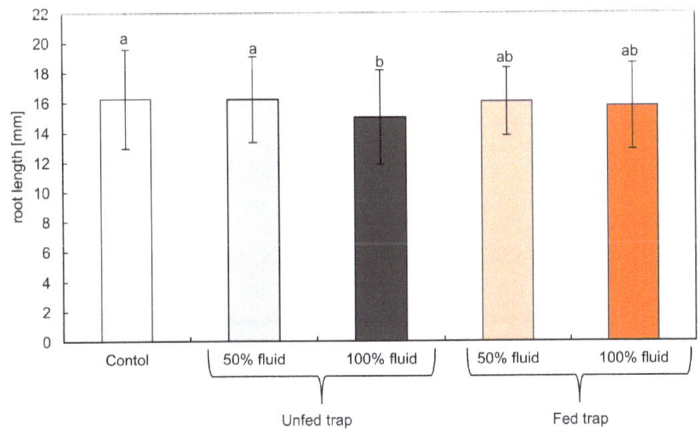


**Figure 2.** Length of roots of tomato seedlings growing for 24 h in water (control) or in phytotoxic cocktails of 100% or 50% digestive fluids from fed and unfed traps of pitcher plants. Due to the lack of significant differences, we did not separate data obtained after treatment, the division into crude and heat-treaded fluids was not included. Values are average ± SD of three replications. Homogenous groups (a, b) were evaluated using Fisher's LSD post hoc test with $p < 0.5$.

**Table 2.** Cell viability (Evans blue test) and cell damage of roots of tomato seedlings cultured in water or treated with digestive fluids from Nepenthes traps (crude, heat-treated, concentrated (100%) or diluted (50%)) after 24 h of the culture.

| | | Evans Blue Uptake to the Roots [mg dye $g^{-1}$ FW] | Cell Damage [%] |
|---|---|---|---|
| Positive control (heat-treated roots) | | 0.476 ± 0.011 c | 100 E |
| Control (seedlings grown in water) | | 0.086 ± 0.021 a | 18.1 A |
| | | Crude fluid | |
| Unfed trap | 50% fluid | 0.122 ± 0.064 b | 25.7 BC |
| | 100% fluid | 0.151 ± 0.053 b | 31.8 D |
| Fed trap | 50% fluid | 0.100 ± 0.048 b | 20.9 B |
| | 100% fluid | 0.140 ± 0.079 b | 29.3 BC |
| | | Heat-treated fluid | |
| Unfed trap | 50% fluid | 0.109 ± 0.056 b | 22.9 BC |
| | 100% fluid | 0.113 ± 0.055 b | 23.7 D |
| Fed trap | 50% fluid | 0.135 ± 0.008 b | 28.4 B |
| | 100% fluid | 0.149 ± 0.084 b | 31.3 BC |

Table includes average values ± SD of three replicated experiments. Homogenous groups (a–c or A–E) were evaluated using Fisher's LSD post hoc test with $p < 0.5$.

### 2.5. *In Situ $H_2O_2$ Localization in Tomato Seedlings Cultured*

$H_2O_2$ was localized using DAB staining as brown precipitates of polymerized DAB (Figure 3). For all tested seedlings, the most visible staining was detected in the root tips. Stronger coloration of the upper part of the roots, on the border with the hypocotyl, was observed in seedlings treated with heat-treated fluid, regardless of the concentration of the fluids or the feeding of the traps (from fed or unfed ones).

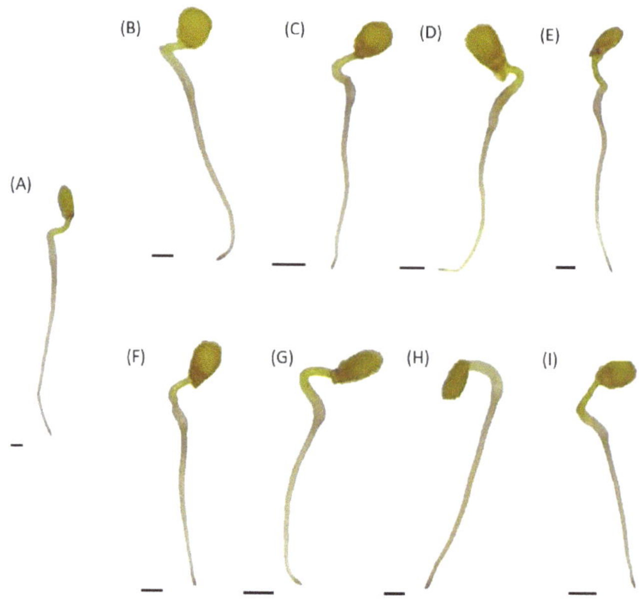


**Figure 3.** In situ $H_2O_2$ localization in tomato seedlings cultured for 24 h in water (the control) or in phytotoxic cocktails of 100% or 50% fed or unfed traps of pitcher plants. Control seedlings (**A**), seedlings growing in crude concentrated fluids of unfed traps (**B**), treated with crude diluted cocktail of unfed traps (**C**), cultured in crude concentrated fluids of fed traps (**D**), exposed to crude diluted cocktails of unfed traps (**E**), growing in heat-treated concentrated fluids of unfed traps (**F**), heat-treated diluted cocktails of unfed traps (**G**), heat-treated concentrated fluids of fed traps (**H**) and heat-treated diluted cocktails of fed traps (**I**). Bar = 2 mm.

### 2.6. *In Situ* $O_2^{\bullet -}$ *Localization*

The histochemical localization of $O_2^{\bullet -}$ was carried out using NBT staining. A dark blue coloration of formazan was observed in the root tips of all the tested seedlings (Figure 4). Only the outer layers of the roots were colored above the tips. The roots of seedlings treated with 50% digestive fluid were characterized by a slightly higher color intensity, regardless of the heating of the phytotoxic cocktails (Figure 4). However, in general, no differences in NBT staining were noticed between the roots of tomato seedlings treated with digestive fluids and those growing in water (Figure 4).

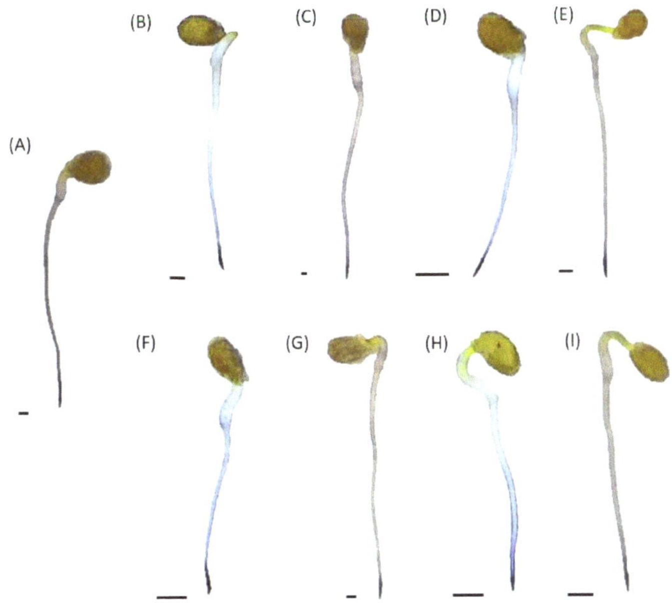


**Figure 4.** In situ $O_2^{\bullet -}$ localization in tomato seedlings cultured for 24 h in water (control) or in phytotoxic cocktails of 100% or 50% fed or unfed traps of pitcher plants. Control seedlings (**A**), seedlings growing in crude concentrated fluids of unfed traps (**B**), treated with crude diluted cocktail of unfed traps (**C**), cultured in crude concentrated fluids of fed traps (**D**), exposed to crude diluted cocktails of unfed traps (**E**), growing in heat-treated concentrated fluids of unfed traps (**F**), heat-treated diluted cocktails of unfed traps (**G**), heat-treated concentrated fluids of fed traps (**H**) and heat-treated diluted cocktails of fed traps (**I**). Bar = 2 mm.

## 3. Discussion

*Nepenthes* is a plant which, by adapting to specific environmental conditions, in the process of evolution, developed a carnivorous syndrome. Although it is known where the components of the fluid are produced and how the substances resulting from the digestion of the prey are absorbed by the plant, knowledge about the composition of the digestive fluid is limited. The phenomenon of carnivorous syndrome in plants has been described for over 150 years; the isolation and identification of enzymes involved in digestion is still only fragmentary. It refers to both the composition of enzymes and other molecules in the digestive fluid. Their identification, structure and biosynthesis may be an interesting target for further research [9]. Until now, the digestive fluid of pitcher plants has been mostly examined in the context of plant nutrition, but its putative toxicity on neighboring plants should not be omitted. Our study is a unique observation of the impact of the digestive fluid on the germination and growth of other plants; acceptors, according to allelopathic terminology.

At the start of this study, we determined the impact of pitcher plant feeding and the inactivation of the fluid by heating on its phytotoxicity. No influence of the temperature inactivation on the toxicity of the digestive fluid on the germination of tomato seeds and the elongation growth of roots suggests temperature-resistant compounds of the fluid, rather than enzymes of the fluid, are responsible for its negative action. The feeding of the pitcher plant resulted in decreased pH of the fluid, which is a typical reaction in the digestion process [21], although it did not affect tomato seed germination. The germination of seeds was inhibited by phytotoxic cocktails with no respect to the pH of the fluid. Tomato seeds similarly germinated in the digestive fluid with a pH range of 3.3–3.8, taken from fed traps and in the digestive fluid of unfed traps (pH 5.5 to 6.1). The low pH of the digestive fluid also did not influence the elongation growth of the tomato roots. The pH value also seems to be correlated with bacterial community composition [22] and feeding. Taking to account no differences in cocktail phytotoxicity in the tomato seedlings before and after heating, it can be concluded that microorganisms from the fluid are not toxic to acceptor tissues; however, perhaps the experiments should be performed longer to observe such effects. The electrical conductivity of the digestive fluid showed no difference in dependence on feeding, nor heating; it only decreased as the dilution of the liquid was performed. Electrical conductivity in a range of 0.8–1.6 mS $cm^{-1}$, observed in the research, indicates moderately saline soils, where only plants resistant to salinity can grow [23,24]. This data confirms the information that the pitcher fluid of *Nepenthes* plants (*N. alata, N. fusca, N.gracilis, N. mirabilis, N. superba, N. thorelii* and *N. ventricosa*) is a 25 mM KCl solution with few additional ions [11].

During the germination tests, solutions with a similar pH, but different digestive fluid concentration, were applied, on which the results of the experiment mainly depended. Undiluted digestive fluid, taken from a pitcher of *N. ventrata* fed with the proteins, inhibited tomato seed germination as compared to the 50% cocktail. Some compounds that may adversely affect the growth and development of other plants have been isolated from carnivorous plants. Studies conducted with the use of Portuguese sundew ((*Drosophyllum lusitanicum* L. (Link)) extracts have shown that the extracts inhibited the germination of lettuce (*Lactuca sativa* L.) and wheat (*Triticum aestivum* L.) seeds. Plumbagin has been identified as the main compound responsible for the inhibition of lettuce sprouting [25]. Other compounds, isolated from carnivorous plants, may show a toxic effect; these include two naphthoquinones, droserone and its derivative 5-O-methyldroserone, which have beem found in the digestive fluid of *N. khasiana* [10] or 7-methyl-juglone isolated from *N. alata* [11]. Previous reports from our laboratory indicated the presence of phenolic compounds in the digestive fluid, the total content of which increased in fed traps [15]. Phenolics are regarded as strong allelochemicals of various modes of action in acceptor plants [26].

Investigating the mode of action of allelopathic compounds is complicated due to the multitude of potential molecular targets. Biological tests using plants or plant tissues successfully detect the biological activity of many synthetic and natural compounds [27]. One of the first visible effects of phytotoxin's action is the reduction of seed germination and/or seedling growth [28]. Diverse phytotoxins (like cyanamide, citral, coumarin) act as inhibitors of root tip cell division, influencing root growth [29–31]. Treatment of tomato seedlings with digestive fluids showed that components of these cocktails had no effect on the growth and development of the young seedlings. Morphology and length of the roots of tomato plants exposed to 100% and 50% digestive fluids of *N. ventrata* traps did not differ and were similar to those observed in control seedlings. It suggests that the impact of the phytotoxic cocktails of the digestive fluids on growth of the roots is weaker than on seed germination. This observation is atypical in allelopathy research, as most allelochemicals applied as the mixture or extract originated from the tissue of allelopathic plant are more toxic in growth tests than germination tests [32]. Many allelochemicals affect seed germination by inhibition of the activity of the enzymes crucial for the process. Extracts from the leaves and flowers of catnip (*Nepeta meyeri* Benth.) decreased α-amylase, ß-1,3 glucanase and protease activities in seeds of field dodder (*Cuscuta campestris* Yunck) [33]. Allelochemicals could disrupt the action of phytohormones in germinating seeds. The inhibition of germination of lettuce (*Lactuca sativa* L.) by myrigalone A, C-methylated dihydrochalcone from sweet gale (*Myrica gale* L.) was accompanied by alterations in gibberellins metabolism by inhibiting GA3 oxidase, as well as by interfering with the gibberellin signaling pathway [34]. Perturbations in ROS metabolism and the induction of oxidative stress were identified as the cause of inhibition of seed germination. Sunflower (*Helianthus annus* L.) extracts increased $H_2O_2$ content in mustard (*Sinapsis alba* L.) seeds, resulting in the restriction of their germination [35].

Although evidence for allelopathic interactions and/or the potential of allelochemicals is based on the evaluation of seed germination and seedling growth of the target species [28], these tests only provide general information regarding the biological effects of phytotoxins. They do not indicate a mechanism of their action [36,37]. In many studies, it has been demonstrated that, for allelopathy stress, as for other stresses, the induction of oxidative stress is the common response of acceptor plants [20,28,29,38]. Such observations are typical for both crude extracts of allelopathic plants, as well as for single allelopathic compounds. An accumulation of ROS, a modification of their localization and a disruption of cellular antioxidant systems were shown for various plants exposed to different allelochemicals (for review, see [20,29,38]. In our study, phytotoxic cocktails of digestive fluids did not lead to increased levels of $H_2O_2$ or $O_2^{\bullet-}$. Moreover, no alteration in the localization of ROS in roots in response to digestive fluids were shown. It may be proposed that compounds in the fluids from *N. ventrata* traps do not impact ROS production. Although investigations of the activity of enzymes of the antioxidant system are still required, the presence of ROS and reactive nitrogen species in the digestion liquid of these plants has been recently revealed [15].

## 4. Materials and Methods

### 4.1. Experimental Model

In our experiments, we used tomato (*Solanum lycopersicum* L. cv Malinowy Ożarowski) seedlings as the test plant. A digestive fluid from pitchers of Nepenthes was applied in the tests as a phytotoxic cocktail.

Pitcher plants *Nepenthes x ventrata* Hort. ex Fleming [=(*N. ventricosa* Blanco × *N. alata* Blanco)] were grown in the greenhouse under conditions of constant high humidity (60%) and temperature (28 °C); light was supplemented with sodium lamps to obtain a 16-/8-h day/night photoperiod. A mixture of acid peat, perlite and sphagnum moss was used as a growing medium and plants were watered with distilled water every other day. The traps of pitcher plants, immediately after opening, were covered with gauze to avoid contamination by accidental insects. Digestive fluid was collected from fed or unfed mature pitchers (aerial type, length approximately 9 cm). Traps were fed with 40 μg hen egg white solution (1 μg $\mu L^{-1}$) introduced with a pipette directly into a pitcher. Digestive fluids from fed traps were collected four days after feeding. The fluids (from fed and unfed pitchers) were shortly centrifuged (5522× *g*, 5 min at 4 °C), and the supernatants were transferred to the sterile tubes, frozen and used for biotests.

Before biotesting, digestive fluids from several traps were combined (fluid separately from fed and unfed traps) to maximize the volume of the phytotoxic cocktail. One portion of the fluid was boiled at 100 °C for 10 min (heat-treated fluid) and the rest was left untreated (crude fluid). Then, part of each fluid (heat-treated or crude) was diluted twice to obtain a 50% solution. The electrical conductivity and pH of phytotoxic cocktails were determined using a pH/conductivity meter (CPC-505 Elmetron, Zabrze, Poland, with suitable electrodes ECF-60 and EPS-1, respectively).

### 4.2. Germination Tests

Tomato seeds (*Solanum lycopersicum* L. cv. Malinowy Ożarowski) (commercially obtained from PNOS Sp. z o.o., Poland) were surface sterilized with 0.5% sodium hypochloride for 10 min at room temperature. Then, seeds were rinsed three times with distilled water, and 8 seeds were placed on Petri dishes (ø 3.5 cm) filled with filter paper wetted with 2.5 mL phytotoxic cocktail or 2.5 mL distilled water (control). The culture was carried out in a growth chamber (Fitotron Versatile Environmental Test Chamber-PAR-10Mn, by Sanyo,

Osaka, Japan, model MLR-350H), in darkness at 20 °C for 3 days. Seeds were considered germinated when the radicle had emerged through the seed coat.

To investigate the impact of pitcher fluids on the growth of tomato seedlings, biotests were performed. Tomato seeds were germinated in water in darkness at 20 °C for 3–4 days. Then, 8 seedlings with roots of equal length (0.5 cm) were selected and transferred to Petri dishes (ø 3.5 cm) filled with filter paper wetted with 2.5 mL phytotoxic cocktails or 2.5 mL distilled water (control). Control seedlings and seedlings treated with digestive fluid were cultured in a growth chamber at 23/20 °C, 12-/12-h day/night regime, and a light intensity of 90 μmol PAR $m^{-2}$ $s^{-1}$ for 24 h as described by Krasuska et al. [39]. The root length of seedlings was measured after 24 h of the culture.

### 4.3. Test of Root Cell Viability

The viability of tomato root cells was determined using Evans blue staining [40]. The whole control seedlings or seedlings treated with pitcher fluids for 24 h were incubated in a 0.25% solution of Evans blue for 30 min at room temperature. Then, seedlings were washed three times in distilled water and roots were isolated, weighed and homogenized in 1 mL of a 1% solution of sodium dodecylsulphate (SDS). After 10 min centrifugation at 21,000× *g* at 4 °C, the supernatant was collected and absorbance was measured at 600 nm (Sunrise, Tecan, Männedorf, Switzerland). For the positive control (100% cell damage), the roots were boiled for 10 min, cooled and then treated as described above. Three roots were used for one repetition. The concentration of the extracted dye was estimated from the standard curve prepared with Evans blue in 1% SDS and expressed as mg $g^{-1}$ FW or % of cell damage. The data were means of three measurements from each of three sets of experiments.

### 4.4. In Situ $H_2O_2$ Localization

The histochemical localization of $H_2O_2$ was carried out with 3,3′-diaminobenzidine (DAB) staining [39]. The roots of the control seedlings and seedlings treated with pitcher fluids for 24 h were washed twice in distilled water and incubated with DAB solution (1 mg $mL^{-1}$) with 2 mM DMSO. Staining was carried out for 4 h at room temperature, in darkness.

### 4.5. In Situ $O_2^{\bullet-}$ Localization

The histochemical localization of $O_2^{\bullet-}$ was performed according to Beyer and Fridovich [41] using nitroblue tetrazolium (NBT) staining. Roots isolated from the control seedlings and seedlings treated with pitcher fluids for 24 h were washed twice in distilled water and incubated for 20 min in darkness at room temperature in 2 mM NBT (Sigma–Aldrich, Tokyo, Japan), freshly prepared in 10 mM Tris-HCl buffer pH 7.4 with 2 mM DMSO. After staining, the roots were cleaned for 24 h in chloral hydrate to avoid artifacts by removing oxidized phenolics [42]. $O_2^{\bullet-}$ was visualized as a deposit of a dark blue insoluble formazan compound.

Images of seedlings stained with DAB and NBT were taken with the TAGARNO FHD TREND digital microscope (magnification x 5.2, F4 diaphragm, enhancement 10.2 dB, exposure time 1/15 s).

Data were obtained in at least three independent experiments with at least three repetitions each. The plants for experiments were randomly selected from 25 individuals. Data were analyzed using Statistica Software. Mean values were calculated and SD was provided. After Anova, homogenous groups were evaluated using Fisher's LSD post hoc test.

## 5. Conclusions

We demonstrated the negative, dose-dependent effect of the digestive fluid of the pitcher plant on tomato seed germination; whereas its impact on root elongation was less evident, but still significant. Application of the digestive fluid decreased cell viability but did not alter ROS ($H_2O_2$ and $O_2^{\bullet-}$) distribution in the roots of tomato seedlings. The explanation of the phytotoxic potential of the digestive fluid requires further study, in which the compounds of the trap fluid, being mainly secondary metabolites, are determined prior to their use in phytotoxicity tests. The context of perturbation in ROS levels in acceptor plants as the target of digestive fluid action needs examination of the activity of the enzymatic antioxidants in the tissue of the acceptor plants.

**Author Contributions:** Conceptualization, P.S. and U.K.; methodology, P.S. and U.K.; validation, P.S. and A.G.; formal analysis, P.S. and A.G.; investigation, A.W., M.P. and P.S.; data curation, P.S.; writing—original draft preparation, P.S. and A.G.; writing—review and editing, P.S., A.W. and A.G.; visualization, P.S. and A.W.; supervision, P.S. All authors have read and agreed to the published version of the manuscript.

**Funding:** This research received no external funding.

**Institutional Review Board Statement:** Not applicable.

**Informed Consent Statement:** Not applicable.

**Data Availability Statement:** Upon request, the data will be provided by the corresponding author.

**Conflicts of Interest:** The authors declare no conflict of interest.

## References

1. Clarke, C. *Nepenthes of Sumatra and Peninsular Malaysia*; Natural History Publications (Borneo): Kota Kinabalu, Malaysia, 2001.
2. Adlassnig, W.; Peroutka, M.; Lendl, T. Traps of Carnivorous Pitcher Plants as a Habitat: Composition of the Fluid, Biodiversity and Mutualistic Activities. *Ann. Bot.* **2011**, *107*, 181–194. [CrossRef] [PubMed]
3. An, C.; Fukusaki, E.I.; Kobayashi, A. Aspartic Proteinases Are Expressed in Pitchers of the Carnivorous Plant *Nepenthes Alata* Blanco. *Planta* **2002**, *214*, 661–667. [CrossRef] [PubMed]
4. Eilenberg, H.; Pnini-Cohen, S.; Schuster, S.; Movtchan, A.; Zilberstein, A. Isolation and Characterization of Chitinase Genes from Pitchers of the Carnivorous Plant Nepenthes Khasiana. *J. Exp. Bot.* **2006**, *57*, 2775–2784. [CrossRef] [PubMed]
5. Płachno, B.J.; Adamec, L.; Lichtscheidl, I.K.; Peroutka, M.; Adlassnig, W.; Vrba, J. Fluorescence Labelling of Phosphatase Activity in Digestive Glands of Carnivorous Plants. *Plant Biol.* **2006**, *8*, 813–820. [CrossRef] [PubMed]
6. Stephenson, P.; Hogan, J. Cloning and Characterization of a Ribonuclease, a Cysteine Proteinase, and an Aspartic Proteinase from Pitchers of the Carnivorous Plant *Nepenthes Ventricosa* Blanco. *Int. J. Plant Sci.* **2006**, *167*, 239–248. [CrossRef]
7. Athauda, S.B.P.; Matsumoto, K.; Rajapakshe, S.; Kuribayashi, M.; Kojima, M.; Kubomura-Yoshida, N.; Iwamatsu, A.; Shibata, C.; Inoue, H.; Takahashi, K. Enzymic and Structural Characterization of Nepenthesin, a Unique Member of a Novel Subfamily of Aspartic Proteinases. *Biochem. J.* **2004**, *381*, 295–306. [CrossRef]
8. Hatano, N.; Hamada, T. Proteome Analysis of Pitcher Fluid of the Carnivorous Plant *Nepenthes alata*. *J. Proteome Res.* **2008**, *7*, 809–816. [CrossRef]
9. Mithöfer, A. Carnivorous Pitcher Plants: Insights in an Old Topic. *Phytochemistry* **2011**, *72*, 1678–1682. [CrossRef]
10. Eilenberg, H.; Pnini-Cohen, S.; Rahamim, Y.; Sionov, E.; Segal, E.; Carmeli, S.; Zilberstein, A. Induced Production of Antifungal Naphthoquinones in the Pitchers of the Carnivorous Plant *Nepenthes khasiana*. *J. Exp. Bot.* **2010**, *61*, 911–922. [CrossRef]
11. Buch, F.; Rott, M.; Rottloff, S.; Paetz, C.; Hilke, I.; Raessler, M.; Mithöfer, A. Secreted Pitfall-Trap Fluid of Carnivorous Nepenthes Plants Is Unsuitable for Microbial Growth. *Ann. Bot.* **2013**, *111*, 375–383. [CrossRef]
12. Likhitwitayawuid, K.; Kaewamatawong, R.; Ruangrungsi, N.; Krungkrai, J. Antimalarial Naphthoquinones from *Nepenthes thorelii*. *Planta Med.* **1998**, *64*, 237–241. [CrossRef] [PubMed]
13. Sandur, S.K.; Ichikawa, H.; Sethi, G.; Ahn, K.S.; Aggarwal, B.B. Plumbagin (5-Hydroxy-2-Methyl-1,4-Naphthoquinone) Suppresses NF-KB Activation and NF-KB-Regulated Gene Products Through Modulation of P65 and IκBα Kinase Activation, Leading to Potentiation of Apoptosis Induced by Cytokine and Chemotherapeutic Agents. *J. Biol. Chem.* **2006**, *281*, 17023–17033. [CrossRef] [PubMed]
14. Shin, K.-S.; Lee, S.-K.; Cha, B.-J. Antifungal Activity of Plumbagin Purified from Leaves of Nepenthes Ventricosa x Maxima against Phytopathogenic Fungi. *Plant Pathol. J.* **2007**, *23*, 113–115. [CrossRef]
15. Wal, A.; Staszek, P.; Pakula, B.; Paradowska, M.; Krasuska, U. ROS and RNS Alterations in the Digestive Fluid of Nepenthes × Ventrata Trap at Different Developmental Stages. *Plants* **2022**, *11*, 3304. [CrossRef] [PubMed]
16. Gaume, L.; Forterre, Y. A Viscoelastic Deadly Fluid in Carnivorous Pitcher Plants. *PLoS ONE* **2007**, *2*, 1185. [CrossRef]
17. Macías, F.A.; Molinillo, J.M.; Varela, R.M.; Galindo, J.C. Allelopathy—A Natural Alternative for Weed Control. *Pest Manag. Sci.* **2007**, *63*, 327–348. [CrossRef]
18. Piesik, D.; Wenda-Piesik, A. Sitophilus Granarius Responses to Blends of Five Groups of Cereal Kernels and One Group of Plant Volatiles. *J. Stored Prod. Res.* **2015**, *63*, 63–66. [CrossRef]

19. Piesik, D.; Wenda-Piesik, A.; Krasińska, A.; Wrzesińska, D.; Delaney, K.J. Volatile Organic Compounds Released by *Rumex Confertus* Following *Hypera Rumicis* Herbivory and Weevil Responses to Volatiles. *J. Appl. Entomol.* **2016**, *140*, 308–316. [CrossRef]
20. Staszek, P.; Krasuska, U.; Wal, A.; Zak, J.; Gniazdowska, A. NO and Metabolic Reprogramming under Phytotoxicity Stress. In *Nitric Oxide in Plant Biology*; Elsevier: Amsterdam, The Netherlands, 2022; pp. 297–318.
21. Chan, X.-Y.; Hong, K.-W.; Yin, W.-F.; Chan, K.-G. Microbiome and Biocatalytic Bacteria in Monkey Cup (*Nepenthes* Pitcher) Digestive Fluid. *Sci. Rep.* **2016**, *6*, 20016. [CrossRef]
22. Bittleston, L.S.; Wolock, C.J.; Yahya, B.E.; Chan, X.Y.; Chan, K.G.; Pierce, N.E.; Pringle, A. Convergence between the Microcosms of Southeast Asian and North American Pitcher Plants. *Elife* **2018**, *7*, e36741. [CrossRef]
23. Hossain, M.S.; Rahman, G.K.M.M.; Solaiman, A.R.M.; Alam, M.S.; Rahman, M.M.; Mia, M.A.B. Estimating Electrical Conductivity for Soil Salinity Monitoring Using Various Soil-Water Ratios Depending on Soil Texture. *Commun. Soil Sci. Plant Anal.* **2020**, *51*, 635–644. [CrossRef]
24. Huliusz, P. Quantitative and Qualitative Diferentiation of Soil Salinity in Poland. *Ber. Dtsch. Bodenkd. Ges.* **2008**, *1*, 1–4.
25. Gonçalves, S.; Ferraz, M.; Romano, A. Phytotoxic Properties of Drosophyllum Lusitanicum Leaf Extracts and Its Main Compound Plumbagin. *Sci. Hortic.* **2009**, *122*, 96–101. [CrossRef]
26. Li, Z.-H.; Wang, Q.; Ruan, X.; Pan, C.-D.; Jiang, D.-A. Phenolics and Plant Allelopathy. *Molecules* **2010**, *15*, 8933–8952. [CrossRef] [PubMed]
27. Macías, F.A.; Castellano, D.; Molinillo, J.M.G. Search for a Standard Phytotoxic Bioassay for Allelochemicals. Selection of Standard Target Species. *J. Agric. Food Chem.* **2000**, *48*, 2512–2521. [CrossRef]
28. Gniazdowska, A.; Bogatek, R. Allelopathic Interactions between Plants. Multi Site Action of Allelochemicals. *Acta Physiol. Plant* **2005**, *27*, 395–407. [CrossRef]
29. Staszek, P.; Krasuska, U.; Ciacka, K.; Gniazdowska, A. ROS Metabolism Perturbation as an Element of Mode of Action of Allelochemicals. *Antioxidants* **2021**, *10*, 1648. [CrossRef]
30. Soltys, D.; Rudzińska-Langwald, A.; Gniazdowska, A.; Wiśniewska, A.; Bogatek, R. Inhibition of Tomato (*Solanum Lycopersicum* L.) Root Growth by Cyanamide Is Due to Altered Cell Division, Phytohormone Balance and Expansin Gene Expression. *Planta* **2012**, *236*, 1629–1638. [CrossRef]
31. Graña, E.; Sotelo, T.; Díaz-Tielas, C.; Araniti, F.; Krasuska, U.; Bogatek, R.; Reigosa, M.J.; Sánchez-Moreiras, A.M. Citral Induces Auxin and Ethylene-Mediated Malformations and Arrests Cell Division in *Arabidopsis Thaliana* Roots. *J. Chem. Ecol.* **2013**, *39*, 271–282. [CrossRef]
32. Haugland, E.; Brandsaeter, L.O. Experiments on Bioassay Sensitivity in the Study of Allelopathy. *J. Chem. Ecol.* **1996**, *22*, 1845–1859. [CrossRef]
33. Shekari, F.; Shekari, F.; Najafi, J.; Abassi, A.; Radmanesh, Z.; Bones, A.M. Phytotoxic Effects of Catnip (Nepeta Meyeri Benth.) on Early Growth Stages Development and Infection Potential of Field Dodder (Cuscuta Campestris Yunck). *Plants* **2022**, *11*, 2629. [CrossRef]
34. Oracz, K.; Voegele, A.; Tarkowská, D.; Jacquemoud, D.; Turečková, V.; Urbanová, T.; Strnad, M.; Sliwinska, E.; Leubner-Metzger, G. Myrigalone A Inhibits Lepidium Sativum Seed Germination by Interference with Gibberellin Metabolism and Apoplastic Superoxide Production Required for Embryo Extension Growth and Endosperm Rupture. *Plant Cell Physiol.* **2012**, *53*, 81–95. [CrossRef] [PubMed]
35. Oracz, K.; Bouteau, H.E.-M.; Farrant, J.M.; Cooper, K.; Belghazi, M.; Job, C.; Job, D.; Corbineau, F.; Bailly, C. ROS Production and Protein Oxidation as a Novel Mechanism for Seed Dormancy Alleviation. *Plant J.* **2007**, *50*, 452–465. [CrossRef] [PubMed]
36. Inderjit; Weston, L.A.; Duke, S.O. Challenges, Achievements and Opportunities in Allelopathy Research. *J. Plant Interact.* **2005**, *1*, 69–81. [CrossRef]
37. Williams, R.; Hoagland, R. Bioassays- Useful Tools for the Study of Allelopathy. In *Allelopathy*; CRC Press: Boca Raton, FL, USA, 2003; pp. 315–351.
38. Gniazdowska, A.; Krasuska, U.; Andrzejczak, O.; Soltys, D. Allelopathic Compounds as Oxidative Stress Agents: Yes or NO. In *Reactive Oxygen and Nitrogen Species Signaling and Communication in Plants, Signaling and Communication in Plants*; Springer: Cham, Switzerland, 2015; Volume 23, pp. 155–176.
39. Krasuska, U.; Andrzejczak, O.; Staszek, P.; Borucki, W.; Gniazdowska, A. Toxicity of Canavanine in Tomato (*Solanum Lycopersicum* L.) Roots Is Due to Alterations in RNS, ROS and Auxin Levels. *Plant Physiol. Biochem.* **2016**, *103*, 84–95. [CrossRef]
40. Baker, C.; Mock, M. An Improved Method for Monitoring Cell Death in Cell Suspension and Leaf Disc Assays Using Evans Blue. *Plant Cell Tissue Organ Cult.* **1994**, *39*, 7–12. [CrossRef]
41. Beyer, W.F.; Fridovich, I. Assaying for Superoxide Dismutase Activity: Some Large Consequences of Minor Changes in Conditions. *Anal. Biochem.* **1987**, *161*, 559–566. [CrossRef]
42. Ciacka, K.; Tyminski, M.; Gniazdowska, A.; Krasuska, U. Cold Stratification-Induced Dormancy Removal in Apple (Malus Domestica Borkh.) Seeds Is Accompanied by an Increased Glutathione Pool in Embryonic Axes. *J. Plant Physiol.* **2022**, *274*, 153736. [CrossRef]

*plants*

MDPI

*Article*

# Phytochemical and Biological Study of Trophic Interaction between *Pseudosphinx Tetrio* L. Larvae and *Allamanda Cathartica* L.

**Linda Matignon [1], Mame Marietou Lo [2], Magneric Monpierre [3], Mauro Vicentini Correia [4], Drochss Pettry Valencia [5], Marie-Noëlle Sylvestre [3], Ludovic Pruneau [3], Muriel Sylvestre [1], Antonio Domenech [7], Zohra Benfodda [2], Patrick Meffre [2] and Gerardo Cebrián-Torrejón [1,*]**

1 COVACHIM-M2E Laboratory EA 3592, Department of Chemistry, Fouillole Campus, University of the French West Indies, UFR SEN, CEDEX, 97157 Pointe-à-Pitre, France
2 CHROME Laboratory, EA7352, University of Nîmes, CEDEX 1, 30021 Nîmes, France
3 Institut de Systématique, Evolution, Biodiversité (ISYEB), Department of Chemistry, Fouillole Campus, University of the French West Indies, UFR SEN, CEDEX, 97157 Pointe-à-Pitre, France
4 Instituto de Química, Campus Universitário Darcy Ribeiro, Universidade de Brasília, Brasília 70910-900, Brazil
5 Departamento de Ciencias Naturales y Matemáticas, Pontificia Universidad Javeriana sede Cali, Calle 18 No. 118-250, Cali 760031, Colombia
6 Instituto de Química, Universidade Federal Fluminense, Outeiro S. João Batista S/N, Niterói 24020-141, Brazil
7 Departament de Química Analítica, Facultat de Química, Universitat de València, Dr. Moliner 50, 46100 Valencia, Spain
* Correspondence: gerardo.cebrian-torrejon@univ-antilles.fr

**Abstract:** In this article, we propose to explore the chemical interaction between *Pseudosphinx tetrio* L. and *Allamanda cathartica* L. using different analytical methods, including an innovative electrochemical approach (called electrochemical ecology) and multivariate analysis, and we investigate the potential antimicrobial effects (antibacterial and antifungal activities) of this interaction in order to gain a better understanding of their specific interaction. The analytical study presents a similar chemical profile between the leaves of healthy and herbivorous *A. cathartica* and the excretions of the caterpillars. The similar analytical profile of the leaves of *A. cathartica* and the excretions of *P. tetrio*, and the difference with the caterpillar bodies, suggests a selective excretion of compounds by the caterpillar. The measured antimicrobial activities support the physicochemical tests. The natural products found selectively in the excretions (rather than in the body) could explain the ability of *P. tetrio* to feed on this toxic Apocynaceae species.

**Keywords:** chemical ecology; electrochemical ecology; aposematism; allelopathy; plant–insect interactions; *Pseudosphinx tetrio*; *Allamanda cathartica*; phytochemical analysis

**Citation:** Matignon, L.; Lo, M.M.; Monpierre, M.; Correia, M.V.; Valencia, D.P.; Palmeira-Mello, M.V.; Sylvestre, M.-N.; Pruneau, L.; Sylvestre, M.; Domenech, A.; et al. Phytochemical and Biological Study of Trophic Interaction between *Pseudosphinx Tetrio* L. Larvae and *Allamanda Cathartica* L.. *Plants* **2023**, *12*, 520. https://doi.org/10.3390/plants12030520

Academic Editors: Margot Schulz and Vincenzo Tabaglio

Received: 6 December 2022
Revised: 13 January 2023
Accepted: 16 January 2023
Published: 23 January 2023



## 1. Introduction

The tetrio sphinx, *Pseudosphinx tetrio* L. (Lepidoptera: Sphingidae), is a moth widely distributed in tropical and subtropical regions of the Americas and the Caribbean basin, where suitable host plants for the development of its larvae (large, conspicuous caterpillars) are present [1–10].

Adult females of *P. tetrio* [11] lay 50–100 eggs on the underside of the host plant's leaves, from which they hatch in about three days [3]. After hatching, the gregarious larvae live in colonies for at least the first three developing stages, feeding initially on the upper surface of leaves and in later stages on all leaf tissues except leaf veins and midribs as they progress to the later instars. Adult larvae (fifth or sixth stages) feed singly or in small groups on entire leaves can reach a length of 63–69 mm [3,4]. The color of larvae is characteristic of aposematism (antipredation strategy: warning predators of bad taste or toxicity). According to an aposematic hypothesis, it becomes toxic to its predators when it ingests toxic phytocomponents from the milky sap of some plants [12]. The body is velvety black with yellow rings on each thoracic and abdominal segment, the head is dark orange-red, and the prothoracic shield, prominent legs and anal segment are orange-red with dark markings. The spine on the eighth abdominal segment is black and emerges from a raised, orange, button-like structure [4,13–15]. The aposematic larvae have few predators due to their venomous nature. However, the squirrel cuckoo, *Piaya cayana* Linn., of Belize, consumes *P. tetrio* by taking larvae, beating them against a branch until the poisonous gut contents are gone, and then swallowing the remains [16]. The larvae wrap themselves in a cocoon of silk or dead leaves and molt into new pupae about 7.0 cm long. The adult moths, colored in shades of gray, hatch from the pupae 53 days after egg laying and have a wingspan of 12.7–14.0 cm (eggs hatch in 3 days or more; average duration of the 5–6 larval stages is 23–4 days; the prepupal stage lasts about 4 days and the pupal stage about 22 days [3]). *P. tetrio* has the ability to eat up to twice its weight in food during a day, hence its name, "glutton caterpillar". The larva of *P. tetrio* feeds preferentially on the leaves of the Apocynaceae family's plants, such as *Allamanda cathartica* L. and *Plumeria alba* L., which are rich in toxic latex [17,18].

*A. cathartica* is commonly known as yellow allamanda, golden trumpet or "*Liane à lait*" [19]. This is a common name for the species. In the review paper by Ghosh and coworkers, it was described as a hermaphroditic, vine-like, woody shrub used primarily in landscaping, more spreading than tall, and with perennial leaves [20]. *A. cathartica* is a fast-growing species that is widely distributed worldwide, but mainly in tropical and subtropical regions, where the caterpillar *P. tetrio* is present [21,22]. *A. cathartica* is one of the fifteen species of the Apocynaceae family according to the "WFO Plant List" [23].

The plant is native to Brazil [24] and its various parts such as leaves, flowers, roots and stems are used in traditional medicine [25] for the treatment of jaundice [26], and have various pharmacological activities such as wound healing [26], antioxidant [27–30], antimicrobial [30–32], antifungal [33], antimalarial [34], anti-inflammatory [35]; anticancer [20,36,37] and gastrointestinal effects [38]. A dichloromethane ($CH_2Cl_2$) extract of the whole plant tested on two pathogenic dermatophytes, *Trichophyton rubrum* and *Microsporum gypseum*, showed moderate activity at a concentration of 50 μg/disk, but very strong activity at a concentration of 200 μg/disk, suggesting that *A. cathartica* may possess antidermatophyte constituents that could be useful in the treatment of ringworm [39,40].

In general, insects are not strictly restricted to the leaves and reproductive parts of living plants. Most studies conducted on strict herbivores [41] indicate that larval hosts of sphingids are concentrated on a few plant families whose foliage is particularly rich in alkaloids, milky sap, essential oils, irritant acids or other small toxic natural products (e.g., Rubiaceae, Euphorbiaceae, Apocynaceae, Vitaceae, Bignoniaceae, etc.).

However, all parts of *A. cathartica* are rich in secondary metabolites, which are exhaustively listed in the review by Petricevich and Abarca-Vargas [42], with plumieride, plumericin, and allamandin being the most characteristic. A total of 151 compounds were distributed as follows: 3 hydrocarbons in flowers; 7 alcohol compounds, 9 esters, 1 ether, 6 aldehydes, and 1 ketone in flowers, leaves, and stems extracts; 37 fatty acids and phospholipids; 43 volatile compounds mostly in flowers and leaves; 5 phenolic compounds and 6 flavonoids in the flowers and stems; 2 alkaloids in stems; 11 steroids and terpenes in leaves, stems and flowers; and 14 lactones in roots, stems, leaves, flowers and bark; 6 carbohydrates in leaves, stems, and nectar. Of the compounds identified, leaves contain: ursolic acid, β-amyrin; β-sitosterol, sesquiterpenes, plumericin, plumieride, long chain esters, flavonoids, polyphenols, allamandin, alkaloids, saponins and carbohydrates; stem and bark contain: ursolic acid, β-amyrin, β-sitosterol, triterpenoids, glucosides, alkaloids, flavonoids and polyphenols; flowers contain: quercetin, quercitrin, kaempferol, hesperetin, flavonoids, polyphenols and polysaccharides; and roots contain: lactones, allamandin, allamandicin, allamdin, plumieride iridoids, triterpenoids, alkaloids and several glucosides [36,38,43] (cited by [44]); [19,21,27,42]. Like *A. cathartica*, various parts of *P. rubra* are widely used in traditional medicine [45]. *P. rubra* contains many chemical constituents such as glycosides, phenolic compounds (phenolic acids and flavonoids), alkaloids, amino acids and terpenoids (iridoids) which give the flower antibacterial and antifungal activities. However, the main chemical constituents responsible for the pharmacological activities of *P. rubra* are: plumieride, fulvoplumierine, lupeol, rubrinol, stigmasterol, oleanolic acid, taraxasteryl acetate, rubranonoside, plumieride-p-E-coumarate, isoplumericin, rubrajalellol and plumericin [46–49]. These molecules form plant may have antimicrobial activities and effects and may be of interest for use against pathogenic microorganisms.

In nature, predatory insects are highly host-specific and exhibit a variety of traits. Direct associations between plants and insects are ubiquitous, and in the context of tropical chemical ecology, many different plant–herbivore interactions are highly specialized [50]. What attracts an egg-laying insect to one plant and prevents it from laying its eggs on another is often an aspect of plant chemistry that is recognized by the insect [51]. Nevertheless, plants can biosynthesize protective secondary metabolites (in the milky sap or via vascular tissue or in specialized tissues) in a self-defense process to reduce herbivory. In turn, herbivores may respond to these compounds and attempt to metabolize them, selectively excrete them, or use them (after ingestion into the body) for their own defense [52,53]. In 2022, McCoy and colleagues showed that for Eocene herbivorous insects that eat leaves with such defense mechanisms, a distinct burrowing or cutting behavior that disrupts the supply of protective compounds distal to the plant tissue allowed the insect to eat the leaf [54].

The coevolution of specialized plant–insect herbivore interactions has been the subject of decades of study [55–57]. Lepidoptera caterpillars, for example, often specialize on toxic plants and are able to either sequester [58–60], metabolize [61,62] or excrete chemical compounds from their hosts in an unmodified form [63]. Understanding how herbivores deal with toxic phytochemicals in their diet is necessary to understanding the evolution of the two most biodiverse groups of multicellular organisms: plants and insects.

In this article, we propose to explore the chemical interaction between *P. tetrio* and *A. cathartica* using different analytical methods, including an innovative electrochemical approach (called electrochemical ecology) and multivariate analysis, and we investigate the potential antimicrobial effects (antibacterial and antifungal activities) of this interaction, in order to gain a better understanding of their specificity.

## 2. Results and Discussion

### 2.1. Phytochemical Tests

***Thin layer chromatography (TLC).*** First, a TLC study was conducted. The different results of this approach are presented in Table 1. In our first hypothesis (Hyp. 1), we propose that the caterpillars take up and store certain metabolites (for example, the metabolite with an Rf (Retention factor) of 0.16 on TLC 3 (orange color)). The second hypothesis proposed (Hyp. 2), also listed in Table 1, refers to the selective excretion of an unidentified molecule by the caterpillars (for example, the metabolite with an Rf of 0.95 on TLCs 2 and 3 (blue color)). Finally, the third hypothesis (Hyp. 3) refers to the response of the healthy plant to herbivory. For example, the metabolite with an Rf of 0.28 on TLC 1 (pink color), since this metabolite is present in healthy leaves and not in predated leaves. The opposite case is observed with the metabolite with an Rf value of 0.18 on TLC 4 (green color), which is present only in predated leaves and could therefore be considered a metabolic marker for herbivores.

**Table 1.** Organic phases obtained with TLC results. (A) Healthy *A. cathartica* leaves, (B) herbivored *A. cathartica* leaves, (C) caterpillar bodies and (D) caterpillars' feces. Solvent percentages are presented as highest polarity in solution (MeOH and EtOAc) *.

| Elution Solvent | % * | TLC | $R_f$ | A (1.2) | B (1.3) | C (1.4) | D (1.5) |
|---|---|---|---|---|---|---|---|
| $CH_2Cl_2$ | 100 | 1 | 0.16 | | | | |
| | | | 0.28 | Hyp. 1 and 3 | | Hyp. 1 | |
| | | | 0.58 | | | | |
| $CH_2Cl_2$/MeOH | 5 | 2 | 0.05 | | | | |
| | | | 0.19 | | | | |
| | | | 0.22 | | | | |
| | | | 0.60 | | | | |
| | | | 0.91 | | | | |
| | | | 0.95 | Hyp. 2 | Hyp. 2 | | Hyp. 2 |
| | 10 | 3 | 0.16 | Hyp. 1 | Hyp. 1 | Hyp. 1 | |
| | | | 0.20 | | | | |
| | | | 0.57 | | | | |
| | | | 0.90 | | | | |
| | | | 0.95 | Hyp. 2 | Hyp. 2 | | Hyp. 2 |
| | 1 | 4 | 0.18 | | Hyp. 1 and 3 | Hyp. 1 | |
| | | | 0.30 | Hyp. 1 and 3 | | Hyp. 1 and 3 | |
| | | | 0.79 | | | | |
| | | | 0.93 | | | | |
| | | | 0.94 | | Hyp. 2 and 3 | | Hyp. 2 |
| $CH_2Cl_2$ | 100 | 5 | 0.08 | | | | |
| | | | 0.17 | | | | |
| | | | 0.37 | | | | |
| | | | 0.62 | | | | |
| | | | 0.93 | | | | |
| $C_6H_{14}$ | 100 | 6 | 0.03 | | | | |
| | | | 0.37 | Hyp. 1 | Hyp. 1 | Hyp. 1 | |
| $C_6H_{14}/C_4H_8O_2$ | 20 | 7 | 0.17 | | | | |
| | | | 0.30 | | | | |
| | | | 0.34 | Hyp. 1 | Hyp. 1 | Hyp. 1 | |
| | | | 0.64 | | | | |
| | | | 0.94 | | Hyp. 2 and 3 | | Hyp. 2 |
| | | | 0.97 | | | | |
| | | | 0.98 | | | | |
| | | | 1 | | | | |
| | 50 | 8 | 0.48 | | Hyp. 1 and 3 | Hyp. 1 | |
| | | | 0.95 | | | | |
| | | | 0.97 | | | | |
| | 80 | 9 | 0.50 | | | | |
| | | | 0.91 | | | | |
| | | | 0.94 | | | | |

* Similarly, metabolites between two extracts or more are described in colors: orange: A, B and C; blue: A, B and D; pink: A and C; yellow: B and D. Hypotheses that can be illustrated by each compound are cited.

***Nuclear magnetic resonance spectroscopy $^1H$ NMR***. The $^1H$ NMR data were obtained only from the organic extracts of the plants and caterpillars using DMSO-$d^6$ as a solvent. Solvent signals from deuterated DMSO and residual water at 2.5 and 3.3 ppm, respectively, were removed (Figure 1). The analysis shows minor differences between the spectra of healthy and predated *Allamanda* leaves. This result is inconsistent with hypothesis 3 (in which a plant response to aggression was observed).

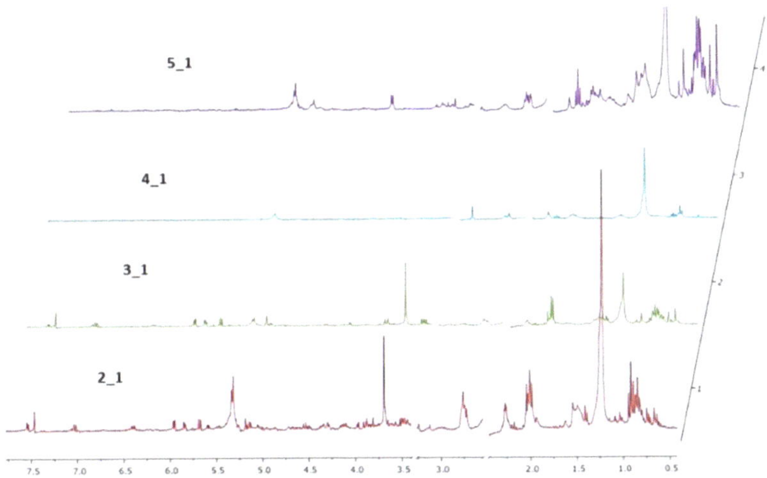


**Figure 1.** $^1$H NMR of organic extracts in DMSO-d$^6$. (2_1) Healthy *Allamanda* leaves; (3_1) predated *Allamanda* leaves; (4_1) caterpillar bodies and (5_1) caterpillar feces.

The $^1$H NMR spectra of caterpillars' bodies and feces show large differences between the samples, and the chemical profile of healthy *Allamanda* leaves and the caterpillar feces is very similar. This result confirms hypothesis 2 and shows the similarity between the chemical profile of *A. cathartica* leaves and caterpillar feces compared to the caterpillar body. These similarities and dissimilarities confirm our hypothesis (Hyp. 3) of the selective excretion of toxic compounds.

***High performance liquid chromatography coupled with mass spectrometry (HPLC-MS).*** In this study, the samples containing the healthy and eaten leaves of *A. cathartica*, as well as the caterpillars and their feces, were analyzed using high-performance liquid chromatography techniques [19,64–66] (Figure 2). The similar profile observed in these spectra indicates the presence of the same main compounds in the healthy (A) and predated (B) *A. cathartica* leaves, with similar retention times (RT) of 20.00 min and 20.50 min, respectively. A second compound can be identified in these spectra with comparable retention times to hypothesis 3 (RTs: 25.52 min and 26.02 min). These results are in contrast to hypothesis 3 (as we can see in the TLCs and $^1$H NMR profiles). The analysis shows the presence of this compound in the caterpillar's feces (D, RT: 25.73 min) but not in its body (C), which also confirms hypothesis 2 (in agreement with the $^1$H NMR and TLC results). Finally, the results show that the compounds found in *P. tetrio*'s bodies (C, RT: 20.43 min and 25.66 min) are significantly different from other compounds found in the feces (also confirming hypothesis 2).

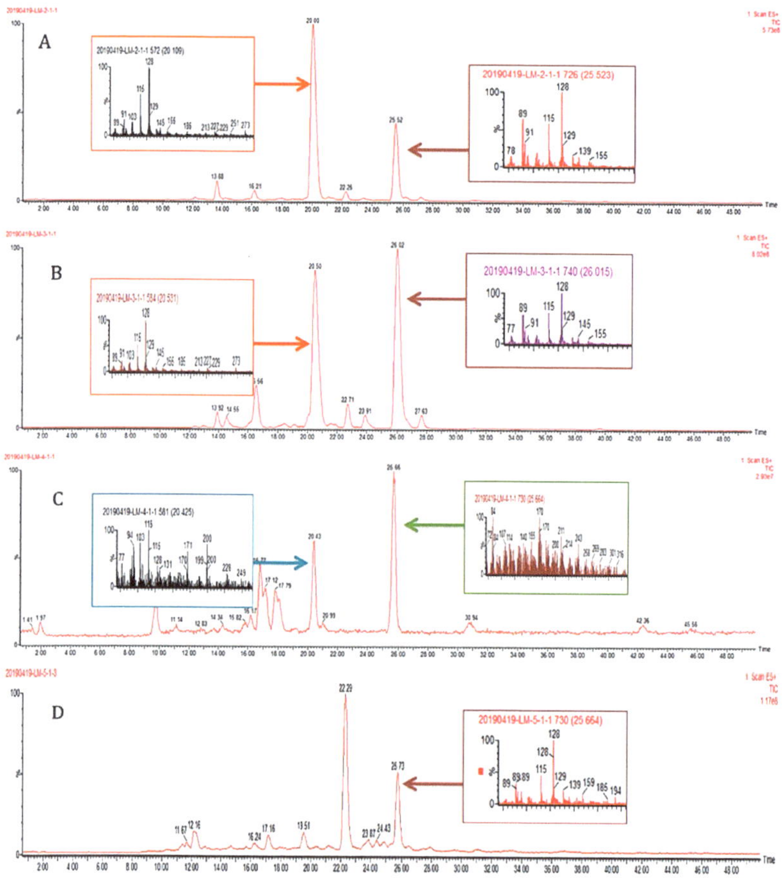


**Figure 2.** HPLC-MS profiles of (**A**) healthy and (**B**) predated leaves of *A. cathartica* and (**C**) caterpillar bodies and (**D**) caterpillar feces.

***Electrochemical investigation.*** Cyclic voltammetry (CV) studies have been used to investigate possible interactions between different compounds and were previously used to monitor plant defenses against external stressors [67–70]. Here, the predation of *A. cathartica* by *P. tetrio* has been monitored electrochemically using CV. We studied the electrochemical response of films (on the surface of a glassy carbon electrode) of organic and aqueous extracts of healthy and predated leaves of the plant and samples of bodies and feces of *P. tetrio* in 0.10 mol $L^{-1}$ phosphate solution buffer at pH 7.0. The reported methodology is ultimately based on the voltammetry of microparticles (VMP) technique [71].

The behavior of films on glassy carbon electrodes of healthy and predated leaves of *A. cathartica* is shown in Figure 3. A series of chemically irreversible oxidation processes: $A_1$, $A_2$ and $A_3$, were observed (0.28 V, 0.65 V and an undefined shoulder at 1.00 V, respectively). While the peaks $A_1$ and $A_2$ decrease with cycling until a fully passivated and stable state is reached at about the second cycle, an increase in the $A_3$ peak was observed. Thus, the variations in the ratio of peaks $A_1$ and $A_3$ suggest differences in the nature of the redox species of *A. cathartica* and in leaves that are strengthened by them. These oxidation processes represent a profile observed in several plant species and are due to the oxidation of polyphenolic organic compounds. Indeed, the voltammogram of the predated leaves exhibits the same signals as healthy leaves, but peak $A_1$ is depleted while the $A_3$ signal is enhanced. Finally, a reduction process can be observed at about −1.0 V when the potential sweep is reversed to less positive potentials. Although these processes are slightly more negative in healthy leaves than in predated leaves, both are consistent with the typical behavior of the oxygen reduction reaction (ORR) in water. This result basically contradicts hypothesis 3 about the chemical response to the herbivory, but using this technique, we can identify slight differences between healthy and predated leaves, possibly related to polyphenols (reaction against oxidative stress) [72].

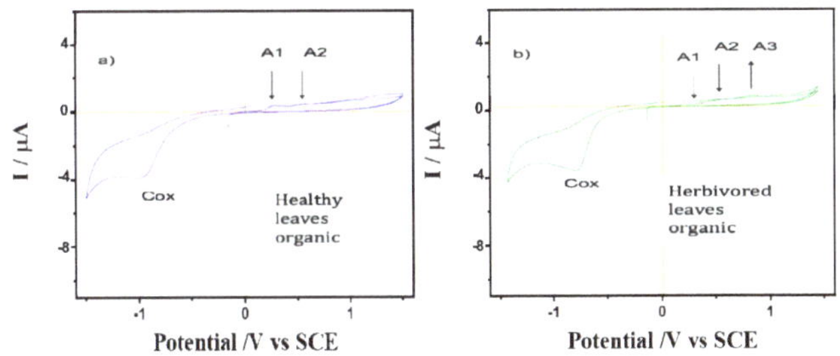


**Figure 3.** Cyclic voltammograms of films from (**a**) healthy and (**b**) predated leaves of *A. cathartica* on glassy carbon electrode in contact with air-saturated 0.10 M phosphate buffer at pH 7.0. Scan rate 10 mV.s$^{-1}$.

The CV of films on glassy carbon electrodes of *P. tetrio*'s bodies and its excrement after predation of leaves of *A. cathartica* are shown in Figure 4. CV shows no clear oxidation process in the initial anodic scan for the body of *P. tetrio*, but three oxidation processes for its excreta at 0.22, 0.45 and 0.78 V for $A_1$, $A_2$ and $A_3$, respectively, which are similar to those found for the *A. cathartica* analysis. Again, a typical oxygen reduction reaction (ORR) in water was observed in the cathodic region in both analyses. In addition, a characteristic signal $C_1$ appears in both samples, indicating the presence of oxidized metabolite of *P. tetrio*. This result confirms hypothesis 2, in agreement with the other analytical approaches.

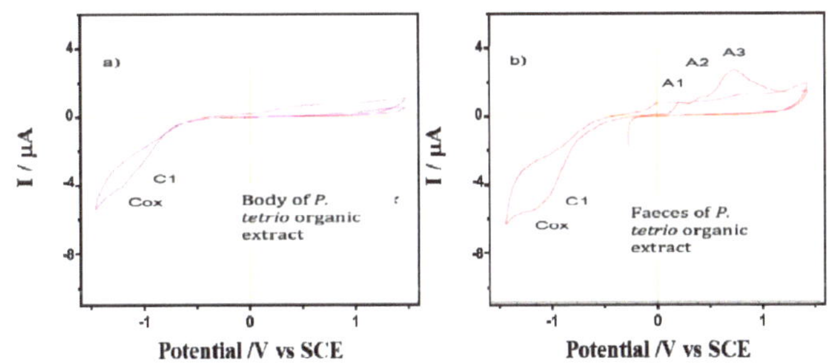


**Figure 4.** Cyclic voltammograms of films from (**a**) *P. tetrio*'s bodies and (**b**) *P. tetrio*'s excrement after predation on leaves of *A. cathartica* on glassy carbon electrode in contact with air-saturated 0.10 M phosphate buffer at pH 7.0. Potential scan rate 10 mV.s$^{-1}$.

A comparison was made between the CV of films from the water extracts of healthy and spoiled leaves of *A. cathartica* in contact with air-saturated 0.10 mol $L^{-1}$ phosphate buffer at pH 7.0 (Figure 5). Here, signal $A_1$ appears clearly recorded in the healthy leaves and is accompanied by a well-defined cathodic peak at—1.25 V ($C_2$). Signal $C_2$ disappears in the CV of the damaged leaves, while signal $A_1$ decreases and signal $A_3$ is clearly visible at 0.78 V. This result confirms hypothesis 3, which shows a reaction of leaves against herbivory; the disappearance of signal $C_2$ and the appearance of signal $A_3$ are a result of herbivory. This CV is reproduced to some extent reproduced in the aqueous extracts of *P. tetrio* and its excrement, as shown in Figure 6, thus suggesting the existence of common electroactive compounds.

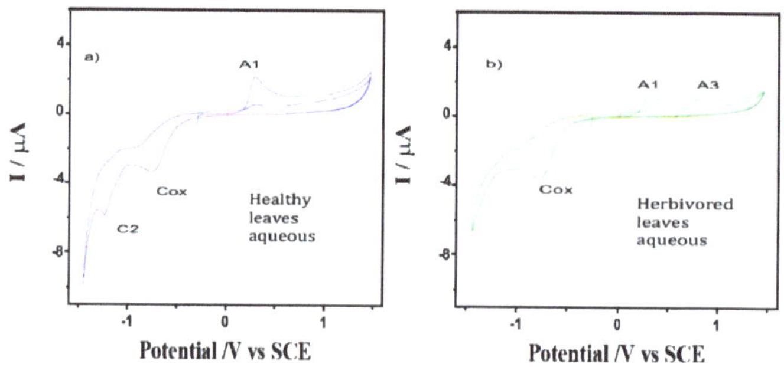


**Figure 5.** Cyclic voltammograms of films from the water extracts of (**a**) healthy and (**b**) predated leaves of *A. cathartica* on glassy carbon electrode in contact with air-saturated 0.10 M phosphate buffer at pH 7.0. Potential scan rate 10 mV.$s^{-1}$.

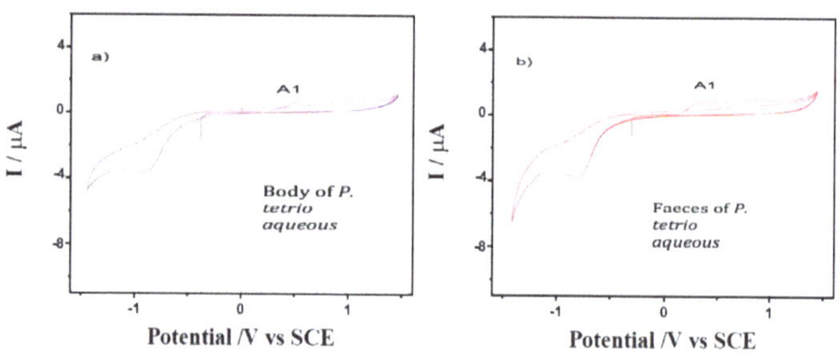


**Figure 6.** Cyclic voltammograms of films from water extracts of (**a**) *P. tetrio*'s bodies and (**b**) its excrement after predation on leaves of *A. cathartica* on glassy carbon electrode in contact with air-saturated 0.10 M phosphate buffer at pH 7.0. Potential scan rate 10 mV.$s^{-1}$.

***Principal Component Analysis (PCA).*** A total of 24 chromatograms were acquired using HPLC-EI-MS, 12 from the aqueous fraction and 12 from the organic fraction (three biological replicates for each species). To identify differences in the metabolites or even in their concentration in the samples, the set of 24 samples was analyzed, obtained from XCMS and used for data analysis. Two spreadsheets were obtained after data processing of the HPLC-MS analysis, with 168 and 412 variables from the organic and aqueous fractions, respectively (retention time m/z). In the PCA analysis, two plots were generated, namely score and loading plots. The first one shows the sample groupings, whereas the second one indicates the contribution of each variable to these samples. The PCA analysis was focused on the detection of any inherent pattern within the data. As observed in Figure 7, samples of healthy and predated *Allamanda* leaves are closely related, with small differences from each other, when compared with the caterpillars' bodies and feces. Further, when all samples are compared, the predated and not predated leaves from *Allamanda* are very similar to each other, and different from the other samples. In addition, the caterpillar body extracts present a great difference. In Figure 8 (loadings plot), the variables that influence the grouping observed are presented.

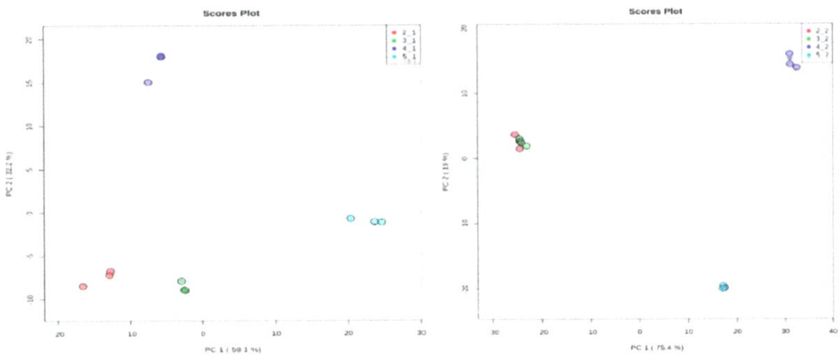


**Figure 7.** Score plot of 12 samples of organic and aqueous extracts of all manipulation, obtained from 168 (**left**) and 412 (**right**) variables, respectively. (2_1and 2_2) red circle, healthy *Allamanda* leaves; (3_1and 3_2) green circle, predated *Allamanda* leaves; (4_1and 4_2) blue circle, caterpillar bodies and (5_1and 5_2) light blue circle, caterpillar feces.

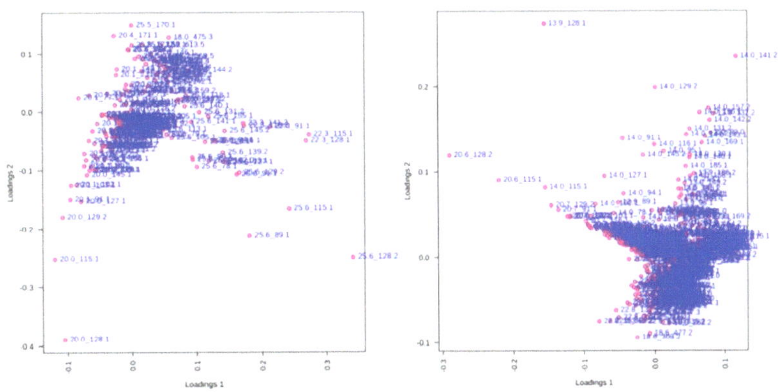


**Figure 8.** Score plots of 12 samples of organic and aqueous extracts of all manipulation, obtained from 168 (**left**) and 412 (**right**) variables, respectively. Each dot represents one variable (retention time m/z).

### *2.2. Microbial Activities*

The potential antimicrobial activities of *P. tetrio/A. cathartica* interaction are shown in Table 2. The yellow boxes show the effects of the consumption of the *A. cathartica* leaves by the caterpillar. The comparison between the healthy leaves (A) and the leaves eaten by the caterpillar (B) shows an increase or occurrence of inhibitory activity in favor of the leaves eaten by the caterpillar (B) on the microorganisms, regardless of the type of extraction (Aqueous ($_A$); Organic ($_O$)), $A_O$ versus $B_O$ for *Escherichia coli* and *Candida albicans* (diameter of inhibition: 7 mm versus 0 mm; 9,5 mm versus 7 mm); and $A_A$ versus $B_A$ for *Escherichia coli* and *Candida albicans* (diameter of inhibition: 7 mm versus 0 mm; 9 mm versus 8 mm)). The occurrence or enhancement of this bioactivity in the predated leaf could be explained by the induction of a chemical or biological defense reaction of the host plant against herbivory (proposed hypothesis 3).

**Table 2.** Microbial activity results of aqueous and organic extracts, obtained from *Allamanda cathartica* (*A. cathartica*) leaves, caterpillar bodies and caterpillar feces on three bacterial (*Escherichia coli; Staphylococcus aureus; Pseudomonas aeruginosa*) and two fungal (*Candida albicans; Aspergillus fumigatus*) strains.

| Extracts (100 µg/disc) | Caterpillar Feces (D) | | Caterpillar Bodies (C) | | Healthy *A. cathartica* Leaves (A) | | Predated *A. cathartica* Leaves (B) | |
|---|---|---|---|---|---|---|---|---|
| **Microorganisms** | $D_A$ | $D_o$ | $C_A$ | $C_o$ | $A_A$ | $A_o$ | $B_A$ | $B_o$ |
| *Escherichia Coli* | - | +++ (11) | + (7) | - | - | - | + (7) | + (7) |
| *Staphylococcus aureus* | - | ++ (9.5) | - | - | - | + (8.5) | - | + (8) |
| *Pseudomonas aeruginosa* | - | - | - | ++ (9) | - | + (7) | - | + (8,5) |
| *Candida albicans* | ++ (8,5) | ++ (9) | + (7) | + (7) | + (8) | + (7) | ++ (9) | ++ (9,5) |
| *Aspergillus fumigatus* | - | +++ (10,5) | - | - | - | +++ (10) | - | +++ (11) |

*Legend:* Aqueous extracts ($_A$); organic ($_O$) extracts; healthy *A. cathartica* leaves (A); predated *A. cathartica* leaves (B); caterpillar bodies (C); caterpillar feces (D), on three bacterial (*Escherichia coli; Staphylococcus aureus; Pseudomonas aeruginosa*) and two fungal (*Candida albicans; Aspergillus fumigatus*) strains. (mm): size of the inhibition halos in millimeters. (-) no inhibitory activity; (+ to +++) more or less intense inhibitory activity.

The green and blue boxes, respectively, represent the non-uptake and the uptake of bioactive compounds from the leaves into the bodies of the caterpillars. The samples obtained after extraction with organic solvents ($_O$) show the same evolution of the inhibitory profile in three of the five microorganisms tested (*Escherichia coli, Staphylococcus aureus* and *Aspergillus fumigatus*). Our results suggest a selective excretion of bioactive compounds from ingested leaves into the feces without being retained or ingested in the caterpillar's body (green boxes). Indeed, the feces of *P. tetrio*'s ($D_O$) show inhibitory activity that is as strong or stronger than that of the eaten *A. cathartica* leaves ($B_O$) [diameter of inhibition fecal matter ($D_O$) versus eaten leaves (Bo): 11 mm versus 7 mm for *Escherichia coli;* 9.5 mm versus 8 mm for *Staphylococcus aureus;* and 10,5 mm versus 11 mm for *Aspergillus fumigatus*) whereas caterpillar body extracts ($C_O$) showed no bio-inhibition (proposed hypothesis 2). The inhibitory effect of the organic and aqueous samples on *Pseudomonas aeruginosa* and *Escherichia coli*, respectively (blue boxes), shows an opposite profile. Indeed, the eaten leaves and the caterpillar body show a bio-inhibition that is not found in the caterpillar feces. This suggests that certain bioactive compounds in the eaten leaves, different from the previous ones, could be selectively taken up and stored specifically in the caterpillar body.

There are few data in the literature on the potential antimicrobial activity of predated leaves and the interaction between caterpillars and plants. Our samples showed higher antimicrobial activity than that reported by Islam et al. (2010) [31] for a concentrated methanol extract of healthy *A. cathartica* leaves fractionated into fractions soluble in petroleum ether, carbon tetrachloride, chloroform and water. The zones of inhibition observed by them have a diameter of less than 10 mm for *E. coli, S. aureus, C. albicans* and *P. aeruginosa,* at a tested concentration of 400 µg $disk^{-1}$ against the 100 µg $disk^{-1}$ in our case. At the same time, they showed higher antimicrobial activity with their methanolic and ethyl acetate extracts from healthy leaves [73]. Quercitrin was explicitly attributed antifungal and antibacterial activity [43].

Our qualitative results on biological activity may explain why *P. tetrio* can feed on this toxic Apocynaceae species. Indeed, the spectral (NMR) profiles of the eaten leaves and the caterpillar droppings are very similar, but very different from those of the caterpillar bodies. There is an association between the plant and caterpillar (specific herbivory). The plant produces organic chemical compounds for defense when the caterpillar attacks, and the caterpillar excretes or assimilates these molecules or derivatives by its own mechanism. The inhibition may be due to a synergistic effect of the different molecules contained in the extracts for all the microorganisms, hence the interest in using different analytical techniques. The genetic and cellular mechanisms by which metabolite diversity arises are becoming better understood, but the evolutionary explanations for the continued diversification of plant secondary metabolites have received less attention. Speed et al. (2019) [74] show a fundamental coevolutionary asymmetry between plants and their herbivores, which is that herbivores must resist all plant toxins, whereas plants must challenge and override only a single resistance trait.

Sequestration likely evolved as a protection from predators [75], [76] because caterpillars with chemical protection are less attractive to predators [77]. *P. tetrio* feeds on toxic species of the Apocynaceae and is aposematically colored, leading to the hypothesis that *P. tetrio* caterpillars may sequester compounds from their host. In many plant species, herbivory leads to the increased production of a secondary metabolite [78]. In particular, herbivores specialized in sequestration are thought to benefit from the induction of intermediate levels of chemical defenses, while plants eaten by such herbivores would benefit most from weak or strong induction. On the other hand, specialists that do not specialize in sequestration may not be deterred by induction unless it is high [55]. Caterpillars also have the ability to metabolize some organic chemical compounds and excrete others intact from the same host plant [63]. This is the case in Monarch butterflies, *Danaus plexippus* Linn. [58]. The study of Ramos et al., 2015 [79], compared the proteolytic system of the gut of *P. tetrio* and *D. plexippus* with the proteolytic system of the milky sap of their respective host plants (*P. rubra* and *Calotropis procera* Aiton). This revealed that the ability of the insect proteolytic systems (serine and cysteine peptidase inhibitors) to digest the milk sap proteins (in vivo) appears to be an important event favoring the caterpillars in overcoming plant chemical defenses.

## 3. Materials and Methods

### 3.1. Plant Material

***Sample preparation.*** Healthy and eaten leaves of *A. cathartica*, as well as *P. tetrio* caterpillars were collected on the island of Guadeloupe (French West Indies), specifically in Le Gosier (16°13′00.5″ N 61°31′09.9″ W). The leaves were cleaned (with distilled water) and lyophilized. The caterpillars were kept in a cage for 24 h, to collect their feces, and starved for 48 h to use their corpse in the evaluation of biomolecule incorporation into the bodies of the caterpillars, excluding the digestive material. Finally, the dried leaves, the caterpillars' bodies and feces were lyophilized and powdered. Afterwards, 50 g of each sample was extracted by maceration extraction for 48 h. Maceration was performed in a ternary mixture of dichloromethane/methanol/distilled water [80,81] (1:1:1 *v/v*, 200 mL). After the complete extraction, the solutions were filtered and extracted by liquid–liquid extraction and two phases were obtained for each manipulation (Table 3). Finally, these phases were dried by rotary evaporation.

**Table 3.** Phases obtained for each manipulation after liquid–liquid extractions.

| | Organic Phase | Aqueous Phase |
|---|---|---|
| Healthy *A. cathartica* leaves | 1.2 | 2.2 |
| Hervivored *A. cathartica* leaves | 1.3 | 2.3 |
| Caterpillars | 1.4 | 2.4 |
| Caterpillar feces | 1.5 | 2.5 |

### 3.2. Phytochemical Tests

***Analysis and quantification.*** Analyses were performed using several techniques such as Thin Layer Chromatography (TLC), Nuclear Magnetic Resonance Spectroscopy (1H-NMR), High Performance Liquid Chromatography coupled with Mass Spectrometry (HPLC-MS) and Cyclic Voltammetry (CV).

***Thin layer chromatography (TLC).*** The thin layer chromatography of all the organic phases was carried out with a gradient of two different mixtures of elution solvents composed of $CH_2Cl_2$/MeOH or nhexane/AcOEt with a volume of 10 mL in different proportions (80/20, 50/50, 90/10, 95/5, 99/1, 50/50). Further, TLCs of all aqueous phases were made on cellulose TLC with a mixture of H2O/MeOH elution solvent in different proportions (50/50–100) as a mobile phase.

***Nuclear magnetic resonance spectroscopy (1H-NMR).*** 15 mg of each extract was solubilized in 650 µL of DMSO and transferred to NMR tubes. 1D 1H nuclear magnetic resonance spectra were recorded with a BRUKER Avance 300 MHz spectrometer equipped with a BBO probe and automatic tube changer. Chemical shifts (δ) were expressed in ppm relative to tetramethylsilane (TMS) taken as the external reference, with internal calibration performed on the solvent signal. All spectra were processed using Topspin 2.1 software. The classical 1D proton with a 90° pulse width was performed. The spectra were acquired using 256 scans and 2 dummy scans of 32 K data points with a spectral width of 5411.255 Hz.

***High performance liquid chromatography coupled with mass spectrometry (HPLC-MS).*** Triplicates of each extract were made and dissolved in 750 µL of methanol (LCMS grade) and 750 µL of ultra-pure water (ElgaPurelab Classic). The mixtures were sonicated in the ultrasonic bath then filtered on 13 mm and 0.45 µm PTFE filters and placed in amber vials. The analysis was performed on a Waters (Milford, MA, USA) Alliance e2695 liquid chromatographic system, equipped with a Waters 2996 photodiode array detector (PDA), coupled with a orthogonal quadrupole mass spectrometer (Micromass ZQ, Manchester, UK). The systems were controlled by MassLynx v.4.1 software (Micromass, Manchester, UK). The mass was equipped with an electrospray ionization ESI (Waters) source; the ionization was performed in positive mode. A double detection was carried out via mass spectrometry in ESI (range 71 to 1200 Da) and using a PDA diode array detector (UV detection between 210 and 400 nm). The analytical column was an XTERRA MS C18 column (2.1 x 100 mm, 3.5 µm) (Waters). The elution was performed with a mobile phase flow rate of 0.2 mL/min consisting of a mixture of ultra-pure water containing 0.1% formic acid (A) and methanol containing 0.1% formic acid (B). The program started at t = 0 min with a ratio (A: B) of 95:5, at t = 2 min (95:5), at t = 5 min (70:30), at t = 15 min (60:40), at t = 40 min (50:50), at t = 55 min (45:55), at t = 60 min (0:100), at t = 65 min (0:100), at t = 75 min (95:5) and at t = 80 min (95:5). The injection volume was 10 µl and detection was at 280 nm and at 320 nm. The ESI-MS parameters were as follows: desolvation gas ($N_2$) flow rate: 650 L/h; cone gas flow rate: 40 L/h; drying gas temperature: 450 °C; source temperature: 120 °C; capillary voltage: 3 kV; cone voltage: 85 V; and RF lens voltage: 0.1 V.

***Cyclic Voltammetry (CV).*** Cyclic voltammograms were recorded at 298 ± 1 K in a conventional three electrode cell using a platinum wire auxiliary electrode and an Ag/AgCl (3M NaCl) reference electrode. Measurements were carried out with CH I660 equipment using 0.10 M potassium phosphate buffer at pH 7.0 as a supporting electrolyte. The working electrode was prepared by evaporating 50 µL of an ethanol (EtOH) suspension of the extract of interest, ground leaves or insect samples, under air on a glassy carbon electrode (GCE, BAS MF 2012, geometrical area 0.071 $cm^2$). In order to mimic the natural environment, no degasification of the electrolyte was performed.

***Principal Component Analysis (PCA).*** The raw data from HPLC-MS were exported as netCDF files, using DataBridge software (Waters, USA), and pre-processed using XCMS Online [82,83] for feature detection, retention time correction and alignment of metabolites detected on HPLC-MS analysis. The dataset was created with 12 samples from each organic and aqueous extract fraction (3 samples from each manipulation (see Table 1)). Peak detection was performed using cent Wave peak detection ($\Delta m/z$ = 10 ppm; minimum peak width, 5 s; maximum peak width, 20 s) and mzwid = 0.015, minfrac = 0.5, and bw = 5 were used for the retention time alignment. The processed data (csv file) were further exported to MetaboAnalyst 4.0 [84]. All data variables were scaled by the pareto method prior to PCA. PCA is an unsupervised method commonly used to identify patterns between multivariate samples [85,86] and was recently employed on the chemical variability of Allamanda cathartica extracts [87].

### 3.3. Antimicrobial Activities

To investigate the potential antimicrobial effects of the interaction between the caterpillar *Pseudosphinx tetrio* L. and one of its host plants, *Allamanda cathartica*, we focused our study on five pathogen microorganisms that are responsible of severe human disease and usually involved in hospital acquired illness: *Escherichia coli*, *Pseudomonas aeruginosa* and *Staphylococcus aureus* for bacteria and *Candida albicans* and *Aspergillus fumigatus* for fungi. All strains were supplied by the ATCC (American Type Culture Collection).

The three bacteria were cultured on the non-selective medium Tryptic Soy Agar, whereas the two fungi were cultured on the selective medium Sabouraud, which is a selective medium for fungi and yeasts. These two media were provided by the manufacturer Grosseron, France, and prepared according to the instructions.

For each microorganism, starting cultures were prepared on Tryptic Soy Agar media for bacteria and Sabouraud media for fungi. From these starting cultures, microbial suspensions were created by picking two colonies from the starting cultures and adding them to 2 mL of sterile water. Finally, 200 µL of these microbial suspensions were used to inoculate the culture media used to test the antimicrobial activities.

Disc diffusion assay was used in order to test the antimicrobial activities of interaction between *P. tetrio* and *A. cathartica*. Sterile filter paper discs of Whatman no.1 (6 mm in diameter) were placed on the surface of the culture media with sterile forceps and gently pressed to ensure good contact with the surface. The different organic extracts were prepared as follows: 5 mg of each extract was mixed in 500 µL of Dimethyl sulfoxide (DMSO) and 10 µL of these mixtures were placed on antibiotic disks (100 µg/disk). The plates were incubated for 24 h to 48 h at 37 °C for bacteria and 30 °C for fungi. The zone of inhibition was calculated by measuring the diameter of the inhibition zone around the well (mm). All tests were conducted in duplicate.

## 4. Conclusions

In conclusion, we investigated the plant–herbivore interaction between the caterpillar *Pseudosphinx tetrio* and the flowering plant *A. cathartica*. In order to better understand this trophic relationship, several techniques were used, such as TLC, 1H NMR, HPLC-MS (analyzed using a 13 multivariate PCA) and an innovative approach using electrochemical methods (electrochemical ecology). The measured antimicrobial activities support the physicochemical tests. The results show a similar profile between the leaves of healthy and predated *A. cathartica* and the excretions of the caterpillars. The similar analytical profile between the leaves of *A. cathartica* and the excretions of *P. tetrio*, and the difference with the caterpillar bodies, suggests a selective excretion of compounds by the caterpillar (proposed hypothesis 2). These organic compounds found selectively in the excretions (rather than in the body) could explain the ability of *P. tetrio* to feed on this toxic Apocynaceae species.

**Author Contributions:** Conceptualization, G.C.-T. and M.S.; methodology, validation, formal analysis, investigation, L.M., M.M.L., M.M., M.V.C., D.P.V., M.V.P.-M., M.-N.S., L.P., A.D., Z.B., P.M. and G.C.-T. All authors have read and agreed to the published version of the manuscript.

**Funding:** The authors would like to acknowledge the financial support of the "AgroEcoDiv" project from the European Union Fund (FEDER) and "Région Guadeloupe". We would also like the Caribaea Initiative association for a two month study grant from Matignon. DPV would like to thank the OMICAS program: Optimización Multiescala In-silico de Cultivos Agrícolas Sostenibles (Infraestructura y validación en Arroz y Caña de Azúcar) Scientific Ecosystem belonging to the Colombia Científica Program, sponsored by The World Bank, The Ministry of Science, Technology and Innovation (MINCIENCIAS), ICETEX, the Colombian Ministry of Education and the Colombian Ministry of Commerce, Industry and Tourism, under GRANT ID: FP44842-217-2018, OMICAS Award ID: 792-61187.

**Data Availability Statement:** Not applicable.

**Acknowledgments:** Thanks are due to Tara Joy Massad (Gorongosa National Park, Mozambique) for her attentive lecture and fruitful discussion.

**Conflicts of Interest:** The authors declare no conflict of interest.

## References

1. Cock, M.J.W. Hawk-moths (Sphingidae) of Trinidad, West Indies: An illustrated and annotated catalogue. *Living World J. Trinidad Tobago Field Nat. Club* **2018**, *2018*, 10–81.
2. Ríos, S.; Drechsel, U. Nuevos registros de Pseudosphinx tetrio (Linnaeus 1771) en el Paraguay (Lepidoptera: Sphingidae). *Parag. Biodivers.* **2017**, *4*, 60–65.
3. Santiago-Blay, J. Notes on *Pseudosphinx tetrio* (L.) (Sphingidae) in Puerto Rico. *J. Lepid. Soc.* **1985**, *39*, 208–214.
4. Dunford, J.; Barbara, K. Tetrio Sphinx, Giant Gray Sphinx, Frangipani Hornworm, *Pseudosphinx tetrio* (Linnaeus) (Insecta: Lepidoptera: Sphingidae)1. *EDIS* **2019**, *2005*, 5. [CrossRef]
5. Cock, M.J. *Pseudosphinx tetrio* (L.) (Lepidotera: Sphingidae) in Trinidad and Tobago. *Living World J. Trinidad Tobago Field Nat. Club* **2008**, *2000*, 49–52.
6. Meurgey, F.; Ramage, T. Challenging the Wallacean shortfall: A total assessment of insect diversity on Guadeloupe (French West Indies), a checklist and bibliography. *Insecta Mundi* **2020**, *786*, 1–183.
7. D'Aguilar, J. Catalogue raisonné des Insectes des Antilles françaises 1. Lépidoptèreq, Sphingidae. *Annales Des Epiphyties 1950* **1966**, *17*, 251–262.
8. Chalumeau, F.; Delplanque, A. Catalogue commenté des Ctenuchidae (Lepidoptera) des Antilles françaises. *Bull. De La Société Linnéenne De Lyon* **1978**, *47*, 176–187. [CrossRef]
9. Sautière, C. Insectes capturés aux abords et dans les limites de Parc national de la Guadeloupe. Cerambycidae, Scarabaeidae, Sphingidae. *Bull. De L'entomologie Tourangelle* **1999**, *20*, 13–34.
10. Meurgey, F. *Les Arthropodes Continentaux de Guadeloupe: Synthèse Bibliographique Pour un État des Lieux Des Connaissances*; Ropport SHNLH pour le Parc national de Guadeloupe; 2011.
11. MNHN & OFB. Fiche de Pseudosphinx tetrio (Linnaeus, 1771). *Inventaire Natl. Du Patrim. Nat. INPN* **2022**, *2003*. Available online: https://inpn.mnhn.fr/espece/cd_nom/641756 (accessed on 5 December 2022).
12. Warrell, D.A. Researching nature's venoms and poisons. *Trans. R. Soc. Trop. Med. Hyg.* **2009**, *103*, 860–866. [CrossRef] [PubMed]
13. De Souza Leão Veiga, A.F.; de Melo, J.P.R.; Moreira, M.D. Aspectos Morfológicos da Forma Imatura de Pseudosphinx tetrio (LINNAEUS, 1771) (LEPIDOP-TERA: SPHINGIDAE). *Jorn. De Ensino Pesqui. E Extensão-JEPEX 9. Recife* **2009**.
14. Haxaire, J.; Rasplus, J.-Y. Contribution à la Connaissance des Sphingidae de Guyane Française. 1e Partie. *Bull. De La Société Entomol. De Fr.* **1986**, *91*, 275–285. [CrossRef]
15. Haxaire, J.; Herbin, D. Les Lépidoptères Sphingidae de Bolivie. Ecologie et Systématique. 2ème Partie: Les Sous-Familles des Smerinthinae et Macroglossinae Pro Parte (1). *Rev. Assoc. Rousillon. Entomol* **2000**, *9*, 4–19.
16. Meerman, J.C. The Annual Outbreak of Colorful Caterpillars of the Frangipani Hawkmoth (Pseudosphinx tetrio). *Biol. Divers. Belize* **2009**. Available online: http://biological-diversity.info/pseudosphinx.htm (accessed on 8 December 2009).
17. Sloan, S.A.; Zimmerman, J.K.; Sabat, A.M. Phenology of Plumeria alba and its Herbivores in a Tropical Dry Forest. *Biotropica* **2007**, *39*, 195–201. [CrossRef]
18. Rajamanickam, K.; Sudha, S.S. In-Vitro Antimicrobial Activity and In-Vivo Toxicity of Moringa Oleifera and Allamanda Cathartica against Multiple Drug Resistant Clinical Pathogens. *Int. J. Pharma. Bio. Sci.* **2013**, *4*, B768–B775.
19. Khanam, M.N.; Anis, M.; Ahmad, S. Establishment of adventitious root cultures of Allamanda cathartica L. for the production of iridoid glycosides and its identification using HPTLC MS. *Ind. Crops Prod.* **2018**, *125*, 198–206. [CrossRef]
20. Wong, S.K.; Lim, Y.; Chan, E. Botany, uses, phytochemistry and pharmacology of selected Apocynaceae species: A review. *Pharmcognosy Commun.* **2013**, *3*, 2–11.
21. Chandreyi, G.; Labani, H.; Sudip, K.N.; Sayantan, S.; Alokila, D.; Swagata, B.; Maitrayee, B.; Pranabesh, G.; Sirshendu Chatterjee Allamanda cathartica Linn. Apocynaceae: A mini review. *Int. J. Herb. Med.* **2019**, *7*, 29–33.
22. Francis, J.K. *Wildland Shrubs of the United States and Its Territories: Thamnic Descriptions, Volume 1*; U.S. Department of Agriculture, Forest Service, International Institute of Tropical Forestry: San Juan, PR, USA, 2004; p. IITF-GTR-26. [CrossRef]
23. WFO. *Allamanda* L. Published on the Internet. 2022. Available online: http://www.worldfloraonline.org/taxon/wfo-4000001228 (accessed on 5 December 2022).
24. Pessoa, C.; Costa-Lotufo, L.V.; Leyva, A.; de Moraes, M.E.A.; de Moraes, M.O. Anticancer potential of Northeast Brazilian plants. In *Advances in Phytomedicine*; Elsevier: Amsterdam, The Netherlands, 2006; Volume 2, pp. 197–211. [CrossRef]

25. Rahman, A.H.M.; Akter, M. Taxonomy and Traditional Medicinal Uses of Apocynaceae (Dogbane) Family of Rajshahi District, Bangladesh. *Res. Rev. J. Bot. Sci.* **2015**, *4*, 5–13.
26. Nayak, S.; Nalabothu, P.; Sandiford, S.; Bhogadi, V.; Adogwa, A. Evaluation of wound healing activity of Allamanda cathartica. L. and Laurus nobilis. L. extracts on rats. *BMC Complement. Altern. Med.* **2006**, *6*, 12. [CrossRef] [PubMed]
27. Ghosh, C.; Banerjee, S. Floral extracts of allamanda blanchetii and allamanda cathartica are comparatively higher resource of anti-oxidants and polysaccharides than leaf and stem extracts. *Int. J. Curr. Pharm. Sci.* **2018**, *10*, 36–39. [CrossRef]
28. Hameed, A.; Nawaz, G.; Gulzar, T. Chemical composition, antioxidant activities and protein profiling of different parts of *Allamanda cathartica*. *Nat. Prod. Res.* **2014**, *28*, 2066–2071. [CrossRef]
29. Sarker, R.; Tasnuva, S.; Farhana, I.; Sharmin, R.C. In vitro antioxidant, total phenolic, membrane stabilizing and antimicrobial activity of Allamanda cathartica L.: A medicinal plant of Bangladesh. *J. Med. Plants Res.* **2014**, *8*, 63–67. [CrossRef]
30. Karunakaran, G.; Jagathambal, M.; Gusev, A.; Kolesnikov, E.; Mandal, A.R.; Kuznetsov, D. Allamanda cathartica flower's aqueous extract-mediated green synthesis of silver nanoparticles with excellent antioxidant and antibacterial potential for biomedical application. *MRS Commun.* **2016**, *6*, 41–46. [CrossRef]
31. Islam, M.R.; Ahamed, R.; Rahman, M.O.; Al-Amin, M.; Alam, K.D.; Lyzu, F. In Vitro Antimicrobial Activities of Four Medicinally Important Plants in Bangladesh. *Eur. J. Sci. Res.* **2010**, *39*, 199–206.
32. Sharmin, M.; Banya, P.D.; Paul, L.; Chowdhury, F.F.K.; Afrin, S.; Acharjee, M.; Rahman, T.; Noor, R. Study of microbial proliferation and the in vitro antibacterial traits of commonly available flowers in Dhaka Metropolis. *Asian Pac. J. Trop. Dis.* **2015**, *5*, 91–97. [CrossRef]
33. Souza, E.; Barcellos, V.D.A.; Sbaraini, N.; Reuwsaat, J.C.V.; Schneider, R.d.O.; da Silva, A.C.; Garcia, A.W.A.; von Poser, G.L.; Barbosa, E.G.; Lima, J.P.M.S.; et al. A Plumieridine-Rich Fraction From Allamanda polyantha Inhibits Chitinolytic Activity and Exhibits Antifungal Properties Against Cryptococcus neoformans. *Front. Microbiol.* **2020**, *11*, 2058. [CrossRef]
34. Conrad, O.A.; Dike, I.P.; Agbara, U. In vivo antioxidant assessment of two antimalarial plants–Allamamda cathartica and Bixa orellana. *Asian Pac. J. Trop. Biomed.* **2013**, *3*, 388–394. [CrossRef]
35. Boeing, T.; de Souza, P.; Bonomini, T.J.; Mariano, L.N.B.; Somensi, L.B.; Lucinda, R.M.; Malheiros, A.; da Silva, L.M.; Andrade, S.F.d. Antioxidant and anti-inflammatory effect of plumieride in dextran sulfate sodium-induced colitis in mice. *Biomed. Pharmacother.* **2018**, *99*, 697–703. [CrossRef] [PubMed]
36. Kupchan, S.M.; Dessertine, A.L.; Blaylock, B.T.; Bryan, R.F. Isolation and structural elucidation of allamandin, and antileukemic iridoid lactone from allamanda cathartica. *J. Org. Chem.* **1974**, *39*, 2477–2482. [CrossRef] [PubMed]
37. Wong, S.; Lim, Y.; Abdullah, N.; Nordin, F. Antiproliferative and phytochemical analyses of leaf extracts of ten Apocynaceae species. *Phcog. Res.* **2011**, *3*, 100. [CrossRef] [PubMed]
38. Akah, P.A.; Offiah, V.N. Gastrointestinal Effects of *Allamanda cathartica* Leaf Extracts. *Int. J. Pharmacogn.* **1992**, *30*, 213–217. [CrossRef]
39. Nithya, K.; Muthumary, J. Bioactive Metabolite Produced by Phomopsis sp., an Endophytic Fungus in Allamanda cathartica Linn. *Recent Res. Sci. Technol.* **2011**, *3*, 44–48.
40. Nahar, A.; Ashrafuzzaman, S.; Islam, M.N.; Alam, M.S. Studies on antidermatophytic effect of Allamanda cathertica. *Bangladesh J. Pharm.* **2010**, *5*, 5–7. [CrossRef]
41. Janzen, D.H. Patterns of Herbivory in a Tropical Deciduous Forest. *Biotropica* **1981**, *13*, 271–282. [CrossRef]
42. Petricevich, V.; Abarca-Vargas, R. Allamanda cathartica: A Review of the Phytochemistry, Pharmacology, Toxicology, and Biotechnology. *Molecules* **2019**, *24*, 1238. [CrossRef]
43. Hema, K.; Krishnaveni, R. Antibacterial and antifungal activities of Allamanda cathartica Linn. *Int. J. Pharma Bio. Sci.* **2014**, *5*, 588–593.
44. Chaithra, A.B.; Satish, S.; Karunakara, H. Therapeutic uses of Allamanda Cathartica Linn. With a note on its pharmacological actions: A Review. *Int. J. Pharma Chem. Res.* **2016**, *2*, 227–232.
45. Bihani, T. Plumeria rubra L.–A review on its ethnopharmacological, morphological, phytochemical, pharmacological and toxicological studies. *J. Ethnopharmacol.* **2021**, *264*, 113291. [CrossRef] [PubMed]
46. Khan, I.A.; Hussain, M.; Syed, S.K.; Saadullah, M.; Alqahtani, A.M.; Alqahtani, T.; Aldahish, A.A.; Asiri, S.; Zeng, L.-H. Pharmacological Justification for the Medicinal Use of Plumeria rubra Linn. in Cardiovascular Disorders. *Molecules* **2021**, *27*, 251. [CrossRef] [PubMed]
47. Shefali, A.; Kanchan, D.B.; Shailey, S.; Mamta, L.; Tanuja, U.S.; Deepak, K. A review on phytopharmacological activity of plumeria species. *Int. J. Eng. Sci. Math.* **2018**, *7*. Available online: http://www.ijma.us (accessed on 5 December 2022).
48. Siti Mohamed Isa; Ablat, A.; Mohamad, J. The Antioxidant and Xanthine Oxidase Inhibitory Activity of Plumeria rubra Flowers. *Molecules* **2018**, *23*, 400. [CrossRef]
49. Thakur, M.; Gupta, P.; Roy, A.; Chandrakar, S.; Sahu, J.; Gupta, U.P. Therapeutic potential of Plumeria rubra plant: A review. *Adv. J. Bioact. Mol.* **2020**, *1*, 40–47.
50. Forister, M.L.; Novotny, V.; Panorska, A.K.; Baje, L.; Basset, Y.; Butterill, P.T.; Cizek, L.; Coley, P.D.; Dem, F.; Diniz, I.R.; et al. The global distribution of diet breadth in insect herbivores. *Proc. Natl. Acad. Sci. USA* **2015**, *112*, 442–447. [CrossRef] [PubMed]
51. Suzuki, H.C.; Ozaki, K.; Makino, T.; Uchiyama, H.; Yajima, S.; Kawata, M. Evolution of Gustatory Receptor Gene Family Provides Insights into Adaptation to Diverse Host Plants in Nymphalid Butterflies. *Genome Biol. Evol.* **2018**, *10*, 1351–1362. [CrossRef]
52. Opitz, S.E.W.; Müller, C. Plant chemistry and insect sequestration. *Chemoecology* **2009**, *19*, 117–154. [CrossRef]

53. Eisner, T.; Meinwald, J. *Chemical Ecology: The Chemistry of Biotic Interaction*; National Academies Press: Washington, DC, USA, 1995; p. 4979. [CrossRef]
54. McCoy, V.E.; Gee, C.T.; Michalski, J.M.; Wings, O. Oldest fossil evidence of latex sabotaging behavior by herbivorous insects. *Rev. Palaeobot. Palynol.* **2022**, *300*, 104631. [CrossRef]
55. Ali, J.G.; Agrawal, A.A. Specialist versus generalist insect herbivores and plant defense. *Trends Plant Sci.* **2012**, *17*, 293–302. [CrossRef]
56. Ehrlich, P.R.; Raven, P.H. Butterflies and plants: A study in coevolution. *Evolution* **1964**, *18*, 586–608. [CrossRef]
57. Bernays, E.A.; Chapman, R.E. *Host-Plant Selection by Phytophagous Insects*; Springer: Boston, MA, USA, 1994. [CrossRef]
58. Jones, P.L.; Petschenka, G.; Flacht, L.; Agrawal, A.A. Cardenolide Intake, Sequestration, and Excretion by the Monarch Butterfly along Gradients of Plant Toxicity and Larval Ontogeny. *J. Chem. Ecol.* **2019**, *45*, 264–277. [CrossRef] [PubMed]
59. Engler-Chaouat, H.S.; Gilbert, L.E. De novo Synthesis vs. Sequestration: Negatively Correlated Metabolic Traits and the Evolution of Host Plant Specialization in Cyanogenic Butterflies. *J. Chem. Ecol.* **2007**, *33*, 25–42. [CrossRef] [PubMed]
60. Lampert, E.C.; Dyer, L.A.; Bowers, M.D. Chemical Defense Across Three Trophic Levels: Catalpa bignonioides, the Caterpillar Ceratomia catalpae, and its Endoparasitoid Cotesia congregata. *J. Chem. Ecol.* **2011**, *37*, 1063–1070. [CrossRef] [PubMed]
61. Winde, I.; Wittstock, U. Insect herbivore counteradaptations to the plant glucosinolate–myrosinase system. *Phytochemistry* **2011**, *72*, 1566–1575. [CrossRef]
62. Berenbaum, M.R.; Zangerl, A.R. Furanocoumarin metabolism in Papilio polyxenes: Biochemistry, genetic variability, and ecological significance. *Oecologia* **1993**, *95*, 370–375. [CrossRef]
63. Frankfater, C.; Schühly, W.; Fronczek, F.R.; Slattery, M. Processing of a Sesquiterpene Lactone by Papilio glaucus Caterpillars. *J. Chem. Ecol.* **2005**, *31*, 2541–2550. [CrossRef]
64. Barny, L.A.; Tasca, J.A.; Sanchez, H.A.; Smith, C.R.; Koptur, S.; Livshultz, T.; Minbiole, K.P.C. Chemotaxonomic investigation of Apocynaceae for retronecine-type pyrrolizidine alkaloids using HPLC-MS/MS. *Phytochemistry* **2021**, *185*, 112662. [CrossRef]
65. Prabhadevi, V.; Sahaya, S.S.; Johnson, M.; Venkatramani, B.; Janakiraman, N. Phytochemical studies on Allamanda cathartica L. using GC–MS. *Asian Pac. J. Trop. Biomed.* **2012**, *2*, S550–S554. [CrossRef]
66. Marques, J.; Alves, J.; Torres-Rêgo, M.; Furtado, A.; Siqueira, E.; Galinari, E.; Araújo, D.; Guerra, G.; Azevedo, E.; Fernandes-Pedrosa, M.; et al. Phytochemical Analysis by HPLC–HRESI-MS and Anti-Inflammatory Activity of Tabernaemontana catharinensis. *IJMS* **2018**, *19*, 636. [CrossRef]
67. Palmeira-Mello, M.V.; Souza, J.L.; Pérez, A.F.; Cavalcanti, A.D.S.; Kahn, S.A.; Passe-Coutrin, N.; Guerra, I.R.; Doménech-Carbó, A.; Jauregui-Haza, U.J.; de Souza, A.M.T.; et al. Insights of Tris(2-pyridylmethyl)amine as anti-tumor agent for osteosarcoma: Experimental and in silico studies. *J. Mol. Struct.* **2021**, *1228*, 129773. [CrossRef]
68. Rozoy, E.; Araya-Farias, M.; Simard, S.; Kitts, D.; Lessard, J.; Bazinet, L. Redox properties of catechins and enriched green tea extracts effectively preserve l-5-methyltetrahydrofolate: Assessment using cyclic voltammetry analysis. *Food Chem.* **2013**, *138*, 1982–1991. [CrossRef] [PubMed]
69. Cebrián-Torrejón, G.; Kablan, L.; Ferreira, M.E.; Rodríguez de la Cruz, D.; Doménech-Carbó, A.; Vera de Bilbao, N.; Rojas de Arias, A.; Figadère, B.; Poupon, E.; Fournet, A. Harvesting canthinones: Identification of the optimal seasonal point of harvest of *Zanthoxylum chiloperone* leaves as a source of 5-methoxycanthin-6-one. *Nat. Prod. Res.* **2015**, *29*, 2054–2058. [CrossRef] [PubMed]
70. Doménech-Carbó, A.; Cebrián-Torrejón, G.; Lopes-Souto, A.; Martins-de-Moraes, M.; Jorge-Kato, M.; Fechine-Tavares, J.; Barbosa-Filho, J.M. Electrochemical ecology: VIMP monitoring of plant defense against external stressors. *RSC Adv.* **2015**, *5*, 61006–61011. [CrossRef]
71. Doménech-Carbó, A.; Labuda, J.; Scholz, F. Electroanalytical chemistry for the analysis of solids: Characterization and classification (IUPAC Technical Report). *Pure Appl. Chem.* **2012**, *85*, 609–631. [CrossRef]
72. Singh, S.; Kaur, I.; Kariyat, R. The Multifunctional Roles of Polyphenols in Plant-Herbivore Interactions. *IJMS* **2021**, *22*, 1442. [CrossRef]
73. Mannan, M.; Alam, M.; Mustari, F.; Kudrat-E-Zahan, M.; Ali, R.; Haque, A.; Zaman, S.; Talukder, D. In vitro Antioxidant, Antimicrobial, Insecticidal and Cytotoxic Activities of the Medicinal Plants: Allamanda cathartica and Mimusops elengi. *EJMP* **2017**, *20*, 1–12. [CrossRef]
74. Speed, M.P.; Fenton, A.; Jones, M.G.; Ruxton, G.D.; Brockhurst, M.A. Coevolution can explain defensive secondary metabolite diversity in plants. *New Phytol.* **2015**, *208*, 1251–1263. [CrossRef]
75. Petschenka, G.; Agrawal, A.A. Milkweed butterfly resistance to plant toxins is linked to sequestration, not coping with a toxic diet. *Proc. R. Soc. B.* **2015**, *282*, 20151865. [CrossRef]
76. Duffey, S.S. Sequestration of Plant Natural Products by Insects. *Annu. Rev. Entomol.* **1980**, *25*, 447–477. [CrossRef]
77. Dyer, L.A. Tasty Generalists and Nasty Specialists? Antipredator Mechanisms in Tropical Lepidopteran Larvae. *Ecology* **1995**, *76*, 1483–1496. [CrossRef]
78. Karban, R. The ecology and evolution of induced resistance against herbivores. *Funct. Ecol.* **2011**, *25*, 339–347. [CrossRef]
79. Ramos, M.V.; Pereira, D.A.; Souza, D.P.; Silva, M.-L.S.; Alencar, L.M.R.; Sousa, J.S.; Queiroz, J.-F.N.; Freitas, C.D.T. Peptidases and peptidase inhibitors in gut of caterpillars and in the latex of their host plants. *Planta* **2015**, *241*, 167–178. [CrossRef] [PubMed]
80. Mushtaq, M.Y.; Choi, Y.H.; Verpoorte, R.; Wilson, E.G. Extraction for Metabolomics: Access to The Metabolome: Extraction for Metabolomics: Access to the Metabolome. *Phytochem. Anal.* **2014**, *25*, 291–306. [CrossRef]

81. Lin, C.Y.; Wu, H.; Tjeerdema, R.S.; Viant, M.R. Evaluation of metabolite extraction strategies from tissue samples using NMR metabolomics. *Metabolomics* **2007**, *3*, 55–67. [CrossRef]
82. Tautenhahn, R.; Patti, G.J.; Rinehart, D.; Siuzdak, G. XCMS Online: A Web-Based Platform to Process Untargeted Metabolomic Data. *Anal. Chem.* **2012**, *84*, 5035–5039. [CrossRef] [PubMed]
83. Mahieu, N.G.; Genenbacher, J.L.; Patti, G.J. A roadmap for the XCMS family of software solutions in metabolomics. *Curr. Opin. Chem. Biol.* **2016**, *30*, 87–93. [CrossRef] [PubMed]
84. Chong, J.; Soufan, O.; Li, C.; Caraus, I.; Li, S.; Bourque, G.; Wishart, D.S.; Xia, J. MetaboAnalyst 4.0: Towards more transparent and integrative metabolomics analysis. *Nucleic Acids Res.* **2018**, *46*, W486–W494. [CrossRef]
85. Jolliffe, I. Principal Component Analysis. In *Encyclopedia of Statistics in Behavioral Science*; Everitt, B.S., Howell, D.C., Eds.; John Wiley & Sons, Ltd.: Chichester, UK, 2005; p. bsa501. [CrossRef]
86. Wold, S.; Esbensen, K.; Geladi, P. Principal component analysis. *Chemom. Intell. Lab. Syst.* **1987**, *2*, 37–52. [CrossRef]
87. Rodrigues, D.; Muller, A.F.; Bonomini, T.; Klein-Júnior, L.; Lucinda-Silva, R.; Malheiros, A. Chemical variability of allamanda cathartica l. flowers assessed by multivariate data analysis. *Quím. Nova* **2020**, *43*, 201–205. [CrossRef]

plants MDPI

Article

# Allelochemicals from the Rhizosphere Soil of Potato (*Solanum tuberosum* L.) and Their Interactions with the Soilborne Pathogens

**Aiyi Xin [1,2], Hui Jin [1], Xiaoyan Yang [1], Jinfeng Guan [3], Heping Hui [1], Haoyue Liu [1], Zengtuan Cui [4], Zhiheng Dun [4] and Bo Qin [1,*]**

1 CAS Key Laboratory of Chemistry of Northwestern Plant Resources and Key Laboratory for Natural Medicine of Gansu Province, Lanzhou Institute of Chemical Physics, Chinese Academy of Sciences (CAS), Lanzhou 730000, China; cpuxay@163.com (A.X.); comefine@licp.cas.cn (H.J.); yangxiaoy@licp.cas.cn (X.Y.); mysy105@163.com (H.H.); liuhaoyue0820@163.com (H.L.)

2 School of Chemistry and Chemical Engineering, Mianyang Normal University, Mianyang 621000, China

3 Institute for Food and Drug Control, Tongliao City, Inner Mongolia Autonomous Region, Tongliao 028000, China; nmtlgjf@sina.com

4 Cultivated Land Quality Construction and Management Station of Gansu Province, Lanzhou 730030, China; konphy@126.com (Z.C.); ruoxi020xw@163.com (Z.D.)

* Correspondence: bqin@licp.cas.cn; Tel.: +86-931-4968371; Fax: +86-931-4968019

**Abstract:** To reveal the allelopathic effects of potato, seven compounds were isolated from the rhizosphere soil: 7-methoxycoumarin (**1**), palmitic acid (**2**), caffeic acid (**3**), chlorogenic acid (**4**), quercetin dehydrate (**5**), quercitrin (**6**), and rutin (**7**). Bioassays showed that compounds **1**, **2**, **4**, and **6** had inhibitory effects on the growth of *L. sativa* and tissue culture seedlings of potato. The existence of the allelochemicals was confirmed by HPLC, and their contents were quantified with a total concentration of 9.02 μg/g in the rhizosphere soil of replanted potato. Approaches on the interactions of the allelochemicals and pathogens of potato including *A. solani*, *B. cinerea*, *F. solani*, *F. oxysporum*, *C. coccodes*, and *V. dahlia* revealed that compound **1** had inhibitory effects but compounds **2**–**4** promoted the colony growth of the pathogens. These findings demonstrated that the autotoxic allelopathy and enhancement of the pathogens caused by the accumulation of the allelochemicals in the continuously cropped soil should be one of the main reasons for the replant problems of potato.

**Keywords:** potato (*Solanum tuberosum* L.); replant problems; allelochemicals; autotoxicity; antifungal effects

**Citation:** Xin, A.; Jin, H.; Yang, X.; Guan, J.; Hui, H.; Liu, H.; Cui, Z.; Dun, Z.; Qin, B. Allelochemicals from the Rhizosphere Soil of Potato (*Solanum tuberosum* L.) and Their Interactions with the Soilborne Pathogens. *Plants* **2022**, *11*, 1934. https://doi.org/10.3390/plants11151934

Academic Editors: Margot Schulz and Vincenzo Tabaglio

Received: 14 June 2022
Accepted: 14 July 2022
Published: 26 July 2022



## 1. Introduction

Tubers of potato (*Solanum tuberosum* L.) are the third most important food crops in terms of human consumption with a population of more than a billion people worldwide consuming them. The global total crop production exceeds 374 million metric tons each year, following wheat (*Triticum aestivum* L.), rice (*Oryza sativa* L.), and maize (*Zea mays* L.) according to the statistics data of the Food and Agriculture Organization of the United Nations (FAO, Rome, Italy) in 2017 [1,2]. Being rich in starch and crude protein, potato is used for both a staple food and a vegetable. Research indicated that potato can provide a great diversity of nutrients such as protein, lipids, minerals, vitamins, and dietary fiber [3]. Owing to the high content of essential amino acids, potato protein is considered as one of the most valuable non-animal proteins [4]. Meanwhile, it is a typical highly productive crop and has been used as a source of starch and alcohol for industrial uses; thus the production of potato has been regarded as a pillar industry for farmers to get rid of poverty and increase income in some major producing areas [5,6].

However, the crop production of potato has often been hampered by replant problems. The occurrence of replant failure not only affects the yield and quality of potato, but also reduces the safety of the product [7]. Therefore, it is urgent to declare the reasons causing the replant failure and explore an efficient way to achieve high and stable production of potato. Replant failure is a phenomenon in which several factors are involved; allelopathy (especially autotoxic allelopathy) and the enhancement of soilborne pathogens coupled with an imbalance in the soil microbial community caused by allelochemicals have been considered as essential factors on this issue [8–11]. A great variety of secondary metabolites produced by the crop and released into the soil environment through leaching, root exudation, and/or residue decomposition have been shown to interact with the replanted plant itself and other organisms [12–16]. Further knowledge indicated that soil-borne pathogens play a primary role in the occurrence of replant disease [17]. It is proposed that the activities of soil borne pathogens would be improved indirectly by the allelochemicals which are released by the crop [18]. The allelochemicals are not only autotoxic compounds for the replanted plant, but also a precipitating factor for changing the composition of the microbial community to lead to the build-up of soil-borne pathogens [19,20]. The accumulation of phytotoxic substances and the decrease in bacterial diversity is attributed to replant failure which was occurred during continuous cropping [21]. Several common diseases of potato were caused by the fungi in major producing regions around the world, such as *Alternaria solani* that may result in early blight, *Botrytis cinerea* that may bring about gray mold, *Fusarium solani* that may increase the risk of dry rot, *Fusarium oxysporum* that may cause root rot, *Colletotrichum coccodes* that may lead to potato black dot, *Verticillium dahliae* that may give rise to potato early dying, etc.

It was reported that water extracts from different organs and root exudates of potato had potential phytotoxicity against potato itself and other plants [22–25]. However, the specific compounds which are responsible for the phytotoxicity still remain unknown, and the relative roles of autotoxic factors and pathogens of potato are unclear as well. Elucidating the chemical reasons for the replant problem is necessary to explor efficient approaches to eliminating the replant failure of potato. Thus, in this work, the allelochemicals from the rhizosphere soil of cultivated potato were isolated and identified for the first time. Further investigations on the interactions of the allelochemicals and pathogens were carried out as well to get more helpful information to understand the chemical basis of the replant failure of potato.

## 2. Results

### 2.1. Allelopathic Activity of the Crude Extract of the Rhizosphere Soil of Potato

The phytotoxic activity of the crude extract was evaluated with *Lactuca sativa* L. (Figure 1a) and potato tissue culture (Figure 1b) seedlings. The results revealed that the crude methanol extract significantly inhibited the growth of the treated seedlings and the effect was in a concentration-dependent manner. The crude extract exhibited a more remarkable inhibitory effect on the growth of roots than that on stems for *L. sativa* seedlings. As Figure 1a showed, the inhibition ratios of roots at the treated concentrations of 100, 200, and 400 μg/mL were 17.82%, 27.39%, and 65.96%, respectively. The growth of potato seedlings was observably inhibited by the crude extract in a similar manner. The inhibitory effect on the growth of the roots was more pronounced than that on the leaves and stems for the potato seedlings, which was in accordance with the growth of *L. sativa*. As shown in Figure 1b, at a concentration of 100 μg/mL, the inhibition ratios of the height of the potato seedlings, the fresh weight of leave and stems, and the fresh weight of the roots were 37.03%, 29.73%, and 50.17%, respectively. The inhibition ratios at the treated concentration of 200 μg/mL reached up to 54.25%, 36.68%, and 55.63%, respectively. At the maximum concentration (400 μg/mL), the inhibition ratios ran up to 61.26%, 48.20%, and 66.28%, respectively.

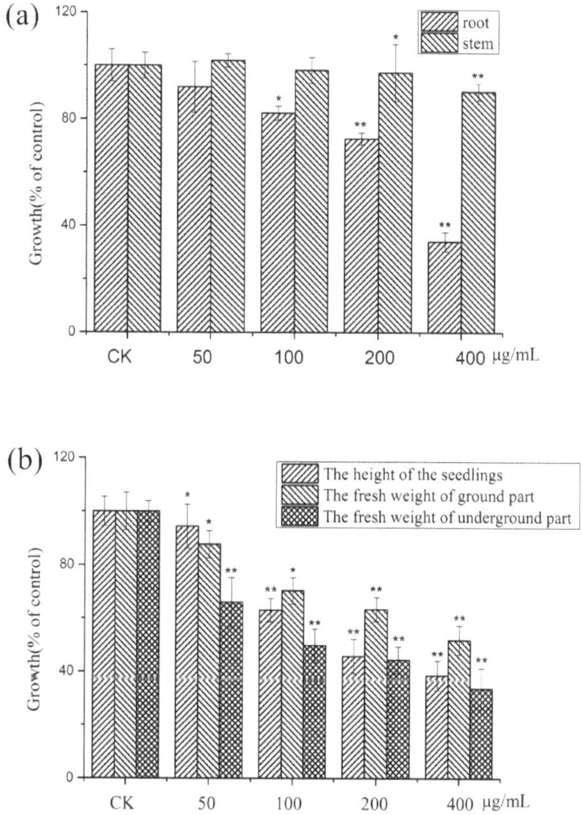


**Figure 1.** Phytotoxic effects of the crude extract of the rhizosphere soil of potato on seedlings of *L. sativa* (**a**) and potato (**b**) at concentrations of 50, 100, 200, and 400 μg/mL, respectively. Values are presented as a percentage of the mean compared to the control. Means significantly lower than the methanol controls are indicated by * (one way ANOVA; $p < 0.05$) or ** ($p < 0.01$). Error bars are one standard error of the mean. $n = 3$.

### 2.2. Isolation of Allelochemicals from the Rhizosphere Soil of Potato

Seven compounds were isolated from the extract of the rhizosphere soil of potato; they were identified as: 7-methoxycoumarin (**1**), palmitic acid (**2**), caffeic acid (**3**), chlorogenic acid (**4**), quercetin dehydrate (**5**), quercitrin (**6**), and rutin (**7**). Their structures were characterized by spectroscopic analysis in comparison with literature data. The structures of compounds **1**–**7** are shown in Figure 2.

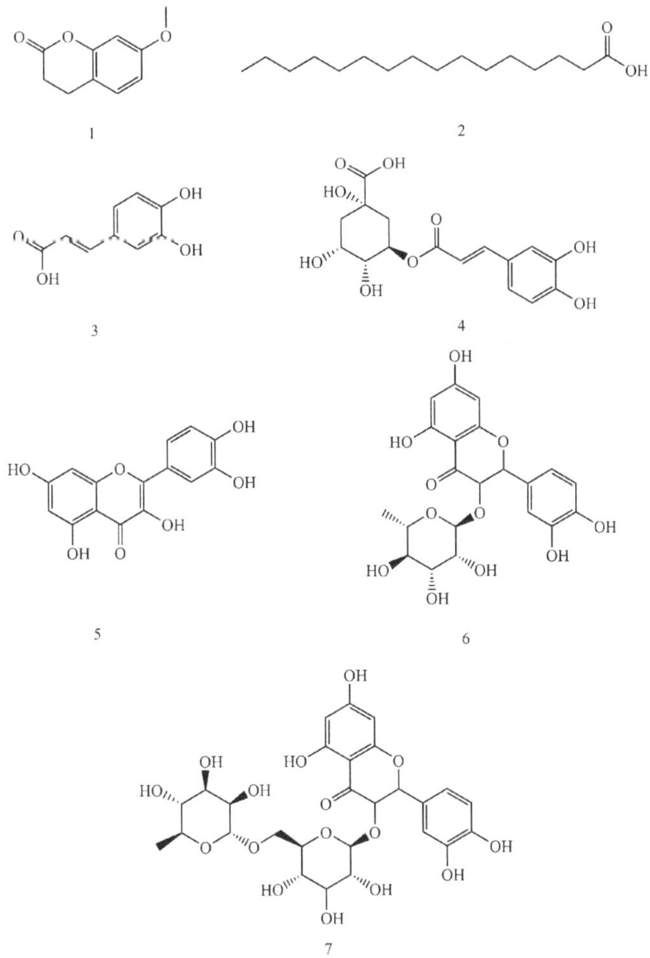

**Figure 2.** Structures of compounds **1–7** isolated from the rhizosphere soil of potato. (**1**. 7-methoxycoumarin, **2**. palmitic acid, **3**. caffeic acid, **4**. chlorogenic acid, **5**. quercetin dehydrate, **6**. quercitrin, and **7**. rutin).

Compound **1**: $C_{10}H_8O_3$

MS: $[M + Na]^+$ $C_{10}H_8NaO_3$, measured m/z 199.0363, calculated m/z 199.0371, err 3.9 ppm.

$^1H$ NMR (400 MHz, $CD_3OD$) δ 7.65 (d, J = 9.5 Hz, 1H), 7.38 (d, J = 8.6 Hz, 1H), 6.85 (dd, J = 8.6, 2.3 Hz, 1H), 6.80 (d, J = 2.1 Hz, 1H), 6.25 (d, J = 9.5 Hz, 1H).

$^{13}C$ NMR (100 MHz, $CD_3OD$) δ 162.57, 160.94, 155.63, 143.21, 128.54, 112.79, 112.30, 100.57, 55.52.

Compound **2**: $C_{16}H_{32}O_2$

MS: $[M + Na]^+$ $C_{16}H_{32}NaO_2$, measured m/z 279.2295, calculated m/z 279.2300, err 1.8 ppm.

$^1$H NMR (400 MHz, $CDCl_3$) δ 2.34 (t, J = 7.5 Hz, 2H), 1.66-1.60 (m, 2H), 1.26 (s, 24H), 0.88 (t, J = 6.7 Hz, 3H).

$^{13}$C NMR (100 MHz, $CDCl_3$) δ 180.57, 34.13, 31.94, 29.71, 29.70, 29.68, 29.67, 29.66, 29.61, 29.45, 29.38, 29.25, 29.08, 24.68, 22.70, 14.10.

Compound **3**: $C_9H_8O_4$

MS: $[M + Na]^+$ $C_9H_8NaO_4$, measured m/z 203.0310, calculated m/z 203.0315, err 2.5 ppm.

$^1$H NMR (400 MHz, $CD_3OD$) δ 7.53 (d, J = 15.9 Hz, 1H), 7.03 (d, J = 1.9 Hz, 1H), 6.92 (dd, J = 8.2, 1.9 Hz, 1H), 6.77 (d, J = 8.2 Hz, 1H), 6.21 (d, J = 15.9 Hz, 1H).

$^{13}$C NMR (100 MHz, $CD_3OD$) δ 169.68, 148.06, 145.69, 145.39, 126.41, 121.50, 115.11, 114.11, 113.71.

Compound **4**: $C_{16}H_{18}O_9$

MS: $[M + Na]^+$ $C_{16}H_{18}NaO_9$, measured m/z 377.0840, calculated m/z 377.0843, err 0.8 ppm.

$^1$H NMR (400 MHz, Acetone) δ 7.56 (d, J = 15.9 Hz, 1H), 7.16 (d, J = 1.9 Hz, 1H), 7.05 (dd, J = 8.2, 1.9 Hz, 1H), 6.88 (d, J = 8.2 Hz, 1H), 6.27 (d, J = 15.9 Hz, 1H), 5.42–5.36 (m, 1H), 4.25 (d, J = 3.3 Hz, 1H), 3.78 (d, J = 3.0 Hz, 1H), 2.29–2.22 (m, 1H), 2.16 (d, J = 3.1 Hz, 1H), 2.05 (d, J = 4.4 Hz, 2H).

$^{13}$C NMR (100 MHz, Acetone) δ 174.20, 166.24, 147.86, 145.42, 144.88, 126.79, 121.65, 115.51, 115.00, 114.34, 75.36, 72.64, 70.76, 70.47, 38.26, 37.03.

Compound **5**: $C_{15}H_{10}O_7$

MS: $[M + Na]^+$ $C_{15}H_{10}NaO_7$, measured m/z 325.0317, calculated m/z 325.0319, err 0.6 ppm.

$^1$H NMR (400 MHz, $CD_3OD$) δ 7.71 (d, J = 2.0 Hz, 1H), 7.61 (dd, J = 8.5, 2.1 Hz, 1H), 6.86 (d, J = 8.5 Hz, 1H), 6.36 (d, J = 2.0 Hz, 1H), 6.15 (d, J = 2.0 Hz, 1H).

$^{13}$C NMR (100 MHz, $CD_3OD$) δ 177.33, 165.57, 162.51, 158.22, 148.76, 147.97, 146.22, 137.24, 124.14, 121.66, 116.21, 115.97, 104.51, 99.21, 94.39.

Compound **6**: $C_{21}H_{20}O_{11}$

MS: $[M + Na]^+$ $C_{21}H_{20}NaO_{11}$, measured m/z 47.0908, calculated m/z 471.0898, err −2.1 ppm.

$^1$H NMR (400 MHz, $CD_3OD$) δ 7.34 (d, J = 1.9 Hz, 1H), 7.32 (dd, J = 8.3, 2.0 Hz, 1H), 6.92 (d, J = 8.3 Hz, 1H), 6.38 (d, J = 2.0 Hz, 1H), 6.21 (d, J = 2.0 Hz, 1H), 5.36 (s, 1H), 4.22 (d, J = 1.5 Hz, 1H), 3.75 (dd, J = 9.3, 3.3 Hz, 1H), 3.43 (dd, J = 9.5, 6.1 Hz, 1H), 3.35 (s, 1H), 0.95 (d, J = 6.1 Hz, 3H).

$^{13}$C NMR (100 MHz, $CD_3OD$) δ 179.45, 165.69, 163.03, 159.11, 158.33, 149.60, 146.22, 136.03, 122.76, 122.64, 116.71, 116.16, 105.69, 103.34, 99.60, 94.49, 73.04, 71.91, 71.83, 71.70, 17.44.

Compound **7**: $C_{27}H_{30}O_{16}$

MS: $[M + Na]^+$ $C_{27}H_{30}NaO_{16}$, measured m/z 633.1435, calculated m/z 633.1426, err −1.5 ppm.

$^1$H NMR (400 MHz, $CD_3OD$) δ 7.66 (s, 1H), 7.62 (d, J = 8.4 Hz, 1H), 6.86 (d, J = 8.4 Hz, 1H), 6.37 (d, J = 1.9 Hz, 1H), 6.18 (d, J = 1.9 Hz, 1H), 5.10 (d, J = 7.4 Hz, 1H), 4.52 (s, 1H), 3.80 (d, J = 10.5 Hz, 1H), 3.64 (d, J = 1.5 Hz, 1H), 3.54 (dd, J = 9.5, 3.3 Hz, 1H), 3.48 (d, J = 9.1 Hz, 1H), 3.45 (d, J = 5.1 Hz, 2H), 3.40 (d, J = 4.8 Hz, 1H), 3.36 (d, J = 4.5 Hz, 1H), 3.33 (s, 1H), 3.27 (d, J = 3.2 Hz, 1H), 1.12 (d, J = 6.2 Hz, 3H).

$^{13}$C NMR (100 MHz, $CD_3OD$) δ 177.98, 164.58, 161.53, 157.92, 157.07, 148.39, 144.41, 134.26, 129.05, 122.18, 121.72, 116.32, 114.66, 104.22, 103.37, 101.02, 98.55, 93.48, 76.78, 75.79, 74.34, 72.55, 70.70, 69.99, 68.31, 67.16, 16.50.

### 2.3. Allelopathic Activities of the Purified Compounds on *L. sativa* Seedlings

As shown in Figure 3, compounds **1**, **2**, **4**, and **6** inhibited the growth of the seedlings of *L. sativa*, while compounds **3**, **5**, and **7** had no effect. The inhibitory effect increased with the increase in treated concentrations. Compound **1** displayed a strong inhibition on the growth of *L. sativa* at all treated concentrations. The inhibition ratios to the roots and stems of *L. sativa* at the concentration of 200 μg/mL were 78.87% and 87.87%, respectively. Compounds **2**, **4**, and **6** showed strong inhibition on the growth of *L. sativa* at higher concentrations (≥50 μg/mL), while there were slight or no effects at low treated concentrations. Meanwhile, the inhibition ratios on roots were more remarkable than that on stems for *L. sativa* seedlings. At the maximum concentration (200 μg/mL), the inhibition ratios of roots reached to 64.29%, 35.50%, and 65.53%, respectively.

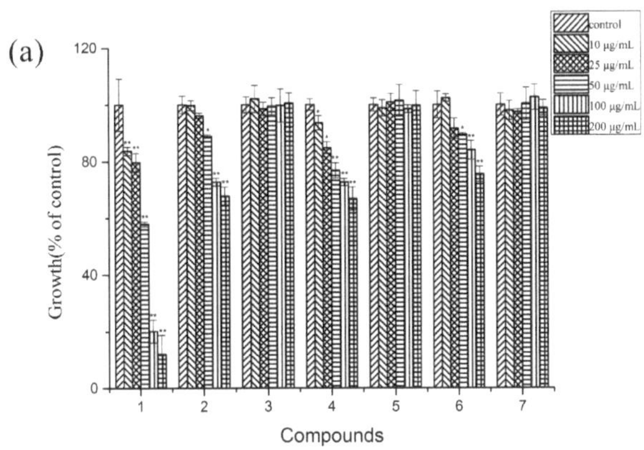


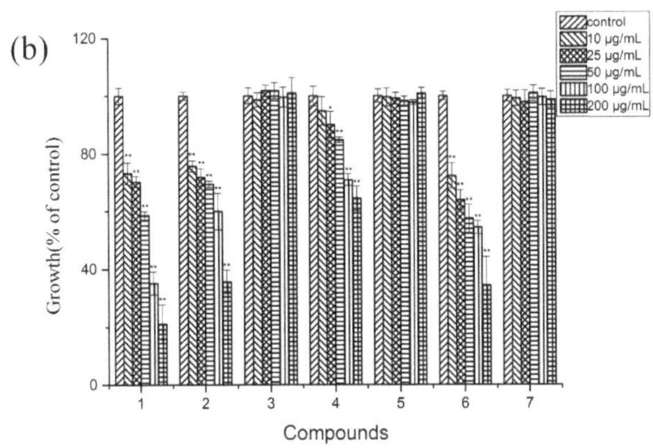


**Figure 3.** Phytotoxic effects of compounds **1–7** on root (**a**) and stems (**b**) lengths of *L. sativa* seedlings at concentrations of 10, 25, 50, 100, and 200 μg/mL, respectively. Values are presented as a percentage of the mean compared to the control. Means significantly lower than the DMSO controls are indicated by * (one way ANOVA; $p < 0.05$) or ** ($p < 0.01$). Error bars are one standard error of the mean. $n = 3$.

### 2.4. Autotoxic Activities of the Purified Compounds on Tissue Culture Seedlings of Potato

The autotoxic activity of the purified compounds was evaluated with tissue culture seedlings of potato. The results revealed that compounds **1**, **2**, **4**, and **6** had an inhibition effect on the growth of the potato seedlings, while compounds **3**, **5**, and **7** had no effect (Figure 4). Compound **1** showed an inhibitory effect on the growth of tissue culture seedlings of potato at the highest treated concentration (200 μg/mL), while there were no effects at lower concentrations. The inhibition ratios at the concentration of 200 μg/mL on the height of the seedlings, the fresh weight of the leaves and stems, and the fresh weight of the roots were 14.06%, 12.67%, and 20.17%, respectively. At higher treated concentrations (≥50 μg/mL), compounds **2**, **4**, and **6** displayed moderate inhibitions on the growth of potato tissue culture seedlings, while there were slight or no effects at lower treated concentrations. Similarly, the autotoxic effects on the fresh weight of the roots of tissue seedlings were more distinguished in a concentration-dependent manner. The inhibition ratios of the fresh weight of the leaves and stems at the maximum concentration (200 μg/mL) reached up to 42.07%, 34.41%, and 43.08%, respectively. The typical patterns of the effects of compounds **1**, **2**, **4**, and **6** on the growth length of *L. sativa* seedlings (a) and potato tissue culture seedlings (b) at concentrations of 0, 10, 25, 50, 100, and 200 μg/mL are shown in Figure 5.

### 2.5. Confirmation and Quantification of the Allelochemicals in the Rhizosphere Soil

High-performance liquid chromatography (HPLC) was performed to quantify the allelochemicals in the rhizosphere soil of replanted potato. The presence of the compounds in the soil was confirmed by comparing the retention times of the standard compounds **1**, **2**, **4**, and **6** under the same chromatographic conditions (Figure 6). At the same time, the standard curve of the content of compounds **1**, **2**, **4**, and **6** was determined at a wavelength of 240 nm (compounds **1**, **2**, and **4**) and 280 nm (compound **6**) (Table 1). The contents of compounds **1**, **2**, **4**, and **6** in the rhizosphere soil were calculated to be 1.46, 6.64, 0.35, and 0.57 μg/g, respectively.

**Table 1.** Regression equations, correlation coefficients, linear range, retention time, and contents for the four allelochemicals.

| Compounds | Linear Equations [a] | $R^2$ | Linear Range (ng/mL) | Retention Time (min) | Content (μg/g) |
|---|---|---|---|---|---|
| 1 | $y = 0.0093x - 343.9$ | 0.9995 | 2000.0–30,000.0 | 23.503 | 1.46 |
| 2 | $y = 0.0133x + 123.7$ | 0.9998 | 2000.0–30,000.0 | 32.605 | 6.64 |
| 4 | $y = 0.0102x + 212.15$ | 0.9999 | 500.0–30,000.0 | 10.687 | 0.35 |
| 6 | $y = 0.0152x + 518.21$ | 0.9993 | 2000.0–30,000.0 | 13.900 | 0.57 |

[a] $y$ represents the peak area, $x$ represents the concentration (ng/mL).

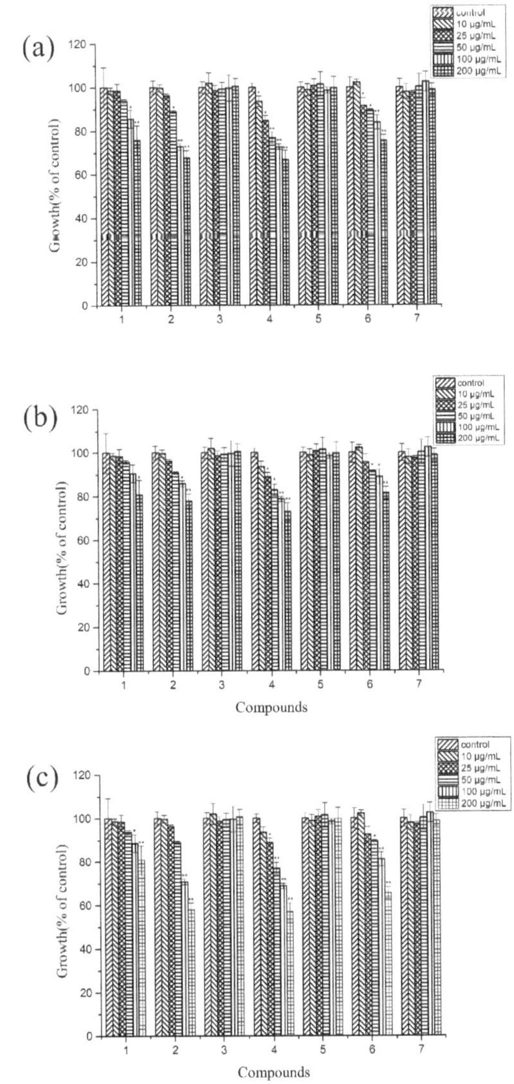


**Figure 4.** Autotoxic effects of compounds **1–7** on the height of the seedlings (**a**), the fresh weight of the leaves and stems (**b**), and the fresh weight of the roots (**c**) at concentrations of 10, 25, 50, 100, and 200 µg/mL, respectively. Values are presented as a percentage of the mean compared to the control. Means significantly lower than the DMSO controls are indicated by * (one way ANOVA; $p < 0.05$) or ** ($p < 0.01$). Error bars are one standard error of the mean. $n = 3$.

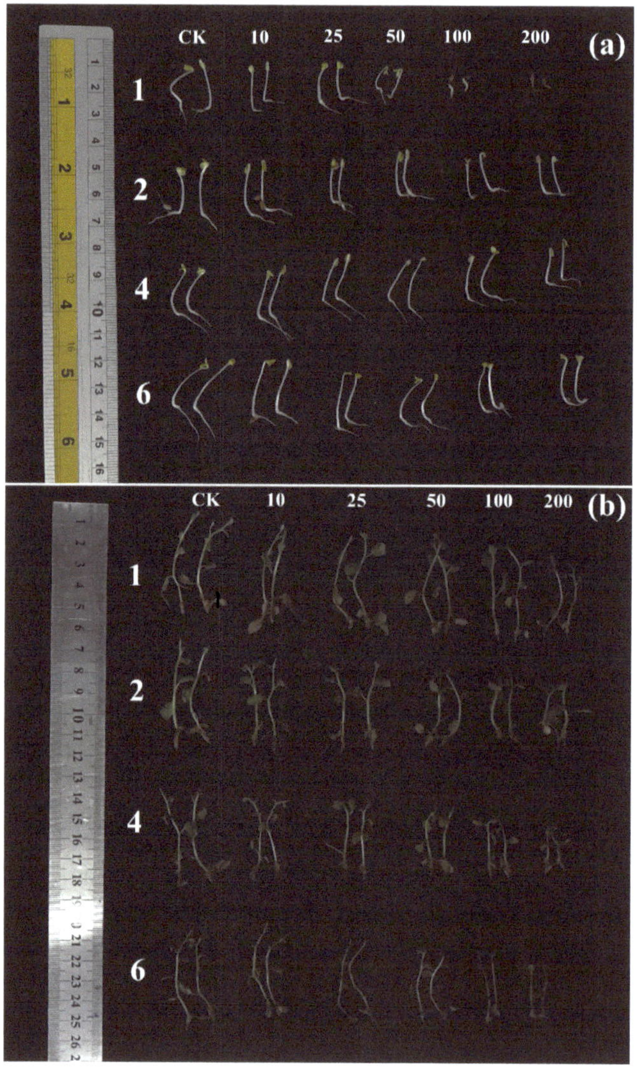


**Figure 5.** Typical pictures of the effects of compounds **1**, **2**, **4** and **6** on the growth of *L. sativa* seedlings (**a**) and potato tissue culture seedlings (**b**) at concentrations of 0, 10, 25, 50, 100, and 200 μg/mL.

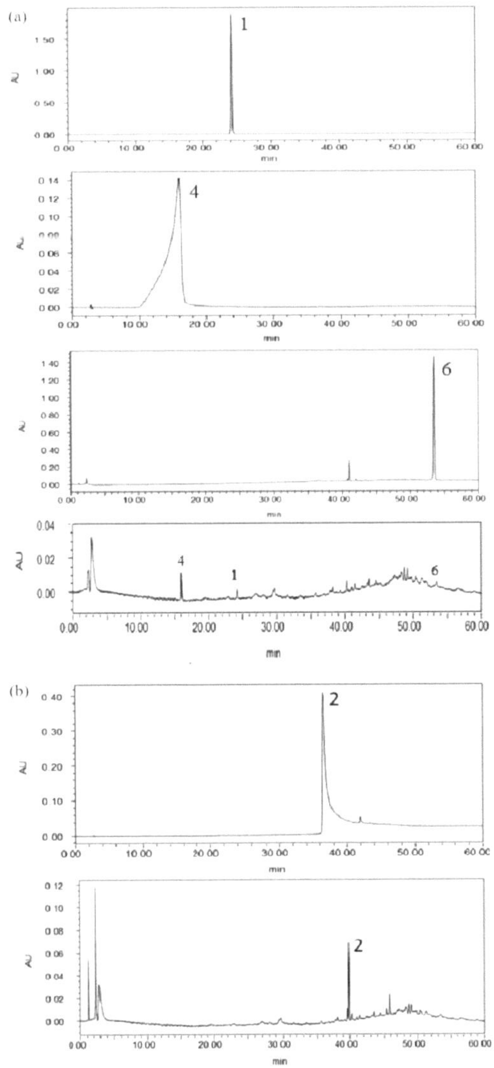


**Figure 6.** HPLC analysis of the allelochemicals in the rhizosphere soil of continuously cropped potato at 240 nm (**a**) and 320 nm (**b**), respectively; purified compounds **1**, **4**, and **6** were detected at 240 nm (**a**) and compound **2** was detected at 320 nm (**b**).

*2.6. Antifungal Activity on Potato Pathogens of the Allelochemicals*

Compounds **1–7** showed different antifungal activity at a treated concentration of 200 μg/mL against pathogens of potato, including *A. solani, B. cinerea, F. solani, F. oxysporum, C. coccodes* and *V. dahlia*, as shown in Figures 7 and 8. The results indicated that compounds **2–4** promoted the growth of the colonies of the six pathogens of potato; only compound **1** showed an inhibitory effect. The promotive indices of compound **2** on *A. solani, B. cinerea*, and *C. coccodes* at 200 μg/mL were 33.8%, 11.5%, and 7.7%, respectively. The promotive indices of compound **3** on *A. solani, B. cinerea, C. coccodes*, and *V. dahlia* at 200 μg/mL were 29.3%, 8.5%, 11.6%, and 7.2%, respectively. The promotive indices of compound **4** on *A. solani, B. cinerea, F. solani, F. oxysporum*, and *V. dahlia* at 200 μg/mL were 20.6%, 7.8%, 7.6%, 8.0%, and 14.9%, respectively.

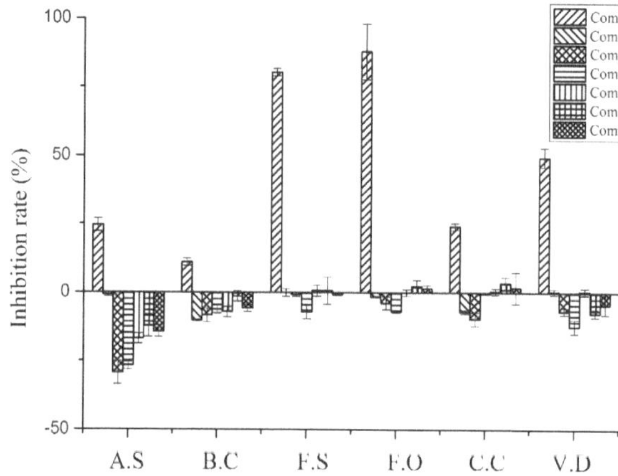


**Figure 7.** The effects of compounds **1–7** against the potato pathogens including *A. solani, B. cinerea, F. solani, F. oxysporum, C. coccodes*, and *V. dahlia* at a concentration of 200 μg/mL.

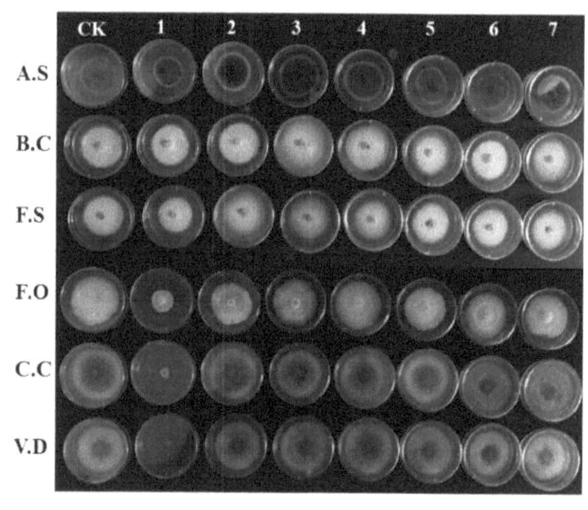


**Figure 8.** Typical pictures of the effects of compounds **1–7** against potato pathogens including *A. solani, B. cinerea, F. solani, F. oxysporum, C. coccodes*, and *V. dahlia* at a concentration of 200 μg/mL.

## 3. Discussion

Negative plant–soil feedback is one of the important factors of the replant problem, which plays an essential role in hindering the sustainable development of agriculture [26]. Investigations indicated that the accumulation of allelochemicals in the soil environment is a crucial factor for the replant failure of large amounts of plants. The growth of replanted plants may be inhibited by the reduction in the number of meristem cells, the reduction in elongation zones, and the accumulation of auxins caused by allelochemicals [27].

The bioassay results of the crude extract in the present study indicated that there were potential allelochemicals in the rhizosphere soil of potato that contributed to the inhibitory effect on the seedling growth of itself and other plants. Nevertheless, the autotoxic effect of the allelochemicals of potato has not been previously clarified.

Hence, in this work, seven compounds were isolated from the rhizosphere soil of potato and bioassays indicated that compounds **1**, **2**, **4**, and **6** had inhibitory effects on the growth of *L. sativa* and potato tissue culture seedlings. Compound **1** belongs to coumarin, which is considered to be one kind of allelochemical by Rice [28]. It was reported that coumarin inhibited the seed germination and plant growth (length and mass of shoots and roots) of several plants [29,30]. The results in this study revealed that it had an inhibitory effect on the growth of lettuce seedlings and tissue culture seedlings of potato at the maximum treatment concentration. Compound **2** is in the range of fatty acids; investigations demonstrate that it has an enormous capacity of phytotoxic activity [31]. The results in this work showed that it inhibited the growth of lettuce seedlings and tissue culture seedlings of potato at high treated concentrations, which are consistent with the previous study. Chlorogenic acid (compound **3**) is abundant in potato peels. It has a broad range of therapeutic properties, including antioxidant activity andantibacterial, anti-inflammatory, and anti-obesity properties [32]. However, phenolic acids are one kind of important allelochemical as well, which generally exist in their cultivated soils [33]. It was reported that chlorogenic acid inhibited the growth of lettuce seedlings at high concentrations, and ROS in lettuce could be accumulated under the stress of chlorogenic acid [34]. The results in the present study indicated that the growth of seedlings of lettuce and potato were suppressed at a high treated concentration of compound **3**. Compound **6** was regarded as a flavonoid; it is reported that flavonoids affect many physiological functions of plants, including the inhibition of auxin transport, phytochemical defense, an allelopathic effect, and an antioxidant effect [35–37]. In the present study, compound **6** only displayed an inhibitory effect on the growth of the *L. sativa* and potato at the maximum treated concentration. Analysis of the characterized compounds in the rhizosphere soil showed that compound **2** had the highest content with a value of 6.64 μg/g, and the total content of the four autotoxic allelochemicals in the rhizosphere soil reached 9.02 μg/g.

Soil microorganisms are critical elements in agricultural ecosystems, and the compositions of soil microbial communities are influenced through rhizodeposition [38]. By this way, beneficial microbes were promoted, but also soil-borne pathogens were built-up [39,40]. The imbalance of soil microbial community has been considered as one of the essential factors for replant problems. Many cultivated plants, which suffer soil sickness, are often connected with soil-borne pathogens [41]. Several research studies suggested that replant disease could be induced directly by the occurrence of pathogens and indirectly by the release of toxic substances which were decomposed by plants [42,43]. Currently, allelochemicals are regarded as a significant cause which influences the microbial community [44]. The accumulation of allelochemicals brings about the increase in harmful pathogens in rhizosphere soil, leads to an unbalance of the structure of the microbial community, and results in replant diseases during continuous cropping [45]. In this work, the antifungal assays showed that compound **1** had an inhibitory effect on the six tested pathogens of potato, but compounds **2–4** promoted the colony growth of the pathogens, suggesting that the release of the autotoxic allelochemicals induced the disequilibrium of the microbial community in the continuously cropped potato soil. The compositions of the allelochemicals affected the composition of the microbial community in the replanted soil and enhanced the feasibility of the outbreak of the soil-borne diseases of potato during continuous cultivation.

## 4. Materials and Methods

### *4.1. General Experimental Instruments and Reagents*

MCI gel CHP20/P120 (Mitsubishi chemical corporation, Tokyo, Japan) and silica gel 60 (200–300 mesh, Qingdao Haiyang Chemical Co., Ltd., Qingdao, China) were used for Column Chromatography (CC). Thin-layer chromatography (TLC) and preparative thin-layer chromatography were carried out on silica gel F254 plates, and the spots were detected under UV detection or by heating after spraying with 5% $H_2SO_4$ in $C_2H_5OH$ (*v*/*v*). By using a Bruker Avance III-400 spectrometer (Bruker AXS GmbH, Karlsruhe, Germany), $^1H$ and $^{13}C$ NMR spectra (400 and 100 MHz, respectively) were recorded. Electrospray ionization quadruple time -of-flight mass spectrometry (ESI-Q-TOF MS) was used to obtain the high-resolution mass data.

The High-Performance Liquid Chromatographic analysis was conducted on a Waters 1525 binary HPLC pump (Waters, Milford, MA, USA) with a Waters 2998 photodiode array detector, coupled with a Waters C18 column (250 mm × 4.6 mm, 5 μm).

### *4.2. Soil Samples*

Soil samples around the roots of potato cultivar Long 7 (within 5 cm) were collected in five different areas of Lanzhou, Gansu Province, China, in October 2018. The collected soil samples were dried in the dark at room temperature and passed through a 1 mm screen sieve. Then, the soil samples were extracted three times (90 min each) in methanol with ultrasonic treatments, and the filtrate was concentrated in vacuum to dryness.

### *4.3. Isolation of Allelochemicals from the Rhizosphere Soil*

The residue of the rhizosphere soil was dissolved in water, then extracted by petroleum ether, chloroform, ethyl acetate, and n-butanol saturated with water, to finally obtain five fractions (Fr. 1–5). Fr. 1 was fractionated by MCI gel column chromatography eluting with methanol/water (3:7, 1:1, 7:3 and 9:1, *v*/*v*), and finally eluted with methanol to get compound **1** (3.6 mg) and compound **2** (12.4 mg), respectively. Fr. 2 was separated by PTLC (petroleum ether/EtOAc, 10:1, *v*/*v*) to yield compound **3** (4.9 mg), compound **4** (2.3 mg), and Fr. 2–3. Fr. 2–3 was subjected on silica gel CC with petroleum ether/EtOAc (3:1) in mobile phase to give compound **5** (3.5 mg). Fr. 3 was submitted to silica gel CC and eluting with chloroform/methanol (10:1, *v*/*v*) to obtain compound **6** (2.5 mg). Fr. 4 was eluted with chloroform/methanol (3:1, *v*/*v*) on silica gel column chromatography to obtain compound **7** (6.3 mg).

### *4.4. Plant Material and Growth Conditions*

Seeds of *Lactuca sativa* L. were purchased from Gansu Academy of Agricultural Sciences. After soaked with 10% sodium hypochlorite for 10 min, the test seeds were washed with distilled sterile water 3 times, then germinated on filter paper in the dark at 25 °C for 1 day.

Healthy potato cultivar Long 7 with strong growth potential and no virus carrying was used for the germination treatment. After germination, the lateral or top buds were cut into a beaker with a scalpel and rinsed with flowing water for 6 h. These materials were soaked with 75% alcohol for 45 s. Then, the buds were sanitized in 0.1% mercuric chloride for 10 min, and washed with sterile water 5 times in order to thoroughly remove residual $Hg^+$ from explant material. The medium for the tissue culture of potatoes was modified on MS medium containing MS medium, agar (7 g/L), sucrose (30 g/L), and 1.5 mg/L naphthaleneacetic acid (NAA). Finally, the tissue culture seedlings (about 1–2 cm length) were cut and inserted into the medium, and placed in a culture chamber for light culture (in the light for 14 h and in the dark for 10 h per day) at 25 °C.

### 4.5. Bioassays

*L. sativa* was selected as the receptor plant, and the allelopathic activities of the crude extract and compounds **1–7** were evaluated by a plate culture method. The crude extract and compounds **1–7** were dissolved in DMSO and diluted with distilled sterile water, with final concentrations of 50, 100, 200, and 400 μg/mL for the crude extract and 10, 25, 50, 100, and 200 μg/mL for compounds **1–7**, respectively. The concentration of DMSO should be ensured not to exceed 1% (*v*/*v*). The same ratio of DMSO was added into distilled sterile water as a control. After germination, the test seedlings were transferred to 6-well plates (Corning, Inc., Corning, NY, USA). 0.5 mL of the solutions was added to each of the wells, and three replicates (six seedlings for each replicate) were set for each treatment. Then, the six-well plates were placed in a constant temperature and humidity chamber in the dark at 25 °C for 2 days. The lengths of the roots and stems were measured and the relative length of the control was calculated.

Tissue culture seedlings of potato were used to evaluate the autotoxic activities of the crude extract and compounds **1–7**. The crude extract and compounds **1–7** were dissolved in DMSO and added into the medium, with final concentrations of 50, 100, 200, and 400 μg/mL for the crude extract and 10, 25, 50, 100, and 200 μg/mL for compounds **1–7**, respectively. The same ratio of DMSO was added into the medium as a control. The tissue culture seedlings with the same growing trend were transferred to the prepared treatment and control medium, and three replicates (six seedlings for each replicate) were set for each treatment. Then, the seedlings were cultured in the same conditions as above for 10 days. The height of the seedlings, the fresh weight of the leaves and stems, and the fresh weight of the roots were measured and the relative ratio of the control was calculated.

### 4.6. High-Performance Liquid Chromatography (HPLC) Analysis

The existence of the allelochemicals in the rhizosphere soil of potato was confirmed by high-performance liquid chromatography (HPLC), and the contents of the allelochemicals were quantified simultaneously. The optimum gradient of the mobile phase was: 20–100% A (A: methanol; B: water) at 0–30 min and 100% (A) at 30–45 min. The detection wavelength was selected as 240 nm for compounds **1**, **2**, and **4**, and 280 nm for compound **6**. The flow rate was 1 mL/min with an injection volume of 20 μL, and the column temperature was 35 °C. The existence of these compounds in the soil was confirmed by comparing the retention times of the standard compounds **1**, **2**, **4**, and **6** under the same chromatographic conditions. By using the linear regression method, the standard curves were achieved. The contents of allelochemicals in the rhizosphere soil of potato could be calculated by using the peak area and linear equations. The results are presented in Table 1.

### 4.7. Antifungal Activity

The antifungal activity of compounds **1–7** was evaluated against *Alternaria solani* Sorauer, *Botrytis cinerea* Persoon, *Fusarium solani* (Mart.) Sacc, *Fusarium oxysporum* Schlecht, *Colletotrichum coccodes* (Wall) Hughes, and *Verticillium dahlia* by a mycelium growth rate test with some modifications [46] using PDA medium. All the plant pathogens were from the CAS Key Laboratory of Chemistry of Northwestern Plant Resources, Lanzhou Institute of Chemical Physics, Chinese Academy of Sciences, Lanzhou, China. The strains were identified by Hui Jin and Xiaoyan Yang from Lanzhou Institute of Chemical Physics, Chinese Academy of Sciences, Lanzhou, China. Compounds **1–7** were dissolved in DMSO and added into the PDA medium with a final concentration of 200 μg/mL; the concentration of DMSO should be ensured not exceed 1% (*v*/*v*). 10 mL of the treatment and control medium were poured into each sterilized Petri dish (60 mm in diameter), and the fungi mycelia disk with a 5.0 mm diameter was placed in the center of the Petri dish and incubated at 25 °C. When the mycelium of the fungi reached the edges of the control plate, the mycelia diameter of each treatment was measured.

### 4.8. Statistical Analysis

All data were subject to an analysis of variance by SPSS 18. The significant differences between the treatment groups and the control group were calculated by the Fisher's least significant difference (LSD) test and one-way analysis of variance (ANOVA). Statistical significance was accepted at * $p < 0.05$, ** $p < 0.01$. The relative ratio (percent) was determined by the formula [treated group/control group] × 100.

## 5. Conclusions

In summary, the isolated compounds from the rhizosphere soil of potato had a close relation to the allelopathy and autotoxicity. The accumulation of the allelochemicals could induce an imbalance of the microbial community in the potato replanted soil and result in replant failure during continuous cropping. These findings are helpful for understanding the allelopathic factors and mechanism that lead to replant failure in the cultivation of potato.

**Author Contributions:** Conceptualization, A.X., X.Y. and B.Q.; validation, J.G., Z.C. and Z.D.; formal analysis, A.X.; investigation, A.X. and X.Y.; resources, X.Y. and H.J.; data curation, A.X.; writing—original draft preparation, A.X.; writing—review and editing, H.J. and B.Q.; visualization, A.X., H.H. and H.L.; supervision, B.Q.; project administration, A.X. and H.J.; funding acquisition, B.Q. All authors have read and agreed to the published version of the manuscript.

**Funding:** This research was funded by the National Natural Science Foundation of China (22076195) and Cooperation Program to Gansu Province of Lanzhou Branch of the Chinese Academy of Sciences (2021).

**Institutional Review Board Statement:** Not applicable.

**Informed Consent Statement:** Not applicable.

**Data Availability Statement:** Not applicable.

**Conflicts of Interest:** The authors declare no conflict of interest.

## Abbreviations

ANOVA—analysis of variance; CC—column chromatography; GC−MS—gas chromatography−mass spectrometry; LSD—least significant difference; MCI—gel, middle chromatogram isolated gel; PTLC—preparative thin-layer chromatography; TLC—Thin-layer chromatography.

## References

1. Lopez, A.; Arazuri, S.; Garcia, I.; Mangado, J.; Jaren, C. A review of the application of near-infrared spectroscopy for the analysis of potatoes. *J. Agric. Food Chem.* **2013**, *61*, 5413–5424. [CrossRef] [PubMed]
2. Food and Agriculture Organization of the United Nations. Available online: https://www.fao.org/about/en (accessed on 1 January 2022).
3. Camire, M.E.; Kubow, S.; Donnelly, D.J. Potatoes and human health. *Crit. Rev. Food Sci. Nutr.* **2009**, *49*, 823–840. [CrossRef] [PubMed]
4. Kondo, Y.; Sakuma, R.; Ichisawa, M.; Ishihara, K.; Kubo, M.; Handa, S.; Mugita, H.; Maruyama, N.; Koga, H.; Ishigami, A. Potato chip intake increases ascorbic acid levels and decreases reactive oxygen species in SMP30/GNL knockout mouse tissues. *J. Agric. Food Chem.* **2014**, *62*, 9286–9295. [CrossRef] [PubMed]
5. Orawetz, T.; Malinova, I.; Orzechowski, S.; Fettke, J. Reduction of the plastidial phosphorylase in potato (*Solanum tuberosum* L.) reveals impact on storage starch structure during growth at low temperature. *Plant Physiol. Biochem.* **2016**, *100*, 141–149. [CrossRef]
6. Sulc, M.; Kotikova, Z.; Paznocht, L.; Pivec, V.; Hamouz, K.; Lachman, J. Changes in anthocyanidin levels during the maturation of color-fleshed potato (*Solanum tuberosum* L.) tubers. *Food Chem.* **2017**, *237*, 981–988. [CrossRef]
7. Qin, Y.; Ma, K.; Liu, P. Effect of potato continuous cropping on genetic diversity of soil microorganisms. *Chin. J. Eco-Agric.* **2015**, *23*, 225–232.
8. Cesarano, G.; Zotti, M.; Antignani, V.; Marra, R.; Scala, F.; Bonanomi, G. Soil sickness and negative plant-soil feedback: A reappraisal of hypotheses. *J. Plant Pathol.* **2017**, *99*, 545–570.

9. Manici, L.M.; Kelderer, M.; Franke Whittle, I.H.; Ruhmer, T.; Baab, G.; Nicoletti, F.; Caputo, F.; Topp, A.; Insam, H.; Naef, A. Relationship between root-endophytic microbial communities and replant disease in specialized apple growing areas in Europe. *Appl. Soil Ecol.* **2013**, *72*, 207–214. [CrossRef]
10. Kardol, P.; Cornips, N.J.; van Kempen, M.M.L.; Bakx-Schotman, J.M.T.; van der Putten, W.H. Microbe-mediated plant soil feedback causes historical contingency effects in plant community assembly. *Ecol. Monogr.* **2007**, *77*, 147–162. [CrossRef]
11. Van de Voorde, T.F.J.; Ruijten, M.; van der Putten, W.H.; Bezemer, T.M. Can the negative plant-soil feedback of *Jacobaea vulgaris* be explained by autotoxicity? *Basic Appl. Ecol.* **2012**, *13*, 533–541. [CrossRef]
12. Liu, J.K.; Yan, Z.Q.; Li, X.Z.; Jin, H.; Yang, X.Y.; Xie, M.; Su, A.X.; Qin, B. Characterization of allelochemicals from the rhizosphere soil of *Pinellia ternate* (Thnub.) and their inhibition activity on protective enzymes. *Appl. Soil Ecol.* **2018**, *125*, 301–306. [CrossRef]
13. Guo, K.; He, X.F.; Yan, Z.Q.; Li, X.Z.; Ren, X.; Pan, L.; Qin, B. Allelochemicals from the Rhizosphere Soil of Cultivated *Astragalus hoantchy* L. *J. Agric. Food Chem.* **2016**, *64*, 3345–3352. [CrossRef] [PubMed]
14. Ren, X.; Yan, Z.Q.; He, X.F.; Li, X.Z.; Qin, B. Allelochemicals from rhizosphere soils of *Glycyrrhiza uralensis* Fisch: Discovery of the autotoxic compounds of a traditional herbal medicine. *Ind. Crops Prod.* **2017**, *97*, 302–307. [CrossRef]
15. Xie, M.; Yan, Z.Q.; Ren, X.; Li, X.Z.; Qin, B. Codonopilate A, a triterpenyl ester as main autotoxin in cultivated soil of *Codonopsis pilosula* (Franch.) Nannf. *J. Agric. Food Chem.* **2017**, *65*, 2032–2038. [CrossRef] [PubMed]
16. Hasegawa, T.; Kato, Y.; Okabe, A.; Itoi, C.; Ooshiro, A.; Kawaide, H.; Natsume, M. Effect of secondary metabolites of tomato (*Solanum lycopersicum*) on chemotaxis of *ralstonia solanacearum*, pathogen of bacterial wilt disease. *J. Agric. Food Chem.* **2019**, *67*, 1807–1813. [CrossRef] [PubMed]
17. Manici, L.M.; Ciavatta, C.; Kelderer, M.; Erschbaumer, G. Replant problems in south tyrol: Role of fungal pathogens and microbial population in conventional and organic apple orchards. *Plant Soil.* **2003**, *256*, 315–324. [CrossRef]
18. Reddy, M.A.; Patrick, Z.A. Colonization of tobacco seedling roots by fluorescent pseudomonad suppressive to black root rot caused by *Thielaviopsis basicola*. *Crop Protection.* **1992**, *11*, 148–154. [CrossRef]
19. Bonanomi, G.; de Filippis, F.; Cesarano, G.; La Storia, A.; Ercolini, D.; Scala, F. Organic farming induces changes in soil microbiota that affect agro-ecosystem functions. *Soil Biol. Biochem.* **2016**, *103*, 327–336. [CrossRef]
20. Xia, Z.C.; Kong, C.H.; Chen, L.C.; Wang, S.L. Allelochemical-mediated soil microbial community in long-term monospecific Chinese fir forest plantations. *Appl. Soil Ecol.* **2015**, *96*, 52–59. [CrossRef]
21. Dong, L.L.; Xu, J.; Li, Y.; Fang, H.L.; Niu, W.H.; Li, X.W.; Zhang, Y.J.; Ding, W.L.; Chen, S.L. Manipulation of microbial community in the rhizosphere alleviates the replanting issues in *Panax ginseng*. *Soil Biol. Biochem.* **2018**, *125*, 64–74. [CrossRef]
22. Soltys-Kalina, D.; Murawska, Z.; Strzelczyk-Zyta, D.; Wasilewicz-Flis, I.; Marczewski, W. Phytotoxic potential of cultivated and wild potato species (*Solanum sp.*): Role of glycoalkaloids, phenolics and flavonoids in phytotoxicity against mustard (*Sinapis alba* L.). *Acta Physiol. Plant.* **2019**, *41*, 41–55. [CrossRef]
23. Wan, N.X.; Yuan, J.C.; He, W.; Long, W.J.; Zhang, Q.; Zhou, S.M.; Zheng, S.L. Autotoxicity of water extracts from different organs of potato. *J. Zhejiang Univ.* **2016**, *42*, 411–418.
24. Zhang, W.M.; Qiu, H.Z.; Zhang, C.H.; Liu, X.; Gao, Y.A.; Shen, Q.R. Identification and autotoxicity of root exudates of continuous cropping potato at different growth stages. *Chin. J. Eco-Agric.* **2015**, *23*, 215–224.
25. Guo, C.P.; Zi, S.H.; Ou-Yang, C.R.; Wu, B.Z. Effect of aboveground aqueous extracts of maize and potato on the maize growth. *J. Maize Sci.* **2016**, *24*, 79–84.
26. Gamiz, B.; Facenda, G.; Celis, R. Nanoengineered sorbents to increase the persistence of the allelochemical carvone in the rhizosphere. *J. Agric. Food Chem.* **2019**, *67*, 589–596. [CrossRef]
27. Zhang, W.; Lu, L.Y.; Hu, L.Y.; Cao, W.; Sun, K.; Sun, Q.B.; Siddikee, A.; Shi, R.H.; Dai, C.C. Evidences for the Involvement of auxin, ethylene and ROS signaling during allelochemical benzoic acid-mediated primary root inhibition of Arabidopsis. *Plant Cell Physiol.* **2018**, *59*, 1889–1904. [CrossRef]
28. Rice, E.L. Allelopathy-Update. *Bot. Rev.* **1979**, *45*, 15–109. [CrossRef]
29. Niro, E.; Marzaioli, R.; de Crescenzo, S.; D'Abrosca, B.; Castaldi, S.; Esposito, A.; Fiorentino, A.; Rutigliano, F.A. Effects of the allelochemical coumarin on plants and soil microbial community. *Soil Biol. Biochem.* **2016**, *95*, 30–39. [CrossRef]
30. Abenavoli, M.R.; Cacco, G.; Sorgona, A.; Marabottini, R.; Paolacci, A.R.; Ciaffi, M.; Badiani, M. The inhibitory effects of coumarin on the germination of durum wheat (*Triticum turgidum* ssp. durum, cv. Simeto) seeds. *J. Chem. Ecol.* **2006**, *32*, 489–506. [CrossRef]
31. Mushtaq, W.; Ain, Q.; Siddiqui, M.B.; Hakeem, K.R. Cytotoxic allelochemicals induce ultrastructural modifications in *Cassia tora* L. and mitotic changes in *Allium cepa* L.: A weed versus weed allelopathy approach. *Protoplasma* **2019**, *256*, 857–871. [CrossRef]
32. Naveed, M.; Hejazi, V.; Abbas, M.; Kamboh, A.A.; Khan, G.J.; Shumzaid, M.; Ahmad, F.; Babazadeh, D.; Xia, F.F.; Modarresi-Ghazani, F.; et al. Chlorogenic acid (CGA): A pharmacological review and call for further research. *Biomed. Pharmacother.* **2018**, *97*, 67–74. [CrossRef] [PubMed]
33. Fu, Y.H.; Quan, W.X.; Li, C.C.; Qian, C.Y.; Tang, F.H.; Chen, X.J. Allelopathic effects of phenolic acids on seedling growth and photosynthesis in *Rhododendron delavayi* Franch. *Photosynthetica* **2019**, *57*, 377–387. [CrossRef]
34. Wang, D.D.; Yang, J.S.; Yan, Z.Q.; Sun, Y.H.; Cui, H.Y.; Ding, L.; Qin, B. Allelopathic effect and mechanism of chlorogenic acid on the growth of lettuce. *Acta Bot. Boreali-Occident. Sin.* **2014**, *34*, 957–962.
35. Yin, R.H.; Han, K.; Heller, W.; Albert, A.; Dobrev, P.I.; Zazimalova, E.; Schaffner, A.R. Kaempferol 3-O-rhamnoside-7-O-rhamnoside is an endogenous flavonol inhibitor of polar auxin transport in Arabidopsis shoots. *New Phytol.* **2014**, *20*, 466–475. [CrossRef]
36. Yang, C.Q.; Yang, W.Y.; Liu, J. Advances on chemical ecology of plant flavonoids. *Nat. Prod. Res. Dev.* **2018**, *30*, 2009–2016.

37. Brunetti, C.; Di Ferdinando, M.; Fini, A.; Pollastri, S.; Tattini, M. Flavonoids as antioxidants and developmental regulators: Relative significance in plants and humans. *Int. J. Mol. Sci.* **2013**, *14*, 3540–3555. [CrossRef] [PubMed]
38. Paterson, E.; Gebbing, T.; Abel, C.; Sim, A.; Telfer, G. Rhizodeposition shapes rhizosphere microbial community structure in organic soil. *New Phytol.* **2007**, *173*, 600–610. [CrossRef]
39. Hayat, R.; Ali, S.; Amara, U.; Khalid, R.; Ahmed, I. Soil beneficial bacteria and their role in plant growth promotion: A review. *Ann. Microbiol.* **2010**, *60*, 579–598. [CrossRef]
40. Huang, L.F.; Song, L.X.; Xia, X.J.; Mao, W.H.; Shi, K.; Zhou, Y.H.; Yu, J.Q. Plant-soil feedbacks and soil sickness: From mechanisms to application in agriculture. *J. Chem. Ecol.* **2013**, *39*, 232–242. [CrossRef]
41. Mazzola, M.; Manici, L.M. Apple replant disease: Role of microbial ecology in cause and control. *Annu. Rev. Phytopathol.* **2012**, *50*, 45–65. [CrossRef]
42. Yang, J.I.; Ruegger, P.M.; McKenry, M.V.; Becker, J.O.; Borneman, J. Correlations between root-associated microorganisms and peach replant disease symptoms in a california soil. *PLoS ONE* **2012**, *7*, e46420. [CrossRef] [PubMed]
43. Bonanomi, G.; D'Ascoli, R.; Antignani, V.; Capodilupo, M.; Cozzolino, L.; Marzaioli, R.; Puopolo, G.; Rutigliano, F.A.; Scelza, R.; Scotti, R.; et al. Assessing soil quality under intensive cultivation and tree orchards in southern Italy. *Appl. Soil Ecol.* **2011**, *47*, 184–194. [CrossRef]
44. Bertin, C.; Yang, X.H.; Weston, L.A. The role of root exudates and allelochemicals in the rhizosphere. *Plant Soil.* **2003**, *256*, 67–83. [CrossRef]
45. Lin, S.; Dai, L.Q.; Chen, T.; Li, Z.F.; Zhang, Z.Y.; Lin, W.X. Screening and identification of harmful and beneficial microorganisms associated with replanting disease in rhizosphere soil of *Pseudostellariae heterophylla*. *Int. J. Agric. Biol.* **2015**, *17*, 458–466. [CrossRef]
46. Wei, L.J.; Tan, W.Q.; Wang, G.; Li, Q.; Dong, F.; Guo, Z.Y. The antioxidant and antifungal activity of chitosan derivatives bearing Schiff bases and quaternary ammonium salts. *Carbohydr. Polym.* **2019**, *226*, 115256. [CrossRef] [PubMed]

plants

MDPI

*Review*

# Novel Cognitions in Allelopathy: Implications from the "Horizontal Natural Product Transfer"

**Laura Lewerenz [1], Sara Abouzeid [2], Mahdi Yahyazadeh [3], Tahani Hijazin [4] and Dirk Selmar [1,*]**

[1] Institut für Pflanzenbiologie, Technische Universität Braunschweig, Mendelssohnstraße 4, D-38106 Braunschweig, Germany
[2] Pharmacognosy Department, Faculty of Pharmacy, Mansoura University, Mansoura 35516, Egypt
[3] Research Institute of Forests and Rangelands, Agricultural Research, Education and Extension Organization (AREEO), Tehran P.O. Box 13185-116, Iran
[4] Biology Department, Faculty of Science, Mutah University, P.O. Box 7, Mutah 61710, Jordan
[*] Correspondence: d.selmar@tu-bs.de

**Abstract:** Whereas the translocation of allelochemicals between plants is well established, a related general transfer of genuine specialized metabolites has not been considered so far. The elucidation of the so-called "Horizontal Natural Product Transfer" revealed that alkaloids, such as nicotine and pyrrolizidine alkaloids, which are leached out from decomposing alkaloid-containing plants (donor plants), are indeed taken up by the roots of plants growing in the vicinity (acceptor plants). Further studies demonstrated that phenolic compounds, such as coumarins or stilbenes, are also taken up by acceptor plants. Contemporary analyses from co-cultivation experiments outlined that natural products are not exclusively transferred from dead and rotting donor plant materials, but also from vital plants. In analogy to xenobiotics, the imported specialized metabolites might also be modified within the acceptor plants. As known from the uptake of xenobiotics, the import of specialized metabolites is also generally due to a simple diffusion of the substances across the biomembranes and does not require a carrier. The uptake depends in stricto sensu on the physicochemical properties of the certain compound. This article presents a current overview of the phenomenon of "Horizontal Natural Product Transfer" and discusses its relevance for our understanding of allelopathic interactions. The knowledge that specialized metabolites might in general be readily translocated from one plant into others should significantly contribute to our understanding of plant–plant interactions and—in particular—to the evolution of typical allelopathic effects, such as inhibition of growth and germination of potential competitors.

**Keywords:** horizontal natural product transfer; allelopathy; alkaloids; uptake

**Citation:** Lewerenz, L.; Abouzeid, S.; Yahyazadeh, M.; Hijazin, T.; Selmar, D. Novel Cognitions in Allelopathy: Implications from the "Horizontal Natural Product Transfer". *Plants* **2022**, *11*, 3264. https://doi.org/10.3390/plants11233264

Academic Editors: Margot Schulz, Vincenzo Tabaglio and Per Kudsk

Received: 5 October 2022
Accepted: 22 November 2022
Published: 28 November 2022



## 1. Background

By their roots, plants take up plenty of inorganic nutrients from the soil, as well as many other compounds. Concerning biochemical ecology, in particular, the uptake of allelochemicals, i.e., active substances, which inhibit germination or growth of putative competitors, is of special interest [1]. In general, these substances are released from donor plants into the soil and exhibit their inhibitory effect on the plants growing in their vicinity [2,3] (see also other chapters of this Special Issue). To execute their inhibitory effects, the allelochemicals have to be taken up by the acceptor plants [1,4]. A further import of natural products is related to Systemic Acquired Resistance (SAR) of plants: it was shown that salicylic acid, which provokes SAR, is also taken up by roots [5,6]. In this context, it has to be emphasized that the uptake of ionic compounds such as salicylic acid, as well as of nutrients such as nitrate, sulfate or metal ions, requires specific transporters [7–9]. As a consequence, by regulating the carrier proteins' number and activity, plants are capable of controlling the import of the related substances by their roots. As opposed to this, the situation is entirely different when considering the uptake of xenobiotics, i.e., systemic herbicides, fungicides [10], or veterinary medicines [11]. Because of their partially hydrophobic character, these substances are able to diffuse smoothly through membranes [12–14]. Thus, these substances are taken up by the roots passively (see below), and, in consequence, the plants cannot control or even prevent the import of these substances. Although these nexuses were well established, corresponding contemplations about common specialized metabolites have not been considered at all. However, this attitude has plainly changed within the last few years due to comprehensive investigations to identify the potential sources of various contaminations of plant-derived commodities.

Triggered by alarming reports of the European Food Safety Authority (EFSA) on contaminations of herbal medicines and phytopharmaceuticals by various toxic alkaloids, i.e., nicotine [15], pyrrolizidine alkaloids [16,17], or tropane alkaloids [18], several studies on the source of these contaminations were conducted. It became apparent that plants take up nicotine [19] and pyrrolizidine alkaloids [20] from the soil. Subsequent field trials demonstrated that nicotine, which is leached out from discarded cigarette butts, is taken up massively by acceptor plants. The related nicotine concentrations in the commodities were around 1 µg/g d.w. [21], thus exceeding the official maximum residue limit (0.01 µg/g d.w.) about a hundred-fold. In the same manner, pyrrolizidine alkaloids (PAs), which are leached out from rotting PA-containing weeds into the soil, e.g., *Senecio jacobaea*, are also taken up by the roots of the acceptor plants and translocated into their leaves [20,22]. Accordingly, such transfer of alkaloids—at least in part—accounts for the numerous and widespread alkaloidal contaminations of spice and medicinal plants reported comprehensively [15,16,23]. Based on these coherences, the so-called "Horizontal Natural Product Transfer" was outlined [24], a so far unrecognized phenomenon which has been studied intensively during the last few years (for review, see [25–27]). It became evident that apart from alkaloids, other natural products, such as coumarins [28], stilbenes [29], or betalains [30], are also taken up by plant roots. In this context, it has to be mentioned that in some cases, the natural products whose import into acceptor plants was verified, i.e., the stilbene resveratrol [29] or the coumarins [27], are known to exhibit allelopathic effects [31,32]. These examples vividly demonstrate that the line between "simple natural products" and "allelochemicals", which are leached out, is quite diffuse. Up to now, this issue has not been taken into consideration when evolutionary aspects of allelopathic effects are discussed.

## 2. Horizontal Natural Product Transfer—Basic Principles and Cognitions

### 2.1. Uptake of Chemicals from the Soil

A vast number of studies on the uptake of xenobiotics showed that by far, most of these substances can smoothly diffuse across membranes [12–14]. The ability for such passive membrane transfer can roughly be deduced from the so-called $K_{OW}$ value [10], which corresponds to the distribution coefficient of a certain substance between octanol and water. In most related publications, its decadal logarithm, denoted as $pK_{OW}$, is outlined [33]. Frequently, this parameter is also denominated as log$P$ [34]. Comprehensive research displayed that substances exhibiting log$P$ values between −1 and 3 are inherently able to diffuse easily through biomembranes [33,35]. It is self-evident that these coherences, which pertain to the uptake of xenobiotics, also apply to all other organic substances. This phenomenon was approved by Hurtado et al. [36], who demonstrated that organic compounds exhibiting appropriate log$P$ values are generally taken up by plants. In consequence, there is no doubt that also all plant-derived natural products exhibiting an appropriate log$P$ value are passively taken up by plants when they are present in the soil.

Nevertheless, an additional factor must be considered when contemplating the membrane permeability of alkaloids, i.e., the pH-dependent protonation of these alkaline specialized metabolites [37]. Whereas the free bases of most alkaloids pass biomembranes smoothly, the protonated forms cannot, since the positive charge strongly increases the hydrophilic character and thus prevents the penetration of biomembranes. This manifestation nicely coincides with the quite negative log$P$ values of charged alkaloid salts. This implies that—apart from the log*P* of the various alkaloids the pH of the medium also strongly determines their membrane permeability and thereby massively influences the extent of the uptake of alkaloids from the soil [38,39]. In acidic soils, due to the high degree of protonation, most alkaloids are unable to cross the plasmalemma of the root cells and accordingly, they are not taken up [10]. In contrast, in soils exhibiting enhanced pH values, protonation is pushed back and the alkaloids exist as free bases, which smoothly penetrate the plasmalemma of the root cells. provoking their strong uptake [39].

### 2.2. Horizontal Natural Product Transfer between Vital Plants

When contemplating the basic coherences of the horizontal natural product transfer, the question arises whether—in analogy to the relocation of natural products from rotting plant material—a corresponding transfer also might occur between living plants. This seems to be obvious because it is well known that allelochemicals are also released into the environment by various mechanisms [40]: they might either be leached out of decomposing plant materials, or they could actively be exuded from vital plants by their roots [2,3] or by their leaves [40,41]. In order to ascertain a putative release of common and typical natural products into the soil and a subsequent transfer into acceptor plants, co-culture experiments have been conducted: *Senecio jacobaea* plants containing high concentrations of pyrrolizidine alkaloids (Pas) were cultivated in the same pot together with parsley plants. After two months of co-cultivation, the plants were harvested and analyzed. Amazingly, in all parsley plants, which had been co-cultivated in the same pot together with a *Senecio* plant, significant concentrations of Pas were present; on average more than 200 µg/kg d.w. [22]. To rule out that the transfer of alkaloids is due to a too intensive contact between the roots of the donor and acceptor plants, a further study employing various distances between the plants was required. Accordingly, in a corresponding field trial, different acceptor plants were co-cultivated with *S. jacobaea*. It turned out that, in all plants grown in the field together with *S. jacobaea*, significant amounts of PAs were also present [22]. Thus, the alkaloids, which previously had been synthesized in the donor plants, are now present in the plants growing in the vicinity. Accordingly, there is no doubt that the PAs indeed had been transferred from vital donor plants via the soil into acceptor plants growing nearby (Figure 1). In further approaches, it could be verified that non-alkaloidal specialized metabolites are also transferred via the soil from donor to acceptor plants, i.e., coumarins [28], stilbenes [29], aristolochic acids [42,43], or betalains [25]. Meanwhile, several studies outlined a corresponding transfer of specialized metabolites from vital donor plants to acceptor plants growing in their vicinity (Table 1). However, up to now, there is no clue concerning the mode of this transfer.

First and foremost, it could be assumed that the described PA-transfer between living plants is due to the shedding of *Senecio* leaves; when the leaves decay, the Pas could be leached out from the rotting plant materials. In principle, this possibility cannot be excluded, but during the pot experiments described above, no leaves had been shed [26]. Thus, at least in these experiments, a transfer via shed leaves could be ruled out. Nonetheless, when referring to the mentioned field experiment, such an option cannot be excluded. These coherences also account for most of the reports on the transfer of specialized metabolites mentioned in Table 1. When considering an entire vegetation period, it has to be regarded that a senescence-induced shedding always takes place. Thus, this option certainly might be relevant, at least to some extent.

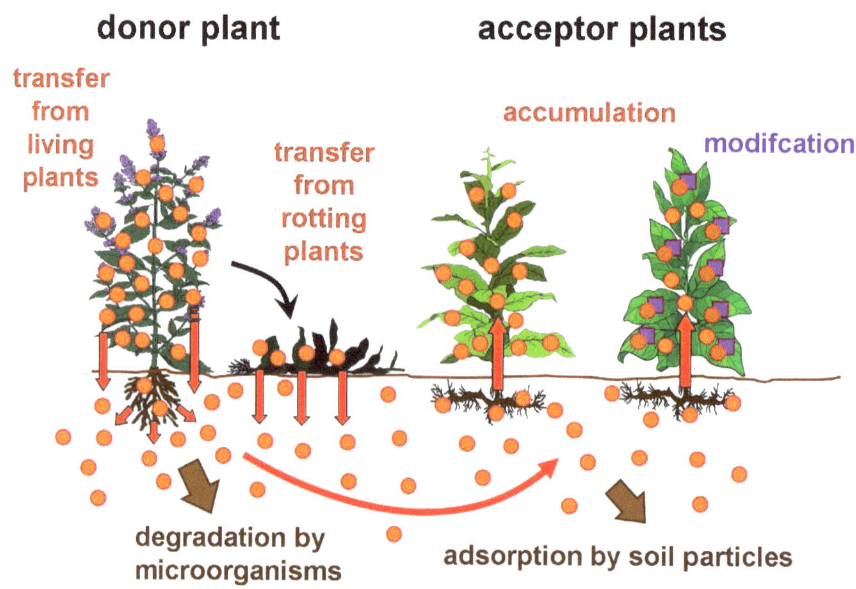


**Figure 1.** Horizontal natural product transfer. The scheme displayed by Selmar et al. [26] is supplemented with the processes occurring in the rhizosphere.

**Table 1.** Transfer of alkaloids via soil between vital donor and acceptor plants.

| Donor Plant | Type of Alkaloid | Acceptor Plant | Authors |
|---|---|---|---|
| *Chromolaena odorata* | Pyrrolizidine alkaloids | *Zea mays* | [44] |
| *Secale cereale* | Benzoxazinoids | *Vicia villosa* | [45] |
| *Senecio jacobaea* | Pyrrolizidine alkaloids | *Matricaria chamomilla* | [20,22] |
| *Senecio jacobaea* | Pyrrolizidine alkaloids | *Melissa officinalis* | [20,22] |
| *Senecio jacobaea* | Pyrrolizidine alkaloids | *Mentha × piperita* | [20,22] |
| *Senecio jacobaea* | Pyrrolizidine alkaloids | *Petroselinum crispum* | [20,22,25] |
| *Senecio jacobaea* | Pyrrolizidine alkaloids | *Tropaeolum majus* | [22] |
| *Solanaceae* | Atropine | *Triticum aestivum* | [46] |

Another option for the transfer of the alkaloids could be due to their bleeding out from minor leaf injuries, which might be caused by herbivore or pathogen attacks. Yet, the plants used in the co-culture experiments had been described as healthy and no marks of herbivory were visible [22]. Thus, it seems unlikely that the observed PA-transfer is related to plain bleeding of the alkaloids from injured leaves. This conclusion is underlined by the massive differences in the PA-spectra of donor and acceptor plants [22]. In case of wound-induced bleeding, all the different PAs accumulated in the donor plant would be leached out and taken up by the acceptor plants to more or less the same extent. The observed differences must be due to a process, whose extent differs for the various alkaloids. In consequence, simple bleeding of the alkaloids from injured leaves can be ruled out. The same deduction is also valid for wound-induced bleeding from putatively injured roots. Thus, we have to suppose that the PAs present in the acceptor plants indeed had been released from vital, healthy and uninjured *Senecio* donor plants.

When bearing in mind the well-established active exudation of allelochemicals [2,3,40], it seems to be obvious that PAs, as well as other alkaloids, are also exuded by the donor plants, either by their roots or by their leaves. When discussing such a release, it readily becomes apparent that in principle there are two possibilities: the alkaloids could either be diffused passively out of the cells, or they could actively be exuded by the roots or shoots. In this context, the finding of García-Jorgensen et al. [47] becomes relevant, which outlined that the carcinogenic phytotoxin ptaquiloside, which is accumulated in the fern *Pteridium aquilinum*, indeed passively diffuses out of its leaves. Consequently, all alkaloids and other specialized metabolites exhibiting appropriate log*P* values might also simply diffuse passively out of leaves or roots into the soil, and accordingly will be taken up passively by the roots of plants growing in the vicinity. Yet, in case of polyphenolic compounds, an uptake might be prevented due to their oxidation to yield quinones, which efficiently bind to proteins, forming insoluble tanning products. The observed differences in the PA spectra of donor and acceptor plants might result from disparities in the log*P*- and $pK_a$-values of the various PAs (see below) and thus, in their ability to diffuse through biomembranes. However, in this context, it has to be considered that in plant cells alkaloids are efficiently trapped in their vacuoles. Already half a century ago, Matile [48] outlined his famous "ion trap mechanism": within the neutral cytosol, most alkaloids are present as free bases and—provided that their log*P*-values are in the range between -1 and 3 (see above), they are able to diffuse through biomembranes, such as the tonoplast. However, due to the acidic conditions in the vacuoles, the alkaloids become protonated. Consequently, they are no longer able to pass the tonoplast and accordingly are trapped and accumulated in the vacuoles. Thus, a passive release out of the cells is quite unlikely. Yet, these coherences only apply to alkaloids revealing a relatively high p*K*a, ensuring a sufficient protonation in the vacuole [39]. In contrast, alkaloids, which reveal a very low p*K*a, e.g., caffeine (p*K*a = 0.7) are not protonated in the acidic vacuole. Since they do not exhibit a positive charge that typically prevents their membrane permeability, these alkaloids are not retained within this compartment. Nevertheless, due to an effective complex formation with chlorogenic acids, caffeine—to a certain extent—is also retained in the vacuole [49], since—in the same manner as protonated alkaloids—the caffeine-chlorogenic acids-complex also cannot pass the tonoplast passively and thus, it is retained in the vacuole.

Most of the literature dealing with the release of alkaloids from vital plant parts is based on organ or cell culture experiments, e.g., harmine and harmaline are exuded from root culture cells of *Oxalis tuberose* [50], the indole alkaloid ajmalicine is secreted from hairy root cultures of *Catharanthus roseus* [51], and nicotine is present in the medium of root cultures from *Nicotiana tabacum* [52]. Based on the coherences outlined above, the occurrence of alkaloids in the culture medium might just be a hint for an active exudation. Nonetheless, Toppel et al. [53] demonstrated that in the culture medium of *Senecio* root cells, senkirkine was exclusively present, although the cultured cells contained a wide variety of PAs. This discrepancy can only be explained by the fact that senkirkine is actively and specifically exuded from the cells into the culture medium [53]. It is evident that such exudation requires specific carriers, which catalyze the transfer of the protonated alkaloids across the tonoplast and thus out of the vacuole. Indeed, numerous alkaloid transporters are described in the literature [54–56], for review see [57]. Unfortunately, in most of these reports, the ability of alkaloids to easily pass biomembranes is entirely ignored, and the authors are not aware that the transporters are required for the membrane transfer of protonated alkaloids rather than for the free bases [27].

Apart from the data on the release of alkaloids into the medium of organ and cell cultures, various data on the liberation of alkaloids from genuine plants into the soil are available. Baumann and Gabriel [58] showed that the roots of coffee seedlings exude caffeine, and Schulz et al. [59] demonstrated that dihydroxybenzoxazinone is released from the roots of *Agropyron repens* into the soil. Analogously, *Oxalis tuberosa* roots liberate carboline alkaloids, i.e., harmine and harmaline, into the soil [60]. Moreover, lupine alkaloids (quinolizidine alkaloids) had been detected in soils well-vegetated by narrow-leaf and yellow lupines [61]. Similarly, Hama and Strobel [62] found PAs in soils, overgrown with PA-containing *Senecio* plants. Apart from the occurrence of various alkaloids in soils, the assumption that alkaloids are released by the roots of various alkaloidal plants is supported by various indirect results, i.e., by detecting them in acceptor plants growing in their vicinity (Table 1). However, when contemplating the mode of release of these alkaloids, any solid proof on the mechanism of the release is lacking. In principle, these alkaloids might be eluted from shed leaves or leached out from injured leaves or roots, respectively. Moreover, they might be released from vital tissues, either by passive diffusion or an active exudation by the means of transporters. Indeed, with respect to the data mentioned above, up to now, no option can ultimately be excluded. Much more research is required to soundly unveil the actual path of alkaloid release into the soil.

### 2.3. *Translocation of Chemicals within the Acceptor Plants*

The alkaloids, which had been taken up by the roots of the acceptor plants, are subsequently present in their leaves [19,20]. Thus, the imported specialized metabolites have to be translocated within the acceptor plants. In principle, there are only two options for such allocation, either via xylem or phloem. In the case of xenobiotics, it is well documented that their transport from root to shoot is accomplished via the xylem [33,63]. Accordingly, it seems to be obvious that analogously also the natural products taken up by acceptor plants are translocated within the xylem. This theory was confirmed by the finding that imported alkaloids accumulated to a high extent in old leaves, whereas the alkaloid concentrations in young leaves were quite lower [19,20]. This different distribution is due to expansion-related differences in the transpiration rates, which in turn drives the xylem transport, and thus is responsible for the different extent of allocation of substances via the xylem. Furthermore, no imported alkaloids had been detected in the flowers of the acceptor plants [20], which represent a major physiological sink. Thus, a source-sink-translocation via phloem can be excluded. Finally, the implication of a xylem-based allocation of imported natural products is verified by the finding that, within the acceptor plants, these substances are also present in guttation droplets [20], whose composition corresponds to that of the xylem sap [64]. From these coherences, it has to be deduced that the imported natural compounds, in particular nicotine and PAs, indeed are translocated within the acceptor plants in the xylem.

When comparing these insights with the transport of PAs in genuine alkaloidal plants, such as *Senecio*, a strong discrepancy becomes evident: In the group of Hartmann, it was soundly verified that the PAs synthesized in the roots of *Senecio* plants are transferred as PA-*N*-oxides via phloem into the physiological sinks, such as flowers and seeds [65–67]. Based on the physicochemical properties of the alkaloids and their corresponding *N*-oxides, this putative contradiction could be elucidated [37]: as outlined above, the free bases of alkaloids readily diffuse through biomembranes. Accordingly, due to the ion trap mechanism already explained for the accumulation of protonated alkaloids within the vacuoles (see above), they are also displaced from the alkaline phloem and trapped within the acidic xylem. In consequence, they are allocated within the xylem into the transpiring leaves—a fact that is fully in accordance with the findings displayed for the alkaloids taken up from the soil. In contrast, the strongly enhanced hydrophilic properties of alkaloid-*N*-oxides or quaternary alkaloids, respectively, are not able to diffuse through biomembranes. Consequently, they would be retained in the alkaline phloem, and thereby enable the option for a long-distance transport to the physiological sinks via phloem as reported by the Hartmann group [65–67].

Since the specialized metabolites are passively taken up by the roots of the acceptor plants, the velocity and the extent of their import should be quite similar in the various species. The only factor which determines the uptake is the corresponding difference in concentration between the soil and the cytosol of the rhizodermis cells. Nevertheless, this gradient between "inside and outside" depends on various additional factors. Apart from the pH, which strongly influences the share of protonated and thus membrane-permeable alkaloids (see above), the most important factor corresponds to the decrease in the concentration of imported compounds within the root cells and thus, how the concentration gradient between "inside and outside" is maintained. In principle, there are two possibilities, either their allocation into other organs or their modification (see below). The velocity of a xylem-based allocation is mainly determined by the rate of transpiration [68]. Indeed, this property varies greatly among different plant species and is therefore responsible for the observed differences in the uptake of a certain natural substance imported into different plants.

Additionally, the gradient of a certain substance between "inside and outside" might also be impacted by a corresponding decrease in its concentration in the soil, either by its adsorption to various soil particles or by a related microbial decomposition or modification, respectively.

In addition to these insights, the transfer of natural products from living donor plants might also open new doors to unveil the beneficial impact of some hitherto not fully understood processes, i.e., co-cultivation of certain vegetables and crop rotations. The findings related to the exchange of natural products among vital plants might provide new approaches for the explanations of these ambiguous phenomena.

### 2.4. *Modification of the Imported Compounds in the Acceptor Plants*

Astonishingly, the contents of alkaloids imported into the acceptor plants decreased over time: a massive decline in concentration was reported for the content of nicotine in peppermint plants [19], as well as for the PAs in various spice plants [20]. Since a complete decomposition of these compounds to $CO_2$ and water seemed to be very unlikely, it was argued that the imported compounds had been modified within the acceptor plants. In this context, it is appropriate to outline that xenobiotics, which are taken up from the soil, are also known to be frequently modified within the acceptor plants (Figure 1). The most abundant modifications comprise oxidations, hydroxylations, and conjugations with glucose [69,70]. Based on these cognitions, the so-called green liver concept—a hypothesis that proposed that these reactions are part of a deliberate detoxification system for xenobiotics—was developed [70,71]. In consequence, it seems to be natural that the time-dependent decrease in the alkaloid content in the acceptor plants might also be due to the modification of the imported natural compounds. The confirmation of this conjecture was elaborated by advanced analyses of PAs present in the acceptor plants: standard quantification of PAs is generally performed based on standard LC-MS methods, quantifying and summing up the individual contents of 27 genuine PAs [20,72]. Thus, in these studies, solely the original already known PAs, which had previously been present in the donor plant, were estimated, whereas their putative derivatives could not be determined. Yet, in a further approach to quantify the PAs in the acceptor plants, an alternative method—denoted as "sum parameter method"—was employed. For this approach, the PAs are degraded to their basic skeleton, the so-called necine base, which subsequently is quantified by HPLC-ESI-MS [73]. In consequence, apart from the genuine Pas, all putative derivatives will also be determined. The related results were really astonishing: in contrast to the putative decline of the alkaloids over time—as estimated by applying the standard method—a further massive increase in the alkaloids content was verified [30]. In parsley, two weeks after the mulching with PA-containing *Senecio* plant material, more than three-quarters of the imported alkaloids had already been modified within the acceptor plants [30], and thus became invisible to the standard LC-MS quantification. Unfortunately, up to now, the structure of these PA derivatives could not be elucidated. There is a massive demand for further research, since the content of alkaloids in contaminated plant-derived commodities is obviously far higher than that previously stated. This especially accounts for PAs to soundly evaluate the actual health risk.

In order to elucidate the basics of the modification of imported natural products in the acceptor plants, fundamental studies employing umbelliferone as a model substance had been performed. In contrast to most alkaloids, due to their high fluorescence, coumarins as well as their putative derivatives could easily be identified. The studies dealing with the uptake of umbelliferone into various acceptor plants clearly unveiled that the metabolic fate of imported natural products strongly depends on the plant species [28]: in various acceptor plants like flax, radish, or pea, the umbelliferone imported by their roots is just accumulated in their leaves. In contrast, in garden cress and barley, it is hydroxylated to yield esculetin. However, in garden cress, the generated esculetin is glucosylated to esculin, whereas in barley, it is methylated to yield scopoletin [28]. Based on the employment of naproxen, an efficient inhibitor of P450 enzymes, it was demonstrated that the oxidative conversion of umbelliferone is catalyzed by cytochrome P450 enzymes [74]. In contrast, the oxidation of harmaline taken up by barley seedlings to yield harmine is not catalyzed by a P450 enzyme [75].

From the coherences mentioned above—in particular that the extent and mode of modification of the imported products strongly vary between plant species—the occurrence of a general detoxification system, hypothesized as "green liver concept" [69,71], has to be doubted. In contrast, the imported substances seem to be accidentally modified by enzymes involved in the inherent specialized metabolism, which are present in some plants and absent in others [27].

## 3. Horizontal Natural Product Transfer and Allelopathy

Allelochemicals released from numerous plants inhibit potential competitors for limited light, water, or nutrient resources [76]. For a number of these allelopathic compounds, their underlying physiological mechanism is related to the inhibition of a wide array of corresponding metabolic processes: allelochemicals can affect photosynthesis by reducing PSII efficiency, might impair nutrient uptake and ATP synthesis, or harm cell cycle and gene expression or the phytohormone metabolism [1,77]. Due to these inhibitory effects, they are already employed in agricultural systems as useful tools for controlling weeds [78,79], inhibiting pests [80,81], and fighting diseases [2,82]. In consequence, the usage of synthetical and potentially toxic plant-protecting agents can significantly be reduced. Indeed, the absorption of some allelochemicals by crop plants might also cause health risks as mentioned for the uptake of PAs. However, in general, the related concentrations are far too low to entail serious consequences for human health.

Apart from that, many plants are able to cope with inhibitory allelochemicals. Whereas seed germination of cucumber, alfalfa, garden cress, or tomato is strongly inhibited by juglone, the germination of seeds from wheat, barley, watermelon, corn, and radish is not affected; and the seedling growth of muskmelon is even enhanced by juglone [83]. Obviously, the sensitivity of seeds for allelochemicals varies strongly between different plant species. As outlined above, the corresponding mechanisms seem to be quite diverse and may pertain to various levels of metabolic processes. In this sense, several primary responses to the presence of allelochemicals are described. One of the most important mechanisms of the inhibitory effect of juglone is due to the generation of reactive oxygen species (ROS) [84]. However, the application of juglone may also enhance the ROS-scavenging systems and thereby reduce radical-related damages [84]. Furthermore, detoxifying enzymes and transporters, which inactivate or eliminate the toxic compounds, can be induced by the allelochemicals. In maize, a glutathione transferase, which modifies juglone, is up-regulated in response to the presence of the allelochemical. As a consequence of this derivatization, its toxic properties are strongly diminished [85]. A comprehensive study on the derivatization of allelochemicals by Schulz et al. [59] outlined that the mode and extent of the detoxification process may vary between different plant species. The authors showed that many acceptor plants detoxify benzoxazinones, such as DIBOA and DIMBO, by glucosylation, whereas others detoxify them by the generation of related carbamates. Furthermore, in several other plant species, some further metabolites of the benzoxazinones had been detected [86]. Apart from varying sensitivities of acceptor plants for allelochemicals based on differences in the detoxification mechanism, the different sensitivities might also be due to quite other causations. In this sense, the actual inhibitory effects of a certain allelochemical could be more or less pronounced in different plant species. In this sense,

Ding et al. [87], unveiled the molecular mechanism, being responsible for the massive differences in the toxicity of cinnamic acid, which is released as an allelochemical from cucumber roots. Even in the roots of *Cucumis sativus*, the cinnamic acid significantly decreases the activity of membrane $H^+$-ATPase, whereas no corresponding inhibition is observed in the roots of fig-leaf gourd (*Cucurbita ficifolia*). Accordingly, it can be argued that observed differences in the sensitivity for a certain allelochemical are indeed related to differences in its direct impact on metabolic events.

These examples outline that more than one factor or mode of action might be responsible for the observed differences in sensitivity. These coherences become even more complex when considering that further environmental factors, e.g., stress, could alter the sensitivity for a certain allelochemical. In this context, the observation of Amari et al. [88] became evident, who showed that the sensitivity for juglone is strongly diminished when reactions involved in the SAR (systemic acquired resistance) are induced. Furthermore, it has to be considered that allelopathy comprises a wide array of interaction between plants by influencing their competition either by the direct effects of allelochemicals, e.g., by inhibiting the germination and growth of potential competitors or by indirect impacts, e.g., by affecting the microbiome, the nutrient availability, and the character of the soil [89].

At this juncture, the question arises whether the observed differences in the sensitivity of the various plant species indeed originate unfailingly from evolutionary adaptations or if some of them are due to random and accidental detoxification processes catalyzed by intrinsic promiscuous enzymes. Depending on the plant species, the specialized metabolism and thus, the composition of immanent enzymes, massively differs. In consequence—in analogy to the proposed random modification of xenobiotics [27]—in some plants the imported allelochemicals might also be modified "accidentally", whereas in others, they are not. However, in contrast to allelopathic interactions which represent quite ancient features, plants had been confronted with xenobiotics, i.e., herbicides or fungicides only for one and a half century. The timespan until today is far too low for the evolutionary generation of a comprehensive detoxification system, which is aimed to "deliberately" detoxify these xenobiotics, i.e., as proposed by the so-called green liver concept [69,71]. Nonetheless, the processes generating the well-known resistances against herbicide can be realized in a very short time, since only one or few mutations are necessary to thwart the toxic effect, i.e., mutations in genes encoding enzyme proteins, non-enzyme proteins, or factors controlling cell division [90]. In consequence, it could be argued that the postulated green liver concept for the detoxification of xenobiotics [69,71] does not represent an adaptation of plants coping with synthetic herbicides or fungicides, but that these detoxification systems had obviously evolved in response to toxic allelochemicals. In consequence, the evolution of the various adaptations of plants to cope with allelochemicals of plants growing in their vicinity ought to be considered as important and principal factors for the deployment and sustaining of a certain plant community. Unfortunately, these insights have not been considered so far, either in plant sociology or in vegetation science.

## 4. Conclusions

The coherences outlined in this treatise display that the horizontal natural product transfer, which represents a quite general mechanism pertaining to all plants, might be the basis for both the evolution of allelochemicals and subsequently, of the corresponding detoxification mechanisms, which in turn currently also include coping with xenobiotics. Moreover, the insights into the differences in the potential detoxification of allelochemicals may open new doors for the understanding of "why and how" the composition of the various plant communities has been evolved and preserved.

**Author Contributions:** All authors contributed on the conceptuation and writing in an eaqual manner. All authors have read and agreed to the published version of the manuscript.

**Funding:** The research received no funding.

**Data Availability Statement:** Not applicable.

**Conflicts of Interest:** The authors declare no conflict of interest.

## References


1. Inderjit, K.; Duke, S.O. Ecophysiological aspects of allelopathy. *Planta* **2003**, *17*, 529–539.
2. Bertin, C.; Yang, X.; West, L.A. The role of root exudates and allelochemicals in the rhizosphere. *Plant Soil* **2003**, *256*, 67–83. [CrossRef]
3. Kalinova, J.; Vrchotova, N.; Triska, J. Exudation of Allelopathic Substances in Buckwheat (*Fagopyrum esculentum* Moench). *J. Agri. Food Chem.* **2007**, *55*, 6453–6459. [CrossRef] [PubMed]
4. Willis, R.J. The Historical Bases of the Concept of Allelopathy. *J. Hist. Biol.* **1985**, *18*, 71–102. [CrossRef]
5. De Meyer, G.; Capieau, K.; Audenaert, K.; Buchala, A.; Métraux, J.P.; Höfte, M. Nanogram Amounts of salicylic acid produced by the Rhizobacterium *Pseudomonas aeruginosa* 7NSK2 activate the systemic acquired resistance pathway in bean. *Mol. Plant Microbe Interact.* **1999**, *12*, 450–458. [CrossRef] [PubMed]
6. Manthe, B.; Schulz, M.; Schnabl, H. Effects of salicylic acid on growth and stomatal movements of *Vicia faba* L.: Evidence for salicylic acid metabolization. *J. Chem. Ecol.* **1992**, *18*, 1525–1539. [CrossRef] [PubMed]
7. Forde, B.G. Review: Nitrate transporters in plants: Structure, function and regulation. *Biochim. Biophys. Acta* **2000**, *1465*, 219–235. [CrossRef] [PubMed]
8. Buchner, P.; Takahashi, H.; Hawkesford, M.J. Plant sulphate transporters: Co-ordination of uptake, intracellular and long-distance transport. *J. Exp. Bot.* **2004**, *55*, 1765–1773. [CrossRef] [PubMed]
9. Kobayashi, T.; Nishizawa, N.K. Iron uptake, translocation, and regulation in higher plants. *Annu. Rev. Plant Biol.* **2012**, *63*, 131–152. [CrossRef] [PubMed]
10. Trapp, S.; Legind, C.N. Uptake of organic contaminants from soil into vegetables and fruits. In *Dealing with Contaminated Sites*; Swartjes, F.A., Ed.; Springer: Heidelberg, The Netherlands, 2011.
11. Boxall, A.B.A.; Johnson, P.; Smith, E.J.; Sinclair, C.J.; Stutt, E.; Levy, L.S. Uptake of veterinary medicines from soils into plants. *J. Agri. Food Chem.* **2006**, *54*, 2288–2297. [CrossRef]
12. Inoue, J.; Chamberlain, K.; Bromilow, R.H. Physicochemical factors affecting the uptake by roots and translocation to shoots of amine bases in barley. *Pest. Manag. Sci.* **1998**, *54*, 8–21. [CrossRef]
13. Nwoko, C.O. Trends in phytoremediation of toxic elemental and organic pollutants. *Afr. J. Biotechnol.* **2010**, *9*, 6010–6016.
14. Sibout, R.; Höfte, H. Plant Cell Biology: The ABC of Monolignol Transport. *Curr. Biol.* **2012**, *22*, R533–R535. [CrossRef] [PubMed]
15. EFSA—European Food Safety Authority. Setting of temporary MRLs for nicotine in tea, herbal infusions, spices, rose hips and fresh herbs. *EFSA J.* **2011**, *9*, 2098. [CrossRef]
16. EFSA—European Food Safety Authority. Scientific Opinion on Pyrrolizidine alkaloids in food and feed. *EFSA J.* **2011**, *9*, 2406. [CrossRef]
17. EFSA—European Food Safety Authority. Risks for human health related to the presence of pyrrolizidine alkaloids in honey, tea, herbal infusions and food supplements. *EFSA J.* **2017**, *15*, 4908. [CrossRef]
18. EFSA—European Food Safety Authority. Human acute exposure assessment to tropane alkaloids. *EFSA J.* **2018**, *16*, 5160. [CrossRef]
19. Selmar, D.; Engelhardt, U.H.; Hänsel, S.; Thräne, C.; Nowak, M.; Kleinwächter, M. Nicotine uptake by peppermint plants as a possible source of nicotine in plant-derived products. *Agron. Sustain. Dev.* **2015**, *35*, 1185–1190. [CrossRef]
20. Nowak, M.; Wittke, C.; Lederer, I.; Klier, B.; Kleinwächter, M.; Selmar, D. Interspecific transfer of pyrrolizidine alkaloids: An unconsidered source of contaminations of phytopharmaceuticals and plant derived commodities. *Food Chem.* **2016**, *213*, 163–168. [CrossRef] [PubMed]
21. Selmar, D.; Radwan, A.; Abdalla, N.; Taha, H.; Wittke, C.; El-Henawy, A.; Alshaal, T.; Amer, M.; Nowak, M.; El-Ramady, H. Uptake of Nicotine from Discarded Cigarette Butts—A so far unconsidered path of contamination of plant derived commodities. *Environ. Pollut.* **2018**, *238*, 972–976. [CrossRef] [PubMed]
22. Selmar, D.; Wittke, C.; Beck-von Wolffersdorff, I.; Klier, B.; Lewerenz, L.; Kleinwächter, M.; Nowak, M. Transfer of pyrrolizidine alkaloids between living plants: A disregarded source of contaminations. *Environ. Pollut.* **2019**, *248*, 456–461. [CrossRef] [PubMed]
23. Mulder, P.P.J.; Sánchez, P.L.; These, A.; Preiss-Weigert, A.; Castellari, M. Occurrence of Pyrrolizidine Alkaloids in food. *EFSA Support. Publ.* **2015**, *12*, 859E. [CrossRef]
24. Selmar, D.; Radwan, A.; Nowak, M. Horizontal Natural Product Transfer: A So Far Unconsidered Source of Contamination of Plant-Derived Commodities. *J. Environ. Anal. Toxicol.* **2015**, *5*, 4. [CrossRef]
25. Nowak, M.; Yahyazadeh, M.; Lewerenz, L.; Selmar, D. Horizontal Natural Product Transfer: A so far unconsidered source of contamination of medicinal. In *Medicinal Plants and Environmental Challenges*; Ghorbanpour, M.M., Varma, A., Eds.; Springer International Publishing: Cham, Switzerland, 2017; pp. 215–226.
26. Selmar, D.; Radwan, A.; Hijazin, T.; Abouzeid, S.; Yahyazadeh, M.; Lewerenz, L.; Kleinwächter, M.; Nowak, M. Horizontal Natural Product Transfer: Intriguing Insights into a Newly Discovered Phenomenon. *J. Agri. Food Chem.* **2019**, *67*, 8740–8745. [CrossRef]
27. Hijazin, T.; Lewerenz, L.; Yahyazadeh, M.; Selmar, D. Horizontal Natural Product Transfer: A Phenomenon Which Is Responsible for the Widespread Alkaloidal Contaminations of Herbal Products. In *Environmental Challenges and Medicinal Plants: Environmental Challenges and Solutions*; Aftab, T., Ed.; Springer Nature: Cham, Switzerland, 2022; pp. 183–201.

28. Hijazin, T.; Radwan, A.; Abouzeid, S.; Dräger, G.; Selmar, D. Uptake and modification of umbelliferone by various seedlings *Phytochemistry* **2019**, *157*, 194–199. [CrossRef]
29. Abouzeid, S.; Beutling, U.; Selmar, D. Stress-induced modification of indole alkaloids: Phytomodificines as a new category of specialized metabolites. *Phytochemistry* **2019**, *159*, 102–107. [CrossRef]
30. Selmar, D.; Abouzeid, S.; Radwan, A.; Hijazin, T.; Yahyazadeh, M.; Lewerenz, L.; Nowak, M.; Kleinwächter, M. Horizontal natural product transfer—A novel attribution in allelopathy. In *Reference Series in Phytochemistry. Co-Evolution of Secondary Metabolite*; Mérillon, J.-M., Ramawat, K.G., Eds.; Springer International Publishing: Cham, Switzerland, 2020; pp. 429–439.
31. Fan, P.; Hostettmann, K.; Lou, H. Allelochemicals of the invasive neophyte *Polygonum cuspidatum* Sieb. & Zucc. (Polygonaceae). *Chemoecology* **2010**, *20*, 223–227. [CrossRef]
32. Pan, L.; Li, X.Z.; Yan, Z.Q.; Guo, H.R.; Qin, B. Phytotoxicity of umbelliferone and its analogs: Structure-activity relationships and action mechanisms. *Plant Physiol. Biochem.* **2015**, *97*, 272–279. [CrossRef]
33. Trapp, S. Modelling uptake into roots and subsequent translocation of neutral and ionizable organic compounds. *Pest Manag. Sci.* **2000**, *56*, 767–778. [CrossRef]
34. Cronin, M.T.D.; Livingstone, J. Calculation of physiochemical properties. In *Predicting Chemical Toxicity and Fate*; Cronin, T.D., Livingstone, J., Eds.; CRC Press: Boca Raton, FL, USA, 2004; pp. 31–40.
35. Limmer, M.A.; Burken, J.G. Plant Translocation of Organic Compounds. Molecularand Physicochemical Predictors. *Environ. Sci. Technol. Lett.* **2014**, *1*, 156–161. [CrossRef]
36. Hurtado, C.; Domínguez, C.; Pérez-Babace, L.; Cãnameras, N.; Comas, J.; Bayona, J.M. Estimate of uptake and translocation of emerging organic contaminants from irrigation water concentration in lettuce grow under controlled conditions". *J. Hazard. Mat.* **2016**, *305*, 139–148. [CrossRef]
37. Nowak, M.; Selmar, D. Cellular distribution of alkaloids and their translocation via phloem and xylem: The importance of compartment pH. *Plant Biol.* **2016**, *18*, 879–882. [CrossRef] [PubMed]
38. Yahyazadeh, M.; Nowak, M.; Kima, H.; Selmar, D. Horizontal natural product transfer: A potential source of alkaloidal contaminants in phytopharmaceuticals. *Phytomedicine* **2017**, *34*, 21–25. [CrossRef]
39. Hijazin, T.; Radwan, A.; Lewerenz, L.; Abouzeid, S.; Selmar, D. The uptake of alkaloids by plants from the soil is determined by rhizosphere pH. *Rhizosphere* **2020**, *15*, 100234. [CrossRef]
40. Nakano, H.; Nakajima, E.; Fujii, Y.; Yamada, K.; Shigemori, H.; Hasegawa, K. Leaching of the allelopathic substance, L-tryptophan from the foliage of mesquite (*Prosopis juliflora* DC.) plants by water spraying. *Plant Growth Regul.* **2003**, *40*, 49–52. [CrossRef]
41. Tukey, H.B. The leaching of substances from plants. *Annu. Rev. Plant Biol.* **1970**, *21*, 305–324. [CrossRef]
42. Pavlović, N.M.; Maksimović, V.; Maksimović, J.D.; Orem, W.H.; Tatu, C.A.; Lerch, H.E.; Bunnell, J.E.; Kostić, E.N.; Szilagyi, D.N.; Paunescu, V. Possible health impacts of naturally occurring uptake of aristolochic acids by maize and cucumber roots: Links to the etiology of endemic (Balkan) nephropathy. *Environ. Geochem. Health* **2013**, *35*, 5–226. [CrossRef] [PubMed]
43. Li, W.; Hu, Q.; Chan, W. Uptake and accumulation of nephrotoxic and carcinogenic aristolochic acids in food crops grown in *Aristolochia clematitis*-contaminated soil and water. *J. Agri. Food Chem.* **2016**, *64*, 107–112. [CrossRef]
44. Letsyo, E.; Adams, Z.S.; Dzikunoo, J.; Asante-Donyinah, D. Uptake and accumulation of pyrrolizidine alkaloids in the tissues of maize (*Zea mays* L.) plants from the soil of a 4-year-old *Chromolaena odorata* dominated fallow farmland. *Chemosphere* **2021**, *270*, 128669. [CrossRef]
45. Hazrati, H.; Fomsgaard, I.S.; Kudsk, P. Root-Exuded Benzoxazinoids: Uptake and translocation in neighboring plants. *J. Agri. Food Chem.* **2020**, *68*, 10609–10617. [CrossRef]
46. Jandrić, Z.; Rathor, M.; Ghhem-Kieth, S.; Adu-Gyamfi, J.; Mayr, L.; Resch, C.; Bado, S.; Švarc-Gajić, J.; Cannavan, A. Uptake of 14C-atropine and/or its transformation products from soil by wheat (*Triticum aestivum* var Kronjet) and their translocation to shoots. *J. Environ. Sci. Health B* **2013**, *48*, 1034–1104. [CrossRef] [PubMed]
47. García-Jorgensen, D.B.; Hansen, H.C.B.; Abrahamsen, P.; Diamantopoulos, E. A novel model concept for modelling the leaching of natural toxins: Results for the case of ptaquiloside. *Environ. Sci. Process. Impacts* **2020**, *22*, 1768–1779. [CrossRef] [PubMed]
48. Matile, P. Localization of alkaloids and mechanism of their accumulation in vacuoles of *Chelidonium majus* laticifers. *Nova Acta Leopold.* **1976**, *7*, 139–156.
49. Waldhauser, S.S.M.; Baumann, T.W. Compartmentation of caffeine and related purine alkaloids depends exclusively on the physical chemistry of their vacuolar complex formation with chlorogenic acids. *Phytochemistry* **1996**, *42*, 985–996. [CrossRef]
50. Bais, H.P.; Vepachedu, R.; Vivanco, J.M. Root specific elicitation and exudation of fluorescent β-carbolines in transformed root cultures of *Oxalis tuberosa. Plant Physiol. Biochem.* **2003**, *41*, 345–353. [CrossRef]
51. Ruiz-May, E.; Galaz-Ávalos, R.M.; Loyola-Vargas, V.M. Differential secretion and accumulation of terpene indole alkaloids in hairy roots of *Catharanthus roseus* treated with methyl jasmonate. *Mol. Biotechnol.* **2009**, *41*, 278–285. [CrossRef] [PubMed]
52. Zhao, B.; Agblevor, F.A.; Ritesh, K.C.; Jelesko, J.G. Enhanced production of the alkaloid nicotine in hairy root cultures of *Nicotiana tabacum. Plant Cell Tissue Organ Cult.* **2013**, *113*, 121–129. [CrossRef]
53. Toppel, G.; Witte, L.; Riebesehl, B.; Borstel, K.V.; Hartmann, T. Alkaloid patterns and biosynthetic capacity of root cultures from some pyrrolizidine alkaloid producing *Senecio* species. *Plant Cell Rep.* **1987**, *6*, 466–469. [CrossRef] [PubMed]
54. Shitan, N.; Bazin, I.; Dan, K.; Obata, K.; Kigawa, K.; Ueda, K.; Sato, F.; Forestier, C.; Yazaki, K. Involvement of CjMDR1, a plant MDR-type ABC protein, in alkaloid transport in *Coptis japonica. Proc. Natl. Acad. Sci. USA* **2003**, *100*, 751–756. [CrossRef] [PubMed]

55. Otani, M.; Shitan, N.; Sakai, K.; Martinoia, E.; Sato, F.; Yazaki, K. Characterization of vacuolar transport of the endogenous alkaloid berberine in *Coptis japonica*. *Plant Physiol.* **2005**, *138*, 1939–1946. [CrossRef] [PubMed]
56. Morita, M.; Shitan, N.; Sawada, K.; Van Montagu, M.C.E.; Inzé, D.; Rischer, H.; Goossens, A.; Oksman-Caldentey, K.-M.; Moriyama, Y.; Yazaki, K. Vacuolar transport of nicotine is mediated by a multidrug and toxic compound extrusion (MATE) transporter in *Nicotiana tabacum*. *Proc. Natl. Acad. Sci. USA* **2009**, *106*, 2447–2452. [CrossRef] [PubMed]
57. Yazaki, K.; Sugiyama, A.; Morita, M.; Shitan, N. Secondary transport as an efficient membrane transport mechanism for plant secondary metabolites. *Phytochem. Rev.* **2008**, *7*, 513–524. [CrossRef]
58. Baumann, T.W.; Gabriel, H. Metabolism and excretion of caffeine during germination of *Coffea arabica* L. *Plant Cell Physiol.* **1984**, *25*, 1431–1436. [CrossRef]
59. Schulz, M.; Knop, M.; Kant, S.; Sicker, D.; Voloshchuk, N.; Gryganski, A. Detoxification of allelochemicals- the case of bezoxazolin-2(3H)-one(BOA). In *Allelopathy: A Physiological Process with Ecological Implications*; Reigosa, R.M.J., Pedrol, N., González, L., Eds.; Springer: Dordrecht, The Netherlands, 2006; pp. 157–170.
60. Bais, H.P.; Park, S.W.; Stermitz, F.R.; Halligan, K.M.; Vivanco, J.M. Exudation of fluorescent β-carbolines from *Oxalis tuberosa* L. roots. *Phytochemistry* **2002**, *61*, 539–543. [CrossRef] [PubMed]
61. Hama, J.; Strobel, B.W. Natural alkaloids from narrow-leaf and yellow lupins transfer to soil and soil solution in agricultural fields. *Environ. Sci. Eur.* **2020**, *32*, 126. [CrossRef]
62. Hama, J.; Strobel, B.W. Occurrence of pyrrolizidine alkaloids in ragwort plants, soils and surface waters at the field scale in grassland. *Sci. Total Environ.* **2021**, *755*, 142822. [CrossRef] [PubMed]
63. Hsu, F.C.; Marxmiller, R.L.; Yang, A.Y.S. Study of root uptake and xylem translocation of cinmethylin and related compounds in detopped soybean roots using a pressure chamber technique. *Plant Physiol.* **1990**, *93*, 1573–1578. [CrossRef]
64. Singh, S. Guttation: Mechanism, Momentum and Modulation. *Bot. Rev.* **2016**, *82*, 149–182. [CrossRef]
65. Ehmke, A.; Borstel, K.V.; Hartmann, T. Alkaloid N-oxides as transport and vacuolar storage compounds of pyrrolizidine alkaloids in *Senecio vulgaris* L. *Planta* **1988**, *176*, 83–90. [CrossRef] [PubMed]
66. Hartmann, T.; Dierich, B. Chemical diversity and variation of pyrrolizidine alkaloids of the senecionine type: Biological need or coincidence? *Planta* **1989**, *206*, 443–451. [CrossRef]
67. Witte, L.; Ehmke, A.; Hartmann, T. Interspecific flow of pyrrolizidine alkaloids: From plants via aphids to ladybirds. *Naturwissenschaften* **1990**, *77*, 540–543. [CrossRef]
68. Riedell, W.E.; Schumacher, T.E. Transport of water and nutrients in plants. In *Agricultural Sciences*; Lal, R., Ed.; EOLSS Publications: Abu Dhabi, United Arab Emirates, 2009; Volume 1, pp. 371–387.
69. Sandermann, H. Higher plant metabolism of xenobiotics: The ´green liver' concept. *Pharmacogenetics* **1994**, *44*, 225–241. [CrossRef] [PubMed]
70. Schäffner, A.; Messener, B.; Langebartels, C.; Sandermann, H. Genes and enzymes for in-planta phytoremediation of air, water and soil. *Acta Biotechnol.* **2002**, *22*, 141–151. [CrossRef]
71. Burken, J.G. Uptake and metabolism of organic compounds: Green-liver model. In *Phytoremediation: Transformation and Control of Contaminants*; McCutcheon, S.C., Schnoor, J.L., Eds.; Wiley: New York, NY, USA, 2003. [CrossRef]
72. Ronczka, S.; These, A.; Bodi, D.; Preiß-Weigert, A. International collaborative study for the determination of pyrrolizidine alkaloids in honey and herbal tea by SPE-LC-MS/MS. *BfR Wiss.* **2015**, *1*, 1–91.
73. Cramer, L.; Schiebel, H.-M.; Ernst, L.; Beuerle, T. Pyrrolizidine alkaloids in the food chain. Development, validation, and application of a new HPLC-ESI-MS/MS sum parameter method. *J. Agri. Food Chem.* **2013**, *61*, 11382–11391. [CrossRef] [PubMed]
74. Miners, J.O.; Coulter, S.; Tukey, R.H.; Veronese, M.E.; Birkett, D.J. Cytochromes P450, 1A2, and 2C9 are responsible for the human hepatic *O*-demethylation of *R*- and *S*-naproxen. *Biochem. Pharmacol.* **1996**, *51*, 1003–1008. [CrossRef] [PubMed]
75. Lewerenz, L.; Hijazin, T.; Abouzeid, S.; Hänsch, R.; Selmar, D. Pilot study on the uptake and modification of harmaline in acceptor plants: An innovative approach to visualize the interspecific transfer of natural products. *Phytochemistry* **2020**, *174*, 102–107. [CrossRef] [PubMed]
76. Bais, H.P.; Vepachedu, R.; Gilroy, S.; Callaway, R.M.; Vivanco, J.M. Allelopathy and exotic plant invasion: From molecules and genes to species interactions. *Science* **2003**, *301*, 1377–1380. [CrossRef] [PubMed]
77. Blum, U. Relationships between phenolic acid concentrations, transpiration, water utilization, leaf area expansion, and uptake of phenolic acids: Nutrient culture studies. *J. Chem. Ecol.* **2005**, *31*, 1907–1932. [CrossRef] [PubMed]
78. Boydston, R.A.; Morra, M.J.; Borek, V.; Clayton, L.; Vaughn, S.F. Onion and weed response to mustard (*Sinapis alba* ) seed meal. *Weed Sci.* **2011**, *59*, 546–552. [CrossRef]
79. Tavella, L.B.; Silva, P.S.L.; Monteiro, A.L.; de Oliveira, V.R.; de Oliveira-Fernandes, P.L. *Gliricidia sepium* intercropping for weed management in immature corn ear production. *Cien. Agron.* **2017**, *48*, 50–656. [CrossRef]
80. Avato, P.; D'Addabbo, T.; Leonetti, P.; Argentieri, M.P. Nematicidal potential of Brassicaceae. *Phytochem. Rev.* **2013**, *12*, 791–802. [CrossRef]
81. Singh, A.; Weisser, W.W.; Hanna, R.; Houmgny, R.; Zytynska, S.E. Reduce pests, enhance production: Benefits of intercropping at high densities for okra farmers in Cameroon. *Pest Manag. Sci.* **2017**, *73*, 2017–2027. [CrossRef] [PubMed]
82. Abdel-Monaim, M.F.; Abo-Elyousr, K.A.M. Effect of preceding and intercropping crops on suppression of lentil damping-off and root rot disease in New Valley—Egypt. *Crop Prot.* **2012**, *32*, 41–46. [CrossRef]

83. Kocaçalikan, I.; Terzi, I. Allelopathic effects of walnut leaf extracts and juglone on seed germination and seedling growth. *J. Hort. Sci. Biotechnol.* **2001**, *76*, 436–440. [CrossRef]
84. Hadrami, A.; Kone, D.; Lepoivre, P. Effect of Juglone on Active Oxygen Species and Antioxidant Enzymes in Susceptible and Partially Resistant Banana Cultivars to Black Leaf Streak Disease. *Eur. J. Plant Pathol.* **2005**, *113*, 241–254. [CrossRef]
85. Sytykiewicz, H. Expression patterns of glutathione transferase gene (GstI) in maize seedlings under juglone-induced oxidative stress. *Int. J. Mol. Sci.* **2011**, *12*, 7982–7995. [CrossRef]
86. Schulz, M.; Wieland, I. Variation in metabolism of BOA among species in various field communities—Biochemical evidence for co-evolutionary processes in plant communities? *Chemoecology* **1999**, *9*, 133–141. [CrossRef]
87. Ding, J.; Sun, Y.; Xiao, C.L.; Shi, K.; Zhou, Y.H.; Yu, J.Q. Physiological basis of different allelopathic reactions of cucumber and figleaf gourd plants to cinnamic acid. *J. Exp. Bot.* **2007**, *58*, 3765–3773. [CrossRef] [PubMed]
88. Amari, L.D.G.E.; Cherif, M.; Kouakou, T.H.; Camara, B.; Konné, D. Salicylic acid and acibenzolar-s-methyl induced resistance against toxic effect of Juglone, a toxin of mycosphaerella fijiensis causal agent of banana black leaf streak disease. *J. Adv. Agric.* **2015**, *3*, 204–217. [CrossRef]
89. Wardle, D.A.; Karban, R.; Callaway, R.M. The ecosystem and evolutionary contexts of allelopathy. *Trends Ecol. Evol.* **2011**, *26*, 655–662. [CrossRef]
90. Powles, S.B.; Yu, Q. Evolution in action: Plants resistant to herbicides. *Ann. Rev. Plant Biol.* **2010**, *61*, 317–347. [CrossRef] [PubMed]

plants

MDPI

*Review*

# Cyperus (*Cyperus esculentus* L.): A Review of Its Compositions, Medical Efficacy, Antibacterial Activity and Allelopathic Potentials

**Shengai Zhang [1,2], Peizhi Li [3], Zunmiao Wei [1], Yan Cheng [1], Jiayao Liu [1], Yanmin Yang [2], Yuyan Wang [1,2] and Zhongsheng Mu [1,*]**

1 Institute of Economic Plants, Jilin Academy of Agricultural Sciences, Gongzhuling 136105, China; wodani999@163.com (S.Z.); miaomiao0825@126.com (Z.W.); chengyan199910@163.com (Y.C.); jiayaoliu@yeah.net (J.L.); wyy6677@126.com (Y.W.)
2 Binzhou Vocational College, Binzhou 256600, China; yanmin107@163.com
3 Jia Sixie Agricultural College, Weifang University of Science and Technology, Weifang 262700, China; llppzz123@126.com
* Correspondence: muzs@163.com

**Abstract:** Cyperus (*Cyperus esculentus* L.) is an edible perennial grass-like plant, which propagates exclusively with underground tubers. Its tubers are rich in starch (20–30%), fat (25–35%), sugar (10–20%), protein (10–15%) and dietary fiber (8–9%). In addition, the tubers also contain alkaloids, organic acids, vitamins (C and E), steroids, terpenoids and other active components. The contents of oleic acid and linoleic acid in Cyperus oil are very high, which have important medicinal value and health-promoting properties. Most of the extracts from the tubers, stems and leaves of Cyperus have allelopathic potential and antibacterial, antioxidant and insecticidal activities. In recent years, the planting area of Cyperus has increased significantly all over the world, especially in China and some other countries. This paper presents the current status of Cyperus and the recent trend in research in this area. Published reports on its nutritional contents, active ingredients, medicinal efficacy, antibacterial activity and allelopathic potential were also reviewed.

**Keywords:** Cyperus; *Cyperus esculentus* L.; bioactive; medicinal efficacy; antibacterial activity; allelopathic potential; phytoinsecticide

**Citation:** Zhang, S.; Li, P.; Wei, Z.; Cheng, Y.; Liu, J.; Yang, Y.; Wang, Y.; Mu, Z. Cyperus (*Cyperus esculentus* L.): A Review of Its Compositions, Medical Efficacy, Antibacterial Activity and Allelopathic Potentials. *Plants* **2022**, *11*, 1127. https://doi.org/10.3390/plants11091127

Academic Editors: Margot Schulz and Vincenzo Tabaglio

Received: 22 March 2022
Accepted: 11 April 2022
Published: 21 April 2022



## 1. Introduction

Cyperus (*Cyperus esculentus* L.) is a perennial herb developed from rhizomes with sweet nut-like tubers, but cultivated species are often annual. It belongs to the genus Cyperus in the family Cyperaceae, and it propagates entirely with underground tubers in soil [1] (Figures 1 and 2). Cyperus is also known by various other names, such as yellow nutsedge, tiger nut, chufa, iron water chestnut, underground chestnut, underground walnut, earth almond, ginseng fruit, ginseng bean, etc. [2,3]. Cyperus is rich in fat, protein, sugar, other nutrients and a variety of active substances. It is a new crop with high quality, high yield and high value [4]. The tuberous rhizomes of Cyperus have been used as food by hunter-gatherers and agricultural societies for millennia.

Varieties and selections of the plant are widely grown in Southern Europe, North Africa and West Africa. Their popular uses as foods, beverage and medicine suggest that these edible tubers may have functional food potential. The ancient Egyptians first recognized the importance of this plant, planting and using it for culinary and medicinal purposes [5]. Later, the application of Cyperus became more and more extensive, from foods and medicine to its use in bioenergy [6]. In addition, there are a variety of active components in Cyperus, such as volatile oil, organic acids, alkaloids, phenols, terpenoids, anthraquinone, steroids, etc., which have antibacterial, antioxidant and antitumor activities. It was reported that the consumption of Cyperus could help prevent heart disease and thrombosis, improve blood circulation and lower the risk of colon cancer [7]. At the same time, a variety of active components in Cyperus have strong allelopathic effects, which have a great impact on intercropping, interplanting and crop rotation. However, due to its grass-like appearance and the poor research on Cyperus, for a long time in the past, some countries had always treated it as a weed, so it had not been fully utilized and investigated [8]. In recent years, it has been widely cultivated in Spain, Africa, Australia, South and North America. The annual value of Cyperus production in Spain has risen to 3.3 million euros, and its production area has also increased significantly in China, Italy, Bulgaria, etc. At present, there is still a lack of understanding in the active components, antibacterial activity and allelopathic potential of Cyperus, which affects the development, utilization and cultivation of Cyperus. Therefore, this paper reviews the chemical composition, medical efficacy and allelopathic potential of Cyperus to provide the references for the in-depth research, further development and utilization of Cyperus.

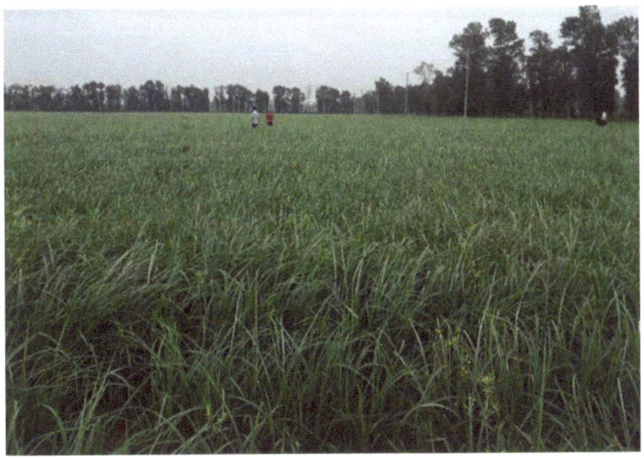

**Figure 1.** Cyperus (*Cyperus esculentus* L.) in growth stage.

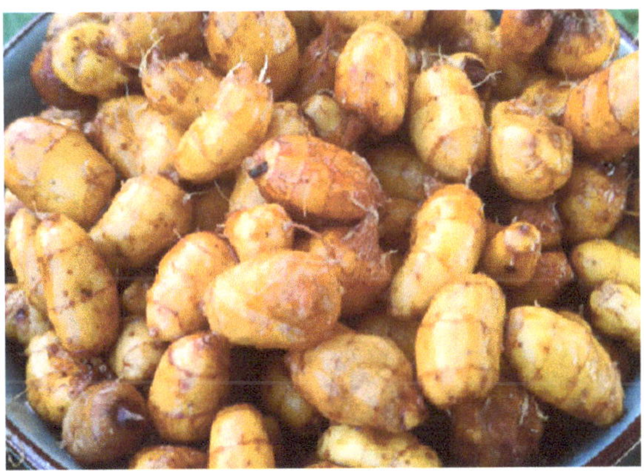

**Figure 2.** Cyperus (*Cyperus esculentus* L.) tubers at maturity.

## 2. Compositions

Cyperus is a new, high-quality oil crop. It is rich in oil, starch and sugar, and it also contains protein, dietary fiber, vitamin C, vitamin E and a variety of minerals (e.g., phosphorus, potassium, magnesium, sodium, calcium, etc.) (Table 1). From Table 1, (i) the content of lipid in Cyperus is higher than that of soybean. It can be used as a new oil crop and has great development potential; (ii) the content of starch in Cyperus is significantly higher than that of common oil crops, up to 23.2–29.9%; (iii) the contents of starch and carbohydrate in Cyperus are significantly higher than that of common oil crops, which indicates that Cyperus is a food of raw materials with high calories.

**Table 1.** Main composition and content of cultivated Cyperus (*Cyperus esculentus* L.) tubers compared to these of key oil crops.

| Product | Cyperus (%) | Peanut (%) | Soybean (%) | Rape (%) | Sunflower (%) | Sesame (%) |
|---|---|---|---|---|---|---|
| Scientific name | *Cyperus esculentus* | *Arachis hypogaea* | *Glycine max* | *Brassica napus* | *Helianthus annuus* | *Sesamum indicum* |
| Starch | 23.2–29.9 | 4.00 | 2.00–6.53 | 0.80–1.18 | 12.0–18.0 | – |
| Lipid | 20.1–34.5 | 39.2–49.8 | 16.0–22.0 | 37.5–46.3 | 49.9–51.2 | 44.9–57.9 |
| Protein | 5.04–8.00 | 20.3–26.7 | 35.0–44.6 | 23.1–32.4 | 15.4–23.9 | 18.4–30.4 |
| Crude Fiber | 8.06–8.91 | 3.30–8.50 | 5.23–15.5 | 5.7–9.6 | 4.90–6.10 | 7.45–12.6 |
| Carbohydrate | 43.3 | 7.48–22.1 | 22.0–30.0 | 15.9–24.8 | 13.0–16.7 | 14.4–31.5 |
| Total sugar | 15.4–23.4 | 3.54–6.53 | 5.06–7.70 | 8.00–12.9 | 16.0–23.0 | 8.44–12.3 |
| Ash | 1.60–2.19 | 2.02–2.27 | 4.35–4.60 | 4.10–5.30 | 3.20–5.40 | 4.77–6.18 |
| Moisture | 6.13–7.27 | 6.20–7.30 | 10.2–11.1 | 8.05 | 3.00–3.82 | 3.06–6.15 |
| References | [9–12] | [13–15] | [16–18] | [19,20] | [14,21,22] | [23,24] |

Note: "–" indicates no report.

In addition, Cyperus also contains a variety of active substances (e.g., alkaloid, saponin, phytosterol, flavone, terpenoid, tannin, etc.) [25]. These active substances are important pharmaceutical components. Most flavonoids have strong biological activities, such as an antioxidant effect, and can be used in pharmacological research (Table 2).

**Table 2.** Main active substances of cultivated Cyperus (*Cyperus esculentus* L.) tubers.

| Ingredient | Concentration | Reference |
|---|---|---|
| Resins | +++ | [7,26] |
| Cyanogenic glycosides | + | [7,26] |
| Alkaloids | +++ | [7] |
| Glycosides | 0 | |
| Flavonoids | +++ | [27,28] |
| Saponins | + | [7] |
| Tannins | + | [7] |
| Sterols | +++ | [7] |
| Cardiac glycosides | 0 | |
| β-sitosterol | +++ | [26] |
| $\delta^5$-avenasterol | + | [26] |
| Vitamin E | + | [26] |

Note: '+++' indicates very high concentration, '++' indicates medium concentration, '+' indicates trace concentration and '0' indicates uncertainty.

Due to the differences in climate, soil and cultivation conditions, the bioactive content in Cyperus varies. It was reported that, under normal conditions, the crude fat content in Cyperus tuber (dry tuber) is 25–35%, crude protein 10–15%, starch 20–30%, sugar 10–20%, vitamin E 0.8–1.4%, and the flavonoids in stems and leaves could reach 13.2 mg/g [11,27]. Chen et al. found that the contents of fat, starch, sugar, protein and water in the tubers of Cyperus were 26.5%, 23.2%, 23.4%, 8.0% and 7.0%, respectively, and other active components (e.g., organic acids, terpenoids, steroids, etc.) were also detected [29].

Liu showed that the basic components of Cyperus were 26.5% fat, 23.2% starch, 23.4% sugar, 8.0% protein and 7.0% water. At the same time, she also detected organic acids, vitamins, steroids and terpenes with health care effects, in which the content of vitamin E was 0.15% and the content of sterols was 0.53% [30]. The test results of Chen et al. and Liu are very similar. It can be concluded that the contents of fat, starch and sugar in Cyperus are indeed very high. In addition, Yan et al. detected the main components in the stems and leaves of Cyperus. The results showed that the stems and leaves of Cyperus contained 2.53% crude fat, 7.08% crude protein, 47.1% crude fiber, 10.5% ash and 7.75% sugar (in glucose) [26]. It also contained peptides, phenols, organic acids and alkaloids. These active ingredients play an important role in the fields of medicine and ecology [31]. Yan et al. conducted a qualitative analysis on the active components of Cyperus. The results showed that Cyperus contained organic acids, alkaloids, amino acids, peptides, polysaccharides, volatile oils, phenols, terpenes, anthraquinones, steroids and other active components [26]. Chukwuma et al. determined the phytochemical composition of Cyperus tubers. The results showed the presence of resins, alkaloids, cyanogenic glycosides, tannins, sterols and saponins were observed in the raw tubers, while only sterols, resins and alkaloids were observed in the roasted tuber. Meanwhile, analysis of the composition yielded saponins (0.88 ± 0.02 mg/100 g), tannins (9.50 ± 0.46 mg/100 g), oxalates (0.25 ± 0.65 mg/100 g), phytate (1.97 ± 0.81 mg/100 g) and cyanogenic glycosides (1.80 ± 0.69 mg/100 g) [7].

Cyperus (*Cyperus esculentus* L.) oil is golden in color, clear and transparent, and has a strong aroma. It is a rare raw material resource in the field of food, health products and cosmetics [32] (Table 3). From Table 3, the oleic acid content of Cyperus oil is significantly higher than that of common vegetable oils, and it does not contain erucic acid. Therefore, it is a healthy edible oil.

**Table 3.** Main fatty acid composition and content of cultivated Cyperus (*Cyperus esculentus* L.) oils compared to those of common vegetable oils (Crude oil).

| Product | Cyperus (%) | Peanut (%) | Soybean (%) | Rape (%) | Sunflower (%) | Sesame (%) |
|---|---|---|---|---|---|---|
| Scientific name | *Cyperus esculentus* | *Arachis hypogaea* | *Glycine max* | *Brassica napus* | *Helianthus annuus* | *Sesamum indicum* |
| Palmitic acid (C16:0) | 11.7–14.2 | 9.7–13.0 | 6.0–9.3 | 5.0 | 5.5 | 8.2 |
| Stearic acid (C18:0) | 1.1–4.9 | 2.7–5.0 | 3.0–5.5 | 3.6 | 2.9 | 1.9 |
| Oleic acid (C18:1) | 67.7–76.6 | 41.0–47.1 | 24.8–36.0 | 14.0–19.0 | 15.0–28.9 | 35.0–49.4 |
| Linoleic acid (C18:2) | 8.8–11.5 | 37.6 | 52.0–65.0 | 12.0–25.4 | 62.0–70.0 | 37.7–49.1 |
| Linolenic acid (C18:3) | 0.2–1.9 | – | 2.0–6.8 | 7.3–10.0 | 0.3 | 0.4 |
| Arachidic acid (C20:0) | 0.4–6.1 | 1.8–8.0 | 0.1–0.4 | 0.4–1.0 | 0.2 | 0.4–1.2 |
| Erucic acid | – | – | 0.23 | 31.0-55.0 | – | – |
| References | [25,33,34] | [35,36] | [35,36] | [35,36] | [35,36] | [35,36] |

Note: "–" indicates no report.

Cyperus oil contains 64–73.3% oleic acid and 11–15.5% linoleic acid, which is similar to olive oil (55–83% oleic acid and 3.5–21% linoleic acid) and is significantly higher than the oil contents in soybean, peanut and rapeseed oils [2,37]. It was found that Cyperus oil also contains active components such as rapeseed sterol, stigmasterol, 7-cholesterol, B-sitosterol, 24 methylene-Δ7-cholesterol, 5-oatsterol and cycloatroxanol. These plant components are important raw materials for the pharmaceutical industry [38,39].

## 3. Medicinal Research

### 3.1. Medicinal Efficacy

It is reported that the tuber of Cyperus (*Cyperus esculentus* L.) possesses an irregular fruit shape, rough surface, pungent smell, bitter taste and cool property. It has important medicinal value [25]. In India, Cyperus tuber is the oldest medicinal material, which can be used to treat critical and serious diseases (e.g., chronic gastritis, lymphatic tuberculosis, burns and scalds, coronary heart disease, acute cholecystitis, acute intracerebral hemorrhage, etc.) [40]. According to the *Xinhua outline of Materia Medica*, the tuber of Cyperus contains a kind of spicy, sweet and warm nature. It has the functions of soothing the liver, aerating and strengthening the spleen and stomach, and it can also prevent many diseases (e.g., obesity, diabetes, gastrointestinal diseases, etc.). The active ingredients of Cyperus can be used to treat chest tightness, dyspepsia, food stasis, female menstrual disorders, and so on. In Indian medical records, Cyperus has similar medicinal effects, too [41,42]. Another study showed that Cyperus contains an active component, anthraquinone (C14H8O2), which has the effects of anti-tumor, anti-oxidation and sterilization [43]. Achoribo et al. found, in their experiment, that the oleic acid contained in Cyperus oil can inhibit the overexpression of "Her-2/neu", thereby promoting the apoptosis of breast cancer cells by using "Her-2/neu" oncogene amplification [44].

Cyperus also has the effects of protecting nerves, the stomach and kidneys, strengthening yang and treating anemia. Wiebe et al. undertook a series of studies in order to indicate the central nervous system activity of the extract (Cyperol) from Cyperus (*Cyperus esculentus* L.). The results showed that Cyperol could induce changes in brain electrical activity (EEG), demonstrating that active ingredients from the extract were absorbed and were bioavailable. In summary, the results of the study indicate calming effects without sedation. The extract (Cyperol) does indeed have functional food potential and can be used to maintain a calm state of mind while dealing with cognitively demanding works [45]. Jing et al. studied the intervention effect of orientin in Cyperus on nerve injury in rats. The results showed that the orientin could significantly improve the neurological function of rats [46]. Elshamy et al. studied the effects of different concentration extracts from Cyperus on gastric ulcers induced by ethanol in rats. The results showed that the protective effect of the extract on gastric epithelial cells increased with the increase in concentration [47]. Imo Chinedu et al. examined the effects of ethanolic extracts from Cyperus (*Cyperus esculentus* L.) on selected indices of kidney function in male albino rats. The results showed the extracts had no apparent toxic effect on the kidney function of the experimental rats. The results also showed the extracts may help to reduce the retention of urea, thereby strengthening kidney functions. This plant material is therefore encouraged for use in general nutrition [48]. Nto et al. studied the intervention effect of Cyperus extracts on testicular dysfunction in Wistar rats. The results showed that Cyperus extracts significantly increased the number and volume of the epithelial cells. This finding indicates that Cyperus extracts can improve the vitality of testis in Wistar rats [49]. Jagpal studied the effects of Cyperus oils on reducing cell sickling in sickle cells anemia in vitro. The results showed that the Cyperus oil treatments resulted in an increase in the antioxidant presence of sickle cell samples when tested in vitro, as well as a morphological decrease in sickle cells and increase in spherical erythrocytes, thereby alleviating the symptoms of anemia [50]. In addition, Cyperus tubers (*Cyperus esculentus* L.) contain various compounds with intestinal health-promoting properties. Moral Anter David et al. studied the effect of Cyperus on *S. enteritidis* agglutination, oxidative stress and lactobacillus plantarum growth. The results revealed that, compared to controls, Cyperus partially restored "TER" in *S. enteritidis* infected cultures and promoted the growth of lactobacillus plantarum [51].

### 3.2. Health-Promoting Properties

Cyperus (*Cyperus esculentus* L.) is rich in fat, and the edible oil (Cyperus oil) can be extracted from it. Cyperus oil has a mellow taste and stable chemical properties, and it is clear and transparent, not easy to corrupt and very easy to be absorbed and utilized by the human body. It is a very high-quality edible oil [52]. The main components of Cyperus oil are unsaturated fatty acids (oleic acid and linoleic acid). Linoleic acid is an essential fatty acid for the human body. It is an important substance for the synthesis of prostaglandins. It can regulate physiological functions of the human body, promote the growth and development of the human body, promote the catabolism of cholesterol in the body, and it can prevent cardiovascular diseases. Cyperus oil is also rich in minerals, but the content of sodium is very low and does not contain cholesterol, which is very close to olive oil, hazelnut oil and avocado oil [53]. It is also reported that the content of sterols in Cyperus oil is about 1000 $\mu g \cdot g^{-1}$, which is significantly higher than that in olive oil (about 100 $\mu g \cdot g^{-1}$). These sterols in Cyperus oil could reduce the absorption of cholesterol and reduce the risk of cardiovascular disease [30]. Bamishaiye et al. studied the effects of Cyperus oil and soybean oil on tissue metabolism in rats. The results showed that, compared with feeding soybean oil, the treatments of feeding Cyperus oil significantly reduced the content of total cholesterol in rats [54]. Moon et al. studied the effect of Cyperus oil meal on lipid metabolism in mice. The results showed that Cyperus oil meal significantly reduced the increase of adipocyte volume, adipose tissue weight and body weight caused by high-fat diet, and it significantly reduced the contents of total cholesterol and triglyceride in serum and triglyceride in liver. The results showed that Cyperus is beneficial in preventing hyperlipidemia caused by diet [55]. Salem M L et al. studied the effects of Cyperus tubers on mice with atherosclerotic disease. The results showed that feeding Cyperus tubers to mice significantly alleviated the symptoms of atherosclerosis in mice [56]. According to research by Oluwajuyitan and others, Cyperus is a food that lowers the glycemic index, and it is suitable for diabetics [57]. Another study showed that Cyperus is a pollution-free and nutritious food raw material with the function of protecting the liver [58]. Onuoha et al. studied the protective effect of Cyperus milk on liver injury induced by acetaminophen (APAP). The results showed that Cyperus milk could significantly improve liver injury induced by acetaminophen (APAP) [59]. Hassanein et al. studied the protective effect of Cyperus essential oil on the hepatotoxicity induced by paracetamol. The results showed that the concentration of the essential oil at 12.5 $\mu g/mL$ has a protective effect on the hepatotoxicity induced by paracetamol [60].

### 3.3. Antibacterial Activity

It is reported that Cyperus (*Cyperus esculentus* L.) contains a variety of active components, and most of its extracts have antibacterial effect [41]. Prakash et al. prepared different extracts of Cyperus, such as acetone, 50% ethanol, chloroform and petroleum ether to evaluate for their antibacterial activity against several human pathogens (*Escherichia coli, Staphylococcus aureus, Salmonella* sp, *Klebsiella pneumoniae, Proteus vulgaris, Pseudomonas aeruginosa* and *Citrobacter freundii*) by using the disc diffusion method. The acetone extract showed the highest inhibitory activity against *S. aureus, ILpneumoniae* and *P. vulgaris*. Furthermore, 50% ethanolic extract showed the maximum activity against *Escherichia coli, S. aureus* and *Salmonella* sp. Chloroform extract maximally inhibited the growth of *S. aureus*, whereas petroleum ether extract showed positive results against *Salmonella* sp., respectively. All extracts were sensitive to *C. freundii* [61]. Abdel et al. evaluated the antibacterial activity of Cyperus (*Cyperus esculentus* L.) oil via cup plate agar diffusion assay against six standard human pathogens (Gram positive: *Staphylococcus aureus* and *Bacillus subtilis*; Gram negative: *Escherichia coli, Pseudomonasa aeruginosa, the fungi Candida albicans* and *Aspergillus niger*). The oil showed different antimicrobial responses against testing organisms. It showed significant activity against the fungus *Candida albicans* and partial activity against *Staphylococcus aureus* [62]. Salem et al. studied the effect of Cyperus tubers on the reduction in atherosclerotic lesions in mice. The results indicated that the ingredients of Cyperus tubers exhibit anti-inflammatory properties upon inflammation and immunostimulatory effects in immunocompetent hosts [56].

### *3.4. Antioxidant Activity*

Some studies showed that Cyperus (*Cyperus esculentus* L.) contains secondary metabolites of flavonoids, which showed antioxidant activity and an anticoagulant effect [63]. Jing et al. studied the antioxidant activity of the extracts from Cyperus. The results showed that the activities of superoxide dismutase (SOD) in liver tissue and serum of mice were significantly increased by different concentrations (high, medium and low) [64]. Willis et al. studied the antioxidant activities of water and methanol extracts from Cyperus. The results showed that both extracts had scavenging effects on free radicals [65]. Badejo et al. mixed Cyperus milk, ginger juice and water (7:1:2) to make a Cyperus mixed beverage, and they studied its effect of scavenging free radical. The results showed that the scavenging rate of free radical (DPPH) was 32.53% [66]. Another study found that the germinated tubers of Cyperus could further improve antioxidant activity [67,68]. Siqun Jing et al. evaluated the antioxidant activity and antibacterial property of the flavonoids from Cyperus (*Cyperus esculentus* L.) leaves. In all the assays, Cyperus leaves flavonoids had pronounced antioxidant activity in vivo that could significantly elevate the content of superoxide dismutase (SOD). Cyperus leaves flavonoids inhibited the growth of both Gram-positive and Gram-negative bacteria. The results indicate that the flavonoids from Cyperus leaves can be taken as a natural antioxidant and bacteriostatic substance in the food and pharmaceutical industry [69].

## 4. Allelopathic Potential

### *4.1. Impacts on Crops*

It is reported that Cyperus has a strong allelopathic effect (inhibition) on many crops [70]. Dirk et al. studied the allelopathic effect of extracts and plant residues of Cyperus (*Cyperus esculentus* L.) on the growth of corn (*Zea mays* L.) and soybean (*Glycine max* L.) and found that tuber residues reduced the dry weight of corn and soybean more than foliage residues. As the concentration increased, the growth decreased, affecting soybean more than corn. Soybean growth was significantly reduced by the addition of tuber extracts. Growth inhibition was greatest when the tuber residue was in contact with the corn or soybean seeds [71]. This shows that extracts and residues of Cyperus have an allelopathic effect on corn and soybean. Reinhardt et al. studied the allelopathic effects of Cyperus (*Cyperus esculentus* L.) tubers on ectomycorrhiza (*Boletus*), lettuce (*Lactuca sativa*) and corn (*Zea mays*), and they further evaluated the allelopathic potential of Cyperus. The results showed that the aqueous extracts from Cyperus tubers significantly reduced the colony diameter of the ectomycorrhiza (*Boletus*) on agar medium. At 2% concentration, the aqueous extracts inhibited the germination of lettuce (*Lactuca sativa*) seeds significantly. The emergence of corn (*Zea mays* L.) was retarded in soil where Cyperus tubers were planted 28 days before planting the crop, irrespective of whether the Cyperus tubers continued to grow or were physically removed at the time the corn was sown. This shows that the root exudates or residues of Cyperus have an inhibitory effect on corn seed germination [72]. Later, H.P. Oamen et al. studied the allelopathic effects of aqueous extracts of *Cyperus esculentus* L. on the germination and seedling growth of *Cajanus cajan* L., *Phaseolus vulgaris* (brown and white varieties) and *Sphenotylis stenocarpa*. The results showed that the extracts have significant positive allelopathic effects on plumule and radicle lengths at $p < 0.05$. The number of root hairs for *C. cajan* was reduced at higher concentrations [73]. Papadi Asimina et al. studied the allelopathic potential of Cyperus (*Cyperus esculentus* L.) on the germination of the seeds of six commonly grown crops (*Zea mays* L., *Citrullus lanatus Thunb*, *Abelmoschus esculentus* (L), *Vigna unguiculata* (L), *Glycine max* (L) and *Arachis hypogaea* (L.).

The results showed that the aqueous extracts from Cyperus reduced the germination counts of the seeds by 10 to 100%. Cyperus shoot extracts were the most phytotoxic. In addition, the decomposing mulches showed varied but less inhibitory effects on the seeds with a trend toward increasing the inhibitory effect with an increasing mulch level and decreasing seed size [70]. Singh C.M. et al. studied the allelopathic effects of Cyperus (*Cyperus esculentus* L.) on the seed germination and seeding growth of wheat. The results showed that the extracts from Cyperus had inhibitory effects on the germination of wheat seeds. The time taken for germination prolonged; root, shoot and leaf developments were seriously inhibited. The findings of this study clearly indicate that before using the Cyperus for manuring in wheat fields, it would be safe to carry out a detailed field experiment to ascertain the allelopathic effects [74]. JJ Sani et al. evaluated the allelopathic effects of extracts from the aerial and underground organs of Cyperus (*Cyperus esculentus* L.) with three levels of extract (5, 10 and 20 percent) on rapeseed germination and growth. The results showed that the extract of Cyperus reduced rapeseed germination and growth. With increasing concentration of extracts, germination rate, germination percent, vigor index, root and shoot length were significantly reduced [75]. M.G. Patterson et al. conducted a series of experiments, from 1976 to 978, to determine the competitive relationship of Cyperus (*Cyperus esculentus* L.) with cotton. In the experiments, Cyperus was left undisturbed or removed from plots to give periods of competition of 2, 4, 6, 8, 10 and 25 weeks. The results showed that the seed cotton yield was reduced in 2 out of the 3 years in a full season (25 weeks) of competition but was unaffected by shorter periods of competition in all years. The main stem diameter of cotton was also reduced 2 out of the 3 years when competing the full season, while the main stem height was reduced in only 1 out of the 3 years in a full season competition [76].

### 4.2. *Phytoinsecticide*

Avicor et al. investigated the larvicidal potential of crude aqueous extracts from two Cyperus (*Cyperus esculentus* L.) varieties (black and yellow) on the mosquitoes *Aedes aegypti* (L.) and Culex *quinquefasciatus* (Say). Differential larvicidal responses were observed in the test mosquitoes, and extracts of black dried Cyperus were more larvicidal than yellow dried Cyperus. The results indicated the potential of Cyperus, particularly black dried Cyperus, as a resource of mosquito insecticide [77]. Based on the research results in this area, Cyperus (*Cyperus esculentus* L.) has great potential in developing phytoinsecticide and reducing people's dependence on synthetic insecticides.

## 5. Future Areas of Research

The following studies need be conducted in the future: (i) Preliminary indications suggest that the extract (Cyperol) from Cyperus (*Cyperus esculentus* L.) may have anxiolytic potential [45], which should be explored in clinical studies. (ii) The extraction and identification of allelochemicals from Cyperus. (iii) The allelopathic effects of extracts and decomposed substances from Cyperus on main crops (e.g., soybeans, corn, wheat, etc.) and its autotoxicity. (iv) The allelopathic effects of extracts and substances from decomposed Cyperus on soil microflora and activity. (v) The development of new allelopathic varieties of Cyperus. (vi) The larvicidal potential and identification of the extracts from Cyperus. Furthermore, (vii) studies on the medicinal efficacy and antibacterial potential of Cyperus should also be conducted in the future.

## 6. Conclusions

Some studies have been carried out on the chemical components, active substances and allelopathy of Cyperus (*Cyperus esculentus* L.), and it has been found that it has medicinal efficacy and antibacterial potential, but these studies are not detailed and in-depth enough. Therefore, it is necessary to study and evaluate its active components and antibacterial and insecticidal potential in more detail, in order to provide a scientific basis for the further development and utilization of Cyperus. In addition, Cyperus has strong allelopathy to many crops, and it inhibits the growth of adjacent crops. At the same time, Cyperus (*Cyperus esculentus* L.) has great potential in developing phytoinsecticide. Research on the allelopathy of Cyperus has a bright future in reducing our reliance on synthetic pesticides and promoting the sustainable development of Cyperus cropping.

**Author Contributions:** Conceptualization, S.Z. and Z.M.; methodology, P.L.; software, Z.W.; validation, Y.W.; formal analysis, P.L.; investigation, Y.C.; resources, J.L.; data curation, Y.Y.; writing—original draft preparation, S.Z. and Z.W.; writing—review and editing, Y.W. and Z.M. All authors have read and agreed to the published version of the manuscript.

**Funding:** Innovation of germplasm resources and breeding of new varieties of Cyperus (*Cyperus esculentus* L.) based on biotechnology (CXGC2021TD013).

**Institutional Review Board Statement:** Not applicable.

**Informed Consent Statement:** Not applicable.

**Data Availability Statement:** Not applicable.

**Acknowledgments:** This work was financially supported by the Agricultural Science and Technology Innovation project of Jilin Province "Innovation of germplasm resources and breeding of new varieties of Cyperus (*Cyperus esculentus* L.) based on biotechnology (CXGC2021TD013)". The authors thank Yuyan Wang and Zhongsheng Mu for their contributions to the preparation and publication of the paper. Compliance with ethical standards.

**Conflicts of Interest:** The authors declare no conflict of interest.

## References

1. Michael, S. Defelice. Yellow nutsedge *Cyperus esculentus* L.: Snack food of the gods. *Weed Technol.* **2002**, *16*, 901–907.
2. Oderinde, R.A.; Tairu, O.A. Evaluation of the properties of yellow nut sedge (*Cyperus esculentus*) tuber oil. *Food Chem.* **1988**, *28*, 233–237. [CrossRef]
3. Yang, Z. Characteristics and Research Progress of *Cyperus esculentus* L. *North. Hortic.* **2017**, *17*, 192–201. (In Chinese)
4. Coskuner, Y.; Ercan, R.; Karababa, E.; Nazlican, A.N. Physical and chemical properties of chufa (*Cyperus esculentus* L.) tubers grown in the C, ukurova region of Turkey. *J. Sci. Food Agric.* **2002**, *82*, 625–631. [CrossRef]
5. Negbi, M. A sweetmeat plant, a perfume plant and their weedy relatives: A chapter in the history of *Cyperus esculentus* L. and *C. rotundus* L. *Econ. Bot.* **1992**, *46*, 64–71. [CrossRef]
6. Li, G.; Yang, L.; Zhu, Z.; Cai, B.; Kang, X. Study on Preparation of Biodiesel from Cyperus Oil. *China Grease* **2012**, *37*, 59–62.
7. Chukwuma, E.R.; Obioma, N.; Cristopher, O.I. The phytochemical composition and some biochemical effects of Nigerian tiger nut (*Cyperus esculentus* L.) tuber. *Pak. J. Nutr.* **2010**, *9*, 709–715. [CrossRef]
8. Femke, T.; de Vries, C. (*Cyperus esculentus, Cyperaceae*): A weedy cultivar or a cultivated weed. *Econ. Bot.* **1991**, *45*, 27–37.
9. Fu, L.; Li, G.; Liu, Y. Analysis and Study on Components of *Cyperus esculentus* Used as Soil, Grain and Feed Crop. *J. Zhengzhou Grain College* **1996**, *7*, 88–90.
10. Mokady, S.H.; Dolev, A. Nutritional evaluation of tubers of *Cyperus esculentus* L. *J. Sci. Food Agric.* **1970**, *21*, 211–214. [CrossRef]
11. Yu, H.; Jing, S. Research Progress on chemical constituents and application of Cyperus. *Food Ind.* **2015**, *36*, 242–245.
12. Yu, Y.; Lu, X.; Zhang, T.; Zhao, C.; Guan, S.; Pu, Y.; Gao, F. Tiger Nut (*Cyperus esculentus* L.): Nutrition, Processing, Function and Applications. *Foods* **2022**, *11*, 601. [CrossRef] [PubMed]
13. Taiyuan, S.; Miao, Y.; Yanqiu, H. Analysis on the Nutrients and Characteristic of Liaoning Peanut Varieties. *Food Res. Dev.* **2017**, *11*, 142–147.
14. Pickett, T.A. Composition of developing peanut seed. *Plant Physiol.* **1950**, *25*, 210–224. [CrossRef]
15. Asare, P.A.; Kpankpari, R.; Adu, M.O.; Afutu, E.; Adewumi, A.S. Phenotypic Characterization of Tiger Nuts (*Cyperus esculentus* L.) from Major Growing Areas in Ghana. *Sci. World J.* **2020**, *1*, 1–11. [CrossRef] [PubMed]
16. Aochen, L. Main Nutrientional Components and Values of Soybean. *Mod. Agric. Sci. Technol.* **2020**, *23*, 213–218.
17. Zhang, Y.; Hu, R.; Lin, G. Preliminary study on the content of soluble sugar and starch in soybean seeds. *Fujian J. Agric. Sci.* **2018**, *33*, 604–607.
18. Guillon, F.; Champ, M.M.-J. Carbohydrate fractions of legumes: Uses in human nutrition and potential for health. *Br. J. Nutr.* **2002**, *88*, 293–306. [CrossRef]
19. Zhenqian, Z.; Biqing, W.; Guohuai, W.; Chunyun, G.; Sheyuan, C. Study on physiological and biochemical characteristics of early maturing rape Varieties. *Crop Res.* **2014**, *28*, 349–353.
20. Yajun, Y.; Xiangyu, Z.; Yu, Z. Study on the changes of main nutrients in rapeseed during ripening. *Food Ind. Technol.* **2015**, *36*, 339–342.

21. Tipoina, H.H.; Yanxia, L. Comparative Analysis on the Composition and Function of Pine Nuts and Several Oil Crops. *J. Jilin Agric. Sci. Technol. Univ.* **2015**, *24*, 4–8.
22. Li, P.-J.; Li, B.-J.; Nan, W.; Mi, Y.; Liao, F.; Li, G. Discriminatory analysis on the morphology and major components of kernels of the edible and oil-type sunflowers. *J. Sichuan Univ. (Nat. Sci. Ed.)* **2017**, *54*, 203–208.
23. Wang, X.; Cui, Y.; Liu, B.; Ma, S. Correlation analysis of various components in sesame. *China Oils Fats* **2015**, *40*, 99–103.
24. Li, T.; Miao, H.; Wang, X.; Wang, D. Changes of main nutritional components and in vitro antioxidant activity of polysaccharide extracts in sesame leaves at different growth periods. *J. Henan Univ. Technol. (Nat. Sci. Ed. )* **2020**, *41*, 42–49.
25. Guo, T.; Wan, C.; Huang, F.; Wei, C.; Hu, Z. Research Progress on main nutritional components and physiological functions of tiger nut (*Cyperus esculentus* L.). *Chin. J. Oil Crop Sci.* **2021**, *43*, 1174–1180.
26. Yan, X.; Ren, Z.; Xiang, H.; Jing, S. Qualitative analysis of active components in Cyperus. *China Brew.* **2010**, *8*, 150–151.
27. Buweizuohere, A.; Deping, W.; Siqun, J.; Yixian, T. Research progress on bioactivity of total flavonoids in *Cyperus esculentus* L. leaves. *Cereals Oils* **2021**, *34*, 21–26.
28. Zhai, H.; Wang, D.; Jing, S. Effects of *Cyperus esculentus* total flavonoids on milk fresh-keeping. *Food Ind. Technol.* **2004**, *25*, 69–70.
29. Chen, X.; Chen, D.; Liu, L. *Cyperus esculentus* whole component analysis. *Food Sci. Technol.* **2009**, *34*, 165–168.
30. Liu, L. Study on the Active Ingredients of *Cyperus Esculentus* and Oil Extraction Technology. Masters's Thesis, Northeast Normal University, Changchun, China, 2008; pp. 1–5.
31. Liu, Z.; Jin, Z.; Zhou, X.; Bian, Y.; Bai, W. Extraction and determination of protein, fat and sugar in Cyperus. *J. Inn. Mong. Norm. Univ. Natl. (Nat. Sci. Ed.)* **1988**, *13*, 62–65.
32. Hu, B.; Zhou, K.; Liu, Y.T. Optimization of microwave-assisted extraction of oil from tiger nut (*Cyperus esculentus* L.) and its quality evaluation. *Ind. Crops Prod.* **2018**, *115*, 290–297. [CrossRef]
33. Linssen, J.P.H.; Kielman, G.M.; Cozijnsen, J.L.; Pilnik, W. Comparison of chufa and olive oils. *Food Chem.* **1988**, *28*, 279–285. [CrossRef]
34. Muhammad, N.O.; Bamishaiye, E.I.; Bamishaiye, O.M.; Usman, L.A.; Salawu, M.O.; Nafiu, M.O.; Oloyede, O.B. Physicochemical properties and fatty acid composition of *Cyperus esculentus* (Tiger Nut) tuber oil. *Biorearch Bull.* **2011**, *5*, 51–54.
35. Ezeh, O.; Gordon, M.H.; Niranjan, K. Tiger nut oil (*Cyperus esculentus* L.): A review of its composition and physic-chemical properties. *Eur. J. Lipid Sci. Technol.* **2014**, *116*, 783–794. [CrossRef]
36. Shi, X.; Tian, L.; Xue, L.; Wang, X.; Zhu, J. Analysis and comparison of main fatty acids among Cyperus oil and other vegetable oils. *Food Ind.* **2016**, *37*, 52–54.
37. Duan, L.; Han, M.; Wei, Z.; Wu, X. Microwave assisted extraction and fatty acid analysis of Cyperus oil. *Cereals Oils* **2021**, *34*, 59–62.
38. Olabiyi, A.A.; Oboh, G.; Adefegha, S.A. Effect of dietary supplementation of tiger nut (*Cyperus esculentus* L.) and walnut (*Tetracarpidium conophorum* müll. Arg.) on sexual behavior, hormonal level, and antioxidant status in male rats. *J. Food Biochem.* **2017**, *41*, 66–75. [CrossRef]
39. Chao, X.; Li, Y.; Jing, S.; Zhai, Y.; Liu, G.; Zhang, J.; Qi, K.; Zhu, X.; Buwizogher, A. Analysis of Nutrient Composition and Bioactivity of *Cyperus esculentus* (*C. esculentus* L.) before and after Germination. *Sci. Technol. Food Ind.* **2021**, *42*, 327–333. (In Chinese)
40. Jebasingh, D.; Venkataraman, S.; Jackson, D.D. Physiochemical and toxicological studies of the medicinal plant *Cyperus rotundus* L. (Cyperaceae). *Int. J. Appl. Res. Nat. Prod.* **2012**, *5*, 1–8.
41. Chen, Z.; Hu, X.; Liu, P.; Bai, C.; Liu, G. Research Progresses on Cultivation and Utilization of *Cyperus esculentus*. *Chin. J. Trop. Agric.* **2017**, *37*, 56–60.
42. Liu, H.; Wang, L.; Liu, Y. Development status of Cyperus products in China. *Farm Prod. Process.* **2021**, *7*, 97–99.
43. Hu, G. Study on Synthesis of Anthraquinones and Their Cytotoxic Activity against Tumor Cells. Master's Thesis, Lanzhou University, Lanzhou, China, 2014; pp. 5–11.
44. Achoribo, E.S.; Ong, M.T. Tiger nut (*Cyperus esculentus*): Source of natural anticancer drug? Brief review of existing literature. *Euromediterranean Biomed. J.* **2017**, *12*, 91–94.
45. Wiebe, J.C.; Lópezríos, L.; Vegamorales, T.; Gericke, N. Neurophysiological effects of a special extract of *Cyperus esculentus* L. (Cyperol). *J. Herb. Med. Res.* **2019**, *4*, 34. [CrossRef]
46. Jing, S.Q.; Wang, S.S.; Zhong, R.M.; Zhang, J.Y.; Wu, J.Z.; Tu, Y.X.; Pu, Y.; Yan, L.J. Neuroprotection of *Cyperus esculentus* L. orientin against cerebral ischemia/reperfusion induced brain injury. *Neural Regen. Res.* **2020**, *15*, 548–556. [CrossRef] [PubMed]
47. Elshamy, A.I.; Farrag, A.R.H.; Ayoub, I.M. UPLC-qTOF-MS phytochemical profile and antiulcer potential of Cyperus conglomeratus rottb. alcoholic extract. *Molecules* **2020**, *18*, 4234. [CrossRef]
48. Imo, C.; Uzochukwuw, C.D.; Mamma, E.; Mayel, M.H.; Kukoyi, A.J.; David Apaj, A. Effects of Ethanolic Extracts of Phoenix dactylifera Fruit, Cyperus esculentus Nut and Cocos nucifera Nut on Selected Indices of Kidney Function in Male Albino Rats. *J. Appl. Sci.* **2018**, *18*, 116–121. [CrossRef]
49. Nto, N.; Hassan, L.; Anyanwu, G.; Obikili, E.; Finbarrs-Bello, E.; Abireh, L. Curative effect of aqueous extract of *Cyperus esculentus* on flutamide-induced testicular dysfunction in male Wistar rats. *J. Exp. Clin. Cancer Res.* **2018**, *17*, 13. [CrossRef]
50. Jagpal, C. The in vitro use of natural antioxidant oils (*Cyperus esculentus; Nigella sativa*) to reduce cell sickling in sickle cell anaemia. *Biochem. Pharmacol.* **2017**, *139*, 134. [CrossRef]

51. Moral-Anter, D.; Campo-Sabariz, J.; Ferrer, R.; Martín-Venegas, R. *Cyperus esculentus* L. Tubers (Tiger Nuts) Protect Epithelial Barrier Function in Caco-2 Cells Infected by Salmonella Enteritidis and Promote Lactobacillus plantarum Growth. *Nutrients* **2020**, *13*, 71. [CrossRef]
52. Huang, M.; Wang, X.; Pang, Z. Research Status and Prospect of *Cyperus esculentus* L. *Crop Res.* **2013**, *27*, 293–301.
53. Gao, Y.; Sun, Y.; Gao, H.; Chen, Y.; Wang, X.; Xue, J.; Jia, X.; Li, R. Correction to: Ectopic overexpression of a type-II DGAT (CeDGAT2-2) derived from oil-rich tuber of *Cyperus esculentus* enhances accumulation of oil and oleic acid in tobacco leaves. *Biotechnol. Biofuels* **2021**, *14*, 51–56. [CrossRef] [PubMed]
54. Bamishaiye, E.I.; Muhammad, N.O.; Bamishaiye, O.M. Histological changes and serum lipid profile of selected rat tissues fed on *Cyperus esculentus* (tiger nut) tuber oil meal-based diet. *Der Pharma Chem.* **2010**, *2*, 90–96.
55. Moon, M.K.; Ahn, J.; Lee, H.; Ha, T.J. Anti-obesity and hypo-lipidemic effects of chufa (*Cyperus esculentus* L.) in mice fed a high-fat diet. *Food Sci. Biotechnol.* **2012**, *21*, 317–322. [CrossRef]
56. Salem, M.L.; Zommara, M.; Imaizumi, K. Dietary supplementation with *Cyperus esculentus* L. (tiger nut) tubers attenuated atherosclerotic lesion in apolipoprotein E knockout mouse associated with inhibition of inflammatory cell responses. *Am. J. Immunol.* **2005**, *1*, 60–67. [CrossRef]
57. Oluwajuyitan, T.D.; Ijarotimi, O.S. Nutritional, antioxidant, glycaemic index and Antihyperglycaemic properties of improved traditional plantain-based (Musa AAB) dough meal enriched with tiger nut (*Cyperus esculentus*) and defatted soybean(*Glycine max*)flour for diabetic patients. *Heliyon* **2019**, *5*, 22–29. [CrossRef] [PubMed]
58. Saheed, S.; Oladipipo, A.E.; Abraham, B.F. Four weeksdaily dose oral administration assessment of *Cyperus esculentus* L. aqueous extract on key metabolic markers of Wistar rats. *Pharmacologia* **2016**, *7*, 125–133. [CrossRef]
59. Onuoha, N.; Ogbusua, N.; Okorie, A.; Ejike, C.E. Tiger nut (*Cyperus esculentus* L.) 'milk' as a potent 'nutri-drink' for the prevention of acetaminophen-induced hepatotoxicity in a murine model. *J. Intercult. Ethnopharmacol.* **2017**, *6*, 290–295. [CrossRef]
60. Hassanein, H.M.; Nazif, N.M.; Aboutabl, E.A.; Hammouda, F.M. In-vitro hepatoprotection study, free radical scavenging activity and gc/ms analysis of *Cyperus esculentus* essential oils from hydrodistillation and mae techniques. *Planta Med.* **2013**, *79*, 312–320. [CrossRef]
61. Prakash, N.; Ragavan, B. Phytochemical observation and antibacterial activity of *Cyperus esculentus* L. *Anc. Sci. Life* **2009**, *28*, 16–20.
62. Abdel Karim, M.; Fath Elrahman, A. GC-MS analysis and antimicrobial activity of sudanese *Cyperus esculentus* (Cyperaceae) fixed oil. *Int. J. Adv. Res.* **1930**, *2016*, 256–263.
63. Su, L.; Wang, S.; Jing, S. Preliminary study on microcirculation and anticoagulant activity of alcohol extract of Cyperus (*Cyperus esculentus* L.). *Food Ind.* **2017**, *38*, 200–203.
64. Jing, S.; Ouyang, W.; Ren, Z.; Ma, Z. In vitro and in vivo antioxidant properties of *Cyperus esculentus* oil from Xinjiang, China. *J. Sci. Food Agric.* **2013**, *93*, 505–509. [CrossRef] [PubMed]
65. Willis, S.; Jackson, C.; Verghese, M. Effects of processing on antioxidant capacity and metabolizing enzyme inhibition of tiger nut tubers. *Food Nutr. Sci.* **2019**, *10*, 1132–1141. [CrossRef]
66. Badejo, A.A.; Olawoyin, B.; Salawu, S.O.; Fasuhanmi, O.S.; Boligon, A.A.; Enujiugha, V.N. Antioxidative potentials and chromatographic analysis of beverages from blends of glutenfree acha (*Digitaria exilis*) and tiger nut (*Cyperus esculentus*) extracts. *J. Food Meas. Charact.* **2017**, *11*, 2094–2101. [CrossRef]
67. Ademosun, A.O.; Oboh, G. Inhibition of carbohydrate hydrolyzing enzymes associated with type 2 diabetes and antioxidative properties of some edible seeds in vitro. *Int. J. Diabetes Dev. Ctries.* **2015**, *35*, 516–521. [CrossRef]
68. Adebayo, S.F.; Arinola, S.O. Effect of germination on the nutrient and antioxidant properties of tiger nut (*Cyperus esculentus*). *Biol. Agric. Healthc.* **2017**, *7*, 88–94.
69. Jing, S.; Wang, S.; Li, Q.; Zheng, L.; Yue, L.; Fan, S.; Tao, G. Dynamic high pressure microfluidization-assisted extraction and bioactivities of *Cyperus esculentus* (*C. esculentus* L.) leaves flavonoids. *Food Chem.* **2016**, *192*, 319–327. [CrossRef]
70. Papadi, A.; Oluwale, B.; Ismail, K. Allelopathic Effect of Some Weeds on the Germination of Seeds of Selected Crops Grown in Akwa Ibom State, Nigeria. *World J. Agric. Res.* **2013**, *1*, 59–64.
71. Drost, D.C.; Doll, J.D. The Allelopathic Effect of Yellow Nutsedge (*Cyperus esculentus*) on Corn (*Zea mays*) and Soybeans (*Glycine max*). *Weed Sci.* **1980**, *28*, 229–233. [CrossRef]
72. Reinhardt, C.F.; Bezuidenhout, S.R. Growth Stage of *Cyperus esculentus* Influences Its Allelopathic Effect on Ectomycorrhizal and Higher Plant Species. *J. Crop Prod.* **2001**, *4*, 323–333. [CrossRef]
73. Oamen, H.P.; Idu, M. Allelopathic effects of aqueous extract of Cyperus esculentus L. on germination and seedling growth of some bean seeds. *Asian J. Microbiol. Biotechnol. Environ. Sci.* **2009**, *11*, 705–710.
74. Singh, C.M.; Angiras, N.N.; Singh, S.D. Allelopathic Effects of Some Weeds on Wheat Seed Germination. *Indian J. Weed Sci.* **1988**, *20*, 63–66.
75. Sani, J.J.; Rahimi, A.; Hosseini, S.M.; Mirik, A.A.M. Allelopathic Effect of Nutsedge Weeds (*Cyperus esculentus* L.) and Redroot Pigweed (*Amaranthus retroflexus* L.) Plants Extracts on Germination and Seedling Growth of Rapeseed (*Brassica napus*). *Weed Sci.* **2012**, *6*, 27–36.

76. Patterson, M.G.; Buchanan, G.A.; Street, J.E.; Crowley, R.H. Yellow Nutsedge (*Cyperus esculentus*) Competition with Cotton (*Gossypium hirsutum*). *Weed Sci.* **1980**, *28*, 327–329. [CrossRef]
77. Avicor, S.W.; Wajidi, M.F.F.; Achoribo, E.S.; Ong, M.T.; Hamzah, S.N. Tiger nut (*Cyperus esculentus*) as a potential phytoinsecticide: Larvicidal activity of crude extracts on Aedes aegypti and Culex quinquefasciatus (Diptera: Culicidae). *Trop. Biomed.* **2021**, *38*, 186–191.

*plants*

MDPI

*Review*

# Allelopathy and Allelochemicals of *Solidago canadensis* L. and *S. altissima* L. for Their Naturalization

**Hisashi Kato-Noguchi * and Midori Kato**

Department of Applied Biological Science, Faculty of Agriculture, Kagawa University, Miki, Kagawa 761-0795, Japan
* Correspondence: kato.hisashi@kagawa-u.ac.jp

**Abstract:** *Solidago canadensis* L. and *Solidago altissima* L. are native to North America and have naturalized many other continents including Europa and Asia. Their species is an aggressive colonizer and forms thick monospecific stands. The evidence of the allelopathy for *S. canadensis* and *S. altissima* has accumulated in the literature since the late 20th century. The root exudates, extracts, essential oil and rhizosphere soil of *S. canadensis* suppressed the germination, growth and the arbuscular mycorrhizal colonization of several plants, including native plant species. Allelochemicals such as fatty acids, terpenes, flavonoids, polyphenols and their related compounds were identified in the extracts and essential oil of *S. canadensis*. The concentrations of total phenolics, total flavonoids and total saponins in the rhizosphere soil of *S. canadensis* obtained from the invasive ranges were greater than those from the native ranges. Allelochemicals such as terpenes, flavonoids, polyacetylene and phenols were also identified in the extracts, essential oil and the rhizosphere soil in *S. altissima*. Among the identified allelochemicals of *S. altissima*, the *cis*-dehydromatricaria ester may be involved in the allelopathy considering its growth inhibitory activity and its concentration in the rhizosphere soil. Therefore, the allelopathy of *S. canadensis* and *S. altissima* may support their invasiveness, naturalization and formation of thick monospecific stands. This is the first review article focusing on the allelopathy of both of *S. canadensis* and *S. altissima*.

**Keywords:** allelochemical; invasive species; monospecific stand; mycorrhizal colonization; *Solidago*; phytotoxicity; rhizosphere soil

**Citation:** Kato-Noguchi, H.; Kato, M. Allelopathy and Allelochemicals of *Solidago canadensis* L. and *S. altissima* L. for Their Naturalization. *Plants* **2022**, *11*, 3235. https://doi.org/10.3390/plants11233235

Academic Editors: Margot Schulz and Vincenzo Tabaglio

Received: 22 October 2022
Accepted: 23 November 2022
Published: 25 November 2022



## 1. Introduction

*Solidago canadensis* sensu lato (s.l.), belonging Asteraceae, is an erect rhizomatous perennial plant, native to North America. *S. canadensis* s.l. was introduced to Europe as an ornamental plant in the 17th to 18th centuries. The species spread from the gardens to the natural environments, and has extended its habitats in Central and Eastern Europe. It expanded its habitat at a rate of 741 $km^2$ per year in Europe [1]. The species has also been introduced and naturalized in many other countries such as Australia, Brazil, China, India, New Zealand and Japan [2–6].

The species expands its habitat though seed distribution and rhizome expansion. The rhizomes arise near the base of the shoots in autumn and produce aerial stems from their apex in the following spring. The stems are not branched, and bear triple-nerved, lanceolate, alternate leaves which are found along the stems and roots at the base of the shoots. The rhizome systems contribute to expanding the species' community and to form thick monospecific stands [7,8]. Shoot density in the established stands of the species was reported to be 309 shoots per $m^2$ [3]. In addition, oil-filled cavities, which contain terpenes and/or lipids, were randomly distributed in the rhizomes [9]. These compounds may have some biological functions such as allelopathy. The species is a prolific seed producer. Its inflorescence forms broad pyramidal panicles, which contain numerous florets (Figure 1). A single plant produces 1000–20,000 light-winged achenes which contain seeds. The achenes disperse easily by wind, water and human activities. The germination rate is 30–75%, depending on the conditions [7,8,10,11]. The seed distribution may contribute to establishing the populations of *S. canadensis* s.l. in new habitats.

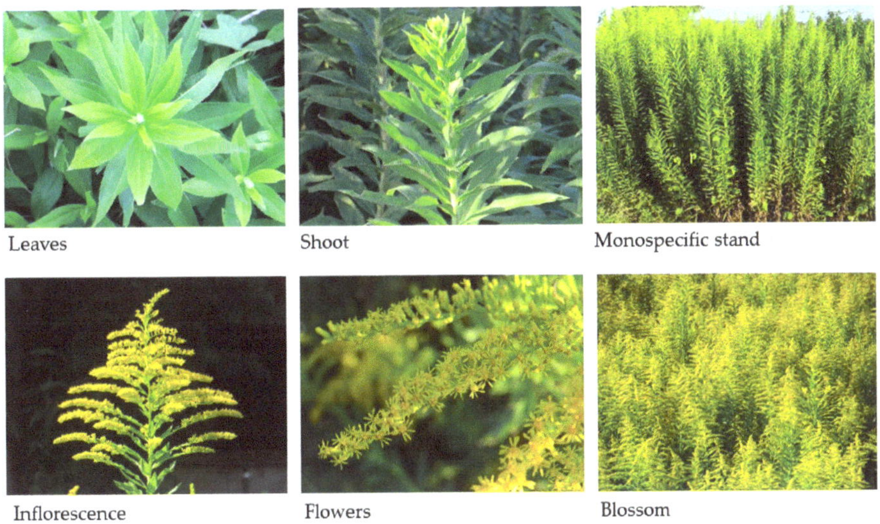


**Figure 1.** *Solidago canadensis* s.l.

This species has adapted to a wide range of soil fertility and water potential [8,11,12], as well as been colonized into disturbed areas such as abandoned fields, roadsides, riverbanks and forest edges [11,13,14]. The species established its population on an agriculture field in two years after the abandonment [15,16]. Once established, the population remained dominant over 30 years [8,17–20]. It was also reported that the species showed great impact on the native plant diversity in the introduced ranges [21–23]. Owing to the potential of the species for the rapid expansion and the formation of thick monospecific stands in the introduced ranges, as well as its impact on the environments, *S. canadensis* s.l. has been designated as a harmful invasive plant species [4,24].

The *S. canadensis* complex is a highly variable species. *S. canadensis* s.l. contains *S. canadensis* L. as *S. canadensis* subsp. *canadensis* (L.), and *S. altissima* L. as *S. canadensis* subsp. *altissima* (L.) O.Bolòs et Vigo [2,25,26]. *S. canadensis* and *S. altissima* are very similar taxa. The field experiments also showed that the competitive abilities of *S. altissima* and *S. canadensis* against other plant species was similar [27]. However, they could be distinguished by their morphological traits such as shoot length and flowering time [2,26,28,29]. The chromosome number between *S. canadensis* (diploid; $2n = 18$) and *S. altissima* (hexaploid; $2n = 54$) is also different [7,29,30]. The native ranges of both species in North America are not exactly the same [8,26]. In addition, the experimental crossing of *S. canadensis* and *S. altissima* could not bear viable seeds [30], which indicates a genetic barrier between both taxa. However, owing to the lack of consistency in the identification of the species, the separation of both species has been considered to be very problematic [2,28,29]. For example, most European populations of both species were described to be *S. altissima* [3,25], although macro-morphological analyses indicate that *S. canadensis* is a common species in Europa [29,31]. *S. altissima* was also mentioned as a synonym of *S. canadensis* [32,33]. There may have been a misidentification of the species.

It was reported that invasive plants are often allelopathic and inhibit the germination and growth of the native plant species in the invasive ranges through specific secondary metabolites defined as allelochemicals [34–43]. *S. canadensis* showed an allelopathic activity on the sugar maple seedlings in the field, greenhouse and laboratory conditions [44]. The *cis*-Dehydromatricaria ester was identified in the extracts of *S. altissima* as its allelochemical [45]. The evidence of the allelopathy of *S. canadensis* and *S. altissima* has been accumulated since the late 20th century, and their allelopathy was often implicated in the potential of their invasiveness and naturalization. However, there has been no review paper focusing on the allelopathy of both *S. canadensis* and *S. altissima*. This review provides an overview of the allelopathy and allelochemicals in *S. canadensis* and *S. altissima*, as well as a discussion on the involvement of allelopathy in the invasiveness and naturalization of the species. Despite the potential misidentification of *S. canadensis* and *S. altissima* described earlier, due to the fact that both species are very similar and the identification of the species is problematic [2,28,29], this paper followed the identification of the species in the publications because it is impossible to confirm their identification.

## 2. Allelopathy of *S. canadensis*

Allelopathy is the chemical interaction between donor plants and recipient plants through allelochemicals. Allelochemicals are produced in some plant parts and released into the vicinity of the donor plants, including their rhizosphere soil either by the root exudation, rainfall leachates, volatilization from the plant parts or decomposition processes of plant residues [46–49]. Several investigations in field conditions showed that *S. canadensis* reduced the number and biodiversity of the native plant community in its invaded ranges [50]. The invasion level of *S. canadensis* correlated negatively with the taxonomic diversity of the native plant community, and positively with the invasibility of the community [51]. Those observations may imply the involvement of allelopathy in the interaction between *S. canadensis* and native plant species to some extent. Many researchers have evaluated the allelopathic activity of the root exudates, rhizosphere soil, residues and plant extracts of *S. canadensis* (Table 1).

### *2.1. Allelopathy of Root Exudate and Plant Residue*

Root exudates of *S. canadensis*, which were obtained from its aeroponic culture, significantly suppressed the growth of two Asian original plant species; *Gnaphalium affine* D.Don and *Xanthium sibiricum* Patrin ex Widder., two of America origin; *Conyza canadensis* (L.) Cronquist and *Celosia argentea* L., two of tropical origin; *Aster subulatus* Michx. and *Sesbania cannabina* (Renz.) Poir. and a cosmopolitan species; *Eclipta prostrata* (L.) L. The suppression rate was similar in all plant species [52]. Root exudates of *S. canadensis* also showed the growth inhibition of *Arabidopsis thaliana* (L.) Heynh. [53]. When the seeds of seven European native plant species were sown into the *S. canadensis* cultivated soils with or without activated carbon, the germination of five species such as *Dactylis glomerata* L., *Lythrum salicaria* L., *Stachys officinalis* (L.) Trevis. and *Trifolium pratense* L. were significantly suppressed in activated carbon-free plots than in activated carbon plots. Although the germination rate was not significantly different between both plots, the biomass of *Arrhenatherum elatius* (L.) P.Beauv. ex J. et C.Presl in the activated carbon plots after three months of sowing was two times greater than that in the activated carbon-free plots [53]. Activated carbon is a widely used material to investigate allelopathy because it adsorbs allelochemicals in the plant rhizosphere soil [34,54]. In addition, aqueous extracts of the rhizosphere soil of *S. canadensis* inhibited the germination and growth of *Digitaria sanguinalis* (L.) Scop. and *Amaranthus retroflexus* L., and the inhibitory activity was greater in the extracts of the soil obtained from the invasive ranges of *S. canadensis* (China) than that from its native ranges (USA) [55]. These observations suggest that certain allelochemicals, which may cause growth inhibition, would be released into the rhizosphere soil as root exudates of *S. canadensis*, and the released allelochemicals in the soil may be greater in the invasive ranges than those in the native ranges.

Crushed stems, leaves and rhizomes of *S. canadensis* were mixed with soil and water and kept at 20/15 °C (12/12 h light/dark condition), and the mixture was filtered after 45 days. The obtained filtrate suppressed the germination and growth of *Raphanus sativus* L. and *Triticum aestivum* L. [56]. This observation also suggests that certain allelochemicals may be released into the rhizosphere soil during the decomposition process of plant residues of *S. canadensis*.

*2.2. Allelopathy of Plant Extract*

Some plant tissues may contain allelochemicals, since allelochemicals are synthesized and stored in certain plant tissues until their release into the environment [46–49]. Many investigations on the allelopathic activity of the extracts from different plant parts of *S. canadensis* have been conducted. Aqueous extracts of the leaves of *S. canadensis* inhibited the germination and root growth of *Raphanus sativus* L. and *Lactuca sativa* L. [57], as well as those of *Triticum aestivum* L. and *Setaria viridis* (L.)P.Beauv. [58]. The extracts also suppressed the germination, growth and chlorophyll content of *Trifolium pratense* L. and *Raphanus sativus* L., and increased their electrolyte leakage from the cell membrane of the seedlings [59,60].

The fresh leaves and stems of *S. canadensis* were soaked in water for 48 h, and the obtained soaking water showed the inhibitory activity on the germination and growth of *Raphanus sativus* L. and *Triticum aestivum* L. [54]. Aqueous extracts of the above-ground parts of *S. canadensis* suppressed the germination and growth of *Lactuca sativa* L. [61], as well as those of *Digitaria sanguinalis* (L.) Scop. and *Amaranthus retroflexus* L. [55]. The inhibitory activity was greater in the plant extracts obtained from the heavily invaded stands than in those obtained from the lightly invaded stands [62], and in the plant extracts obtained from the invasive ranges than those from the native ranges [55].

Aqueous extracts of the above-ground parts and roots of *S. canadensis* inhibited the germination and growth of *Zoysia japonica* Steud, and the extracts of the above-ground parts significantly stimulated malondialdehyde and peroxidase activity [62]. The extracts of the stems, roots, blossoms and seeds of *S. canadensis* suppressed the germination and growth of *Brassica napus* L. and *Lolium perenne* L. [63], and the extracts of the roots and rhizomes of *S. canadensis* also inhibited the root growth of *Raphanus sativus* L. and *Lactuca sativa* L. [57].

Aqueous ethanol extracts of the roots and rhizomes of *S. canadensis* inhibited the germination and growth of *Trifolium repens* L., *Trifolium pratense* L., *Medicago lupulina* L., *Suaeda glauca* (Brunge) Brunge, *Plantago virginica* L., *Kummerowia stipulacea* (Maxium.) Makino, *Festuca arundinacea* Schreb., *Ageratum conyzoides* L., *Portulaca oleracea* L. and *Amaranthus spinosus* L. [64]. Aqueous ethanol extracts of the above- and below-ground parts of *S. canadensis* suppressed the germination of *Kummerowia striata* (Thunb.) Schindl., and the inhibitory activity was greater in the plant extracts collected from the invasive ranges of *S. canadensis* than those from its native ranges [65]. Aqueous and ethanol extracts of the leaves, stems and rhizomes of *S. canadensis* inhibited the germination and growth of *Morus alba* L., *Pharbitis nil* (L.) Roth, *Triticum aestivum* L. and *Brassica campestris* L., and the inhibition was grater in the ethanol extracts than in the aqueous extracts [66].

Investigations on the aqueous and ethanol extracts of every part of *S. canadensis* showed the allelopathic activity on the germination, growth, chlorophyll content, electrolyte leakage and/or some enzyme activities of several plant species, including the native plant species. The inhibitory activity was greater in the plant extracts obtained from the invasive ranges of *S. canadensis* than in those from its native ranges, and in the extracts collected from the heavily invaded stands than in those collected from the lightly invaded stands. These observations suggest that whole parts of *S. canadensis* may contain water and ethanol extractable allelochemicals, which may cause the inhibition. In addition, the plants grown in the invasive ranges and heavily invaded stands may contain more allelochemicals than the plants in the native ranges and lightly invaded stands.

### 2.3. *Effects of the Extract on Arbuscular Mycorrhizal Fungi*

The rhizomes of *S. canadensis* were soaked in water for 24 h, and the obtained soaking water caused the suppression of the arbuscular mycorrhizal colonization of *Echinochloa crus-galli* (L.) P.Beauv., *Kummerowia striata* (Thnb.) Schindl. and *Ageratum conyzoides* L. [67]. The field and greenhouse investigations also showed that *S. canadensis* altered the composition of the arbuscular mycorrhizal fungal population in its rhizosphere soil through the inhibition of some dominant species and the stimulation of other species. The established arbuscular mycorrhizal community increased the competitive ability and the biomass of *S. canadensis* [67–71]. This altered arbuscular mycorrhizal community also increased the mycorrhizal-mediated $^{15}N$ uptake in *S. canadensis*, as well as decreased the $^{15}N$ uptake in the native species *Kummerowia statrica* (Thunb.) Schindl. [72]. In addition, the aqueous ethanol extract of the roots and rhizomes of *S. canadensis* also suppressed the population of the soilborne pathogens, namely *Pythium ultimum* Trow and *Rhizoctonia solani* J.G. Kühn [73]. These observations indicate that the aqueous extracts *of S. canadensis* may alter the arbuscular mycorrhizal population and suppress the colonization of the native plant species. The established arbuscular mycorrhizal community enhanced the competitive ability of *S. canadensis*. Certain compounds in the extracts may be involved in the alteration of the arbuscular mycorrhizal community.

**Table 1.** Allelopathic activities of exudates, rhizosphere soil, residues and plant extracts of *S. canadensis*.

| Source | Inhibition | | | | Target Plant Species | Reference |
|---|---|---|---|---|---|---|
| | Germination | Growth | Chlorophyll | Mycorrhizal colonization | | |
| **Root exudate** | | ✓ | | | *Gnaphalium affine, Xanthium sibiricum, Conyza canadensis, Celosia argentea, Aster subulatus, Sesbania cannabina, Eclipta prostrata* | [52] |
| | | ✓ | | | *Arabidopsis thaliana,* | [53] |
| **Rhizosphere soil** | ✓ | ✓ | | | *Dactylis glomerata, Lythrum salicaria, Stachys officinalis, Trifolium pratense* | [53] |
| **Soil extract** | ✓ | ✓ | | | *Digitaria sanguinalis, Amaranthus retroflexus* | [55] |
| **Residue** | ✓ | ✓ | | | *Raphanus sativus, Triticum aestivum* | [56] |
| **Plant extract** | | | | | | |
| Whole part | ✓ | ✓ | | | *Kummerowia striata* | [65] |
| Leaf | ✓ | ✓ | | | *Raphanus sativus, Lactuca sativa* | [57] |
| | ✓ | ✓ | | | *Triticum aestivum, Setaria viridi* | [58] |
| | | | ✓ | | *Raphanus sativus* | [59] |
| | | | ✓ | | *Trifolium pratense* | [60] |
| Leaf and stem | ✓ | ✓ | | | *Raphanus sativus, Triticum aestivum* | [56] |
| Above-ground part | ✓ | ✓ | | | *Lactuca sativa* | [61] |
| | ✓ | ✓ | | | *Digitaria sanguinalis (L.) Scop. and Amaranthus retroflexus* | [55] |
| Above-ground part, root | ✓ | ✓ | | | *Zoysia japonica* | [62] |
| Stem, root, blossom, seed | ✓ | ✓ | | | *Brassica napus, Lolium perenne* | [63] |

**Table 1.** *Cont.*

| Source | Inhibition | | | Target Plant Species | Reference |
|---|---|---|---|---|---|
| Leaf, stem, rhizome | ✓ | ✓ | | *Morus alba, Pharbitis nil, Triticum aestivum, Brassica campestris* | [66] |
| Root, rhizome | | ✓ | | *Raphanus sativus, Lactuca sativa* | [57] |
| | ✓ | ✓ | | *Trifolium repens, Trifolium pratense, Medicago lupulina, Suaeda glauca, Plantago virginica, Kummerowia stipulacea, Festuca arundinacea, Ageratum conyzoides, Portulaca oleracea, Amaranthus spinosus* | [69] |
| Rhizome | | | ✓ | *Echinochloa crus-galli, Kummerowia striata, Ageratum conyzoides* | [67] |

### 2.4. Allelochemicals

As described above, the inhibitory activity of the extracts of the plants and rhizosphere soil of *S. canadensis* obtained from the invasive ranges was greater than that obtained from the native ranges [55,65]. The concentrations of total phenolics, total flavones and total saponins in *S. canadensis* and its rhizosphere soil obtained from the invasive ranges were also greater than those from the native ranges [55,65]. These concentrations in the soil obtained from *S. canadensis*-infested stands were also greater than those in the soil obtained from *S. canadensis*-free stands [74].

Major compounds identified in the aqueous methanol extracts of the leaves and inflorescences of *S. canadensis* were chlorogenic acid, quercitrin and rutin (quercetin-3-*O*-β-rutinoside) (Figure 2) [75]. A fatty acid, *n*-hexadecanonic acid, was isolated from the aqueous ethanol extract of the stems and leaves of *S. canadensis* as an allelopathic agent. *n*-Hexadecanonic acid significantly inhibited the growth of *Triticum aestivum* L. [56]. A flavonoid, kaempferol-3-*O*-D-glucoside, was isolated from the aqueous ethanol extract of the *S. canadensis* straw, and the compound inhibited the growth of *Echinochloa colona* (L.) Link [75]. In addition, the concentration of rutin in the leaves of *S. canadensis* was greater than that of other *Solidago* species [76,77]. Some flavonoids were also identified in the aerial parts of *S. canadensis* [78].

The essential oil of many plant species was reported to have several biological activities, and to comprise volatile compounds such as terpenoids [79]. These volatile compounds often exhibited several biological activities including allelopathic activity [80,81]. Therefore, the involvement of the essential oil of *S. canadensis* in allelopathy was also investigated. The production of the essential oil was greater in *S. canadensis* obtained from the heavily invaded stands than that from mildly invaded stands [82]. The main components of the essential oil in the leaves and inflorescences of *S. canadensis* were α-pinene, trans-verbenol, limonene, bornyl acetate and β-cubebene [83], and those in the aerial parts of *S. canadensis* were α-pinene, β-pinene, germacrene D, limonene, thymol, (+)epi-bicyclosesquiphellandrene, β-cadinene, γ-cadinene, δ-cadinene, α-muurolene, γ-muurolene, α-cubebene and β-elemene [84,85]. The essential oil in the inflorescences of *S. canadensis* showed antimicrobial activity, antioxidant activity and free-radical scavenging activity, and its main components were α-pinene, germacrene D and limonene [86]. α-Pinene and β-pinene were reported to disturb the cell division through the interference of DNA synthesis, and cause membrane peroxidation [87–89]. Several monoterpenes were reported to alter soil microflora [90]. It was also reported that the essential oil of the aerial parts of *S. canadensis* inhibited the germination and radical growth of *Raphanus sativus* L. and *Lepidium sativum* L. [84].

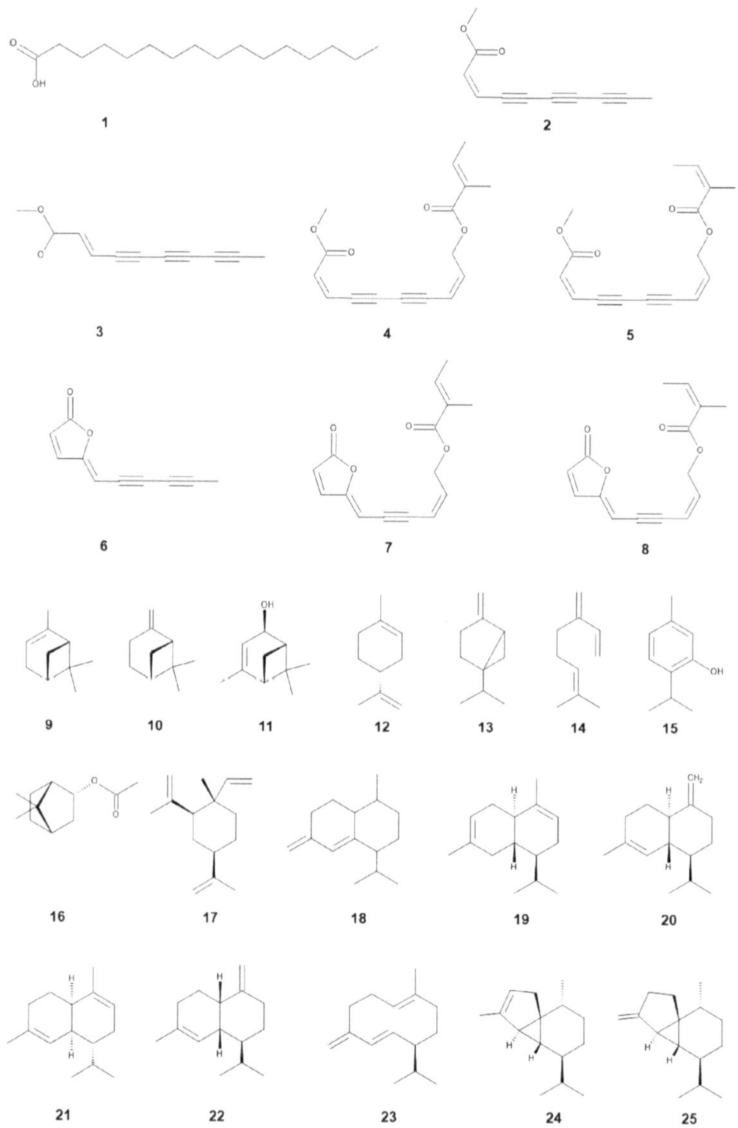


**Figure 2.** *Cont.*

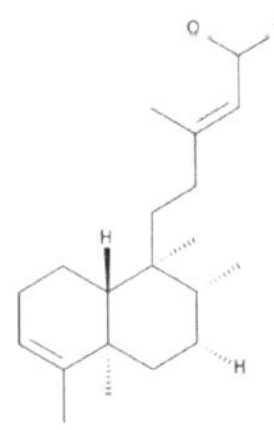

**26**

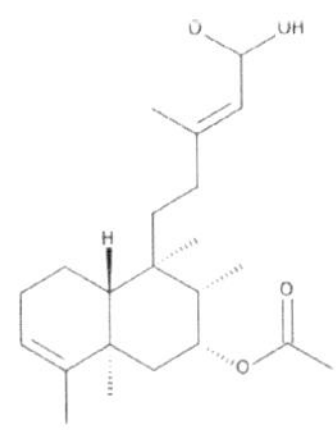

**27**

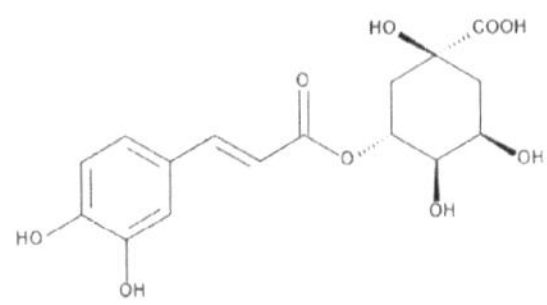

**28**

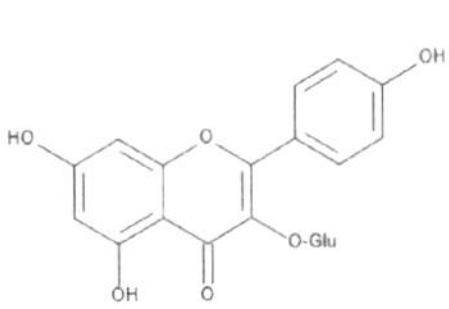

**29**

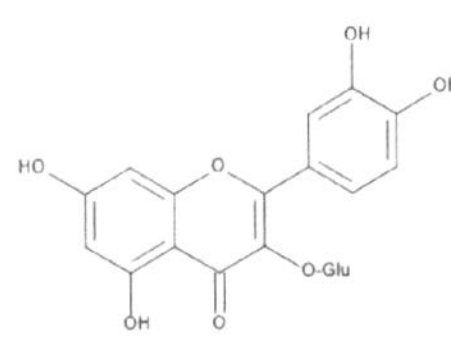

**30**

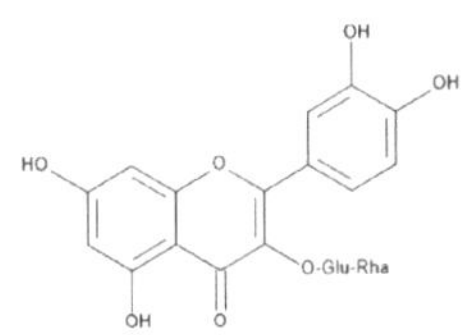

**31**

**Figure 2.** Allelochemicals identified in *S. canadensis* and *S. altissima*. Compound number and name were listed in Table 2.

*2.5. Contribution of Allelopathy of S. canadensis to Its Invasiveness*

All parts of the extracts of *S. canadensis,* including its rhizosphere soils, the root exudates, residues and essential oil, inhibited the germination and growth of several plant species (Table 1). These observations suggest that *S. canadensis* produces and accumulates allelochemicals in its plant tissues, and that it releases those allelochemicals into the surrounding environments of *S. canadensis,* including its rhizosphere soils through the root exudation, decomposition process of plant residues and volatilization from its essential oil. Several allelochemicals such as fatty acids, terpenes, flavonoids and polyphenols (Table 2) were identified in the extracts and essential oil of *S. canadensis.* Some of these compounds were reported to inhibit the germination and growth of other plants species, including the native plant species.

The extracts of *S. canadensis* and its rhizosphere soil obtained from its invasive ranges had greater inhibitory activity compared to the extracts and rhizosphere soil obtained from its native ranges [55,65]. The total phenolics, flavones and saponins in *S. canadensis* in the invasive ranges were also greater than those in the native ranges [55,65,74]. These observations suggest that *S. canadensis* in the invasive ranges may enhance the competitive ability through the increased production of some of these compounds. The novel weapons hypothesis suggests that the competitive ability of the invasive plants is superior to that of the native plant species due to its allelochemicals. Those allelochemicals are new to the indigenous plant species, and those indigenous plants are susceptible to the compounds [34,91]. However, there has been no available information on the specific compounds of which the production is increased in *S. canadensis* in the invasive ranges, as well as the reasons for which those productions are increased in the invasive ranges.

*S. canadensis* showed the alteration of the composition of the arbuscular mycorrhizal population and suppressed the mycorrhizal colonization of the native plant species in the field and greenhouse experiments. The extracts of *S. canadensis* also suppressed the mycorrhizal colonization of the native plant species. These investigations suggest that certain compounds in the extracts may be involved in the suppression. The authors also indicated the involvement of allelochemicals in the suppression. Arbuscular mycorrhizal fungi are important mycorrhiza for the most territorial plants, and their colonization enhances the ability of the host plants to absorb mineral nutrients and water, as well as increase the defense functions against pathogen attacks and stress conditions [92–94]. The suppression of the colonization reduces the potential of the native plants for nutrient and water absorption, as well as the defense function, which may cause the reduction in growth and vigor of the native plant species.

All the literature described above indicates that *S. canadensis* may suppress the regeneration process of the native plant species directly by the suppression of their germination and growth, and indirectly by the degradation of the mycorrhizal fungal mutualism of the native plant species through its allelopathy. Therefore, the allelopathy of *S. canadensis* may contribute to its increasing competitive ability and make the plant invasive. However, it is necessary to identify the allelochemicals involved in the suppression of the fungal mutualism of the native plant species. Investigations into the specific inhibitory activity of the identified allelochemicals on the native plant species, as well as their concentrations in the rhizosphere soil and/or surrounding environments are necessary to evaluate the contribution of these allelochemicals to the invasiveness of *S. canadensis*.

## 3. Allelopathy of *S. altissima*

There has been limited information on the allelopathic activity of the root exudates, extracts and residues of *S. altissima*, unlike *S. canadensis*, as well as its allelopathy in the field conditions. The available information is the inhibitory effect of the *n*-hexane extracts of the underground parts of *S. altissima* on the growth of *Lactuca sativa* L. [95]. However, phytochemical investigations suggest that *S. altissima* contains polyacetylenes [96,97], monoterpene and sesquiterpenes [98], diterpenes [95,98–102], triterpenes [103,104], flavonoid glycosides [105,106] and polyphenols [107]. Some of them may act as allelopathic agents of the species.

### *3.1. Terpene*

13*E*-7α-acetoxyl kolavenic acid (solidagonic acid) was isolated from the aqueous acetone extract of *S. altissima* [95,108], and the compound showed the growth inhibitory activity on the seedlings of *Lactuca sativa* L. and *Lolium multiflorum* Lam. [95,108]. 13*E*-kolavenic acid was also isolated from its *n*-hexane extracts [95]. Although 13*E*-kolavenic acid did not show any growth inhibitory activity, it exhibited antifungal activity and insect antifeedant activity [109,110]. These activities may help the species to protect itself from fungal pathogens and insect damage, as well as to establish its stands. It was reported that young rhizomes contained many more terpenes than old rhizomes, and α-pinene, β-pinene, limonene and germacrene D were identified in the rhizomes by GC-MS analysis [98]. α-Pinene, β-pinene, sabinene, myrcene, limonene, bornyl acetate and germacrene D were also found in the essential oil of *S. altissima*. However, the species was identified as a synonym of *S. canadensis* [33].

**Table 2.** Allelochemicals identified in *S. canadensis* and *S. canadensis* and their sources.

| Chemical Class | Compound | *Solidado canadensis* | | Reference | *Solidado altissima* | | | Reference |
|---|---|---|---|---|---|---|---|---|
| | | Extract | Essential oil | | Extract | Soil | Essential oil | |
| Fatty acid | **1**: *n*-Hexadecanonic acid | ✓ | | [56] | | | | |
| Polyacetylene | **2**: *cis*-Dehydromatricaria ester | | | | ✓ | ✓ | | [45,96,98,104] |
| | **3**: *trans*-Dehydromatricaria ester | | | | | ✓ | | [45] |
| | **4**: (2Z,8Z)-10-Tigloyloxy matricaria ester | | | | ✓ | | | [95] |
| | **5**: (2Z,8Z)-10-Angeloyloxy matricaria ester | | | | ✓ | | | [95,96] |
| | **6**: Dehydromatricaria lactone | | | | ✓ | | | [95,104,111] |
| | **7**: (4Z,8Z)-10-Trigloyloxy matricaria lactone | | | | ✓ | | | [95,111] |
| | **8**: (4Z,8Z)-10-Angeloyloxy matricaria lactone | | | | ✓ | | | [95] |
| Monoterpene | **9**: α-Pinene | | ✓ | [83–86] | ✓ | | ✓ | [33,98] |
| | **10**: β-Pinene | | ✓ | [84] | ✓ | | ✓ | [33,98] |
| | **11**: *trans*-Verbenol | | ✓ | [83] | | | | |
| | **12**: Limonene | | ✓ | [83–86] | ✓ | | ✓ | [33,98] |
| | **13**: Sabinene | | | | | | ✓ | [33] |
| | **14**: Myrcene | | | | | | ✓ | [33] |
| | **15**: Thymol | | ✓ | [84] | | | | |
| | **16**: Bornyl acetate | | ✓ | [83] | | | ✓ | [33] |
| Sesquiterpene | **16**: β-Elemene | | ✓ | [84] | | | | |
| | **17**: (+)epi-Bicyclosesquiphellandrene | | ✓ | [84] | | | | |
| | **18**: β-Cadinene | | ✓ | [84] | | | | |
| | **19**: γ-Cadinene | | ✓ | [84] | | | | |
| | **20**: *δ-Cadinene* | | ✓ | [84] | | | | |
| | **21**: α-muurolene | | ✓ | [84] | | | | |
| | **22**: γ-muurolene | | ✓ | [84] | | | | |
| | **23**: Germacrene D | | ✓ | [84,86] | ✓ | | ✓ | [33,98] |
| | **24**: α-cubebene | | ✓ | [84] | | | | |
| | **25**: β-Cubebene | | ✓ | [83,84] | | | | |
| Diterpene | **26**: 13*E*-kolavenic acid | | | | ✓ | | | [95] |
| | **27**: 13*E*-7α-acetoxyl kolavenic acid | | | | ✓ | | | [95,108] |
| Polyphenol | **28**: Chlorogenic acid | ✓ | | [76] | | | | |
| Flavonoid | **29**: Kaempferol-3-*O*-D-glucoside | ✓ | | [75] | | | | |
| | **30**: Quercitrin | ✓ | | [76,77] | | | | |
| | **31**: Rutin | ✓ | | [76] | | | | |

### 3.2. Polyacetylene

Several polyacetylenes, such as *cis*-dehydromatricaria ester (*cis*-DME), dehydromatricaria lactone, (2Z,8Z)-10-tigloyloxy matricaria ester, (4Z,8Z)-10-trigloyloxy matricaria lactone, (2Z,8Z)-10-angeloyloxy matricaria ester (methyl10-[(Z)-2-methyl-2-butenoyloxy]-(2Z,8Z)-2,8-decadiene-4,6-diynoate) and (4Z,8Z)-10-angeloyloxy matricaria lactone were isolated from the stems, roots and/or rhizomes of *S. altissima* [45,95,96,98,104,111]. Polyacetylenes in Asteraceae plants were reported to be synthesized from crepenynic acid, which is formed oleic acid with linoleic acid, introducing the first acetylene bond [95,112].

Among the polyacetylenes found in *S. altissima*, *cis*-DME, dehydromatricaria lactone and the (2Z,8Z)-10-angeloyloxy matricaria ester were reported to inhibit the coleoptile growth of *Panicum crus-galli* L. var. *frumentaceum* Trin. up to 77.4–93.5%, 81.7% and 80.0% that of the control, respectively, at the concentration of 1 ppm [96,111]. The (2Z,8Z)-10-Tigloyloxy matricaria ester also inhibited the growth of *Lolium multiflorum* Lam. [95]. However, *cis*-DME among those polyacetylenes was the most studied.

The bioactive concentration of *cis*-DME caused the growth inhibition, which was of 1–20 ppm in laboratory conditions [45,95,96,98,108,111,113]. *cis*-DME suppressed the germination of *Asclepias syriaca* L., *Ambrosia artemisiifolia* L. and *Miscanthus sinensis* Anderson; the germination and growth of *Poa pratensis* L. and *Oryza sativa* L.; and the growth of *Lactuca sativa* L. and *Panicum crus-galli* L. var. *frumentaceum* Trin. Their germination was inhibited up to 20–95% that of the control by 32–60 ppm *cis*-DME, and their growth was inhibited up to 10–56% that of the control by 48–100 ppm *cis*-DME (Table 3). *Asclepias syriaca* and *Miscanthus sinensis*, respectively, are competitive species with *S. altissima* in the native range of the USA and in the invasive range of Japan. *Ambrosia artemisiifoli* and *Poa pratensis* are the invasive plant species from North America, Europa and North Asia [45,98,114,115]. However, the effectiveness of *cis*-DME on those plant species was not evidently different.

**Table 3.** Growth inhibitory activity of *cis*-dehydromatricaria ester.

| *cis*-DME Concentration (ppm) | Target Plant | Germination | Growth | Reference |
|---|---|---|---|---|
| | | (% of Control) | | |
| 32 | *Asclepias syriaca* | 5 | | [98] |
| 48 | *Poa pratensis* | 20 | 50 | [113] |
| 50 | *Oryza sativa* | 88 | 10–15 | [45] |
| 50 | *Ambrosia artemisiifolia* | 25 | | [45] |
| 50 | *Miscanthus sinensis* | 22 | | [45] |
| 100 | *Lactuca sativa* | | 30–56 | [108] |
| 100 | *Panicum crus-galli* | | 18 | [111] |

The concentration of *cis*-DME was reported to be of 250–400 ppm in the roots of *S. altissima*, of 6.3 ppm in the soil under *S. altissima* [45] and of 0–17.3 ppm in the soil [116]. The concentrations in the soil varied depending on the soil properties and microbial activities [117–119]. The existence of *cis*-DME in the soil under *S. altissima* suggests that *cis*-DME may be released from *S. altissima* into the soils through the root exudation, rainfall leachates and/or the decomposition processes of plant residues. In addition, considering the bioactive concentration (1–20 ppm) described above and the soil concentration (0–17.3 ppm) of *cis*-DME, which is the same in laboratory conditions, the *cis*-DME in the soil may have some ecological function.

*trans*-DME was also in the soil under *S. altissima*, and its inhibitory activity was comparable of that of *cis*-DME [45]. When the ethanol solution (1%) of *cis*-DME was kept at 29 °C under 2000 lux for 2 days, 50% of *cis*-DME was isomerized into *trans*-DME, since the *cis*-form of the unsaturated ester is easily isomerized by light, pH or other conditions into the more stable *trans*-form [120]. In addition, *trans*-DME was not found in the roots and rhizomes of *S. altissima* [45]. Therefore, *cis*-DME may be isomerized by light and other environmental factors into *trans*-DME after the exudation from the plants into the soil. When we consider the involvement of DME in the allelopathy of *S. altissima*, the concentration of both *cis*-DME and *trans*-DME in the rhizosphere soil should be counted.

It was also reported that the aqueous extracts of the below-ground parts of *S. altissima* killed a pine wilt nematode (*Bursaphelenchus lignicolous* Mamiya and Kiyohara), and an active compound involved in it was determined as *cis*-DME. *cis*-DME at 10–11 ppm increased 50% of the molarity of the pine wilt nematode and a root-knot nematode (*Meloidogyne incognita* Kofild and White) [121]. The methanol extracts of the *S. altissima* rhizomes suppressed the hatching of fruit flies (*Drosophila melanogaster* Meigen), and an active compound was also determined as *cis*-DME [97]. The defense capacity of the invasive plants with natural enemies, such as pathogens, parasites and herbivores, contributes their establishment and naturalization into introduced ranges [37,122,123]. Therefore, the nematicidal and insecticidal activities of *cis*-DME may contribute to the establishment and naturalization of *S. altissima* in the introduced ranges.

### 3.3. *Contribution of Allelopathy of* S. altissima *to Its Invasiveness*

Unlike *S. canadensis*, the information on the allelopathic activity of *S. altissima* extracts, root exudates and residues is limited. However, polyacetylenes, monoterpene and sesquiterpenes, diterpenes, triterpenes and flavonoid glycosides were identified in its extracts and essential oil as allelopathic agents. Most potential compounds among them involved in the allelopathy may be *cis*-DME. *cis*-DME inhibited the germination and growth of several plant species at the concentration of 1–20 ppm [45,95,98,108,111,113]. Its concentration in the roots of *S. altissima* and in its rhizosphere soil was of 250–400 ppm and 0–17.3 ppm, respectively [45,116]. These observations suggest that *cis*-DME may be released into the rhizosphere soil by root exudation, rainfall leachates and/or decomposition processes of plant residues. *trans*-DME was also formed by the isomerization of *cis*-DME in the soil, and its inhibitory activity was the same as *cis*-DME. Although there has been no information of the concentration of *trans*-DME in the rhizosphere soil of *S. altissima*, the concentration of only *cis*-DME in several soils was over the concentration which was able to cause the growth inhibition [45,116]. In addition, *cis*-DME possesses nematicidal and insecticidal activities [97,113,121,124] Some flavonoids were also identified in the aerial parts of *S. canadensis* [78]. 13*E*-kolavenic acid also showed antifungal activity and insect antifeedant activity [109,110]. Therefore, these compounds including *trans*-DME may be involved in allelopathy and/or defense function against natural enemies, such as fungal pathogens, parasites and herbivores, and may contribute to their establishment and naturalization into the introduced ranges. However, it is necessary to determine the concentration of *trans*-DME in the rhizosphere soil of *S. altissima*, as well as to investigate the allelopathy of *S. altissima* in greenhouse and field conditions. It is also worth investigating the effect of *S. altissima* on the arbuscular mycorrhizal colonization of the native plant species due to the fact that *S. altissima* and *S. canadensis* are very close species.

## 4. Conclusions

*S. canadensis* and *S. altissima* are harmful invasive species naturalized in many countries, and form thick monospecific stands. Based on the literature, both species are allelopathic. The root exudate, residues, extracts, essential oil and rhizosphere soil of *S. canadensis* showed allelopathic activity on several plant species, including native plants, and suppressed the arbuscular mycorrhizal mutualism of the native plant species. Several allelochemicals were also identified in its extracts and essential oil. The concentrations of total phenolics, total flavones and total saponins in the rhizosphere soil of *S. canadensis* obtained from the invasive ranges were greater than those obtained from the native ranges. Therefore, the allelopathy of *S. canadensis* may contribute the interruption of the regeneration process of native plant species directly through the suppression of their germination and growth, and indirectly through the suppression of the mycorrhizal fungal mutualism of the native plant species. Several allelochemicals of *S. altissima* were also identified in its extracts and essential oil. Among them, *cis*-DME inhibited the germination and growth of several plant species at a concentration of 1–20 ppm, and its extractable concentration in the rhizosphere soil of *S. altissima* was of 0–17.3 ppm. *cis*-DME also exhibited nematicidal and insecticidal activities. *trans*-DME was formed by the isomerization of *cis*-DME in the soil, and its inhibitory activity was similar to that of *cis*-DME. Therefore, *cis*-DME, including *trans*-DME, may also cause the suppression of the regeneration process of the native plant species through the inhibition of their germination and growth. The allelopathy of *S. canadensis* and *S. altissima* may provide the species with competitive advantage against native plant species, and contribute to their invasiveness and naturalization.

**Funding:** This research received no external funding.

**Institutional Review Statement:** Not applicable.

**Informed Consent Statement:** Not applicable.

**Conflicts of Interest:** The authors declare no conflict of interest.

## References


1. Weber, E. The dynamics of plant invasions: A case study of three exotic goldenrod species (*Solidago* L.) in Europe. *J. Biogeogr.* **1998**, *25*, 147–154. [CrossRef]
2. Weber, E. Morphological variation of the introduced perennial *Solidago canadensis* L. *sensu lato* (Asteraceae) in Europe. *Bot. J. Linn. Soc.* **1997**, *123*, 197–210. [CrossRef]
3. Weber, E. Biological flora of Central Europe: *Solidago altissima* L. *Flora* **2000**, *195*, 123–134. [CrossRef]
4. Invasive Species Compendium, Solidago canadensis. Available online: https://www.cabi.org/isc/datasheet/50599 (accessed on 12 September 2022).
5. Royal Botanical Gardens, Kew, Solidago canadensis. *Solidago altissima* L. Available online: https://powo.science.kew.org/taxon/urn:lsid:ipni.org:names:249454-1 (accessed on 12 September 2022).
6. Royal Botanical Gardens, Kew, *Solidago altissima* L. Available online: https://powo.science.kew.org/taxon/urn:lsid:ipni.org:names:285347-2 (accessed on 12 September 2022).
7. Croat, T. *Solidago canadensis* complex of the great plains. *Brittonia* **1972**, *24*, 317–326. [CrossRef]

8. Werner, P.A.; Bradbury, I.K.; Gross, R.S. The biology of Canadian weeds. 45. *Solidago canadensis* L. *Can. J. Plant Sci.* **1980**, *60*, 1393–1409. [CrossRef]
9. Curtis, J.D.; Lersten, N.R. Oil reservorirs in stem, rhizomes, and root of *Solidago canadensis* (Asteraceas, tribe Astereae). *Nor. J. Bot.* **1990**, *10*, 443–449. [CrossRef]
10. Meyer, A.H.; Schmid, B. Seed dynamics and seedling establishment in the invading perennial *Solidago altissima* under different experimental treatments. *J. Ecol.* **1999**, *87*, 28–41. [CrossRef]
11. Cornelius, R. The strategies of *Solidago canadensis* L. in relation to urban habitats. I. Resource requirements. *Acta Oecol.* **1990**, *11*, 19–34.
12. Huang, H.; Guo, S.; Chen, G. Reproductive biology in an invasive plant *Solidago canadensis*. *Front. Biol. China* **2007**, *2*, 196–204. [CrossRef]
13. Follak, S.; Eberius, M.; Essl, F.; Fürdös, A.; Sedlacek, N.; Trognitz, F. Invasive alien plants along roadsides in Europe. *EPPO Bull.* **2018**, *48*, 256–265. [CrossRef]
14. Park, J.S.; Choi, D.; Kim, Y. Potential Distribution of Goldenrod (*Solidago altissima* L.) during Climate Change in South Korea. *Sustainability* **2020**, *12*, 6710. [CrossRef]
15. Kotowska, D.; Pärt, T.; Żmihorski, M. Evaluating google street view for tracking invasive alien plants along roads. *Ecol. Indi.* **2021**, *121*, 107020. [CrossRef]
16. Shimoda, M.; Nakamoto, M. Vegetation and threatened plant dynamics of wet abandoned rice fields in Nakaikemi, Fukui, Prefecture, Japan. *Jpn. J. Ecol.* **2003**, *53*, 197–217.
17. Shimoda, S.; Wagai, R. Ecosystem dynamics after abandonment of rice paddy fields; Does aaien plant invasion enhance carbon storage? *Ecosystems* **2020**, *23*, 617–629. [CrossRef]
18. Newell, S.J.; Tramer, E.J. Reproductive strategies in herbaceous plant communities during succession. *Ecology* **1978**, *59*, 228–234. [CrossRef]
19. Bakelaar, R.G.; Odum, E.P. Community and population level response to fertilization in an old-field ecosystem. *Ecology* **1978**, *59*, 660–665. [CrossRef]
20. Maddox, G.D.; Cook, R.E.; Wimberger, P.H.; Gardescu, S. Clone structure in four *Solidago altissima* (Asteraceae) population: Rhizome connections within genotypes. *Am. J. Bot.* **1989**, *76*, 318–326. [CrossRef]
21. Dong, L.J.; Yu, H.W.; He, W.M. What determines positive, neutral and negative impacts of *Solidago canadensis* invasion on native plant species richness? *Sci. Rep.* **2015**, *5*, 16804. [CrossRef]
22. Fenesi, A.; Vágási, C.I.; Beldean, M.; Földesi, R.; Kolcsár, L.P.; Shapiro, J.T.; Török, E.; Kovács-Hostyánszki, A. *Solidago canadensis* impacts on native plant and pollinator communities in different-aged old fields. *Basic Appl. Ecol.* **2015**, *16*, 335–346. [CrossRef]
23. Zagurskaya, Y.V. Study issues of invasive species of the genus *Solidago*. *Ecosyst. Transform.* **2022**, *5*, 42–54. [CrossRef]
24. EPPO. PQR database. Paris, France: European and Mediterranean Plant Protection Organization. Available online: https://gd.eppo.int/taxon/SOOCA (accessed on 12 September 2022).
25. Weber, E.; Schmid, B. Latitudinal population differentiation in two species of *Solidago* (Asteraceae) introduced into Europe. *Am. J. Bot.* **1998**, *85*, 1110–1121. [CrossRef] [PubMed]
26. iNatuarist, Identifying Solidago altissima & Solidago canadensis. Available online: https://www.inaturalist.org/posts/19288-identifying-solidago-altissima-solidagocanadensis (accessed on 12 September 2022).
27. Szymura, M.; Szymura, T.H. Interactions between alien goldenrods (*Solidago* and *Euthamia* species) and comparison with native species in Central Europe. *Flora* **2016**, *218*, 51–61. [CrossRef]
28. Semple, J.C.; Rahman, H.; Bzovsky, S.; Sorour, M.K.; Kornobis, K.; Laphitz, R.L.; Tong, L. A multivariate morphometric study of the *Solidago altissima* complex and *S. canadensis* (Asteraceae: Astereae). *Phytoneuron* **2015**, *10*, 1–31.
29. Verloove, F.; Zonneveld, B.J.M.; Semple, J.C.S. First evidence for the presence of invasive *Solidago altissima* (Asteraceae) in Europe. *Willdenowia* **2017**, *47*, 69–75. [CrossRef]
30. Melville, M.R.; Morton, J.K. A biosystematics study of the *Solidago canadensis* (Compositae) complex. I. The Ontario populations. *Can. J. Bot.* **1982**, *60*, 976–997. [CrossRef]
31. Szymura, M.; Szymura, T.H.; Kreitschitz, A. Morphological and cytological diversity of goldenrods (*Solidago* L. and *Euthamia* Nutt.) from south-western Poland. *Biodiv. Res. Conserv.* **2015**, *38*, 41–49. [CrossRef]
32. Pisula, N.; Meiners, S.J. Allelopatyhic effcts of goldenrod species on turnover in successional communities. *Am. Midl. Nat.* **2010**, *163*, 161–172. [CrossRef]
33. Lawson, S.K.; Sharp, L.G.; Powers, C.N.; McFeeters, R.L.; Satyal, P.; Setzer, W.N. Volatile Compositions and Antifungal Activities of Native American Medicinal Plants: Focus on the Asteraceae. *Plants* **2020**, *9*, 126. [CrossRef]
34. Callaway, R.M.; Aschehoug, E.T. Invasive plants versus their new and old neighbors: A mechanism for exotic invasion. *Science* **2000**, *290*, 521–523. [CrossRef]
35. Callaway, R.M.; Ridenour, W.M. Novel weapons: Invasive success and the evolution of increased competitive ability. *Front. Ecol. Environ.* **2004**, *2*, 419–426. [CrossRef]
36. Cappuccino, N.; Arnason, J.T. Novel chemistry of invasive exotic plants. *Biol. Lett.* **2006**, *2*, 189–193. [CrossRef] [PubMed]
37. Chengxu, W.; Mingxing, Z.; Xuhui, C.; Bo, Q. Review on allelopathy of exotic invasive plants. *Procedia. Engin.* **2011**, *18*, 240–246. [CrossRef]

38. Meiners, S.J.; Kong, C.H.; Ladwig, L.M.; Pisula, N.L.; Lang, K.A. Developing an ecological context for allelopathy. *Plant. Ecol.* **2012**, *213*, 1861–1867. [CrossRef]
39. Kato-Noguchi, H. Involvement of allelopathy in the invasive potential of *Tithonia diversifolia*. *Plants* **2020**, *9*, 766. [CrossRef]
40. Kato-Noguchi, H.; Kurniadie, D. Allelopathy of *Lantana camara* as an invasive plant. *Plants* **2021**, *10*, 1028. [CrossRef]
41. Kato-Noguchi, H. Allelopathy of knotweeds as invasive plants. *Plants* **2022**, *11*, 3. [CrossRef]
42. Kato-Noguchi, H.; Kurniadie, D. Allelopathy and allelochemicals of *Leucaena leucocephala* as an invasive plant species. *Plants* **2022**, *11*, 1672. [CrossRef]
43. Kato-Noguchi, H. Allelopathy and Allelochemicals of *Imperata cylindrica* as an invasive plant species. *Plants* **2022**, *11*, 2551. [CrossRef]
44. Fisher, R.F.; Woods, R.A.; Glavicic, M.R. Allelopathic effects of golderrod and aster on young sugar maple. *Can. J. Forest Res.* **1978**, *8*, 1–9. [CrossRef]
45. Kobayashi, A.; Morimoto, S.; Shibata, Y.; Yamashita, K.; Numata, M. $C_{10}$-Polyacetylenes as allelopathic substances in dominants in early stages of secondary succession. *J. Chem. Ecol.* **1980**, *6*, 119–131. [CrossRef]
46. Rice, E.L. *Allelopathy*, 2nd ed.; Academic Press: Orlando, FL, USA, 1984; pp. 1–422.
47. Bais, H.P.; Weir, T.L.; Perry, L.G.; Gilroy, S.; Vivanco, J.M. The role of root exudates in rhizosphere interactions with plants and other organisms. *Annu. Rev. Plant Biol.* **2006**, *57*, 233–266. [CrossRef] [PubMed]
48. Bonanomi, G.; Sicurezza, M.G.; Caporaso, S.; Esposito, A.; Mazzoleni, S. Phytotoxicity dynamics of decaying plant materials. *New Phytol.* **2006**, *169*, 571–578. [CrossRef] [PubMed]
49. Belz, R.G. Allelopathy in crop/weed interactions—An update. *Pest. Manag. Sci.* **2007**, *63*, 308–326. [CrossRef] [PubMed]
50. Bielecka, A.; Borkowska, L.; Królak, E. Environmental changes caused by the clonal invasive plant *Solidago canadensis*. *Ann. Bot. Fennici.* **2019**, *57*, 33–48. [CrossRef]
51. Wang, C.; Cheng, H.; Wanga, S.; Weia, M.; Du, D. Plant community and the influence of plant taxonomic diversity on community stability and invasibility: A case study based on *Solidago canadensis* L. *Sci. Total Environ.* **2021**, *768*, 144518. [CrossRef]
52. Yang, B.; Li, J. Phytotoxicity of toot exudates of invasive *Solidago canadensis* on co-occurring native and invasive plant species. *Pak. J. Bot.* **2022**, *54*, 1019–1024. [CrossRef]
53. Abhilasha, D.; Quintana, N.; Vivanco, J.; Joshi, J. Do allelopathic compounds in invasive *Solidago canadensis* s.l. restrain the native European flora? *J. Ecol.* **2008**, *96*, 993–1001. [CrossRef]
54. Weißhuhn, K.; Prati, D. ; Activated carbon may have undesired side effects for testing allelopathy in invasive plants. *Basic Appl. Ecol.* **2009**, *10*, 500–507. [CrossRef]
55. Yang, X.; Cheng, J.; Yao, B.; Lu, H.; Zhang, Y.; Xu, J.; Song, X.; Qiang, S. Polyploidy-promoted phenolic metabolism confers the increased competitive ability of *Solidago canadensis*. *Oikos* **2021**, *130*, 1014–1025. [CrossRef]
56. Zhang, D.; Ye, Y.; Li, L.; Domg, L. Allelopathic pathways, isolation and identification of an allelopathic substance from *Solidago canadensis* L. *Allelopath. J.* **2014**, *33*, 201–212.
57. Butcko, V.M.; Jensen, R.J. Evidence of tissue-specific allelopathic activity in *Euthamia graminifolia* and *Solidago canadensis* (Asteraceae). *Am. Midl. Nat.* **2002**, *148*, 253–262. [CrossRef]
58. Li, S.L.; Li, Z.H.; Wang, Y.F.; Xiao, R.; Pan, C.D.; Wang, Q. Preliminary study for the allelopathic effect of water extracts from *Solidago canadensis* leaves. *Adv. Mater. Res.* **2013**, *699*, 340–348. [CrossRef]
59. Możdżeń, K.; Barabasz-Krasny, B.; Zandi, P.; Kliszcz, A.; Puła, J. Effect of aqueous extracts from *Solidago canadensis* L. Leaves on germination and early growth stages of three cultivars of *Raphanus Sativus* L. var. *Radicula* Pers. *Plants* **2020**, *9*, 1549. [CrossRef] [PubMed]
60. Zandi, P.; Barabasz-Krasny, B.; Stachurska-Swakoń, A.; Puła, J.; Możdżeń, K. Allelopathic effect of invasive Canadian goldenrod (*Solidago canadensis* L.) on early growth of red clover (*Trifolium pratense* L.). *Not. Bot. Horti. Agrobo.* **2020**, *48*, 2060–2071. [CrossRef]
61. Yu, Y.; Cheng, H.; Xu, Z.; Zhong, S.; Wang, C.; Guo, E. Invasion intensity modulates the allelopathic impact of *Solidago canadensis* L. leaves and roots against *Lactuca sativa* L. during germination and early seedling stage. *Int. J. Environ. Res.* **2022**, *16*, 48. [CrossRef]
62. Sun, J.F.; Liang, Q.J.; Wu, N.; Javed, Q.; Huang, P.; Du, D.L. Allelopathic effects of aqueous extracts from different plant parts of Canada goldenrod (*Solidago canadensis* L.) on seed germination and seedling growth of Korean lawngrass (*Zoysia japonica* Steud.). *Appl. Ecol. Environ. Res.* **2022**, *20*, 1009–1022. [CrossRef]
63. Baležentien, L. Secondary metabolite accumulation and phytotoxicity of invasive species *Solidago canadensis* L. during the growth period. *Allelopath. J.* **2015**, *35*, 217–226.
64. Yang, R.Y.; Mei, L.X.; Tang, J.J.; Chen, X. Allelopathic effects of invasive *Solidago canadensis* L. on germination and growth of native Chinese plant species. *Allelopath. J.* **2007**, *19*, 241–248.
65. Yuan, Y.; Wang, B.; Zhang, S.; Tang, J.; Tu, C.; Hu, S.; Yong, J.W.H.; Chen, X. Enhanced allelopathy and competitive ability of invasive plant *Solidago canadensis* in its introduced range. *J. Plant Ecol.* **2013**, *6*, 253–263. [CrossRef]
66. Sun, B.Y.; Tan, J.Z.; Wan, Z.G.; Gu, F.G.; Zhu, M.D. Allelopathic effects of extracts from *Solidago canadensis* L. against seed germination and seedling growth of some plants. *J. Environ. Sci.* **2006**, *18*, 304–309.
67. Zhang, Q.; Yao, L.J.; Yang, R.Y.; Yang, X.Y.; Tang, J.J.; Chin, X. Potential allelopathic effects of an invasive species *Solidago canadensis* on the mycorrhizae of native plant species. *Allelopath. J.* **2007**, *20*, 71–78.
68. Sun, Z.K.; He, W.M. Evidence for enhanced mutualism hypothesis: *Solidago canadensis* plants from regular soils perform better. *PLoS ONE* **2010**, *5*, e15418. [CrossRef]

69. Betekhtina, A.A.; Mukhacheva, T.A.; Kovaleva, S.Y.; Gusevb, A.P.; Veselkin, D.V. Abundance and diversity of arbuscular mycorrhizal fungi in invasive *Solidago canadensis* and indigenous *S. virgaurea*. *Russ. J. Ecol.* **2016**, *47*, 575–579. [CrossRef]
70. Dong, L.J.; Ma, L.N.; He, W.M. Arbuscular mycorrhizal fungi help explain invasion success of *Solidago canadensis*. *Appl. Soil. Ecol.* **2021**, *167*, 103763. [CrossRef]
71. Řezáčová, V.; Řezáč, M.; Gryndler, M.; Hršelová, H.; Gryndlerová, H.; Michalová, T. Plant invasion alters community structure and decreases diversity of arbuscular mycorrhizal fungal communities. *Appl. Soil. Ecol.* **2021**, *167*, 104039. [CrossRef]
72. Yang, R.; Zhou, G.; Zan, S.; Guo, F.; Su, N.; Li, J. Arbuscular mycorrhizal fungi facilitate the invasion of *Solidago canadensis* L. in southeastern China. *Acta Oecol.* **2014**, *61*, 74–77. [CrossRef]
73. Zhang, S.; Jin, Y.; Tang, J.; Chen, X. The invasive plant *Solidago canadensis* L. Suppresses local soil pathogens through allelopathy. *Appl. Soil. Ecol.* **2009**, *41*, 215–222. [CrossRef]
74. Zhang, S.; Zhu, W.; Wang, B.; Tang, J.; Chen, X. Secondary metabolites from the invasive *Solidago canadensis* L. Accumulation in soil and contribution to inhibition of soil pathogen *Pythium ultimum*. *Appl. Soil. Ecol.* **2011**, *48*, 280–286. [CrossRef]
75. Jun, L.; Yonghao, Y.; Hongwu, H.; Liyao, D. Kaempferol-3-O-β-D-glucoside, a potential allelochemical isolated from *Solidago canadensis*. *Allelopath. J.* **2011**, *28*, 259–266.
76. Radusiene, J.; Marska, M.; Ivanauskas, L.; Jakstas, J.; Karpaviciene, B. Assessment of phenolic compound accumulation in two widespread goldenrods. *Ind. Crops Prod.* **2015**, *63*, 158–166. [CrossRef]
77. Likhanov, A.; Oliinyk, M.; Pashkevych, N.; Churilov, A.; Kozyr, M. The role of flavonoids in invasion strategy of *Solidago canadensis* L. *Plants* **2021**, *10*, 1748. [CrossRef]
78. Shelepova, O.; Vinogradova, Y.; Vergun, O.; Grygorieva, O.; Brindza, J. Assessment of flavonoids and phenolic compound accumulation in invasive *Solidago canadensis* L. in Slovakia. *Slovak J. Food Sci.* **2020**, *14*, 587–594.
79. Sharifi-Rad, J.; Sureda, A.; Tenore, G.C.; Daglia, M.; Sharifi-Rad, M.; Valussi, M.; Tundis, R.; Sharifi-Rad, M.; Loizzo, M.R.; Ademiluyi, A.O.; et al. Biological activities of essential oils: From plant chemoecology to traditional healing systems. *Molecules* **2017**, *22*, 70. [CrossRef] [PubMed]
80. Jassbi, A.R.; Zare, S.; Firuzi, O.; Xiao, J. Bioactive phytochemicals from shoots and roots of *Salvia* species. *Phytochem Rev.* **2016**, *15*, 829–867. [CrossRef]
81. Macías, F.A.; Mejías, F.J.R.; Molinillo, J.M.G. Recent advances in allelopathy for weed control: From knowledge to applications. *Pest Manag. Sci.* **2019**, *75*, 2413–2436. [CrossRef] [PubMed]
82. Baranová, B.; Troščáková-Kerpčárová, E.; Gruľová, D. Survey of the *Solidago canadensis* L. morphological traits and essential oil production: Aboveground biomass growth and abundance of the invasive goldenrod appears to be reciprocally enhanced within the invaded dtands. *Plants* **2022**, *11*, 535. [CrossRef]
83. Radušienė, J.; Karpavičienė, B.; Marksa, M.; Ivanauskas, L.; Raudonė, L. Distribution patterns of essential oil terpenes in native and invasive *Solidago* species and their comparative assessment. *Plants* **2022**, *11*, 1159. [CrossRef]
84. Gruľová, D.; Baranová, B.; Ivanova, V.; De Martino, L.; Mancini, E.; De Feo, V. Composition and bio activity of essential oils of *Solidago* spp. and their Impact on radish and garden cress. *Allelopath. J.* **2016**, *39*, 129–141.
85. Shelepova, O.; Vinogradova, Y.; Zaitchik, B.; Ruzhitsky, A.; Grygorieva, O.; Brindza, J. Constituents of the essential oil in *Solidago canadensis* L. from Eurasia. *Slovak J. Food Sci.* **2018**, *12*, 20–25. [CrossRef]
86. Marinas, I.C.; Oprea, E.; Buleandra, M.; Bleots, C.; Badea, I.R.; Anastasiu, P.; Lazar, V.; Gardus, I.D.; Chifiric, M.C. Chemical, antimicrobial, antioxidant and anti-proliferative features of the essential oil extracted from the invasive plant *Solidago canadensis* L. *Rev. Chim.* **2020**, *71*, 255–264. [CrossRef]
87. Nishida, N.; Tamotsu, S.; Nagata, N.; Saito, C.; Sakai, A. Allelopathic effects of volatile monoterpenoids produced by *Salvia leucophylla*: Inhibition of cell proliferation and DNA synthesis in the root apical meristem of *Brassica campestris* seedlings. *J. Chem. Ecol.* **2005**, *31*, 1187–1203. [CrossRef]
88. Chowhan, N.; Singh, H.P.; Batish, D.R.; Kohli, R.H. Phytotoxic effects of β-pinene on early growth and associated biochemical changes in rice. *Acta Physiol. Plant.* **2011**, *33*, 2369–2376. [CrossRef]
89. Chowhan, N.; Singh, H.P.; Batish, D.R.; Kaur, S.; Ahuja, N.; Kohli, R.K. β-Pinene inhibited germination and early growth involves membrane peroxidation. *Protoplasma* **2013**, *250*, 691–700. [CrossRef] [PubMed]
90. Yun, K.W.; Kil, B.S.; Han, D.M. Phytotoxic and antimicrobial activity of volatile constituents of *Artemisia princeps* var. *orientalis*. *J. Chem. Ecol.* **1993**, *19*, 2757–2766. [CrossRef] [PubMed]
91. Bais, H.P.; Vepachedu, R.; Gilroy, S.; Callaway, R.M.; Vivanco, J.M. Allelopathy and exotic plant invasion: From molecules and genes to species interaction. *Science* **2003**, *301*, 1377–1380. [CrossRef]
92. Smith, S.E.; Read, D.J. *Mycorrhizal Symbiosis*, 3rd ed.; Academic Press: London, UK, 2008; pp. 1–815.
93. Diagne, N.; Ngom, M.; Djighaly, P.I.; Fall, D.; Hocher, V.; Svistoonoff, S. Roles of Arbuscular Mycorrhizal Fungi on Plant Growth and Performance: Importance in Biotic and Abiotic Stressed Regulation. *Diversity* **2020**, *12*, 370. [CrossRef]
94. Tang, H.; Hassan, M.U.; Feng, L.; Nawaz, M.; Shah, A.N.; Qari, S.H.; Liu, Y.; Miao, J. The critical role of arbuscular mycorrhizal fungi to improve drought tolerance and nitrogen use efficiency in crops. *Front. Plant Sci.* **2022**, *13*, 919166. [CrossRef] [PubMed]
95. Nishidono, Y.; Tanaka, K. Comprehensive characterization of polyacetylenes and diterpenes from the underground parts of *Solidago altissima* L. and their contribution to the overall allelopathic activity. *Phytochemistry* **2022**, *193*, 112986. [CrossRef]
96. Ichihara, K.; Kawai, T.; Kaji, M.; Noda, M. A mew polyacetylene from *Solidago altissima* L. *Agric. Biol. Chem.* **1976**, *40*, 353–358. [CrossRef]

97. Kawazu, K.; Ariwa, M.; Kii, Y. An ovicidal substance, *cis*-dehydromatricaria ester from *Solidago altissima*. *Agric. Biol. Chem.* **1977**, *41*, 223–224.
98. Johnson, R.H.; Halitschke, R.; Kessler, A. Simultaneous analysis of tissue- and genotype-specific variation in *Solidago altissima* (Asteraceae) rhizome terpenoids, and the polyacetylene dehydromatricaria ester. *Chemoecology* **2010**, *20*, 255–264. [CrossRef]
99. Nishino, C.; Manabe, S.; Kazui, M.; Matsuzaki, T. Piscicidal *cis*-clerodane diterpenes from *Solidago altissima*. L.: Absolute configurations of 5α, 10α-*cis*-clerodanes. *Tetrahedron Lett.* **1984**, *25*, 2809–2812. [CrossRef]
100. Bohlmann, F.; Singh, P.; Singh, R.K.; Joshi, K.C.; Jakupovic, J. A diterpene with a new carbon skeleton from *Solidago altissima*. *Phytochemistry* **1985**, *24*, 1114–1115. [CrossRef]
101. Tori, M.; Katto, A.; Sono, M. Nine new clerodane diterpenoids from rhizomes of *Solidago altissima*. *Phytochemistry* **1999**, *52*, 487–493. [CrossRef]
102. Nishidono, Y.; Tanaka, K. New clerodane diterpenoids from *Solidago altissima* and stereochemical elucidation via $^{13}C$ NMR chemical shift analysis. *Tetrahedron* **2022**, *110*, 132691. [CrossRef]
103. Okano, A.; Nomura, Y.; Tezuka, T. Identification of bauerenol in *Solidago altissima*. *J. Nat. Prod.* **1983**, *46*, 750–751. [CrossRef]
104. Sawabe, A.; Minemoto, K.; Minematsu, T.; Ouchi, S.; Okamoto, T.; Morita, M.; Ouchi, S.; Okamoto, T. Characterization of the *Z* and *E* isomers of dehydromatricaria lactones. *J. Jpn. Oil Chem. Soc.* **1997**, *46*, 413–417. [CrossRef]
105. Jin, H.; Tanaka, T.; Kouno, I.; Ishimaru, K. A new kaempferol trioside from *Solidago altissima* L. *J. Nat. Med.* **2007**, *61*, 351–354. [CrossRef]
106. Wu, B.; Takahashi, T.; Kashiwagi, T.; Tebayashi, S.; Kim, C.S. New flavonoid glycosides from the leaves of *Solidago altissima*. *Chem. Pharm. Bull.* **2007**, *55*, 815–816. [CrossRef]
107. Jin, H.; Ogino, K.; Fujioka, T.; Yoshida, M.; Ishimaru, K. A new acylphloroglucinol glycoside from *Solidago altissima* L. *J. Nat. Med.* **2008**, *62*, 199–201. [CrossRef]
108. Sawabe, A.; Minemoto, K.; Ouchi, S.; Okamoto, T. Effects of acetylenes and terpenoids from *Solidago altissima* L. on seed germination. *J. Jpn. Oil Chem. Soc.* **1999**, *48*, 139–142. [CrossRef]
109. Salah, M.A.; Bedir, E.; Toyang, N.J.; Khan, I.A.; Harries, M.D.; Wedge, D.E. Antifungal clerodane diterpenes from *Macaranga monandra* (L) Muell. et Arg. (Euphorbiaceae). *J. Agric. Food Chem.* **2003**, *51*, 7607–7610. [CrossRef] [PubMed]
110. Morimoto, M. Chemical defense against insects in *Heterotheca subaxillaris* and three Orobanchaceae species using exudates from trichomes. *Pest Manag. Sci.* **2019**, *75*, 2474–2481. [CrossRef] [PubMed]
111. Ichihara, K.; Kawai, T.; Noda, M. Polyacetylenes of *Solidago altissima* L. *Agric. Biol. Chem.* **1978**, *42*, 427–431. [CrossRef]
112. Minto, R.E.; Blacklock, B.J. Biosynthesis and function of polyacetylenes and allied natural products. *Prog. Lipid Res.* **2008**, *47*, 233–306. [PubMed]
113. Uesugi, A.; Kessler, K. Herbivore exclusion drives the evolution of plant competitiveness via increased allelopathy. *New Phytol.* **2013**, *198*, 916–924. [CrossRef]
114. Carson, W.; Root, R. Herbivory and plant species coexistence: Community regulation by an outbreaking phytophagous insect. *Ecol. Monogr.* **2000**, *70*, 73–99. [CrossRef]
115. Yamada, T. Miscanthus. In *Industrial Crops. Handbook of Plant Breeding*; Cruz, V.M.V., Dierig, D.A., Eds.; Springer: New York, NY, USA, 2015; Volume 9, pp. 43–66.
116. Uesugi, A.; Johnson, R.; Kessler, K. Context-dependent induction of allelopathy in plants under competition. *Oikos* **2019**, *128*, 1492–1502. [CrossRef]
117. Ito, I.; Kobayashi, K.; Yoneyama, T. Fate of dehydromatricaria ester added to soil and its implications for the allelopathic effect of *Solidago altissima* L. *Ann. Bot.* **1998**, *82*, 625–630. [CrossRef]
118. Kaur, H.; Kaur, R.; Kaur, S.; Baldwin, I.T.; Inderjit. Taking ecological function seriously: Soil microbial communities can obviate allelopathic effects of released metabolites. *PLoS ONE* **2004**, *4*, e4700. [CrossRef]
119. Kobayashi, K.; Koyama, H.; Shim, I. Relationship between behaviour of dehydromatricaria ester in soil and the allelopathic activity of *Solidago altissima* L. in the laboratory. *Plant Soil* **2004**, *259*, 97–102. [CrossRef]
120. Tsao, R.; Eto, M. Light-activated plant growth inhibitory activity of *cis*-dehydromatricaria ester, rose bengal and fluoren-9-one on lettuce (*Lactuca sativa* L.). *Chemosphere* **1996**, *32*, 1307–1317. [CrossRef]
121. Sakai, H.; Yoneda, K. Possible dual roles of an allelopathic compound, *cis*-dehydromatricaria ester. *J. Chem. Ecol.* **1981**, *8*, 185–193. [CrossRef] [PubMed]
122. Mack, R.M. Predicting the identity and fate of plant invaders: Emergent and emerging approaches. *Biol. Conserv.* **1996**, *78*, 107–121. [CrossRef]
123. Keane, R.M.; Crawley, M.J. Exotic plant invsions and the enemy release hypothesis. *Trends Ecol. Evol.* **2002**, *17*, 164–169. [CrossRef]
124. Ismail, M.; Kowsar, A.; Javed, S.; Choudhary, M.I.; Khan, S.W.; Abbas, Q.; Tang, Y.; Wang, W. The antibacterial, insecticidal and nematocidal activities and toxicity studies of *Tanacetum falconeri* Hook.f. Turk. *J. Pharm. Sci.* **2021**, *18*, 744–751.

plants

MDPI

*Review*

# *Abutilon theophrasti*'s Resilience against Allelochemical-Based Weed Management in Sustainable Agriculture – Due to Collection of Highly Advantageous Microorganisms?

**Vincenzo Tabaglio [1], Andrea Fiorini [1], Tracy M. Sterling [2] and Margot Schulz [3,*]**

[1] Department of Sustainable Crop Production DI.PRO.VE.S., Section Agronomy and Plant Biotechnologies, Università Cattolica del Sacro Cuore, Via Emilia Parmense 84, 29122 Piacenza, Italy
[2] Department of Land Resources & Environmental Sciences, Montana State University, Bozeman, MT 59717, USA
[3] IMBIO Institute of Molecular Physiology and Biotechnology of Plants, University of Bonn, Karlrobert-Kreiten Str. 13, 53115 Bonn, Germany
* Correspondence: ulp509@uni-bonn.de

**Abstract:** *Abutilon theophrasti* Medik. (velvetleaf) is a problematic annual weed in field crops which has invaded many temperate parts of the world. Since the loss of crop yields can be extensive, approaches to manage the weed include not only conventional methods, but also biological methods, for instance by microorganisms releasing phytotoxins and plant-derived allelochemicals. Additionally, benzoxazinoid-rich rye mulches effective in managing common weeds like *Amaranthus retroflexus* L. have been tested for this purpose. However, recent methods for biological control are still unreliable in terms of intensity and duration. Rye mulches were also ineffective in managing velvetleaf. In this review, we present the attempts to reduce velvetleaf infestation by biological methods and discuss possible reasons for the failure. The resilience of velvetleaf may be due to the extraordinary capacity of the plant to collect, for its own survival, the most suitable microorganisms from a given farming site, genetic and epigenetic adaptations, and a high stress memory. Such properties may have developed together with other advantageous abilities during selection by humans when the plant was used as a crop. Rewilding could be responsible for improving the microbiomes of *A. theophrasti*.

**Keywords:** *Abutilon theophrasti*; biological control; allelopathy; fungi; bacteria; secondary metabolites; benzoxazinoids; rye mulch

**Citation:** Tabaglio, V.; Fiorini, A.; Sterling, T.M.; Schulz, M. *Abutilon theophrasti*'s Resilience against Allelochemical-Based Weed Management in Sustainable Agriculture – Due to Collection of Highly Advantageous Microorganisms? *Plants* **2023**, *12*, 700. https://doi.org/10.3390/plants12040700

Academic Editor: Mónica Fernández-Aparicio

Received: 20 December 2022
Revised: 30 January 2023
Accepted: 1 February 2023
Published: 4 February 2023



## 1. Introduction

While its center of origin is uncertain, *Abutilon theophrasti* Medik. (velvetleaf) is thought to be native to China and India [1]. It was introduced across the Northern hemisphere as a fiber crop or protein food source and may have spread as a seed contaminant [1–4]. It is now a troublesome weed in major agricultural crops, such as in maize, soybeans, and cotton, and also grows in crops such as citrus, peach, and asparagus [5]. It has expanded its range to Africa, Australia, and New Zealand [6–9], and was recently identified as naturalized in Libya [10]. The species has regained interest as a fiber crop [7,11], taking up one of its old uses in Asia and for a short time in the USA, aside from its use as a medicinal plant [1,12]. In China and Kashmir, the seed is a valuable food because of its high protein content [2,8,9,13]. With the first archeological find of 7000-year-old velvetleaf seeds in a storage jar in southern Hungary, there is now evidence that velvetleaf was harvested, prepared, and stored by the Tisza culture, further supporting velvetleaf's use as food, fiber, and medicine [14].

However, velvetleaf remains a very competitive weed. Depending on water availability, velvetleaf density, and herbicide efficacy, maize yield loss can range up to 80% [5,15,16], up to 50% in cotton [17], and up to 70% in soybean [15,18,19], causing large economic losses [2,6,20]. Competitive maize hybrids have been evaluated as a strategy to manage velvetleaf [21–23]; nevertheless, velvetleaf must be controlled within maize's V3 to V8 growth stages to avoid negative effects on crop yield. Therefore, mixtures of synthetic herbicides are instead commonly recommended as pre- and post-treatments to manage velvetleaf [10,20,22]. However, herbicides can be expensive, and may persist in the environment or create selection pressures which result in the evolution of resistant biotypes. Four velvetleaf biotypes resistant to PSII herbicides have been independently reported to date [24].

Several *A. theophrasti* characteristics contribute to its competitive abilities and include its relatively large, hard-coated seeds, fast germination and emergence of the seedlings throughout the growing season, vigorous growth and large leaves, and high seed production, with long viability leading to persistent soil seed banks [2,25]. One plant can produce 8,000 seeds, with a significant percentage of them still viable for more than 50 years [2,13,25]. Moreover, velvetleaf is better colonized by arbuscular mycorrhizal fungi than other weeds, allowing velvetleaf greater access to nitrogen [26,27]. When in competition with maize, the genes of hexaploid velvetleaf involved in carbon utilization, photosynthesis, red light signaling, cell division, secondary metabolism, and phosphate availability are preferentially and more highly expressed [28]. In turn, numerous genes are downregulated in maize when grown near velvetleaf, such as those involved in photosynthesis, nutrient utilization, or signal transduction [29]. In addition, velvetleaf releases allelochemicals which are inhibitory to alfalfa, maize, and other crops (see below). In the 1980s, seed-associated endophytic microorganisms were suspected of enhancing velvetleaf´s fitness [30].

Therefore, in this article emphasizing sustainable agriculture, we shortly review results that underpin the hypothesis that *Abutilon* may organize its variable seed-coat and root-associated microbiomes with high flexibility. Additionally, this dependency on microbial diversity in site-specific soils allows for velvetleaf survival across diverse environments, for instance in those rich in benzoxazinoids and related allelochemicals.

## 2. Biological Control of *Abutilon theophrasti* by Microorganisms

Approaches to biological control of *A. theophrasti* include the use of microorganisms, plant-derived allelochemicals, mycoherbicides, or other microbial secondary metabolites. Fungi like *Verticillium dahliae, Alternaria abutilonis, Cercospora abutilonis, Cladosporium herbarum, Colletotrichum malvarum, Fusarium lateritium*, and others have been studied for this purpose [2,30–36], (Table 1). However, many of these fungi are not host specific and also infest crops (for instance, *Cercospora* leaf spot disease of sugar beet). In other cases, any biological activity damaging the weed is dependent on environmental conditions, and therefore, an unreliable tool for weed management. For instance, *F. lateritium*, a pathogenic agent of velvetleaf, reduced its growth in greenhouse experiments and in the field, but velvetleaf suppression varied from year to year, ranging from 46 to only 27% [35].

Similarly, an *Abutilon*-specific pathovar of *Colletotrichum coccodes* was genetically engineered to overexpress the oxaloacetate acetylhydrolase gene, creating a hypervirulent strain which was active at lower humidity and lethal to velvetleaf, but only through its three-leaf stage just after emergence [37]. Oxalate inhibits callose synthase by chelating the co-factor calcium, leading to less callose which weakens plant defenses [37]. Infection by other phytopathogens was also facilitated by higher oxalate levels and by exogenously applied oxalate [38–42]. Moreover, high oxalate amounts change the physicochemical properties of the soil, which may influence adjacent crops [43].

Another example in which pathogen efficacy for biological control of weeds was enhanced includes work which introduced the necrosis-inducing extracellular protein Nep1 from *Fusarium oxysporum*. This protein induces necrosis via ethylene synthesis and has been described as a successful biological control agent against weeds, including *A. theophrasti* [44,45]. However, genetically upgraded phytopathogens are generally not allowed anywhere in organic agriculture systems, nor in conventional agriculture in most EU countries.

Microbial secondary metabolites with phytotoxic properties against *Abutilon* produced by *Streptomyces* species [46] are able to inhibit velvetleaf germination and seedling growth by 100%. Even so, the velvetleaf seeds used in this study were surface-sterilized, disallowing any degradation or inactivation of bioherbicides by seed-surface-colonizing microorganisms, most likely reduced, if not eliminated under sterile conditions. Thus, the inhibition of velvetleaf growth found in laboratory experiments may not occur under field conditions. In other studies, hydrogen cyanide-producing *Pseudomonas putida* ATH-1RI/9 and *Acidovorax delafieldii* ATH2-2RS/1 suppress the growth of velvetleaf [47,48], though it is not known whether the bacterial-produced hydrogen cyanide was in concentrations lethal to soil organisms. It is important to note that many microorganisms can degrade hydrogen cyanide [49,50], which would remove any phytotoxic effects in the soil environment.

Overall, biological control of velvetleaf is not commonly used. Accordingly, velvetleaf is not mentioned as a target for biological control in relevant recent reviews [51,52]. As implied by Chee-Sanford et al. [53], a detailed knowledge of the entire ecosystem is a prerequisite when microorganisms will be used for the weed management. In general, it can be said that these biological control methods are still unreliable in terms of intensity and consistency, especially against weeds with gradual emergence in the field, like *A. theophrasti*.

**Table 1.** Microorganisms with biocidal effects on velvetleaf.

| Microorganisms | Mode of Action | Note | Reference |
|---|---|---|---|
| **Fungi** | | | |
| *Alternaria abutilonis* | leaf spot | | [2] |
| *Cercospora abutilonis*<br>*Cerospora* spec. complex? | Leaf spot | species needs<br>additional identification | [2] |
| *Cercospora althaeina* Sac. | Leaf rot | | [2] |
| *Cladosporium herbarum* | secondary leaf spot | | [2] |
| *Colletotrichum coccodes* | foliar pathogen, plant death;<br>suppression of plant defences | enhancement of virulence by mannose and oxalic acid, NEP1 for hypervirulent transgenic strain | [2,39,40,45] |
| *Colletotrichum malvarum* | leaf spot | | [2] |
| *Fusarium lateritium* | growth<br>suppression | | [2,35] |
| *Fusarium oxysporum* | 24-kDa protein Nep1 induces<br>necrosis | | [44] |
| *Macrophomina phaseoli* | stem rot | | [2] |
| *Phyllosticta althaeina* Sacc. | Leaf rot | | [2] |
| *Phymatotrichum omnivorum* | root rot | | [2] |
| *Puccinia heterospora* | rust | possible mycoherbicide | [2] |
| *Verticillium dahliae, V. nigrescens* | wilt | suggested as a biocontrol<br>agent, unspecific | [2] |
| **Bacteria** | | | |
| *Acidovorax delafieldii* ATH2-2RS/1 | inhibits growth | | [48] |
| *Pseudomonas putida* ATH-1RI/9 | inhibits growth | | [48] |
| *Pseudomonas* spec isolates Pp001<br>and Pf239 | Reduction of seedlings emergence<br>weaken seedlings | | [32] |
| *Streptomyces isolates* | inhibits germination, growth | | [46] |

*Natural Compounds—Monoterpenoids, Benzyl-Isothiocyanate, Phenolics, and Sorgoleone in the Management of Abutilon theophrasti*

Monoterpenes can be phytotoxic when applied in high dosage [54,55]. Vaughn and Spencer tested several volatile monoterpenes from the essential oils of aromatic plants for velvetleaf control in comparison to crops like maize, wheat, alfalfa, cucumber, and soybean [56]. While seed germination of Italian ryegrass (*Lolium multiflorum* Lam.), large crabgrass, (*Digitaria sanguinalis* (L.) Scop.), and redroot pigweed (*Amaranthus retroflexus* L.) was completely inhibited by many of the essential oils, velvetleaf exhibited a tolerance similar to that found with maize and cucumber. Only fenchone, citronellol, and citral totally suppressed velvetleaf germination, but fenchone was non-selective, also inhibiting maize, wheat, and alfalfa germination. The monoterpenes also inhibited growth of maize seedlings less than cucumber and alfalfa, but greater than soybean. Consistently, most volatile monoterpenes were not specific enough to only inhibit velvetleaf germination or seedling growth.

Wolf et al. described inhibitory effects of benzyl isothiocyanate from *Carica papaya* L. seeds on velvetleaf germination and seedling growth [57]. The *C. papaya* seeds contain not only the glucosinolate glucotropaeolin but also cyanogenic glycosides; in this study, the velvetleaf seeds were surface-sterilized. The inhibition of velvetleaf by benzyl isothiocyanate was also reported by Tollsten and Bergstrom [58]. In a study of Shettle and Balke [59], effects of salicylic acid, p-hydroxybenzoic acid, caffeine, hydroquinone, and umbelliferone on shoot dry-weight accumulation of several weeds and crops were investigated in a greenhouse trial. Except for hydroquinine, velvetleaf growth was only inhibited by the compounds when exposed to high amounts (56.0 kg $ha^{-1}$). Exudates from roots of competitive soybean cultivars have been studied for velvetleaf suppression as well; just 20 of 280 tested cultivars were able to reduce the dry weight of velvetleaf plants and did so up to 15% [60]. Dayan et al. demonstrated negative effects of sorgoleone, an allelochemical of *Sorghum bicolor* (L.) Moench on velvetleaf seedling emergence and rates of photosynthetic electron transfer in leaf discs [61]; however, the seedlings were again grown from surface-sterilized seeds. Apparently, there are presently no plant-derived compounds or extracts available which have sufficient allelopathic potential to manage velvetleaf in the field, including the benzoxazinoid-derived compounds (see below) and others [62].

Many secondary metabolites can modulate, even impoverish, species abundancies and the biodiversity of the original soil microbiome. Therefore, the use of plant and microbial allelochemicals as potential bioherbicides can lead to unexpected negative effects on valuable soil microorganisms. This consequence can be a problem when other crops relying on microbial species are subsequently cropped. Plant secondary metabolites such as glucosinolate breakdown products, p-coumaric acid, vanillic acid, salicylic acid, the flavonoids catechin and quercetin, and benzoxazinoids, gramine, and others affect microbe growth in laboratory and field studies [63–72]. Recovery of a rich biodiversity of microbial communities, for instance after fallow periods, is of utmost importance, not only for soil quality and fertility [73], but also to catalyze the complete metabolization of important plant and microbial allelochemicals such as catechol and polyphenols, including catechin and dihydroquercetin (see below) by specialized microorganisms and under special soil conditions [74].

## 3. Resilience of *Abutilon theophrasti* against Benzoxazinoid Allelochemicals from Rye (*Secale cereale* L.) Mulches

Benzoxazinoids are characteristic compounds found in maize and other gramineous species, including rye or wheat. Benzoxazinoids and phenoxazinone spontaneously produced from 2-aminophenol, a microbial degradation of benzoxazolinone, are phytotoxic [75,76]. These allelochemicals have the potential to help manage defined weed species [77–79]. Furthermore, rye cultivation as cover crop is increasingly gaining ground, both in conventional and, even more, in organic farming systems, due to agro-environmental benefits [80]. For instance, benzoxazinoids contained in rye mulch can manage numerous weeds such as *Chenopodium album* (L.), *Amaranthus retroflexus* (L.), *Portulaca oleracea* (L.), and others. At the same time, benzoxazinoid content in rye biomass depends on cultivar and growth stage [81–83]. In this respect, the termination timing of rye cover crop may influence the allelochemical concentrations in rye mulches which decrease with plant age [83], but, if delayed, also allow more biomass production and a concomitant physical control of weed seedlings emergence [84].

Therefore, several approaches have been undertaken to manage *A. theophrasti* using rye mulch. Mulches were prepared from different rye cultivars differing in their benzoxazinoid content, ranging from about 200 to 550 μg $g^{-1}$, and were used for pot experiments [83,85] (Figure 1). The mulches effectively reduced seedling growth of three weeds (*C. album*, *A. retroflexus*, *P. oleracea*); however, none of the mulches inhibited the growth of velvetleaf seedlings (Figure 1). Interestingly, the number of emerged velvetleaf seedlings in the mulched pots was 35% higher than in the control pots on average, though not statistically different. These results corroborate previous outcomes in other pot and field studies [82,85]. The failure to manage velvetleaf with rye mulches and velvetleaf's subsequent success in maize fields point to efficient strategies of the plant to cope with benzoxazinoid allelochemicals.

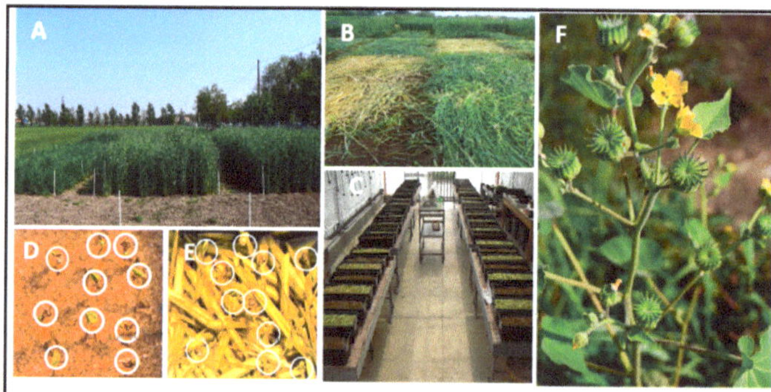


**Percentage of velvetleaf seedlings emerged 30 days after sowing, in presence of rye mulches or not control**

| Cultivar | Born | Fasto | For | Mat | Nik | Prim | Pro | Tri | C |
|---|---|---|---|---|---|---|---|---|---|
| % em. | 118 | 106 | 125 | 142 | 120 | 123 | 120 | 106 | 100 |
| **Cultivar** | **Duk.** | **Fasto** | **Fore** | **Hell** | **Hym** | **Prim.** | **Pro** | **Sito** | **C** |
| % em. | 70 | 65 | 63 | 69 | 61 | 69 | 63 | 68 | 49 |

**Figure 1.** (**A**,**B**): Preparation of rye mulches at the Università Cattolica del Sacro Cuore research station in Piacenza, Italy. (**C**): Rye mulch covered and control planter boxes for velvetleaf germination experiments in the greenhouse. (**D**,**E**): Emergence of velvetleaf seedlings (white circles) in pots with rye mulch (**E**), only seedlings overtopping the rye mulch cover are circled) in comparison to the control (**D**). (**F**): Flowering velvetleaf plant in a maize field. Table—Abbreviations: % em: percentage of emerged velvetleaf seedlings; cultivars: For, Forestier; Mat, Matador; Nik, Nikita, Prim, Primizia; Pro, Protector; Tri, Treviso; Duk, Dukato; Fore, Forestal; Hell, Hellvus; Hym, Hymonta; Sito, Sito70; C: control.

### 3.1. *Microorganisms Associated with Abutilon theophrasti and Microbial Role in Benzoxazinoid Tolerance*

A number of fungal species are known to colonize the seed coat of *A. theophrasti*, including *Cordyceps sinensis*, *Cephaliophora tropica*, *Mandurella mycetomatis*, *Actinomucor elegans*, *Aspergillus flavus*, *Trichoderma viridae*, *Penicillium* spp., *Fusarium* spp., *Alternaria alternata*, and *Verticillium* spp. [30,31,53], while *Cladosporium cladosporioides* and *Epicoccum purpurascens* are seed-borne fungi (Table 2). Bacteria isolated from the seed surface were identified as species belonging to the genera *Bacillus*, *Flavobacterium*, and *Pseudomonas*. More than half of the seeds contained seed-borne bacteria belonging to the genera *Pseudomonas*, *Alcaligenes*, and *Flavobacteria* [30]. There is also evidence for site-specific composition of seed-colonizing microorganisms. For example, velvetleaf seeds collected from three sites (Meleti, Pralboino, and Gambara) in Northern Italy were tested to verify the presence of endophytic fungi [86]. Seeds were surface-sterilized and then incubated at 25 °C for germination. *Alternaria alternata* was identified in 27% of the radicles and *Fusarium* spp. was identified in 36% of the radicles from seeds collected at Meleti site. In 42% of radicles from seeds collected at the Pralboino site, *Fusarium* species were present. Seeds from the Gambara site led to seedlings without these fungal endophytes. The isolation of fungi from 6-day-old radicles suggests migration from the seed to the root system. *Alternaria alternata* and *Fusarium* species, frequently associated with *A. theophrasti* seeds, are often endophytic [87,88].

**Table 2.** Microorganisms known to be associated with velvetleaf. Locations: 1 Missouri Agronomy Research Center, 2 Osage County, MO, USA; 3 Meleti, 4 Gambara, 5 Pralboino, Italy; 6 Gradiste, Serbia; 7 ASSET agricultural fields IL, USA; 8 USSEU undisturbed site IL, USA.

| Microorganisms | Seed Surface | Within Seeds | Location | Activity | Reference |
|---|---|---|---|---|---|
| **Fungi** | | | | | |
| *Actinomucor elegans*,<br>strain AF157119 | x<br>x | | 6<br>7 | protects *Abutilon* seedlings | [53,89–91] |
| *Alternaria alternata* | x | x | 1, 2, 3 | | [30,86] |
| *Aspergillus flavus* | x | | 7 | | [53] |
| *Cephaliophora tropica* strains | x | | 8 | | [53] |
| *Cladosporium cladosporioides* | x | | 1, 2 | | [30] |
| *Cordyceps sinensis* | x | | 7, 8 | | [53] |
| *Epicoccumpurpurascens* | x | | 1, 2 | inhibits seed-borne bacteria | [30] |
| *Fusarium* spp. | x | x | 1, 2, 3, 4, 5 | moderate antagonism toward test fungi | [30,86] |
| *Madurella mycetomatis* | x | | 8 | | [53] |
| **Bacteria** | | | | | |
| *Alcaligenes* spec. isolates | | | 1, 2 | highly antagonistic to seed fungi | [30] |
| *Bacillus* spec. isolates | | | 1, 2 | | [30] |
| *Bacillus subtilis* | | | 1, 2 | | [30] |
| *Flavobacterium* spec. | | | 1, 2 | | [30] |
| *Pseudomonas* spec. isolates | | | 1, 2 | | [30] |

*Actinomucor elegans* was found on velvetleaf seeds purchased from Herbiseed (Twyford, UK), which were harvested from the Herbiseed farm Gradiste, Serbia, in 2011 and 2012. *Actinomucor elegans* was not found on seeds harvested in 2013 from another Herbiseed farm site. These findings support the assumption that the habitat of the parent plant is crucial for the variable microbial species composition associated with *A. theophrasti* seeds. It is known that root microbiomes contain microorganisms attracted from the soil microbial community [89]. *Actinomucor elegans*, re-isolated from velvetleaf roots, was identified as a "consortium", harboring numerous bacteria, for instance, *Pantoea ananatis* and *Stenotrophomonas maltophilia* and the yeast *Papiliotrema baii*. This consortium has a larger metabolic potential than its isolated members [90].

Incubations of the *A. elegans* consortium with benzoxazolinone (BOA), the first degradation product of benzoxazinone, did not inhibit fungal growth or lead to any degradation or detoxification products within one week. Additionally, phenoxazinone, a phytotoxin derived from 2-aminophenol, a microbial degradation product of BOA, did not impair fungal growth. Even under nutrient deficiencies, the consortium did not use these compounds as a C or N source [91,92]. Nevertheless, the consortium responded to high BOA concentrations by enhancing the glucosyl ceramide content of membranes isolated from the consortium [93]. The consortium released tryptophan as the most prominent compound into the medium. Tryptophan release increased in the presence of BOA during the first week of incubation but dropped below the control level with increasing incubation times over four weeks [92]. It is doubtful that the released tryptophan is used for auxin production by the Trp-dependent IAA biosynthetic pathway when the consortium colonizes velvetleaf roots, since its root exudates have the potential to reduce IAA production significantly. This possibility is important since high IAA amounts are deleterious to velvetleaf growth [94]. The consortium had no inhibitory effect of germination or seedling growth (Figure 2). In contrast, *A. elegans* hyphae seems to protect the seedlings ([90,95], and see below).

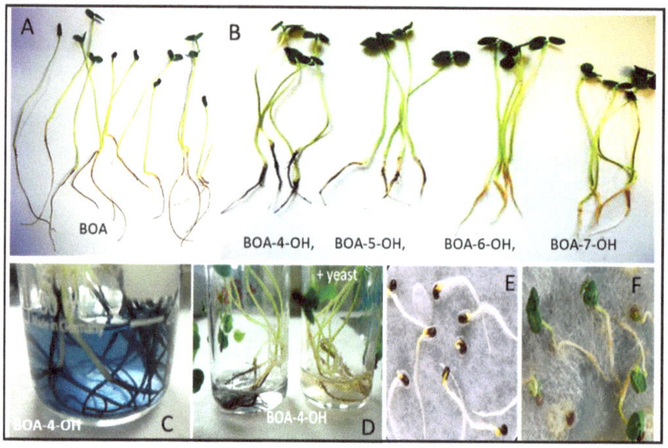


**Figure 2.** (**A**): Seedlings after 24 h BOA incubation, leaves are not impaired. (**B**): Incubations of seedlings with the four BOA-OH isomers. Seedlings are shown after the incubation: Only BOA-4-OH led to roots covered with a bluish-black polymer. (**C**): Roots exposed to BOA-4-OH during incubation. (**D**): Addition of the yeast *Papiliotrema baii*, a member of the *Actinomucor elegans* consortium, prevents polymer covers on the root surfaces. (**E**): *A. elegans* consortium has no damaging effects on germinating velvetleaf. (**F**): Healthy velvetleaf seedlings are cocooned by *A. elegans* hyphae.

Isolated *P. ananatis* and the entire consortium, but not the isolated yeast, are able to nitrate the plant-produced detoxification intermediate BOA-6-OH, resulting in 6-hydroxy-5-nitrobenzo[*d*]oxazol-2(3*H*)-one (NO2-BOA-6-OH). In contrast, *P. baii* formed only a dimer of BOA-6-OH [90,96]. NO2-BOA-6-OH was produced by velvetleaf root surface proteins and was also identified in the incubation media of velvetleaf when supplemented with BOA-6-OH. This nitroaromatic compound in concentrations of 8 to 86 μM enhanced *A. theophrasti* root growth at pH 5 but had no effect on shoot growth. The $I_{50}$ value was 300 μM for root growth at pH 5 and 700 μM for shoot growth at pH range of 4 to 6. Velvetleaf root surface proteins that included microbial sources were able to reduce NO2-BOA-6-OH up to 90% when assayed in vitro with the compound. In contrast, *Lepidium sativum* (L.) root and shoot growth was inhibited by 50% and 90%, respectively, with 86 μM NO2-BOA-6-OH [96].

NO2-BOA-6-OH? $I_{50}$ values were 20 μM at pH 6.0 for *L. sativum* root growth and 10 μM for its shoot growth [96]. Thus, NO2-BOA-6-OH can be deleterious for other plants, but apparently not for velvetleaf grown from non-sterilized seeds.

### 3.2. Defense Strategies against Benzoxazolinone (BOA)—Uptake, Detoxification, Membrane Repair, and Polymerizations at the Root Surface

Velvetleaf detoxifies benzoxazolinone (BOA) differently than other important summer weeds, such as *Chenopodium album*, *Amaranthus retroflexus*, and *Portulaca oleracea*, but also many others. While BOA uptake by velvetleaf roots was similar to uptake by *C. album*, *A. retroflexus* and *P. oleracea*, velvetleaf roots produced remarkably fewer detoxification products when 20 to 40 μmol BOA was applied. Additionally, less BOA was transported to the shoots where almost no detoxification products were found in velvetleaf shoots, in contrast to the above-mentioned weed species [97].

Velvetleaf seedlings not colonized by the *A. elegans* consortium exhibited a different detoxification behavior by accumulating higher amounts of BOA-6-O-glucoside in roots and shoots during incubation with 500 μM BOA [90,97]. When colonized by the consortium, more BOA-5-O-glucoside than BOA-6-O-glucoside accumulated in velvetleaf roots, suggesting that the consortium influences the position of BOA hydroxylation. Without the fungus, velvetleaf seedling length was affected by BOA-6-OH and BOA-5-OH in comparison to the control, while BOA-6-OH led to a higher inhibition than BOA-5-OH. Velvetleaf seedlings grown from seeds not associated with *A. elegans* from the Meleti field also had more BOA-6-O-glucoside than BOA-5-O-glucoside.

The responsible glucosyltransferase activity could be extracted from plant cell wall material whereas the cytosolic fraction was inactive. The plant-produced intermediates BOA-6-OH and BOA-5-OH, as well as the synthetic isomers BOA-4- and -7-OH, led to brownish and black roots but otherwise had no effect on the phenotype, although all these compounds also induced $H_2O_2$ production, indicated by high catalase activity at the root surfaces [90] (Figure 2). High catalase activity was found in the bacterial isolates and a yeast belonging to the *A. elegans* consortium (see above). On root surfaces, peroxidase, laccase, and phenol oxidase activities could also be measured, so at least a portion of these activities are from root-colonizing microorganisms [90]. Acting in concert, the activities are responsible for BOA-OH polymer formation at the root surface (Figure 2). It is unknown whether these polymers permanently cover roots under natural conditions, because microorganisms, for instance the yeast *P. baii*, associated with the consortium, remove BOA-4-OH over time, also preventing its polymerization.

Incubation of velvetleaf seedlings with BOA-6-OH, which has a higher toxicity than BOA, damages membrane lipids and fatty acids in the root tips. Decreased content of α-linoleic acid (18:2), phosphatidylinositol, and phosphatidylcholine were measured in root tips within 30 min of incubation. However, membrane repair was as rapid as found with maize root tips and control levels were reestablished within one hour after exposure to the compound [98]. Thus, even when BOA-6-OH would accumulate in velvetleaf root tips, which had not yet been observed, the plant has powerful mechanisms for rapid membrane repair.

Like many other natural compounds, benzoxazinoids are considered templates for the design of new herbicides. Substitutions such as hydroxylation, especially in position 6, activate BOA, allowing further substitutions, for instance, in the case of 6-hydroxylation, in which nitration in position 5 reduces the phytotoxicity for *Abutilon*.

## 4. Secondary Metabolites of Velvetleaf

The allelopathic activity of aqueous and methanolic extracts from all parts of *A. theophrasti* has often been studied. In particular, exudates of the glandular trichomes of *Abutilon* are phytotoxic [18,99]. Inhibitory effects of aqueous extracts from velvetleaf plants on maize, tomato, sugar beet, oilseed rape, oats, cucumber, radish, soybean, and sunflower have also been described [100–102]. Paszkowski and Kremer [103] identified the flavonoids delphinidin, cyanidin, quercetin, myricetin, (+), (−)- catechin, and -epicatechin in extracts from velvetleaf seed coats. Kaempferol 3-O-β-(6″-p-coumaroyl) glucopyranoside was identified in methanolic extracts of above-ground velvetleaf tissue [104]. Tian et al. [105] reported gallic acid, protocatechuic acid, tannin, catechin, vanillic acid, caffeic acid, ferulic acid, rutin, and quercetin in extracts from the root, stem, leaves, seeds, and exocarp. Hibiscuslide C isolated from velvetleaf above-ground tissue had antifungal activity in *Candida albicans* [106]. In addition, Mamadalieva et al. [107] isolated (6S,9R)-roseoside and (6S,9S)-roseoside from the aerial parts of the plant (Figure 3).

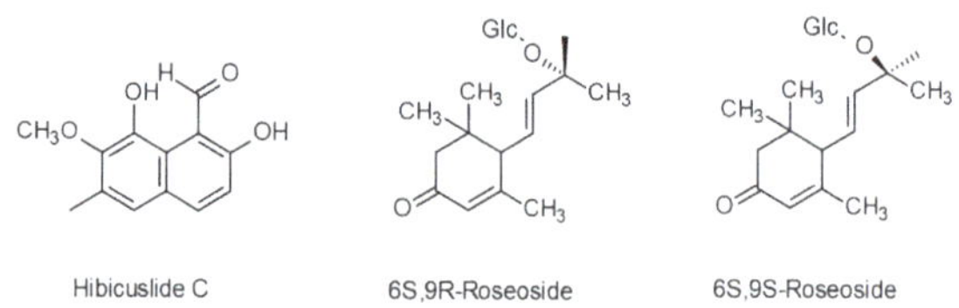


**Figure 3.** Less known secondary metabolites found in extracts of *A. theophrasti:* hibiscuslide C and roseosides, identified by Hwang et al. and Mamadalieva et al. [106,107].

Aqueous extracts of velvetleaf seed coats can inhibit multiple soil fungi. Single flavonoids from velvetleaf leaves and stems had negative effects on fungi with seed-decomposing properties [104]. It is possible that not all bioactive secondary metabolites of velvetleaf are yet identified, but almost all of those known are widespread across plants and can act as allelochemicals. Additionally, the more recently identified roseosides are not specific to velvetleaf. They have been found in *Adina* and a *Polygonum* species and in *Centella erecta* [108–110]. Except for the roseosides and hibiscuslide C, all the identified phenolic compounds are known for complete degradation by bacteria (Figure 4).

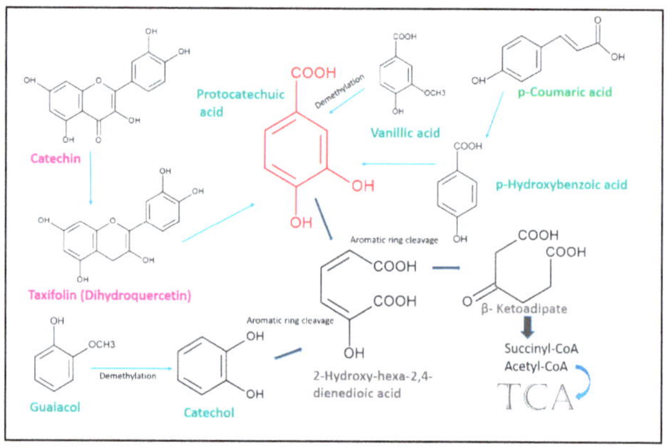


**Figure 4.** Some steps of the microbial degradation of catechin and taxifolin as members of the flavonoids (magenta), p-coumaric acid, a cinnamic acid derivative (green), and several simple phenolic compounds (petrol). Many phenolic compounds are degraded via the central intermediate protocatechuic acid, and others via catechol. Catechol and protocatechuic acid (red structure) undergo either ortho- or meta- cleavage of the aromatic ring, resulting in 2-hydroxy-hexa-2,4-dienedioic acid and β-ketoadipate. These compounds are converted to succinyl-CoA and acetyl-CoA for entering the citrate cycle (TCA).

Consistently, these compounds in their monomeric form do not accumulate appreciably in the soil, but perhaps do so within the rhizosphere in amounts that are sufficient for allelopathic inhibitions or other functions. More likely, the compounds in their specific combination and amount may have defined chemotactic properties, attracting microorganisms valuable for velvetleaf fitness at a given growing site. Additionally, degradation intermediates, when sufficiently stable, may have defined functions, as was shown for protocatechuic acid derived from catechin [69]. Protocatechuic acid is phytotoxic, but the compound also has antioxidant activity [111]. Microbial conversions and degradation products of the parental phenolic secondary metabolites increase the number of bioactive derivatives dramatically, at least temporarily, but their roles, particularly short-term ones, in the plant–microbe interaction are understudied. Is the production of common and unusual microbial conversion products one reason for the deleterious impacts on other plants, although these plants synthesize the same compounds and exude them? Presently, this question cannot be answered. Since many phenolic compounds have antioxidant properties, they may also protect beneficial, root-colonizing microorganisms against oxidative stress when attacked by pathogens or when faced with antibiotics produced by competitive species used for allelopathic activity. When highly concentrated, the protection provided by phenolic compounds with antioxidant properties will reverse and become toxic.

## 5. Considerations and Further Perspective

This short review demonstrates the extraordinary capability of *A. theophrasti* to withstand attempts for its biological control, for instance by allelochemicals. Velvetleaf seems equipped with a combination of highly efficient, unique strategies, in addition to those mentioned in the introduction, for high tolerance against allelochemicals such as benzoxazinoids. One of these strategies is certainly featured by attracting the most suitable soil microorganisms, thus avoiding competitive conflicts among the attracted species and the already established species. This strategy allows enormous flexibility and an optimal adaptation to different growing sites with specific pedo-climatic conditions and interspecific interactions between micro- and macro-biota. The mode of attraction is unclear, but the exuded secondary metabolites, perhaps specific mixtures of them, are certainly involved. The microbe-*Abutilon* interactions may be of crucial importance for the success of the plant.

Another strategy encompasses the translocation of allelochemical detoxification and elimination into the cell wall compartment and to the root surface, where microorganisms take over the work. This strategy seems to be highly developed in velvetleaf and presents a distinctive difference to many other weeds and crops. The assumption is in line with the finding that bentazon metabolites were not detected in velvetleaf cells prepared from calli produced in axenic culture, in the velvetleaf hypocotyl sections, or in the media used for incubations. In contrast, soybean cells from suspension cultures detoxified bentazon to 6-*O*-ß-glucose-bentazon and 8-*O*-ß-glucose-bentazon [112]. It can also be hypothesized that the plant has evolved mechanisms for suppressing the release of phytotoxins produced by microorganisms that intrude the rhizosphere. The inhibition of bacterial IAA production points in this direction.

Other reasons for *Abutilon's* fitness may be related to its old use as a crop, where plants with desired new properties were selected by humans for further cultivation [1], while escapes of the cultured plant to the wild might allow velvetleaf more opportunity to select suitable microorganisms from its soil. During rewilding, domesticated *Abutilon* could reestablish or even improve its microbiomes for re-attaining biodiversity levels previously lost or diminished during domestication. Diminished microbiome diversity as a result of cultivation is a known phenomenon for some crops [113,114], and rewilding to improve microbiomes is being explored to strengthen modern crops [115], if such restoration is still possible given the loss of microbial biodiversity due to human activities [116]. When experiencing stress conditions during rewilding, *Abutilon* might have also evolved a strong transgenerational stress memory that includes epigenetics, overaccumulation of proteins involved in managing stress, in dynamic proteome modulation and rapid protein interactions to adapt quickly to stress conditions [117], while concurrently maintaining high seed production. Presently speculative, *Abutilon* may collect preferentially microorganisms with a well-developed stress memory [118], although the molecular mechanisms of selective capture are enigmatic.

Ghanizadeh and James studied the establishment of velvetleaf in different regions of New Zealand and found that the invasion dynamics depend on climate niches with different local temperatures and daily solar radiation [9]. For this reason, velvetleaf is problematic only in one region in the North Island where temperatures are higher, suggesting that there are limiting factors for velvetleaf and its ability to adapt [9], although the influence of soil microbiomes was not included in the study. It is certainly worthwhile to study the genetic, biochemical, and physiological traits of this weed more intensively to disclose vulnerable features and strong attributes important for survival. In this sense, *A. theophrasti* could be a role model for the development of new strategies and environmentally acceptable technologies that strengthen crops when in competition with weeds.

**Author Contributions:** Conceptualization, M.S. and V.T.; data curation, V.T., M.S. A.F. and T.M.S.; writing, M.S., V.T. and T.M.S. All authors have read and agreed to the published version of the manuscript.

**Funding:** This research received no external funding.

**Data Availability Statement:** Not applicable.

**Conflicts of Interest:** The authors declare no conflict of interest.

## References


1. Cardina, J. *Lives of Weeds: Opportunism, Resistance, Folly*; Cornell University Press: Ithaca, NY, USA, 2021; Chapter 3; pp. 73–100, ISBN 9781501758980.
2. Warwick, S.I.; Black, L.D. The biology of Canadian Weeds. 90. *Abutilon theophrasti*. *Can. J. Plant Sci.* **1988**, *68*, 1069–1085. [CrossRef]
3. Stegink, S.J.; Spencer, N.R. Using Protein Electrophoresis to Investigate the Phylogeny of Velvetleaf (*Abutilon theophrasti*). *Weed Sci.* **1988**, *36*, 172–175. Available online: https://www.jstor.org/stable/4044866 (accessed on 31 January 2023). [CrossRef]
4. Rojas-Sandoval, J. Abutilon theophrasti (Velvet Leaf). Available online: https://cabidigitallibrary.org/terms-and-conditions (accessed on 3 March 2022).
5. Cortés, J.A.; Mendiola, M.A.; Castejón, M. Competition of velvetleaf (*Abutilon theophrasti*) weed with cotton (*Gossypium hirsutum* L.). Economic damage threshold. *Span. J. Agric. Res.* **2010**, *8*, 391–399. [CrossRef]
6. Rain, A.S.; Cârciu, G. *Abutilon theophrasti* L. (velvetleaf): A problem-weed for grain maize. *J. Hortic. Sci. Biotechnol.* **2018**, *22*, 124–127. Available online: https://journal-hfb.usab-tm.ro/2018/Volum%2022(3)%20PDF/21Rain%20A.%202.pdf (accessed on 31 January 2023).
7. Follak, S.; Aldrian, U.; Schwarz, M. Spread dynamics of *Abutilon theophrasti* in Central Europe. *Plant Protect. Sci.* **2014**, *50*, 157–163. [CrossRef]
8. Tanji, A.; Taleb, A. New weed species recently introduced into Morocco. *Weed Res.* **1997**, *37*, 27–31. [CrossRef]
9. Ghanizadeh, H.; James, T.K. Behaviour of *Abutilon theophrasti* in Different Climatic Niches: A New Zealand Case Study. *Front. Plant Sci.* **2022**, *13*, 885779. [CrossRef]
10. Mahklouf, M.H.; El-Ahamir, S.M. The First Record of *Abutilon theophrasti* (Malvaceae) in the Flora of Libya. *Phytotaxa* **2019**, *402*, 259–264. [CrossRef]
11. Scheliga, M.; Brand, U.; Türk, O.; Gruber, S.; Petersen, J. Field Trials Indicating the Potential of *Abutilon theophrasti* (Medic.) as a New Fibre Crop in Southwest Germany. *J. Adv. Agric.* **2019**, *10*, 1726–1739. [CrossRef]
12. Bensky, D.; Gamble, A.; Kaptchuk, T.J. *Chinese Herbal Medicine: Materia Medica*; Eastland Press: Seattle, WA, USA, 1993; pp. 142–143. ISBN 0939616157.
13. Spencer, N.R. Velvetleaf, *Abutilon theophrasti* (Malvaceae). History and Economic Impact in the United States. *Econ. Bot.* **1984**, *38*, 407–416. Available online: https://www.jstor.org/stable/4254678 (accessed on 31 January 2023). [CrossRef]
14. Medovic, A.; Horvath, F. Content of a Storage Jar from the Late Neolithic Site of Hódmezővásárhely-Gorzsa, South Hungary: A Thousand Carbonized Seeds of *Abutilon theophrasti* Medic. *Veg. Hist. Archaeobot.* **2012**, *21*, 215–220. [CrossRef]
15. Vaughn, L.G.; Bernards, M.L.; Arkebauer, T.J.; Lindquist, J.L. Corn and Velvetleaf (*Abutilon theophrasti*) Growth and Transpiration Efficiency under Varying Water Supply. *Weed Sci.* **2016**, *64*, 596–604. Available online: https://www.jstor.org/stable/26420728 (accessed on 31 January 2023). [CrossRef]
16. Lindquist, J.L.; Mortensen, D.A. Tolerance and Velvetleaf (*Abutilon theophrasti*) Suppressive Ability of Two Old and Two Modern Corn (*Zea mays*) Hybrids. *Weed Sci.* **1998**, *46*, 569–574. [CrossRef]
17. Ma, X.; Yang, J.; Wu, H.; Jiang, W.; Ma, Y.; Ma, Y. Growth Analysis of Cotton in Competition with Velvetleaf (*Abutilon theophrasti*). *Weed Technol.* **2016**, *30*, 123–136. [CrossRef]

18. Sterling, T.M.; Putnam, A.R. Possible role of glandular trichome exudates in interference by velvetleaf (*Abutilon theophrasti*). *Weed Sci.* **1987**, *35*, 308–314. Available online: https://www.jstor.onarg/stable/4044589 (accessed on 31 January 2023). [CrossRef]
19. De Sanctis, J.; Jhala, A. Interaction of dicamba, fluthiacet-methyl, and glyphosate for control of velvetleaf (*Abutilon theophrasti*) in dicamba/glyphosate–resistant soybean. *Weed Technol.* **2021**, *35*, 761–767. [CrossRef]
20. Striegel, A.; Eskridge, K.M.; Lawrence, N.C.; Knezevic, S.Z.; Kruger, G.R.; Proctor, C.A.; Hein, G.L.; Jhala, A.J. Economics of herbicide programs for weed control in conventional, glufosinate, and dicamba/glyphosate-resistant soybean across Nebraska. *Agron. J.* **2020**, *112*, 5158–5179. [CrossRef]
21. Travlos, I.; Kanatas, P.; Economou, G.; Kotoulas, V.; Chachalis, D.; Tsioros, S. Evaluation of velvetleaf interference with maize hybrids as influenced by relative time of emergence. *Exp. Agric.* **2012**, *48*, 127–137. [CrossRef]
22. Tataridas, A.; Kanatas, P.; Chatzigeorgiou, A.; Zannopoulos, S.; Travlos, I. Sustainable Crop and Weed Management in the Era of the EU Green Deal: A Survival Guide. *Agronomy* **2022**, *12*, 589. [CrossRef]
23. Barnes, E.R.; Lawrence, N.C.; Knezevic, S.Z.; Rodriguez, O.; Irmak, S.; Jhala, A.J. Weed control and response of yellow and white popcorn hybrids to herbicides. *Agron. J.* **2020**, *112*, 458–469. [CrossRef]
24. Heap, I. The International Survey of Herbicide Resistant Weeds. Available online: www.weedscience.org (accessed on 12 December 2022).
25. Cardina, J.; Norquay, H.M. Seed Production and Seedbank Dynamics in Subthreshold Velvetleaf (*Abutilon theophrasti*) Populations. *Weed Sci.* **1997**, *45*, 85–90. Available online: https://www.jstor.org/stable/4045717 (accessed on 31 January 2023). [CrossRef]
26. Vatovec, C.; Jordan, N.; Huerd, S. Responsiveness of certain agronomic weed species to arbuscular mycorrhizal fungi. *Renew. Agric. Food Syst.* **2005**, *20*, 181–189. [CrossRef]
27. O'Neil, C.M.; Nash, J.; Tiemann, L.K.; Miesel, J.R. Mycorrhizal Symbioses Enhance Competitive Weed Growth in Biochar and Nutrient-Amended Soils. *Front. Agron.* **2021**, *3*, 731184. [CrossRef]
28. Horvath, D.P.; Llewellyn, D.; Clay, S.A. Heterologous Hybridization of Cotton Microarrays with Velvetleaf (*Abutilon theophrasti*) Reveals Physiological Responses due to Corn Competition. *Weed Sci.* **2007**, *55*, 546–557. Available online: https://www.jstor.org/stable/4539616 (accessed on 31 January 2023). [CrossRef]
29. Horvath, D.; Gulden, R.; Clay, S. Microarray analysis of late-season velvetleaf (*Abutilon theophrasti*) effect on corn. *Weed Sci.* **2006**, *54*, 983–994. [CrossRef]
30. Kremer, R.J.; Hughes, L.B., Jr.; Aldrich, R.J. Examination of Microorganisms and Deterioration Resistance Mechanisms Associated with Velvetleaf Seed. *Agron. J.* **1984**, *76*, 745–749. [CrossRef]
31. Kremer, R.J. Antimicrobial Activity of Velvetleaf (*Abutilon theophrasti*) Seeds. *Weed Sci.* **1986**, *34*, 617–622. [CrossRef]
32. Kremer, R.J.; Kennedy, A.C. Rhizobacteria as biocontrol agents of weeds. *Weed Technol.* **1996**, *10*, 601–609. [CrossRef]
33. Boyetchko, S. Impact of soil microorganisms on weed biology and ecology. *Phytoprotection* **1996**, *77*, 41–56. [CrossRef]
34. Kremer, R.J.; Spencer, N.R. Impact of a Seed-Feeding Insect and Microorganisms of Velvetleaf (*Abutilon theophrasti*) Seed Viability. *Weed Sci.* **1989**, *37*, 211–216. Available online: https://www.jstor.org/stable/4044846 (accessed on 31 January 2023). [CrossRef]
35. Boyette, C.; Walker, H. Evaluation of *Fusarium lateritium* as a Biological Herbicide for Controlling Velvetleaf (*Abutilon theophrasti*) and Prickly Sida (*Sida spinosa*). *Weed Sci.* **1986**, *34*, 106–109. [CrossRef]
36. Chee-Sanford, J.C.; Williams, M.M.; Davis, A.S.; Sims, G.K. Do microorganisms influence seed-bank dynamics? *Weed Sci.* **2006**, *54*, 575–587. [CrossRef]
37. Meir, S.; Larroche, C.; Al-Ahmad, H.; Gressel, J. Fungal transformation of *Colletotrichum coccodes* with bacterial oahA to suppress defenses of *Abutilon theophrasti*. *Crop. Prot.* **2009**, *28*, 749–755. [CrossRef]
38. Gressel, J.; Michaeli, D.; Kampel, V.; Amsellem, Z.; Warshawsky, A. Ultralow calcium requirements of fungi facilitate use of calcium regulating agents to suppress host calcium-dependent defenses, synergizing infection by a mycoherbicide. *J. Agric. Food Chem.* **2002**, *50*, 6353–6360. [CrossRef]
39. Ahn, B.; Paulitz, T.; Jabaji-Hare, S.; Watson, A. Enhancement of *Colletotrichum coccodes* virulence by inhibitors of plant defense mechanisms. *Biocontrol Sci. Technol.* **2005**, *15*, 299–308. [CrossRef]
40. Dutton, M.V.; Evans, C.S. Oxalate production by fungi: Its role in pathogenicity and ecology in the soil environment. *Can. J. Microbiol.* **1996**, *42*, 881–895. [CrossRef]
41. Briere, S.C.; Watson, A.K.; Hallett, S.G. Oxalic acid production and mycelia biomass yield of *Sclerotinia minor* for the formulation enhancement of a granular turf bioherbicide. *Biocontrol Sci. Technol.* **2000**, *10*, 281–289. [CrossRef]
42. Watson, A.K.; Ahn, E.S. *Better Control of Weeds with Enhanced Bioherbicides. Enhancing Biocontrol Agents and Handling Risks*; Vurro, M., Gressel, J., Butt, T., Harman, G., Pilgeram, A., Leger, R.S., Nuss, D., Eds.; IOS Press: Amsterdam, The Netherlands, 2001; pp. 106–113.
43. Syed, S.; Buddolla, V.; Lian, B. Oxalate Carbonate Pathway—Conversion and Fixation of Soil Carbon—A Potential Scenario for Sustainability. *Front. Plant Sci.* **2020**, *11*, 591297. [CrossRef]
44. Jennings, J.C.; Apel-Birkhold, P.C.; Bailey, B.A.; Anderson, J.D. Induction of Ethylene Biosynthesis and Necrosis in Weed Leaves by a *Fusarium oxysporum* Protein. *Weed Sci.* **2000**, *48*, 7–14. Available online: http://www.jstor.org/stable/4046151 (accessed on 31 January 2023). [CrossRef]
45. Amsellem, Z.; Cohen, B.C.; Gressel, J. Engineering hypervirulence in a mycoherbicidal fungus for efficient weed control. *Nat. Biotechnol.* **2002**, *10*, 1035–1039. [CrossRef]

46. Šantrić, L.; Radivojević, L.; Gajić Umiljendić, J.; Sarić-Krsmanović, M. Allelopathic effects of actinobacterial isolates on seed germination and early seedling growth of velvetleaf (*Abutilon theophrasti* Medik.). *Pestic. Phytomed.* **2022**, *37*, 41–48. [CrossRef]
47. Kremer, R.J.; Begonia, M.F.T.; Stanley, L.; Lanham, E.T. Characterization of rhizobacteria associated with weed seedlings. *Appl. Environ. Microbiol.* **1990**, *56*, 1649–1655. [CrossRef] [PubMed]
48. Owen, A.; Zdor, R. Effect of cyanogenic rhizobacteria on the growth of velvetleaf (*Abutilon theophrasti*) and corn (*Zea mays* L.) in autoclaved soil and the influence of supplemental glycine. *Soil Biol. Biochem.* **2001**, *33*, 801–809. [CrossRef]
49. Siegien, I.; Bogatek, R. Cyanide action in plants-from toxic to regulatory. *Acta Physiol. Plant.* **2006**, *28*, 483–497. [CrossRef]
50. Silva-Avalos, J.; Richmond, M.G.; Nagappan, O.; Kunz, D.A. Degradation of the metal-cyano complex tetracyanonickelate(II) by cyanide-utilizing bacterial isolates. *Appl. Environ. Microbiol.* **1990**, *56*, 3664–3670. [CrossRef]
51. Harding, D.P.; Raizada, M.N. Controlling weeds with fungi, bacteria and viruses: A review. *Front. Plant Sci.* **2015**, *6*, 659. [CrossRef] [PubMed]
52. Cheng, L.; DiTommaso, A.; Kao-Kniffin, J. Opportunities for Microbiome Suppression of Weeds Using Regenerative Agricultural Technologies. *Front. Soil Sci.* **2022**, *2*, 838595. [CrossRef]
53. Chee-Sanford, J.C. Weed Seeds as Nutritional Resources for Soil Ascomycota and Characterization of Specific Associations Between Plant and Fungal Species. *Biol. Fertil. Soils* **2008**, *44*, 763–771. [CrossRef]
54. Verdeguer, M.; Sánchez-Moreiras, A.M.; Araniti, F. Phytotoxic Effects and Mechanism of Action of Essential Oils and Terpenoids. *Plants* **2020**, *9*, 1571. [CrossRef]
55. Preusche, M.; Vahl, M.; Riediger, J.; Ulbrich, A.; Schulz, M. Modulating Expression Levels of TCP Transcription Factors by *Mentha x piperita* Volatiles—An Allelopathic Tool to Influence Leaf Growth? *Plants* **2022**, *11*, 3078. [CrossRef]
56. Vaughn, S.; Spencer, G. Monoterpenes as parent structures for herbicides. *Weed Sci.* **1993**, *41*, 114–119. [CrossRef]
57. Wolf, R.B.; Spencer, G.F.; Kwolek, W.F. Inhibition of Velvetleaf (*Abutilon theophrasti*) Germination and Growth by Benzyl Isothiocyanate, a Natural Toxicant. *Weed Sci.* **1984**, *32*, 612–615. [CrossRef]
58. Tollsten, L.; Bergstrom, G. Headspace volatiles of whole plants and macerated plant parts of *Brassica* and *Sinapis*. *Phytochemistry* **1988**, *27*, 4013–4018. [CrossRef]
59. Shettle, N.; Balke, E.N. Plant Growth Response to Several Allelopathic Chemicals. *Weed Sci.* **1983**, *31*, 293–298. [CrossRef]
60. Rose, S.J.; Burnside, O.C.; Specht, J.E.; Swisher, B.A. Competition and Allelopathy Between Soybeans and Weeds. *Agron. J.* **1984**, *76*, 523–528. [CrossRef]
61. Dayan, F.E.; Howell, J.L.; Weidenhamer, J.D. Dynamic root exudation of sorgoleone and its in planta mechanism of action. *J. Exp. Bot.* **2009**, *60*, 2107–2117. [CrossRef]
62. Godlewska, K.; Ronga, D.; Michalak, I. Plant extracts—Importance in sustainable agriculture. *Ital. J. Agron.* **2021**, *16*, 1851. [CrossRef]
63. Lebeis, S.L.; Paredes, S.H.; Lundberg, D.S.; Breakfield, N.; Gehring, J.; McDonald, M.; Malfatti, S.; Glavina del Rio, T.; Jones, C.D.; Tringe, S.G.; et al. Salicylic acid modulates colonization of the root microbiome by specific bacterial taxa. *Science* **2015**, *349*, 860–864. [CrossRef]
64. Siebers, M.; Rohr, T.; Ventura, M.; Schütz, V.; Thies, S.; Kovacic, F.; Jaeger, K.E.; Berg, M.; Dörmann, P.; Schulz, M. Disruption of microbial community composition and identification of plant growth promoting microorganisms after exposure of soil to rapeseed-derived glucosinolates. *PLoS ONE* **2018**, *13*, e0200160. [CrossRef]
65. Hansen, J.C.; Schillinger, W.F.; Sullivan, T.S.; Paulitz, T.C. Soil microbial biomass and fungi reduced with canola introduced into long-term monoculture wheat rotations. *Front. Microbiol.* **2019**, *10*, 1488. [CrossRef]
66. Hu, P.; Hollister, E.B.; Somenahally, A.C.; Hons, F.M.; Gentry, T.J. Soil bacterial and fungal communities respond differently to various isothiocyanates added for biofumigation. *Front. Microbiol.* **2015**, *5*, 729. [CrossRef] [PubMed]
67. Zhou, X.; Wu, F. Vanillic acid changed cucumber (*Cucumis sativus* L.) seedling rhizosphere total bacterial, *Pseudomonas* and *Bacillus* spp. communities. *Sci. Rep.* **2018**, *8*, 4929. [CrossRef] [PubMed]
68. Zhou, X.; Zhang, J.; Pan, D.; Xin, G.; Jin, X.; Chen, S.; Wu, F. p-Coumaric can alter the composition of cucumber rhizosphere microbial communities and induce negative plant-microbial interactions. *Biol. Fert. Soils* **2018**, *54*, 363–372. [CrossRef]
69. Wang, C.-M.; Li, T.-C.; Jhan, Y.-L.; Weng, J.-H.; Chou, C.-H. The Impact of Microbial Biotransformation of Catechin in Enhancing the Allelopathic Effects of *Rhododendron formosanum*. *PLoS ONE* **2013**, *8*, e85162. [CrossRef] [PubMed]
70. Hu, L.; Robert, C.A.M.; Cadot, S.; Zhang, X.; Ye, M.; Li, B.; Manzo, D.; Chervet, N.; Steinger, T.; Van der Heijden, M.G.A.; et al. Root exudate metabolites drive plant-soil feedbacks on growth and defense by shaping the rhizosphere microbiota. *Nat. Comm.* **2018**, *9*, 2738. [CrossRef]
71. Kudjordjie, E.N.; Sapkota, R.; Steffensen, S.K.; Fomsgaard, I.S.; Nicolaisen, M. Maize synthesized benzoxazinoids affect the host associated microbiome. *Microbiome* **2019**, *7*, 59. [CrossRef]
72. Schütz, V.; Frindte, K.; Cui, J.; Zhang, P.; Hacquard, S.; Schulze-Lefert, P.; Knief, C.; Schulz, M.; Dörmann, P. Differential Impact of Plant Secondary Metabolites on the Soil Microbiota. *Front. Microbiol.* **2021**, *12*, 666010. [CrossRef]
73. Lehman, R.M.; Cambardella, C.A.; Stott, D.E.; Acosta-Martinez, V.; Manter, D.K.; Buyer, J.S.; Maul, J.E.; Smith, J.L.; Collins, H.P.; Halvorson, J.J.; et al. Understanding and Enhancing Soil Biological Health: The Solution for Reversing Soil Degradation. *Sustainability* **2015**, *7*, 988–1027. [CrossRef]
74. McGivern, B.B.; Tfaily, M.M.; Borton, M.A.; Kosina, S.M.; Daly, R.A.; Nicora, C.D.; Purvine, S.O.; Wong, A.R.; Lipton, M.S.; Hoyt, D.W.; et al. Decrypting bacterial polyphenol metabolism in an anoxic wetland soil. *Nat. Commun.* **2021**, *12*, 2466. [CrossRef]

75. Macías, F.A.; Marín, D.; Oliveros-Bastidas, A.; Castellano, D.; Simonet, A.M.; Molinillo, J.M. Structure-activity relationships (SAR) studies of benzoxazinones, their degradation products and analogues. Phytotoxicity on standard target species (STS). *J. Agric. Food Chem.* **2005**, *53*, 538–548. [CrossRef]
76. Krogh, S.; Mensz, S.; Nielsen, S.; Mortensen, A.; Christophersen, C.; Fomsgaard, I. Fate of Benzoxazinone Allelochemicals in Soil after Incorporation of Wheat and Rye Sprouts. *J. Agric. Food Chem.* **2006**, *54*, 1064–1074. [CrossRef] [PubMed]
77. Schulz, M.; Marocco, A.; Tabaglio, V.; Macias, F.A.; Molinillo, J.M.G. Benzoxazinoids in rye allelopathy—From discovery to application in sustainable weed control and organic farming. *J. Chem. Ecol.* **2013**, *39*, 154–174. [CrossRef] [PubMed]
78. La Hovary, C.; Baerson, S.R.; Williamson, J.D.; Danehower, D.A.; Ma, G.; Pan, Z.; Mask, M.M.; Burton, J.D. Phytotoxicity and benzoxazinone concentration in field grown cereal rye (*Secale cereale* L.). *Int. J. Agron.* **2016**, *2016*, 6463826. [CrossRef]
79. Hussain, M.I.; Araniti, F.; Schulz, M.; Baerson, S.; Vieites-Álvarez, Y.; Rempelos, L.; Bilsborrow, P.; Durán, A.G.; Chinchilla, N.; Macías, F.A.; et al. Benzoxazinoids in wheat allelopathy—From discovery to application for sustainable weed management. *Environ. Exp. Bot.* **2022**, *202*, 101997. [CrossRef]
80. Fiorini, A.; Maris, S.C.; Abalos, D.; Amaducci, S.; Tabaglio, V. Combining no-till with rye (*Secale cereale* L.) cover crop mitigates nitrous oxide emissions without decreasing yield. *Soil Tillage Res.* **2020**, *196*, 104442. [CrossRef]
81. Gavazzi, C.; Schulz, M.; Marocco, A.; Tabaglio, V. Sustainable weed control by allelochemicals from rye cover crops: From the greenhouse to field evidence. *Allelopath. J.* **2010**, *25*, 259–274.
82. Tabaglio, V.; Marocco, A.; Schulz, M. Allelopathic cover crop of rye for integrated weed control in sustainable agroecosystems. *Ital. J. Agron.* **2013**, *8*, 35–40. [CrossRef]
83. Boselli, R.; Anders, N.; Fiorini, A.; Ganimede, C.; Faccini, N.; Marocco, A.; Schulz, M.; Tabaglio, V. Improving weed control in sustainable agroecosystems: Role of cultivar and termination timing of rye cover crop. *Ital. J. Agron.* **2021**, *16*, 1807. [CrossRef]
84. Reberg-Horton, S.C.; Burton, J.D.; Danehower, D.A.; Ma, G.; Monks, D.W.; Murphy, J.P.; Ranells, N.N.; Williamson, J.D.; Creamer, N.G. Changes over time in the allelochemical content of ten cultivars of rye (*Secale cereale* L.). *J. Chem. Ecol.* **2005**, *31*, 179–193. [CrossRef]
85. Tabaglio, V.; Gavazzi, C.; Schulz, M.; Marocco, A. Alternative weed control using the allelopathic effect of natural benzoxazinoids from rye mulch. *Agron. Sustain. Dev.* **2008**, *28*, 397–401. [CrossRef]
86. Ganimede, C.; Marocco, A.; Schulz, M.; Tabaglio, V. Investigation of Endophytic Fungi Associated to *Abutilon theophrasti* Root. In Proceedings of the 7th World Congress on Allelopathy, Vigo, Spain, 28 July–1 August 2014.
87. DeMers, M. *Alternaria alternata* as endophyte and pathogen. *Microbiology* **2022**, *168*, 001153. [CrossRef]
88. Toghueo, R.M.K. Bioprospecting endophytic fungi from *Fusarium* genus as sources of bioactive metabolites. *Mycology* **2019**, *11*, 1–21. [CrossRef] [PubMed]
89. Prudence, S.; Newitt, J.; Worsley, S.F.; Macey, M.C.; Murrell, J.C.; Lehtovirta-Morley, L.E.; Hutchings, M.I. Soil, senescence and exudate utilisation: Characterisation of the Paragon var. spring bread wheat root microbiome. *Environ. Microbiome* **2021**, *16*, 12. [CrossRef]
90. Schulz, M.; Sicker, D.; Schackow, O.; Hennig, L.; Yurkov, A.; Siebers, M.; Hofmann, D.; Disko, U.; Ganimede, C.; Mondani, L.; et al. Interspecies-Cooperations of *Abutilon theophrasti* with Root Colonizing Microorganisms Disarm BOA-OH Allelochemicals. *Plant Signal. Behav.* **2017**, *12*, e1358843. [CrossRef]
91. Haghi Kia, S. Unraveling *Abutilon theophrasti's* Tolerance to the Allelochemical Benzoxazolinone. Master's Thesis, Rheinische Friedrich-Wilhelms-Universität, Bonn, Germany, 2013.
92. Kia, S.H.; Schulz, M.; Ayah, E.; Schouten, A.; Müllenborn, C.; Paetz, C.; Schneider, B.; Hofmann, D.; Disko, U.; Tabaglio, V.; et al. *Abutilon theophrasti*'s defense against the allelochemical benzoxazolin-2(3H)-one: Support by *Actinomucor elegans*. *J. Chem. Ecol.* **2014**, *40*, 1286–1298. [CrossRef] [PubMed]
93. Kia, S.H.; Wewer, V.; Hölzl, G.; Schulz, M. Assessing the Effect of Benzoxazolinone on the Plant–Associated Zygomycete *Actinomucor elegans* and Its Possible Role in a Weed's Tolerance to Allelochemicals. In Proceedings of the 10th International Mycological Congress (Imc10), Bangkok, Thailand, 3–8 August 2014; Available online: http://www.imc10.com (accessed on 31 January 2023).
94. Nadane, A. Effect of Velvetleaf Root Exudates on Indole-3-Acetic Acid Production by *Rhizobium rubi* AT3-4RS/6. Ph.D. Thesis, Andrews University, Berrien Springs, MI, USA, 2012. Available online: https://digitalcommons.andrews.edu/honors/24 (accessed on 31 January 2023).
95. Schulz, M. (University of Bonn, Bonn, Germany); Hofmann, D. (Forschungszentrum Jülich GmbH, Jülich, Germany). Personal communication, 2022.
96. Schulz, M.; Sicker, D.; Schackow, O.; Hennig, L.; Hofmann, D.; Disko, U.; Ventura, M.; Basyuk, K. 6-Hydroxy-5-nitrobenzo[d]oxazol- 2(3H)-one—A degradable derivative of natural 6-hydroxybenzoxazolin-2(3H)-one produced by *Pantoea ananatis*. *Commun. Integr. Biol.* **2017**, *10*, e1302633. [CrossRef] [PubMed]
97. Schulz, M.; Marocco, A.; Tabaglio, V. BOA detoxification of four summer weeds during germination and seedling growth. *J. Chem. Ecol.* **2012**, *38*, 933–946. [CrossRef]
98. Laschke, L.; Schütz, V.; Schackow, O.; Sicker, D.; Hennig, L.; Hofmann, D.; Dörmann, P.; Schulz, M. Survival of Plants during Short-Term BOA-OH Exposure: ROS Related Gene Expression and Detoxification Reactions Are Accompanied with Fast Membrane Lipid Repair in Root Tips. *J. Chem. Ecol.* **2022**, *48*, 219–239. [CrossRef]

99. Sterling, T.M.; Houtz, R.L.; Putnam, A.R. Phytotoxic Exudates from Velvetleaf (*Abutilon theophrasti*) Glandular Trichomes. *Am. J. Bot.* **1987**, *74*, 543–550. [CrossRef]
100. Radivojević, L.; Sarić-Krsmanović, M.; Umiljendić, J.G.; Šantrić, L. Allelopathic effects of invasive weed species *Abutilon theophrasti* Medik., *Ambrosia artemisiifolia* L., *Datura stramonium* L. and *Xanthium strumarium* L. on tomato. *Pestic. Fitomed.* **2019**, *34*, 183–191. [CrossRef]
101. Tian, M.; Li, Q.; Zhao, W.; Qiao, B.; Shi, S.; Yu, M.; Li, X.; Li, C.; Zhao, C. Potential Allelopathic Interference of *Abutilon theophrasti* Medik. Powder/Extract on Seed Germination, Seedling Growth and Root System Activity of Maize, Wheat and Soybean. *Agronomy* **2022**, *12*, 844. [CrossRef]
102. Novak, N.; Novak, M.; Barić, K.; Šćepanović, M.; Ivić, D. Allelopathic potential of segetal and ruderal invasive alien plants. *J. Cent. Eur. Agric.* **2018**, *19*, 408–422. [CrossRef]
103. Paszkowski, W.L.; Kremer, R.J. Biological activity and tentative identification of flavonoid components in velvetleaf (*Abutilon theophrasti* Medik.) seed coats. *J. Chem. Ecol.* **1988**, *14*, 1573–1582. [CrossRef] [PubMed]
104. Balah, M.A.; Nassar, M.I. Allelopathic Constituents from *Abutilon theophrasti* Aerial Parts to Other Weeds. *Res. J. Agric. Sci.* **2011**, *7*, 243–250.
105. Tian, C.; Yang, C.; Zhang, D.; Han, L.; Liu, Y.; Guo, W.; Fan, R.; Liu, M. Antibacterial and antioxidant properties of various solvent extracts of *Abutilon theophrasti* Medic. leaves. *Pak. J. Pharm. Sci.* **2017**, *3*, 767–772.
106. Hwang, J.H.; Jin, Q.; Woo, E.R.; Lee, D.G. Antifungal property of hibicuslide C and its membrane-active mechanism in *Candida albicans*. *Biochimie* **2013**, *95*, 1917–1922. [CrossRef]
107. Mamadalieva, N.Z.F.; Sharopov, F.; Girault, J.-P.; Wink, M.; Lafont, R. Phytochemical analysis and bioactivity of the aerial parts of *Abutilon theophrasti* (Malvaceae), a medicinal weed. *Nat. Prod. Res.* **2014**, *28*, 1777–1779. [CrossRef]
108. Itoh, A.; Fujii, K.; Tomatsu, S.; Takao, C.; Tanahashi, T.; Nagakura, N.; Chen, C.-C. Six secoiridoid glucosides from *Adina racemosa*. *J. Nat. Prod.* **2003**, *66*, 1212–1216. [CrossRef]
109. Murai, Y.; Kashimura, S.; Tamezawa, S.; Hashimoto, T.; Takaoka, S.; Asakawa, Y.; Kiguchi, K.; Murai, F.; Tagawa, M. Absolute Configuration of (6S,9S)-Roseoside from *Polygonum hydropiper*. *Planta Med.* **2001**, *67*, 480–481. [CrossRef]
110. Rumalla, C.S.; Ali, Z.; Weerasooriya, A.D.; Smillie, T.J.; Khan, I.J. A new triterpene glycoside from *Centella erecta*. *Fitoterapia* **2010**, *81*, 751–754. [CrossRef]
111. Zhang, S.; Gai, Z.; Gui, T.; Chen, J.; Chen, Q.; Li, Y. Antioxidant Effects of Protocatechuic Acid and Protocatechuic Aldehyde: Old Wine in a New Bottle. *Evid. Based Complement Alternat. Med.* **2021**, *8*, 6139308. [CrossRef]
112. Sterling, T.M.; Balke, N.E. Use of Soybean (*Glycine max*) and Velvetleaf (*Abutilon theophrasti*) Suspension-Cultured Cells to Study Bentazon Metabolism. *Weed Sci.* **1988**, *36*, 558–565. Available online: https://www.jstor.org/stable/4044806 (accessed on 31 January 2023). [CrossRef]
113. Reese, A.T.; Chadaideh, K.S.; Caroline, E.; Diggins, C.E.; Schell, L.D.; Beckel, M.; Callahan, P.; Ryan, R.; Thompson, E.M.; Carmody, R.N. Effects of domestication on the gut microbiota parallel those of human industrialization. *eLife* **2021**, *10*, e60197. [CrossRef]
114. Soldan, R.; Fusi, M.; Cardinale, M.; Daffonchio, D.; Preston, G.M. The effect of plant domestication on host control of the microbiota. *Commun. Biol.* **2021**, *4*, 936. [CrossRef] [PubMed]
115. Raaijmakers, J.M.; Kiers, E.T. Rewilding plant microbiomes. *Science* **2022**, *378*, 599–600. [CrossRef] [PubMed]
116. Berg, G.; Cernava, T. The plant microbiota signature of the Anthropocene as a challenge for microbiome research. *Microbiome* **2022**, *10*, 54. [CrossRef]
117. García-Campa, L.; Guerrero, S.; Lamelas, L.; Meijon, M.; Hasbún, R.; Cañal, M.J.; Valledor, L. Chloroplast proteomics reveals transgenerational cross-stress priming in *Pinus radiata*. *Environ. Exp. Bot.* **2022**, *202*, 105009. [CrossRef]
118. Lagage, V.; Uphoff, S. Pulses and delays, anticipation and memory: Seeing bacterial stress responses from a single-cell perspective. *FEMS Microbiol. Rev.* **2020**, *44*, 565–571. [CrossRef] [PubMed]

plants MDPI

Review

# The Potential of Allelochemicals from Microalgae for Biopesticides

Livia Marques Casanova [1,*], Andrew Macrae [2], Jacqueline Elis de Souza [1], Athayde Neves Junior [1] and Alane Beatriz Vermelho [1,*]

[1] Biotechnology Center-Bioinovar, Institute of Microbiology Paulo de Goes, Universidade Federal do Rio de Janeiro (UFRJ), Rio de Janeiro 21941-902, RJ, Brazil
[2] Sustainable Biotechnology and Microbial Bioinformatics Laboratory, Institute of Microbiology Paulo de Goes, Universidade Federal do Rio de Janeiro (UFRJ), Rio de Janeiro 21941-902, RJ, Brazil
* Correspondence: liviacasanova@micro.ufrj.br (L.M.C.); abvermelho@micro.ufrj.br (A.B.V.)

**Abstract:** Improvements in agricultural productivity are required to meet the demand of a growing world population. Phytopathogens, weeds, and insects are challenges to agricultural production. The toxicity and widespread application of persistent synthetic pesticides poses a major threat to human and ecosystem health. Therefore, sustainable strategies to control pests are essential for agricultural systems to enhance productivity within a green paradigm. Allelochemicals are a less persistent, safer, and friendly alternative to efficient pest management, as they tend to be less toxic to non-target organisms and more easily degradable. Microalgae produce a great variety of allelopathic substances whose biocontrol potential against weeds, insects, and phytopathogenic fungi and bacteria has received much attention. This review provides up-to-date information and a critical perspective on allelochemicals from microalgae and their potential as biopesticides.

**Keywords:** bioherbicide; biocide; biopesticide; allelochemical; microalgae

**Citation:** Casanova, L.M.; Macrae, A.; de Souza, J.E.; Neves Junior, A.; Vermelho, A.B. The Potential of Allelochemicals from Microalgae for Biopesticides. *Plants* **2023**, *12*, 1896. https://doi.org/10.3390/plants12091896

Academic Editors: Margot Schulz and Vincenzo Tabaglio

Received: 10 February 2023
Revised: 3 May 2023
Accepted: 4 May 2023
Published: 6 May 2023



## 1. Introduction

Allelopathy is an ecological phenomenon in which allelochemicals are produced under certain environmental conditions. The term 'allelopathy' was introduced by Molisch in 1937 and originated from the Greek words 'allelon' (mutual) and "pathos" (harm). The term means one organism influences others through a chemical mode [1].

Allelochemicals are toxic secondary metabolites produced by plants, microalgae, bacteria, and fungi that influence the development of other organisms. These substances can be harmful to humans, other microalgae, and organisms, including phytoplankton, animals, and submerged macrophytes. Photosynthesis and enzyme activity inhibition, damage to cell structures, and other physiological alterations such as inhibition of respiration, protein synthesis, and gene expression have been observed [2,3].

Allelopathy is much studied in plants, but allelochemicals started to be reviewed in microalgae by Inderjit and Dakshini in 1994 [2,4]. Microalgae are a widely diversified group of prokaryotic and eukaryotic photosynthetic microorganisms. More than 50,000 microalgae species are distributed in rivers, lakes, oceans, and even in terrestrial ecosystems. Cyanobacteria are prokaryotic microalgae in which membrane-bound organelles such as plastids and mitochondria are missing, while eukaryotic microalgae rely on these structures to control cellular functions [5,6]. Many common microalgae taxa are included in the latter group, such as Chlorophyta (green algae) and Bacillariophyta (diatoms) [5,6]. Pyrrophyta (dinoflagellates) are mostly microplankton, they are eukaryotic and live in aquatic environments, be it salt, brackish or fresh water. Around half of all dinoflagellates are photosynthetic, while the other half are heterotrophic; some live as mixotrophic and obligate symbionts/parasites. They are usually reported as microalgae;

indeed, the most toxic microalgae are dinoflagellates [7] The non-algal dinoflagellates are primarily predators of other microorganisms or parasites of animals or giant protists [8].

One of the fields of study for allelochemicals in microalgae began with harmful algal blooms (HABs). HABs are a consequence of an ecosystem imbalance in marine and freshwater systems worldwide [9]. HABs affect water usage, including fisheries, water resources, and recruitment. The poisoning caused by the allelochemicals affects different organisms and leads to economic losses [10]. The use of allelochemicals as biocontrol agents has been suggested as a means of improving microalgae cultivation and controlling contamination [11]. An example of a mode of action is the generation of reactive oxygen species (ROS). *Nostoc spongiaeforme* produces a pigment named nostocine A; this pigment is highly cytotoxic for several microalgae. The compound accelerates ROS formation in *Chlorella reinhardtii.* Nostocine A penetrates the target and is reduced by NADPH; when oxygen levels are high, reduced nostocine A is oxidated, generating superoxide radical anion ($O^{2-}$) that may cause cytotoxicity [12].

The bioactivity of allelochemicals and their toxic or beneficial effects have also been the focus of research in medicine and agriculture [13], and for their anticancer [14] and antimicrobial properties (Figure 1) [15].

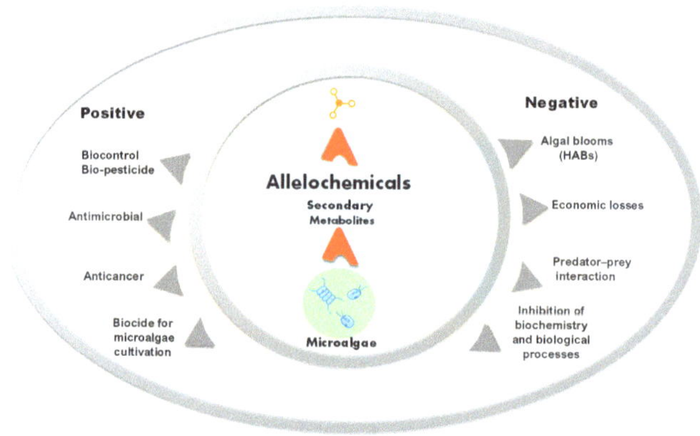


**Figure 1.** Schematic representation of positive and negative aspects of allelochemicals from microalgae.

Toxic compounds that are used to protect crops, and to control weeds, insects and disease, are known as pesticides. The extensive and widespread use of synthetic pesticides, however, poses several long-term health and environmental risks. Often, pesticides are also toxic to humans and animals, resulting in carcinogenicity, teratogenicity, and the disruption of hormonal systems. Pesticides that persist in the environment for years result in the contamination of water and food sources [16,17]. Another challenging problem for agriculture is the emergence of pesticide resistance in target species [18]. In a scenario of increasing pollution on the planet and of climate changes triggering environmental problems, it is urgent that sustainable, green methods for the biocontrol of pests are found. Environmentally-friendly allelochemicals from microalgae have been described as bioherbicides. These compounds arise as an alternative source of natural biocides to reduce the use of toxic synthetic biocides/herbicides [19].

This review aims to examine allelopathy in microalgae, focusing on the potential applications of allelochemicals as herbicides, insecticides, and in their action against phytopathogens.

## 2. Allelopathy in Microalgae

As mentioned previously, the term allelopathy was originally used to describe biomolecules produced by plants. However, it is now openly used with other organisms and has been studied in microalgae [19,20]. Microalgae organisms produce numerous secondary metabolites, including fatty acids, alkaloids, amino acids, and peptides, which are investigated and characterized as natural products by chemists and described as novel bio compounds. In the environment, these molecules are secreted for communication, defence, and adaptation purposes [21]. More knowledge is needed in order to understand the complexity of these bioactive chemicals and their interaction with and effect on ecosystems [19,22].

A recent review paper showed that *Microcystis, Nodularia, Karenia, Alexandrium (A. catenella, A. fundyense*, and others species), *Skeletonema*, *Chlorella* (*C. vulgaris*, *C. sorokiniana*, *C. ellipsoidea*), *Chlamydomonas*, and *Dunaliella* displayed allelopathic activity against other microalgae and cyanobacteria [23]. One strategy to study the allelopathic effects of different microalgae agents is to analyse the biochemicals present in mono- and co-cultures [24]. Wang et al. [24] observed that the dinoflagellate *Scrippsiella* acuminata had its growth significantly inhibited when in co-cultivation and/or in the presence of exudates (cell-free and sonicated-cell filtrates) from three diatoms (*Chaetoceros curvisetus*, *Phaeodactylum tricornutum* and *Skeletonema dohrnii*), suggesting the diatoms developed significant competitive advantage over other antagonists. Furthermore, the authors detected several types of volatile organic compounds (VOCs) in the sonicated cell-free filtrates. Polyunsaturated aldehydes (PUAs) were found in all three diatoms that showed inhibitory effects on the growth of *S. acuminata* and the diatoms themselves. Generally, the production of microalgae VOCs is influenced by environmental conditions, such as nutrient availability, temperature, and light incidence [25,26].

Studies show that allelochemicals of microalgae have either a positive or negative impact on other organisms. Those which can cause inhibitory effects are suitable for application as biopesticides, and as a new source of antimicrobials or bio-herbicide agents [19,23], especially because these biocompounds present increased target specificity [27]. The liberation of species-specific allelochemicals is desired in agriculture and is an important focus for future studies because they can be responsible for modulating the ecosystem under favourable conditions to an allelopathic microalgae. An example of this was observed in a study where, by alternating the nutrients conditions and balance of nitrogen and phosphorus sources, the allelopathic interaction between strains of *Anabaena* spp. and *Microcystis* spp. seemed to control their relative abundance and their dominance in that habitat [28].

An interesting point to remark upon here is that one of several new applications of microalgae is as a bioenergy source and an alternative to fossil fuels [29–31]. Nevertheless, one of the elements that industry must be alert to is the accumulation of allelopathic molecules released into the water by microalgae themselves. These compounds, when in high concentrations due to high biomass, along with other biomolecules can trigger positive or negative effects on other cells, leading to auto-stimulation or self-inhibition [32–34]. Lu and colleagues (2020) described studies that focused on water reuse for microalgae cultivation, and stated that several factors, including allelopathy mechanisms, cause cell damage, aggregation, and programmed cell death (PCD) (negative effects) or, on the other hand, the liberation of growth regulators and removal of growth inhibitors (positive effects). Bacterial agents can have a significant influence on allelopathy affecting microalgae biomass tanks [33,35].

Some allelopathic molecules have been characterized in the scientific literature as having a role in algal community growth regulation. Satake et al. [36] described a 19 membered ring-structured molecule called alexandrolide, which was isolated from dinoflagellate *Alexandrium catenella* and inhibited diatoms (*Skeletonema costatum* and *Chattonella antiqua*) but did not inhibit other dinoflagellates. Marennine, a blue-green polyphenolic pigment produced by diatom *Haslea ostrearia*, was described as being responsible for inhibiting the growth of other diatom species and self-stimulating the producer species in oyster-ponds [37]. By elucidating the properties of these compounds, more studies can be performed to apply these chemicals for industrial and human purposes, such as in additives in agricultural technology [38].

## 3. Allelochemicals from Microalgae

Microalgae are the source of a remarkable diversity of biologically active compounds, which can be involved in allelopathic interactions. The main chemical classes of microalgal allelochemicals are: alkaloids, fatty acids and derivatives, polyketides, peptides, phenolics, and terpenoids.

### 3.1. *Alkaloids*

Alkaloids are a prominent class of allelochemicals with biocidal properties. They consist of nitrogen-containing heterocyclic substances, in which the nitrogen atom is usually derived from an amino acid [39,40]. Alkaloids have been reported mainly in cyanobacteria and dinoflagellates. In the former, indole alkaloids are the most frequent. For instance, 12-*epi*-hapalindole E isonitrile (Figure 2A; **1**), from *Fischerella* sp., is an indole alkaloid with activity against green microalgae and other microorganisms [41]. Another example is the toxin calothrixin A (Figure 2A; **2**) from *Calothrix* sp [41].

Domoic acid (Figure 2A; **3**) is a well-known biotoxin from the bloom-generating diatom *Pseudo-nitzschia* sp. which has a pyrrolidine skeleton derived from glutamic acid [42–44]. Another example of an alkaloid from diatoms is saxitoxin (Figure 2A; **4**), a potent neurotoxin with a complex skeleton whose nitrogen atoms are derived from arginine. It has been reported in cyanobacterial species as well [45–48].

### 3.2. *Fatty acids and Derivatives*

Extracellular free fatty acids from microalgae have a possible allelopathic effect, controlling the growth of other microalgae and harmful organisms. Green microalgae, such as *Chlorella* sp. and *Botryococcus braunii*, are reported to secrete mixtures of common fatty acids (e.g., oleic and linoleic acids; Figure 2B) under certain conditions, which may favor their dominance [49,50]. Additionally, unsaturated fatty acids are reported to possess antimicrobial activity [51].

Substances derived from fatty acids can also act as allelochemicals. Polyunsaturated fatty acids (PUFAs), after various oxidative transformations, originate polyunsaturated aldehydes (PUAS) (e.g., 2*E*,4*E*-decadienal, 2*E*,4*E*-heptadienal, and 2*E*,4*E*-octadienal; Figure 2B), which play a role in communication and chemical defense in diatoms [11,39,52]. They exert a deleterious effect on grazers and competing microalgal species, and stimulate organic-matter-recycling bacteria [52].

### 3.3. *Polyketides*

Polyketides are a large group of structurally diverse substances biosynthesized from carboxylic acid precursors through repeated cycles of condensation, reduction and dehydration reactions catalyzed by multifunctional enzymatic complexes called polyketide synthases (PKS). These substances are found mainly in dinoflagellates and cyanobacteria and are frequently associated with harmful blooms [39,53]. Examples include maitotoxin from the dinoflagellate *Gambierdiscus* sp., the largest and most toxic known polyketide [54,55], and also brevetoxins from *Karenia brevis* (e.g., brevetoxin A; Figure 2C; **10**), a dinoflagellate associated with "red tides" [56]. Another remarkable example are trichophycins (e.g., trichophycin A; Figure 2C; **11**), linear chlorinated polyketides from cyanobacteria from the genus *Trichodesmium*, which produce frequent blooms in the Pacific Ocean [57,58].

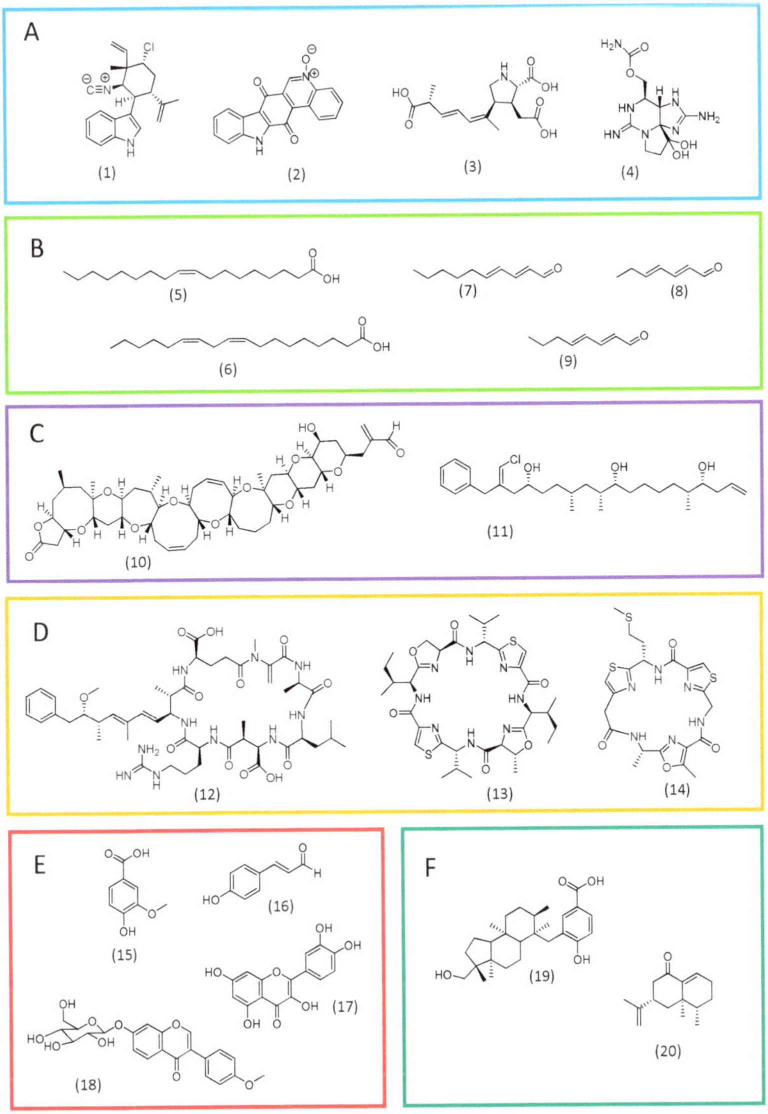

**Figure 2.** Examples of allelochemicals from microalgae. Alkaloids (**A**): 12-*epi*-hapalindole E isonitrile (**1**), calothrixin A (**2**), domoic acid (**3**), and saxitoxin (**4**). Fatty acids and derivatives (**B**): oleic acid (**5**), linoleic acid (**6**), 2*E*,4*E*-decadienal (**7**), 2*E*,4*E*-heptadienal (**8**), and 2*E*,4*E*-octadienal (**9**). Polyketides (**C**): brevetoxin A (**10**) and trichophycin A (**11**). Peptides (**D**): microcystin-LR (**12**), patellamide A (**13**), and tenuecyclamide C (**14**). Phenolic substances (**E**): vanillic acid (**15**), p-coumaric acid (**16**), quercetin (**17**) and ononin (**18**). Terpenoids (**F**): comnostin A (**19**) and eremophilone (**20**).

### 3.4. *Peptides*

A significant amount of cyanobacterial allelochemicals are peptides. Most of them belong to the group of non-ribosomal peptides, which are biosynthesized by multifunctional enzyme complexes, the non-ribosomal peptide synthases (NRPS). NPRS are similar to PKS and assemble sequentially common amino acids but also unusual amino acids [12,39,59]. For example, microcystins are cyclic non-ribosomal peptides produced by cyanobacteria of the genus *Anabaena*, *Microcystis*, *Planktothrix*, *Oscillatoria*, and others. They are toxic for microalgae, aquatic plants, and for mammals and birds as well [12,60]. Microcystin-LR (Figure 2D; **12**) is the most frequent of them [60].

Ribosomal peptides also occur in cyanobacteria. For instance, cyanobactins are small cyclic peptides formed solely from proteinogenic amino acids and reported in many genus, such as *Anabaena*, *Lyngbya*, *Microcystis*, *Nostoc*, and *Trichodesmium* [59,61]. They possess antimicrobial activity and probably have the function of inhibiting the growth of competing and harmful microorganisms. Patellamide A, from *Prochloron*, and tenuecyclamide C, from *Trichodesmium erythraeum*, are representatives of the group (Figure 2D; **13** and **14**) [61].

### 3.5. *Phenolic Compounds*

Phenolic compounds represent a large group of secondary metabolites, which play multiple roles in photosynthetic organisms, including in defense strategies and in communication with interacting species [62,63]. Phenolic substances are biosynthesized mainly by the phenylpropanoid pathway, having phenylalanine or tyrosine as precursors. In microalgae, knowledge about their biosynthetic pathways is still scarce, however, a recent study has shown that the enzymatic apparatus for key phenolic biosynthetic intermediates is well conserved in all major algal divisions, although the ability to biosynthesize some subclasses of phenolics seems to be restricted to some groups [62]. For instance, phenolic acids such as vanillic, ferulic, and coumaric acids are widespread. Flavonoids are frequent in green algae (e.g., quercetin and apigenin) and cyanobacteria, in which unusual structures have been reported (e.g., ononin from *Synechocystis*) (Figure 2E) [62].

### 3.6. *Terpenoids*

Terpenoids are a prominent family of organic substances biosynthesized from $C_5$ precursors, which are present in all living organisms [64]. Substances belonging to this group can also act as allelochemicals. Examples are comnostins, extracellular antibacterial diterpenoids produced by cyanobacteria *Nostoc* sp. [65], and the sesquiterpene eremophilone (Figure 2F), produced by cyanobacteria *Calothrix* sp. and toxic to invertebrates [66].

### 3.7. *Volatile Organic Compounds*

A specific group of allelochemicals is the volatile organic compounds (VOCs). VOCs are a broad group of compounds that encompass substances from different chemical classes, ranging from small molecules such as methane, to terpenoids and compounds derived from PUFAs including hydrocarbons, aldehydes, and ketones [25]. With a complex classification, the World Health Organization (WHO) defines VOCs as having boiling point ranges that have to fall between 50 °C and 100 °C up to 240–260 °C [67].

VOCs produced by microalgae have been widely demonstrated to have different ecological functions, including allelopathy. Environmental factors such as light, temperature, nutrition, and abiotic stresses affect VOCs emission [68]. Functions such as defense mechanisms, stress response, intra- and inter-species communication, modulating predator-prey interaction, and affecting biochemistry, metabolism, and physiology processes are described. These emissions from microalgae occur in vivo, in cells undergoing senescence or apoptosis, or when they are perishing under predator attack [69,70]. The role and the possible impact that these compounds have has been extensively studied and, in the future, they could be exploited for industrial purposes [67].

## 4. Allelochemicals from Microalgae for Biopesticides

Allelochemicals are considered safer and eco-friendly alternatives for efficient pest management as they have different and diversified modes of action compared with synthetic pesticides and are more easily degradable and less toxic to non-target organisms [71–74]. The potential use of allelochemicals from microalgae as biopesticides has attracted much attention lately [19,74–77]. In this section, we will present and discuss the potential use of allelochemicals from microalgae for the biocontrol of insects, weeds, and phytopathogens.

### *4.1. Allelochemicals against Phytopathogens*

Allelochemicals from microalgae are known for their activity against a large spectrum of microorganisms, as evidenced by several reports [78–81]. Examples include hapalindole T, an antibacterial alkaloid from *Fischerella* sp. [82], nostofungicine, a lipopeptide with fungicide activity isolated from *Nostoc* sp. [83], and eicosapentaenoic acid (EPA), an antimicrobial fatty acid from *Phaeodactylum tricornutum* [84]. For this reason, extracts from microalgae have been evaluated for their potential against phytopathogens with encouraging outcomes.

Senousy et al. [85] evaluated the methanolic extracts of ten microalgal strains against phytopathogenic fungi. Among them, three stood out: the cyanobacteria *Anabaena* sp. HSSASE11 and *Oscillatoria nigroviridis* HSSASE 15, which were active against the fungi *Botryodiplodia theobromae* and *Pythium ultimum*, respectively, and the Chlorophyta *Dunaliella* sp. HSSASE13 which was active against *Fusarium solani* [85]. Similarly, Schmid et al. [86] assayed aqueous extracts from five microalgae for their activity against fungal phytopathogens. The Chlorophyta *Scenedesmus obliquus* showed the best results, inhibiting *Sclerotium rolfsii* by 32% [86]. Another Chlorophyta, *Chlorella vulgaris*, was active against the phytopathogenic bacteria *Stenotrophomonas maltophilia*, which affects potato and green vegetables. The researchers evaluated three types of extracts: aqueous, ethanolic, and methanolic. Only the latter was active against the bacteria [87].

Interestingly, microalgae can also be active against phytopathogenic nematodes. Suspended algal cultures from *Scenedesmus obliquus*, *Chlorella vulgaris*, and *Anabaena oryzae* were able to inhibit the root-knot nematode (*Meloidogyne incognita*), a pathogen for banana cultures [88].

The activity of microalgae extracts against phytopathogenic organisms is frequently attributed to metabolites such as phenolics, alkaloids, and peptides [86,87,89]; however, few have conducted a thorough investigation to identify these compounds. In the study of Senousy et al. [85] mentioned above, the authors observed a positive correlation between the activity of the microalgal extracts against *Fusarium solani* and their phenolics and flavonoid content. These results indicate the probable chemical class of the bioactive substances. Phenolic substances also seem to be responsible for the antifungal activity of *Nannochloropsis* sp and *Spirulina* sp. Extracts composed of free phenolic acids from both microalgae exhibited significant inhibitory activity of *Fusarium* complex fungal pathogens. Both extracts had chlorogenic acid, a cinnamic acid derivative, (Figure 3; **21**) as their major component [90]. In another study, a phenolic substance isolated from culture filtrates of the cyanobacteria *Calothrix elenkinii* was reported as bioactive against the oomycete *Pythium debaryanum*. This substance, identified as 3-acetyl-2-hydroxy-6-methoxy-4-methyl benzoic acid (Figure 3; **22**), induced multiple morphological abnormalities in the hyphae of the microorganism [91].

Even though the antifungal mechanisms of the phenolic compounds mentioned above are not known, mechanistic studies on cinnamic and benzoic acid derivatives have been reported in the scientific literature. The antifungal activity of trans-cinnamaldehyde is related to the biosynthesis of cell wall components (glucan and chitin) [92,93]. In addition, methyl trans-cinnamate acts as an inhibitor of tyrosinase enzymes, which makes it interesting as a food anti-browning agent, but it also presented antimicrobial activity against bacteria and fungi [94]. Moreover, benzoic acid and its derivatives generally have multiple effects on fungal cells such as, for example, against *Alternaria solani* and *Eutypa lata* phytopathogens and other fungal genera. Several authors have discussed the fact that these phenolic substances generally affect cell respiration by altering cytochrome pathways, causing energy reduction by unbalancing intracellular benzoate levels, and inducing intracellular acidification, leading to protein aggregation and oxidative stress, for example. It is important to highlight that the effect of antifungal action depends on the concentration and molecular arrangement of these compounds [95–97].

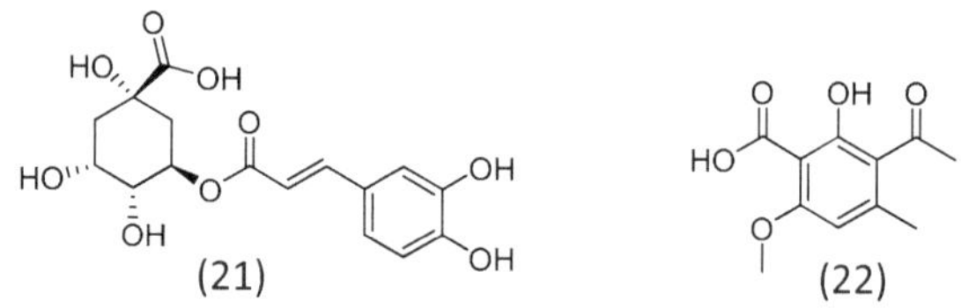

**Figure 3.** Phenolic substances active against phytopathogens: chlorogenic acid (**21**) and 3-acetyl-2-hydroxy-6-methoxy-4-methyl benzoic acid (**22**).

*4.2. Allelochemicals as Herbicides*

The focus on the herbicide potential of metabolites from microalgae has also had some promising results. Allelochemicals identified as having phytotoxic activity belong to different chemical classes, but most of them were detected in cyanobacteria. Examples are depicted in Figure 4 and will be explored in this section. This is the case for cyanobacterin (Figure 4; **23**), a phenolic substance isolated from *Scytonema hofmanni* in 1982. The substance was demonstrated to be a potent inhibitor of the photosynthetic electron transport in photosystem II. The inhibition of photosynthesis is a potential mechanism of herbicides [98,99]. The peptide nostocyclamide (Figure 4; **24**), from *Nostoc* sp., and the alkaloids fischerellins (Figure 4; **26**), from *Fischerella*, were also shown to inhibit photosystem II [99].

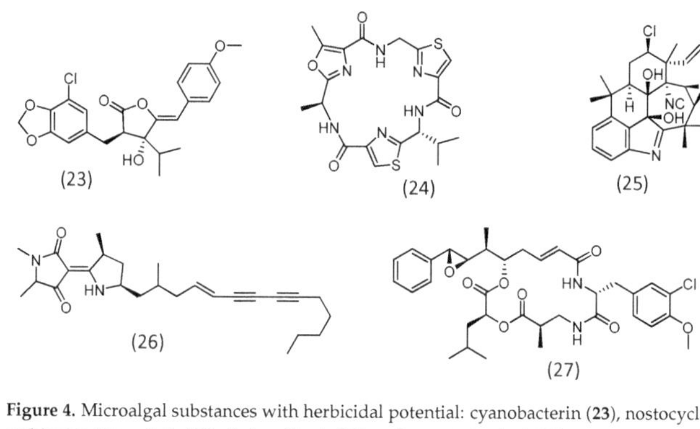

**Figure 4.** Microalgal substances with herbicidal potential: cyanobacterin (**23**), nostocyclamide (**24**), ambiguine D isonitrile (**25**), fischerellin A (**26**), and cryptophycin A (**27**).

The peptidic cyanobacterial toxins, the microcystins, on the other hand, are inhibitors of serine/threonine protein phosphatases, which results in cell growth suppression. They are phytotoxic due to their negative effects on plant physiology [99,100]. These substances, however, also represents a risk for human health and can bioaccumulate in vegetables, which hinders their application as herbicides [100]. Another substance with cell growth inhibitory activity is ambiguine D isonitrile (Figure 4; **25**), isolated from *Hapalosiphon* spp. This indole alkaloid was shown to suppress lettuce growth, an effect probably related to cell death induction by the overproduction of reactive oxygen species (ROS) and mitosis inhibition. Its potential as an herbicide remains to be further investigated [101].

Other substances with cell growth inhibitory activity may also exert herbicidal effects. For instance, cryptophycins (Figure 4; **27**), polyketides from *Nostoc* strains, which suppress microtubule polymerization. Methanolic extracts of a cryptophycin producer *Nostoc* strain hindered the growth of the stems and, in particular, the roots of a grass mixture [102], an effect that may be related to the cryptophycin content. Microalgae, especially cyanobacteria, are a rich source of cell division inhibitors, which have been primarily assessed for their antitumor or antimicrobial properties. These compounds, however, could also be useful as herbicides and represent an almost unexplored research field [99].

Metabolites from eukaryotic microalgae have been scarcely investigated for their herbicidal activity. However, some studies can be found, for example, VOCs from the green microalgae *Chlorella vulgaris* have evidenced a phytotoxic effect against barley. The mixture of volatiles consisted of hydrocarbons, carboxylic acids, aldehydes, alcohols, and ketones [103].

### 4.3. Allelochemicals as Insecticides

Allelochemicals produced by microalgae may be useful in the defense against plant predators. Thus, microalgae have been proposed as a source of allelochemicals with insecticide properties [104,105]. The good larvicidal performance of microalgae has also stimulated new technologies, such as the exploitation of the insecticide properties of *Chlamydomonas reinhardtii* extracts in the development of preparations based on nano/microparticles. The extract of the microalgae combined with microparticles of zinc oxide was able to double the mortality of mealworm beetle larvae (*Tenebrio molitor*) compared to zinc oxide alone [106].

Biofilm-forming cyanobacteria showed defense mechanisms against insects that hinder feeding, such as the formation of colonies, filaments, mucilage, spines, and production of allelochemicals. The chemical compounds produced by their biofilm is considered more effective than other defense mechanisms. *Fischerella* strain 43,239 was selected in a cyanobacterial screening for insecticidal activity against the larvae of dipteran *Chironomus riparius* (harlequin fly). The toxic active fraction from *Fischerella* 43,239 had its chemical profile assessed by mass spectrometry, which provided evidence of the presence of indole compounds, considered possible bioactive substances [107]. Later, another study with *Fischerella* 43,239 identified indole alkaloids (Figure 5; **28–31**) with insecticide activity against the larvae of *Chironomus riparius*. Among the isolated hapalindoles, 12-*epi*-hapalindole J isonitrile was able to increase the larvae mortality at 26 μM within 48 h [108].

Extracts from cyanobacteria were tested against larvae of *Aedes aegypti*. Among the samples tested, *Microcystis aeruginosa* 205 and *Anabaena circinalis* 86 were the most active. The fractionation of these extracts showed the presence of anatoxin A and microcystins, which were toxic for *Aedes aegypti* larvae [109]. Microcystins are cyclic peptides isolated from cyanobacteria that exhibit high toxicity to insects [110]. These compounds were shown to form lesions in the midgut epithelial cells of *Aedes aegypt* larvae [111]. Anatoxin-A (Figure 5; **32**) is another insecticidal secondary metabolite from cyanobacteria that acts as an acetylcholine analogue. The action mechanisms of these compounds is similar to organophosphate and carbamate insecticides; the inhibition of the acetylcholinesterase enzyme (AchE) thus disrupts the nervous system of the insects [112]. An extract of cyanobacteria rich in anatoxin- A exhibited potential insecticide activity against *Nauphoeta cinerea* cockroaches. It is speculated that the compound caused cholinergic intoxication affecting the insect locomotion [113].

The insecticide potential of *Amphora coffeaeformis* (diatom) and *Scenedesmus obliquus* (Chlorophyta) were investigated against *Culex pipiens* mosquito larvae. The acetonic extract of these microalgae showed larvicidal activity. Among them, the extracts of *Amphora coffeaeformis* was the most active ($LC_{50}$ = 513.63 μg/mL), while the lethal concentration of *Scenedesmus obliquus* was 855.66 μg/mL. The analysis of the extracts by HPLC-DAD detected the presence of phenolic compounds such as benzoic acids (gallic acid, methyl gallate, and syringic acid), cinnamic acids (caffeic acid and cinnamic acids), and flavonoids (taxifolin, kaempferol, and naringenin) [114]. The insecticidal properties of some of the phenolic compounds identified have already been described. Gallic acid (Figure 5; **33**) affects the growth of *Spodoptera litura* (tobacco cutworm) larvae and is toxic to *Aphis craccivora* (an aphid) [115,116]. Caffeic acid (Figure 5; **34**), a cinnamic acid derivative, inhibits the digestive protease of *Helicoverpa armigera* (polyphagous pest) [117]. Moreover, kaempferol (Figure 5; **35**) was able to cause 82% mortality of *Mythimna separata* (pest of cereal crops) in the concentration of 1 mg/mL [118].

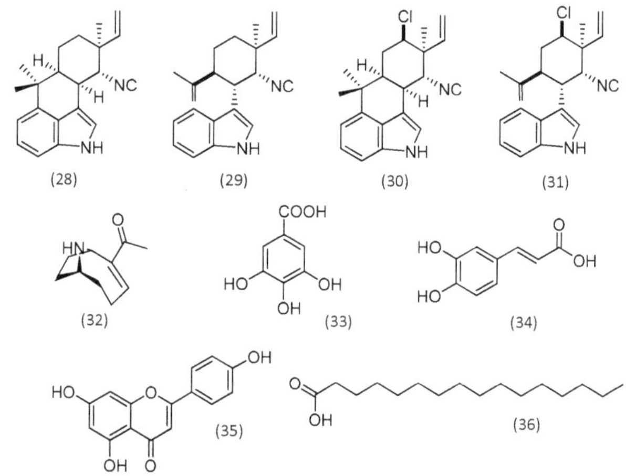

**Figure 5.** Microalgal substances with larvicidal or insecticidal activity. 12-*epi*-hapalindole J isonitrile (**28**), 12-*epi*-hapalindole C isonitrile (**29**), hapalindole L (**30**), 12-*epi*-hapalindole E isonitrile (**31**), anatoxin- A (**32**), gallic acid (**33**), caffeic acid (**34**), kaempferol (**35**), and *n*-hexadecenoic acid (**36**).

Unsaturated fatty acids were also detected in *Amphora coffeaeformis* and *Scenedesmus obliquus* extracts by gas chromatography coupled with mass spectrometry (CG/MS). Fatty acids can also act against insects. Hexadecanoic acid methyl ester, 7- hexadecanoic acid methyl ester, and 9-octadecenoic acid (Z)-methyl ester were detected as major compounds in *Amphora coffeaeformism*, while in *Scenedesmus obliquus* extract (Z)-9-octadecenoic acid methyl ester, hexadecanoic acid (Figure 5; **36**) methyl ester, and 7-hexadecenoic acid methyl ester were the major compounds. It is speculated that the high content of phenolics compounds and unsaturated fatty acids in these extracts are responsible for their larvicidal activity. [114].

A study described unsaturated and saturated fatty acids as being responsible for the insecticidal activity of ethanolic extracts from microalgae against *Spodoptera littoralis* (cotton leafworm) larvae [119]. The bioassay-guided fractionation of chloroform and methanol extracts from *Chlorella* sp. showed that fatty acids (*n*-hexadecanoic acid, di-*N*-octyl phthalate, 1-hexacosanol, oleic acid, and 1-docosene) are among the larvicidal compounds in the active fractions. Some fatty acids detected in these fractions had their insecticidal activity reported [120]. Additionally, another study described *n*-hexadecanoic (Figure 5; **36**) acid as a potent larvicidal against *Culex quinquefasciatus*, *Anopheles stephensi*, and *Aedes aegypti* mosquitoes [121]. Fatty acids have also been evaluated in vitro against *Melanaphis sacchari* (an aphid) Zehntner larvae. Among them, linoleic acid showed 85% of mortality rate ($LC_{50}$ = 1181 ppm) [122].

The possible mechanism of larvicidal activity of fatty acids was investigated by Perumalsamy et al. [123]. The authors evaluated some fatty acids for two common modes of insecticidal activity: the inhibition of AchE and the interference with the octopamine signaling pathways (cAMP level enhancement). While linoleic and linolenic acids were able to both inhibit AchE and enhance cAMP levels, palmitic and oleic acid inhibited AchE and had no significant effects on cAMP levels. Elaidic and arachidic acids where ineffective as AchE inhibitors but considerably enhanced cAMP levels. These results indicate that linoleic and linolenic acids might have a dual mode of action [123].

## 5. Safety and Toxicity of Allelochemicals and Synthetic Pesticides

The herbicide resistance (HR) plant list continues to grow and is listed on the site: www.weedscience.org (accessed on 1 May 2023) [124]. New herbicides and pesticides are necessary to feed the world's population and even more so as pests become resistant to currently available pesticides. Pesticides are, by nature, toxic and the challenge is to increase their specificity and reduce their persistence. Pesticides can cause adverse effects on the quality of the agricultural products they are used to protect. Pesticide residues can produce long-term adverse effects on the health of humans and animals and the stability of ecosystems by poisoning water sources. These chemicals can be the cause of neurotoxicity, endocrine disruption, Parkinson's disease, cancers, and type 2 diabetes [125]. For instance, organochlorine pesticides, used in agriculture since the 1950s, are listed as a persistent organic pollutant (POP) and forbidden in most countries. Nevertheless, high concentrations of these pesticides and their transformation products (TPs) and degradation products, such as dichlorodiphenyltrichloroethane (DDT), are very persistent and have long half-lives. All of them are still detected in agricultural soils [126]. Modern formulations, called current-use pesticides (CUPs), are relatively safe to non-target species. The objective of modern formulations is to avoid persistent compounds that bioaccumulate and reduce their non-target toxic properties. However, they are capable of migrating over long distances and CUPs have been reported in air and surface water samples in the Arctic [127].

Allelochemicals as a source of biopesticides have been studied in greater detail from plants than from microalgae. However, several compounds found in plants with potential use as biopesticides are extensively present and described in microalgae, such as organic acids, esters, alkaloids, flavonoids, and terpenoids [19,76,128]. The multi-kingdom effects of some secondary allelopathic plant metabolites are known. Despite the original definition, that addresses plant–plant interactions, several compounds exhibit allelopathy and toxicity to other organisms. Currently, the term allelopathy is now used in this broader context by the International Society of Allelopathy and has been since the 1990s [129].

Plant allelochemicals typically present partial water solubility enabling easy application without surfactants and some of them are known to have similar modes of action to synthetic herbicides. Non-halogenated molecules decrease the environmental half-life while preventing soil accumulation. They have eco-environmental chemical structures with a higher nitrogen and oxygen content [130]. Modern technologies allow for their effective use and management and confer fewer environmental problems in soil due to the faster degradability of allelochemicals. However, rapid degradation of one of the chemical groups can decrease the compound's bioactivity [131].

The diversity of allelochemicals makes them promising targets for discovering novel, specific target sites in plants or other organisms. Besides this, allelochemicals are also characterized by multi-site action, which differs from the synthetic pesticides, and affords them high specificity. In the case of synthetic herbicides, before they are licensed for use, they are tested to evaluate that their phytotoxic activity is in the range between $10^{-5}$ and $10^{-7}$ M. The chemical characterization of the molecular structure, the study of the mode/s of action, and their half-life in soil need to be established. It is also necessary to evaluate their influence on microbial ecology and other organisms, their potential toxic properties on human health, and the economic viability of their production on commercial scales [132]. Allelochemical toxicity depends on the concentration and compounds involved. Several secondary metabolites of other natural substance groups from plants and microalgae, such as glycosides, polyphenols, polysaccharides, terpenes, flavones, and alkaloids, have shown to be ecologically safe and biodegradable [133–136]. Triketones are one of the most important herbicide classes developed from an allelochemical triketone. These compounds inhibit invasive plants. Another example is cryptophycin-1, a depsipeptide from the cyanobacterium *Nostoc* sp. Cryptophycin-1 has an antiproliferative and antimitotic activity, inhibiting the cell cycle during the metaphase of mitosis, mainly in yeasts of the genus *Cryptococcus* [74,137].

## 6. Microalgae Allelochemicals: Gaps and Opportunities

Even though the prospects for the application of microalgal allelochemicals as biopesticides seem promising, there are still many knowledge gaps about these compounds. For instance, the action mechanisms of most of them is poorly understood. Some allelochemicals are known to have modes of action similar to synthetic pesticides, such as the insecticidal compound anatoxin A (inhibition of acetylcholinesterase) and the herbicidal molecule cyanobacterin (inhibition of photosystem II). However, many others are likely to exhibit new mechanisms and multi-target actions, which should be elucidated [132].

Moreover, their persistence and biodegradation in the environment needs further study. Once released into the soil, allelochemicals are more readily microbially degraded than xenobiotic persistent synthetics compounds. Their biodegradation depends on the soil composition and on the structure and population of the soil microbial community. Most assays conducted to investigate pesticide properties of allelochemicals are conducted under artificial laboratory conditions. Thus, to further estimate their potential in agricultural applications and to assess their environmental impact, in-field bioassays are necessary [129,131]. Studies on their possible toxic effects to non-target organisms, including humans, are also mandatory. These steps are important for any biopesticide candidate and require a great amount of interdisciplinary research [129].

The research and application of plant allelochemicals in agriculture is undoubtedly far more advanced than those from microalgae. However, concerning the production process, microalgal allelochemicals may have multiple advantages. Microalgae outdoor cultivation systems can be implemented in non-arable lands employing wastewater from agricultural or industrial activities, thus avoiding competition with food production. Their cultivation is also possible in closed bioreactors. In this case, the most important advantage is the possibility of having good control of the chemical and physical conditions of the whole process, which enables a high reproducibility and high yield [30,138]. The mass cultivation of microalgae for the production of food and chemicals on a commercial scale has already been established. The carotenoid, astaxanthin, for instance, which can be obtained from different microalgae, annually moves approximately 2 billion dollars in the global market [138–140]. For the industrial production of astaxanthin, *Haematococcus pluvialis* is cultivated in a two-step process. In the first stage, the microalgae grow in photobioreactors with a culture-rich medium for biomass accumulation. The second stage, in which the production of the carotenoid is induced by nutrient starvation, can be carried out in larger bioreactors or in open ponds. This process is energy-intensive and costly; however, improvements have been intensively researched and their implementation can substantially reduce the prices of the product [140,141].

Thus, since it is already possible to achieve bioactive substances from microalgae on a large scale, the obtaining of other compounds, such as allelochemicals, employing similar biotechnological processes can be envisaged. Nevertheless, the costs of biopesticide production through microalgae cultivation are still higher than the production of synthetic pesticides. However, the production of microalgae-derived biopesticides could be integrated with the production of biofuels and other valuable compounds within a biorefinery concept. This integrated approach is expected to lower the overall costs and enable better energy utilization as well as a reduction in the generation of residues [30,142–145].

Synthetic biology also has the potential to modify microalgal allelochemicals to improve activity, increase productivity and decrease non-specific toxicity [146].

The literature shows progress is being made in developing natural products from microalgae as biopesticides. Studies are in progress to reach commercial biopesticides from microalgae; in the future, they can complement or be an alternative to synthetic pesticides. At the moment, several promising less toxic and biodegradable allelochemicals have been identified and are worthy of further investigation into their application.

## 7. Perspectives

Much has been reported on the ecological effects of allelochemicals from plants and microbes but less so from algae and microalgae. All studies have highlighted the importance of the secondary "special" metabolism that is crucial for plant productivity and the biocontrol of pests in natural, agricultural, and anthropogenic environments. Studies on microalgae, while they have not received as much attention as agricultural crop plants, are equally important and present a new and promising low-cost source of bioactive compounds of increasing economic importance. As previously discussed, microalgae can be employed as bio-factories not only as a source of green energy but also a low-cost source of bioactive molecules, which can be useful for agriculture with minimal negative environmental impact. In this light, the future for using algae within a circular economic context is strengthened and the value of the algal production is increased by separating the differing components of their metabolism. The mechanisms of algal allelopathy require further study and specifically at the genetic level. It seems highly likely that gene editing with CRISPR will only increase the production of molecules of interest in a directed way. Given that secondary metabolism often occurs in response to a stress, be that competitive or environmental, genetic studies involving the algal holobiont (algae + bacteria + virus) and the role of interference RNAs will help us manage the algal bio-factory. The increased use of bioactive compounds from algae is promising. Here, we have described the potential of the interesting allelopathic compounds from microalgae. We have made the case for more intensive research on microalgae and hinted that microalgal bio-factories warrant industrial investment.

**Author Contributions:** Conceptualization, L.M.C. and A.B.V.; writing—original draft preparation, L.M.C.; J.E.d.S.; A.N.J.; A.M. and A.B.V.; writing—review and editing, L.M.C.; J.E.d.S.; A.N.J.; A.M. and A.B.V. All authors have read and agreed to the published version of the manuscript.

**Funding:** This work was financially supported by the Brazilian National Council for Scientific and Technological Development (MCT-CNPq), Carlos Chagas Filho Foundation for Research Support in the State of Rio de Janeiro (FAPERJ), Coordination for the Improvement of Higher Education Personnel (CAPES), and the Brazilian Society of Microbiology (SBM).

**Data Availability Statement:** No new data were generated in this review article.

**Conflicts of Interest:** The authors declare no conflict of interest.

## References

1. Molisch, H. Der Einfluss einer Pflanze auf die Andere, Allelopathie. *Nature* **1938**, *141*, 493. [CrossRef]
2. Tan, K.; Huang, Z.; Ji, R.; Qiu, Y.; Wang, Z.; Liu, J. A review of allelopathy on microalgae. *Microbiology* **2019**, *165*, 587–592. [CrossRef] [PubMed]
3. Gomes, M.P.; Garcia, Q.S.; Barreto, L.C.; Pimenta, L.P.S.; Matheus, M.T.; Figueredo, C.C. Allelopathy: An overview from micro- to macroscopic organisms, from cells to environments, and the perspectives in a climate-changing world. *Biologia* **2017**, *72*, 113–129. [CrossRef]
4. Inderjit; Dakshini, K.M.M. Algal allelopathy. *Bot. Rev.* **1994**, *60*, 182–196. [CrossRef]
5. Hemaiswarya, S.; Raja, R.; Ravikumar, R.; Carvalho, I.S. Microalgae Taxonomy and Breeding. In *Biofuel Crops: Production, Physiology and Genetics*; CABI: Wallingford, UK, 2013; pp. 44–53.
6. Sajjadi, B.; Chen, W.-Y.; Raman, A.A.A.; Ibrahim, S. Microalgae lipid and biomass for biofuel production: A comprehensive review on lipid enhancement strategies and their effects on fatty acid composition. *Renew. Sustain. Energy Rev.* **2018**, *97*, 200–232. [CrossRef]

7. Gallardo-Rodríguez, J.; Sánchez-Mirón, A.; García-Camacho, F.; López-Rosales, L.; Chisti, Y.; Molina-Grima, E. Bioactives from microalgal dinoflagellates. *Biotechnol. Adv.* **2012**, *30*, 1673–1684. [CrossRef]
8. Stevens, P.F. Angiosperm Phylogeny and Diversification. In *Encyclopedia of Evolutionary Biology*; Elsevier: Amsterdam, The Netherlands, 2016; pp. 78–83. ISBN 978-0-12-800426-5.
9. Watson, S.B.; Whitton, B.A.; Higgins, S.N.; Paerl, H.W.; Brooks, B.W.; Wehr, J.D. Harmful Algal Blooms. In *Freshwater Algae of North America*; Elsevier: Amsterdam, The Netherlands, 2015; pp. 873–920. ISBN 978-0-12-385876-4.
10. Mathieu, A. Advances in Bioengineering Study of Microalgae. *J. Pet. Environ. Biotechnol.* **2022**, *13*, 1000453.
11. Mendes, L.B.B.; Vermelho, A.B. Allelopathy as a potential strategy to improve microalgae cultivation. *Biotechnol. Biofuels* **2013**, *6*, 152. [CrossRef]
12. Leflaive, J.; Ten-Hage, L. Algal and cyanobacterial secondary metabolites in freshwaters: A comparison of allelopathic compounds and toxins. *Freshw. Biol.* **2007**, *52*, 199–214. [CrossRef]
13. Shahbaz, A.; Hussain, N.; Saba, S.; Bilal, M. Actinomycetes, Cyanobacteria, and Fungi: A Rich Source of Bioactive Molecules. In *Microbial Biomolecules*; Elsevier: Amsterdam, The Netherlands, 2023; pp. 113–133. ISBN 978-0-323-99476-7.
14. Luesch, H.; Yoshida, W.Y.; Moore, R.E.; Paul, V.J.; Mooberry, S.L. Isolation, Structure Determination, and Biological Activity of Lyngbyabellin A from the Marine Cyanobacterium *Lyngbya majuscula*. *J. Nat. Prod.* **2000**, *63*, 611–615. [CrossRef]
15. Legrand, C.; Rengefors, K.; Fistarol, G.O.; Granéli, E. Allelopathy in phytoplankton—Biochemical, ecological and evolutionary aspects. *Phycologia* **2003**, *42*, 406–419. [CrossRef]
16. Ali, S.; Ullah, M.I.; Sajjad, A.; Shakeel, Q.; Hussain, A. Environmental and Health Effects of Pesticide Residues. In *Sustainable Agriculture Reviews 48*; Inamuddin, Ahamed, M.I., Lichtfouse, E., Eds.; Sustainable Agriculture Reviews; Springer International Publishing: Cham, Switzerland, 2021; Volume 48, pp. 311–336. ISBN 978-3-030-54718-9.
17. Riyaz, M.; Ahmad Shah, R.; Sivasankaran, K. Pesticide Residues: Impacts on Fauna and the Environment. In *Biodegradation Technology of Organic and Inorganic Pollutants*; Ferreira Mendes, K., Nogueira de Sousa, R., Cabral Mielke, K., Eds.; IntechOpen: London, UK, 2022; ISBN 978-1-83968-895-9.
18. Gould, F.; Brown, Z.S.; Kuzma, J. Wicked evolution: Can we address the sociobiological dilemma of pesticide resistance? *Science* **2018**, *360*, 728–732. [CrossRef] [PubMed]
19. Chaïb, S.; Pistevos, J.C.A.; Bertrand, C.; Bonnard, I. Allelopathy and allelochemicals from microalgae: An innovative source for bio-herbicidal compounds and biocontrol research. *Algal Res.* **2021**, *54*, 102213. [CrossRef]
20. Molisch, H.; Narwal, S.S. *The Influence of One Plant on Another, Allelopathy*; Published by Scientific Publishers (India) for International Allelopathy Foundation, Hisar: Jodhpur, India, 2001; ISBN 978-81-7233-285-3.
21. Caruana, A.M.N.; Amzil, Z. Microalgae and Toxins. In *Microalgae in Health and Disease Prevention*; Elsevier: Amsterdam, The Netherlands, 2018; pp. 263–305. ISBN 978-0-12-811405-6.
22. Cembella, A.D. Chemical ecology of eukaryotic microalgae in marine ecosystems. *Phycologia* **2003**, *42*, 420–447. [CrossRef]
23. Śliwińska-Wilczewska, S.; Wiśniewska, K.; Konarzewska, Z.; Cieszyńska, A.; Felpeto, A.B.; Lewandowska, A.U.; Latała, A. The current state of knowledge on taxonomy, modulating factors, ecological roles, and mode of action of phytoplankton allelochemicals. *Sci. Total. Environ.* **2021**, *773*, 145681. [CrossRef]
24. Wang, Z.; Wang, C.; Li, W.; Wang, M.; Xiao, L. Interspecies competition between *Scrippsiella acuminata* and three marine diatoms: Growth inhibition and allelopathic effects. *Aquat. Toxicol.* **2021**, *237*, 105878. [CrossRef]
25. Kumari, P.; Cna'ani, A.; Didi-Cohen, S.; Tzin, V.; Khozin-Goldberg, I. Nitrogen Deprivation-Induced Production of Volatile Organic Compounds in the Arachidonic-Acid-Accumulating Microalga *Lobosphaera incisa* Underpins Their Role as ROS Scavengers and Chemical Messengers. *Front. Mar. Sci.* **2020**, *7*, 410. [CrossRef]
26. Sartori, R.B.; Siqueira, S.F.; Maroneze, M.M.; Fagundes, M.B.; Wagner, R.; Zepka, L.Q.; Jacob-Lopes, E. Microalgal secondary metabolites: Effect of climatic variables, seasons, and photocycles on the biogeneration of volatile organic compounds (VOCs). *J. Appl. Phycol.* **2021**, *33*, 1457–1472. [CrossRef]
27. Grabski, K.; Tukaj, Z. Autoinduction activity of a conditioned medium obtained from high density cultures of the green alga *Scenedesmus subspicatus*. *J. Appl. Phycol.* **2007**, *20*, 323–330. [CrossRef]
28. Chia, M.A.; Jankowiak, J.G.; Kramer, B.J.; Goleski, J.A.; Huang, I.-S.; Zimba, P.V.; do Carmo Bittencourt-Oliveira, M.; Gobler, C.J. Succession and toxicity of *Microcystis* and *Anabaena* (Dolichospermum) blooms are controlled by nutrient-dependent allelopathic interactions. *Harmful Algae* **2018**, *74*, 67–77. [CrossRef]
29. Ali, S.S.; Mastropetros, S.G.; Schagerl, M.; Sakarika, M.; Elsamahy, T.; El-Sheekh, M.; Sun, J.; Kornaros, M. Recent advances in wastewater microalgae-based biofuels production: A state-of-the-art review. *Energy Rep.* **2022**, *8*, 13253–13280. [CrossRef]
30. Casanova, L.M.; Mendes, L.B.B.; Corrêa, T.D.S.; da Silva, R.B.; Joao, R.R.; Macrae, A.; Vermelho, A.B. Development of Microalgae Biodiesel: Current Status and Perspectives. *Microorganisms* **2022**, *11*, 34. [CrossRef] [PubMed]
31. Oliveira, C.Y.B.; Jacob, A.; Nader, C.; Oliveira, C.D.L.; Matos, Â.P.; Araújo, E.S.; Shabnam, N.; Ashok, B.; Gálvez, A.O. An overview on microalgae as renewable resources for meeting sustainable development goals. *J. Environ. Manag.* **2022**, *320*, 115897. [CrossRef]
32. Loftus, S.E.; Johnson, Z.I. Cross-study analysis of factors affecting algae cultivation in recycled medium for biofuel production. *Algal Res.* **2017**, *24*, 154–166. [CrossRef]
33. Lu, Z.; Loftus, S.; Sha, J.; Wang, W.; Park, M.S.; Zhang, X.; Johnson, Z.I.; Hu, Q. Water reuse for sustainable microalgae cultivation: Current knowledge and future directions. *Resour. Conserv. Recycl.* **2020**, *161*, 104975. [CrossRef]

34. Thomas, P.K.; Hietala, D.C.; Cardinale, B.J. Tolerance to allelopathic inhibition by free fatty acids in five biofuel candidate microalgae strains. *Bioresour. Technol. Rep.* **2023**, *21*, 101321. [CrossRef]
35. Qixin, L.; Xuan, F.; Zhiya, S.; Wenxin, S.; Shuo, W.; Ji, L. Enhanced wastewater treatment performance by understanding the interaction between algae and bacteria based on quorum sensing. *Bioresour. Technol.* **2022**, *354*, 127161. [CrossRef]
36. Satake, M.; Honma, D.; Watanabe, R.; Oshima, Y. Alexandrolide, a diatom growth inhibitor isolated from the dinoflagellate *Alexandrium catenella*. *Tetrahedron Lett.* **2019**, *60*, 1341–1344. [CrossRef]
37. Pouvreau, J.-B.; Housson, E.; Le Tallec, L.; Morançais, M.; Rincé, Y.; Fleurence, J.; Pondaven, P. Growth inhibition of several marine diatom species induced by the shading effect and allelopathic activity of marennine, a blue-green polyphenolic pigment of the diatom *Haslea ostrearia* (Gaillon/Bory) Simonsen. *J. Exp. Mar. Biol. Ecol.* **2007**, *352*, 212–225. [CrossRef]
38. Kapoore, R.V.; Wood, E.E.; Llewellyn, C.A. Algae biostimulants: A critical look at microalgal biostimulants for sustainable agricultural practices. *Biotechnol. Adv.* **2021**, *49*, 107754. [CrossRef]
39. Sasso, S.; Pohnert, G.; Lohr, M.; Mittag, M.; Hertweck, C. Microalgae in the post-genomic era: A blooming reservoir for new natural products. *FEMS Microbiol. Rev.* **2012**, *36*, 761–785. [CrossRef] [PubMed]
40. Lichman, B.R. The scaffold-forming steps of plant alkaloid biosynthesis. *Nat. Prod. Rep.* **2020**, *38*, 103–129. [CrossRef] [PubMed]
41. Doan, N.T.; Rickards, R.W.; Rothschild, J.M.; Smith, G.D. Allelopathic actions of the alkaloid 12-epi-hapalindole E isonitrile and calothrixin A from cyanobacteria of the genera *Fischerella* and *Calothrix*. *J. Appl. Phycol.* **2000**, *12*, 409–416. [CrossRef]
42. Brunson, J.K.; McKinnie, S.M.K.; Chekan, J.R.; McCrow, J.P.; Miles, Z.D.; Bertrand, E.M.; Bielinski, V.A.; Luhavaya, H.; Oborník, M.; Smith, G.J.; et al. Biosynthesis of the neurotoxin domoic acid in a bloom-forming diatom. *Science* **2018**, *361*, 1356–1358. [CrossRef]
43. Quilliam, M.A.; Wright, J.L.C. The Amnesic Shellfish Poisoning Mystery. *Anal. Chem.* **1989**, *61*, 1053A–1060A. [CrossRef]
44. Takemoto, T.; Daigo, K. Constituents of *Chondria Armata*. *Chem. Pharm. Bull.* **1958**, *6*, 578–580. [CrossRef]
45. Orr, R.J.S.; Stüken, A.; Murray, S.A.; Jakobsen, K.S. Evolution and Distribution of Saxitoxin Biosynthesis in Dinoflagellates. *Mar. Drugs* **2013**, *11*, 2814–2828. [CrossRef]
46. Murray, S.A.; Mihali, T.K.; Neilan, B.A. Extraordinary Conservation, Gene Loss, and Positive Selection in the Evolution of an Ancient Neurotoxin. *Mol. Biol. Evol.* **2011**, *28*, 1173–1182. [CrossRef]
47. Schantz, E.J.; Lynch, J.M.; Vayvada, G.; Matsumoto, K.; Rapoport, H. The Purification and Characterization of the Poison Produced by *Gonyaulax catenella* in Axenic Culture. *Biochemistry* **1966**, *5*, 1191–1195. [CrossRef]
48. Jackim, E.; Gentile, J. Toxins of a Blue-Green Alga: Similarity to Saxitoxin. *Science* **1968**, *162*, 915–916. [CrossRef]
49. Chiang, I.-Z.; Huang, W.-Y.; Wu, J.-T. Allelochemicals of *Botryococcus braunii* (Chlorophyceae). *J. Phycol.* **2004**, *40*, 474–480. [CrossRef]
50. DellaGreca, M.; Zarrelli, A.; Fergola, P.; Cerasuolo, M.; Pollio, A.; Pinto, G. Fatty Acids Released by *Chlorella vulgaris* and Their Role in Interference with *Pseudokirchneriella subcapitata*: Experiments and Modelling. *J. Chem. Ecol.* **2010**, *36*, 339–349. [CrossRef]
51. Benkendorff, K.; Davis, A.R.; Rogers, C.N.; Bremner, J.B. Free fatty acids and sterols in the benthic spawn of aquatic molluscs, and their associated antimicrobial properties. *J. Exp. Mar. Biol. Ecol.* **2005**, *316*, 29–44. [CrossRef]
52. Cózar, A.; Morillo-García, S.; Ortega, M.J.; Li, Q.P.; Bartual, A. Macroecological patterns of the phytoplankton production of polyunsaturated aldehydes. *Sci. Rep.* **2018**, *8*, 12282. [CrossRef] [PubMed]
53. Demay, J.; Bernard, C.; Reinhardt, A.; Marie, B. Natural Products from Cyanobacteria: Focus on Beneficial Activities. *Mar. Drugs* **2019**, *17*, 320. [CrossRef] [PubMed]
54. Yokoyama, A.; Murata, M.; Oshima, Y.; Iwashita, T.; Yasumoto, T. Some Chemical Properties of Maitotoxin, a Putative Calcium Channel Agonist Isolated from a Marine Dinoflagellate. *J. Biochem.* **1988**, *104*, 184–187. [CrossRef]
55. Reyes, J.G.; Sánchez-Cárdenas, C.; Acevedo-Castillo, W.; Leyton, P.; López-González, I.; Felix, R.; Gandini, M.A.; Treviño, M.B.; Treviño, C.L. Maitotoxin: An Enigmatic Toxic Molecule with Useful Applications in the Biomedical Sciences. In *Seafood and Freshwater Toxins*; Botana, L.M., Ed.; CRC Press: Boca Raton, FL, USA, 2014; pp. 677–694. ISBN 978-0-429-09621-1.
56. Baden, D.G.; Bourdelais, A.J.; Jacocks, H.; Michelliza, S.; Naar, J. Natural and Derivative Brevetoxins: Historical Background, Multiplicity, and Effects. *Environ. Health Perspect.* **2005**, *113*, 621–625. [CrossRef]
57. McManus, K.M.; Kirk, R.D.; Via, C.W.; Lotti, J.S.; Roduit, A.F.; Teta, R.; Scarpato, S.; Mangoni, A.; Bertin, M.J. Isolation of Isotrichophycin C and Trichophycins G–I from a Collection of *Trichodesmium thiebautii*. *J. Nat. Prod.* **2020**, *83*, 2664–2671. [CrossRef]
58. Bertin, M.J.; Wahome, P.G.; Zimba, P.V.; He, H.; Moeller, P.D.R. Trichophycin A, a Cytotoxic Linear Polyketide Isolated from a *Trichodesmium thiebautii* Bloom. *Mar. Drugs* **2017**, *15*, 10. [CrossRef]
59. Micallef, M.L.; D'Agostino, P.M.; Al-Sinawi, B.; Neilan, B.A.; Moffitt, M.C. Exploring cyanobacterial genomes for natural product biosynthesis pathways. *Mar. Genom.* **2014**, *21*, 1–12. [CrossRef]
60. Rastogi, R.P.; Sinha, R.P.; Incharoensakdi, A. The cyanotoxin-microcystins: Current overview. *Rev. Environ. Sci. Bio/Technol.* **2014**, *13*, 215–249. [CrossRef]
61. Sivonen, K.; Leikoski, N.; Fewer, D.P.; Jokela, J. Cyanobactins—Ribosomal cyclic peptides produced by cyanobacteria. *Appl. Microbiol. Biotechnol.* **2010**, *86*, 1213–1225. [CrossRef] [PubMed]
62. Del Mondo, A.; Smerilli, A.; Ambrosino, L.; Albini, A.; Noonan, D.M.; Sansone, C.; Brunet, C. Insights into phenolic compounds from microalgae: Structural variety and complex beneficial activities from health to nutraceutics. *Crit. Rev. Biotechnol.* **2021**, *41*, 155–171. [CrossRef]

63. Del Mondo, A.; Sansone, C.; Brunet, C. Insights into the biosynthesis pathway of phenolic compounds in microalgae. *Comput. Struct. Biotechnol. J.* **2022**, *20*, 1901–1913. [CrossRef]
64. Oldfield, E.; Lin, F.-Y. Terpene Biosynthesis: Modularity Rules. *Angew. Chem. Int. Ed.* **2011**, *51*, 1124–1137. [CrossRef]
65. Jaki, B.; Orjala, J.; Heilmann, J.; Linden, A.; Vogler, B.; Sticher, O. Novel Extracellular Diterpenoids with Biological Activity from the Cyanobacterium *Nostoc commune*. *J. Nat. Prod.* **2000**, *63*, 339–343. [CrossRef] [PubMed]
66. Höckelmann, C.; Becher, P.G.; von Reuß, S.H.; Jüttner, F. Sesquiterpenes of the Geosmin-Producing Cyanobacterium Calothrix PCC 7507 and their Toxicity to Invertebrates. *Z. Naturforsch C. J. Biosci.* **2009**, *64*, 49–55. [CrossRef] [PubMed]
67. Pozzer, A.C.; Gómez, P.A.; Weiss, J. Volatile organic compounds in aquatic ecosystems—Detection, origin, significance and applications. *Sci. Total. Environ.* **2022**, *838*, 156155. [CrossRef] [PubMed]
68. Zuo, Z. Why Algae Release Volatile Organic Compounds—The Emission and Roles. *Front. Microbiol.* **2019**, *10*, 491. [CrossRef]
69. Achyuthan, K.E.; Harper, J.C.; Manginell, R.P.; Moorman, M.W. Volatile Metabolites Emission by In Vivo Microalgae—An Overlooked Opportunity? *Metabolites* **2017**, *7*, 39. [CrossRef]
70. Xie, Y.; Tian, L.; Han, X.; Yang, Y. Research Advances in Allelopathy of Volatile Organic Compounds (VOCs) of Plants. *Horticulturae* **2021**, *7*, 278. [CrossRef]
71. Liu, X.; Cao, A.; Yan, D.; Ouyang, C.; Wang, Q.; Li, Y. Overview of mechanisms and uses of biopesticides. *Int. J. Pest Manag.* **2021**, *67*, 65–72. [CrossRef]
72. Kumar, J.; Ramlal, A.; Mallick, D.; Mishra, V. An Overview of Some Biopesticides and Their Importance in Plant Protection for Commercial Acceptance. *Plants* **2021**, *10*, 1185. [CrossRef] [PubMed]
73. Farooq, M.; Jabran, K.; Cheema, Z.A.; Wahid, A.; Siddique, K.H. The role of allelopathy in agricultural pest management. *Pest Manag. Sci.* **2011**, *67*, 493–506. [CrossRef] [PubMed]
74. Costa, J.A.V.; Freitas, B.C.B.; Cruz, C.G.; Silveira, J.; Morais, M.G. Potential of microalgae as biopesticides to contribute to sustainable agriculture and environmental development. *J. Environ. Sci. Health Part B* **2019**, *54*, 366–375. [CrossRef]
75. Berthon, J.-Y.; Michel, T.; Wauquier, A.; Joly, P.; Gerbore, J.; Filaire, E. Seaweed and microalgae as major actors of blue biotechnology to achieve plant stimulation and pest and pathogen biocontrol—A review of the latest advances and future prospects. *J. Agric. Sci.* **2021**, *159*, 523–534. [CrossRef]
76. Pattanayak, S.; Das, S.; Biswal, G. Crop Disease Control through Application of Algal Biopesticides: Alternate Route Map in Organic Farming. In *Biopesticides in Organic Farming*; CRC Press: Boca Raton, FL, USA, 2021; pp. 123–126. ISBN 978-0-367-46017-4.
77. Gonçalves, A.L. The Use of Microalgae and Cyanobacteria in the Improvement of Agricultural Practices: A Review on Their Biofertilising, Biostimulating and Biopesticide Roles. *Appl. Sci.* **2021**, *11*, 871. [CrossRef]
78. Bratchkova, A.; Alexander, D. Kroumov Microalgae as Producers of Biologically Active Compounds with Anti-bacterial, Antiviral, Antifungal, Antialgal, Antiprotozoal, Antiparasitic and Anticancer Activity. *Acta Microbiol. Bulg.* **2020**, *36*, 79–89.
79. Stirk, W.A.; van Staden, J. Bioprospecting for bioactive compounds in microalgae: Antimicrobial compounds. *Biotechnol. Adv.* **2022**, *59*, 107977. [CrossRef]
80. Swain, S.S.; Paidesetty, S.K.; Padhy, R.N. Antibacterial, antifungal and antimycobacterial compounds from cyanobacteria. *Biomed. Pharmacother.* **2017**, *90*, 760–776. [CrossRef]
81. Hernández-Carlos, B.; Gamboa-Angulo, M.M. Metabolites from freshwater aquatic microalgae and fungi as potential natural pesticides. *Phytochem. Rev.* **2011**, *10*, 261–286. [CrossRef]
82. Asthana, R.K.; Srivastava, A.; Singh, A.P.; Deepali; Singh, S.P.; Nath, G.; Srivastava, R.; Srivastava, B.S. Identification of an antimicrobial entity from the cyanobacterium *Fischerella* sp. isolated from bark of *Azadirachta indica* (Neem) tree. *J. Appl. Phycol.* **2006**, *18*, 33–39. [CrossRef]
83. Kajiyama, S.-I.; Kanzaki, H.; Kawazu, K.; Kobayashi, A. Nostofungicidine, an antifungal lipopeptide from the field-grown terrestrial blue-green alga *Nostoc commune*. *Tetrahedron Lett.* **1998**, *39*, 3737–3740. [CrossRef]
84. Desbois, A.P.; Mearns-Spragg, A.; Smith, V.J. A Fatty Acid from the Diatom *Phaeodactylum tricornutum* is Antibacterial Against Diverse Bacteria Including Multi-resistant *Staphylococcus aureus* (MRSA). *Mar. Biotechnol.* **2009**, *11*, 45–52. [CrossRef]
85. Senousy, H.H.; El-Sheekh, M.M.; Saber, A.A.; Khairy, H.M.; Said, H.A.; Alhoqail, W.A.; Abu-Elsaoud, A.M. Biochemical Analyses of Ten Cyanobacterial and Microalgal Strains Isolated from Egyptian Habitats, and Screening for Their Potential against Some Selected Phytopathogenic Fungal Strains. *Agronomy* **2022**, *12*, 1340. [CrossRef]
86. Schmid, B.; Coelho, L.; Schulze, P.S.C.; Pereira, H.; Santos, T.; Maia, I.B.; Reis, M.; Varela, J. Antifungal properties of aqueous microalgal extracts. *Bioresour. Technol. Rep.* **2022**, *18*, 101096. [CrossRef]
87. Almalki, M.A.; Khalifa, A.Y.Z.; Alkhamis, Y.A. In vitro Antibiosis of Chlorella vulgaris Extract against the Phytopathogen, *Stenotrophomonas maltophilia*. *J. Pure Appl. Microbiol.* **2022**, *16*, 630–637. [CrossRef]
88. Ragaa, A.; Hamouda, M.S.M. El-Ansary Potential of Plant-Parasitic Nematode Control in Banana Plants by Micro-algae as a New Approach Towards Resistance. *Egypt. J. Biol. Pest Control.* **2017**, *27*, 165–172.
89. Righini, H.; Francioso, O.; Quintana, A.M.; Roberti, R. Cyanobacteria: A Natural Source for Controlling Agricultural Plant Diseases Caused by Fungi and Oomycetes and Improving Plant Growth. *Horticulturae* **2022**, *8*, 58. [CrossRef]
90. Scaglioni, P.T.; Pagnussatt, F.A.; Lemos, A.C.; Nicolli, C.P.; Del Ponte, E.M.; Badiale-Furlong, E. *Nannochloropsis* sp. and *Spirulina* sp. as a Source of Antifungal Compounds to Mitigate Contamination by *Fusarium graminearum* Species Complex. *Curr. Microbiol.* **2019**, *76*, 930–938. [CrossRef]

91. Natarajan, C.; Prasanna, R.; Gupta, V.; Dureja, P.; Nain, L. Characterization of the fungicidal activity of *Calothrix elenkinii* using chemical methods and microscopy. *Appl. Biochem. Microbiol.* **2012**, *48*, 51–57. [CrossRef]
92. Bang, K.-H.; Lee, D.-W.; Park, H.-M.; Rhee, Y.-H. Inhibition of Fungal Cell Wall Synthesizing Enzymes by *trans*-Cinnamaldehyde. *Biosci. Biotechnol. Biochem.* **2000**, *64*, 1061–1063. [CrossRef] [PubMed]
93. Wang, S.-Y.; Chen, P.-F.; Chang, S.-T. Antifungal activities of essential oils and their constituents from indigenous cinnamon (*Cinnamomum osmophloeum*) leaves against wood decay fungi. *Bioresour. Technol.* **2005**, *96*, 813–818. [CrossRef] [PubMed]
94. Huang, Q.-S.; Zhu, Y.-J.; Li, H.-L.; Zhuang, J.-X.; Zhang, C.-L.; Zhou, J.-J.; Li, W.-G.; Chen, Q.-X. Inhibitory Effects of Methyl *trans*-Cinnamate on Mushroom Tyrosinase and Its Antimicrobial Activities. *J. Agric. Food Chem.* **2009**, *57*, 2565–2569. [CrossRef] [PubMed]
95. Amborabé, B.-E.; Fleurat-Lessard, P.; Chollet, J.-F.; Roblin, G. Antifungal effects of salicylic acid and other benzoic acid derivatives towards *Eutypa lata*: Structure–activity relationship. *Plant Physiol. Biochem.* **2002**, *40*, 1051–1060. [CrossRef]
96. Berne, S.; Kovačič, L.; Sova, M.; Kraševec, N.; Gobec, S.; Križaj, I.; Komel, R. Benzoic acid derivatives with improved antifungal activity: Design, synthesis, structure–activity relationship (SAR) and CYP53 docking studies. *Bioorganic Med. Chem.* **2015**, *23*, 4264–4276. [CrossRef] [PubMed]
97. Nehela, Y.; Taha, N.A.; Elzaawely, A.A.; Xuan, T.D.; Amin, M.A.; Ahmed, M.E.; El-Nagar, A. Benzoic Acid and Its Hydroxylated Derivatives Suppress Early Blight of Tomato (*Alternaria solani*) via the Induction of Salicylic Acid Biosynthesis and Enzymatic and Nonenzymatic Antioxidant Defense Machinery. *J. Fungi* **2021**, *7*, 663. [CrossRef] [PubMed]
98. D'agostino, P.M.; Seel, C.J.; Ji, X.; Gulder, T.; Gulder, T.A.M. Biosynthesis of cyanobacterin, a paradigm for furanolide core structure assembly. *Nat. Chem. Biol.* **2022**, *18*, 652–658. [CrossRef]
99. Berry, J. Marine and Freshwater Microalgae as a Potential Source of Novel Herbicides. In *Herbicides and Environment*; Kortekamp, A., Ed.; InTech: London, UK, 2011; ISBN 978-953-307-476-4.
100. Zhang, Y.; Whalen, J.K.; Sauvé, S. Phytotoxicity and bioconcentration of microcystins in agricultural plants: Meta-analysis and risk assessment. *Environ. Pollut.* **2020**, *272*, 115966. [CrossRef]
101. Koodkaew, I.; Sunohara, Y.; Matsuyama, S.; Matsumoto, H. Isolation of ambiguine D isonitrile from *Hapalosiphon* sp. and characterization of its phytotoxic activity. *Plant Growth Regul.* **2012**, *68*, 141–150. [CrossRef]
102. Biondi, N.; Piccardi, R.; Margheri, M.C.; Rodolfi, L.; Smith, G.D.; Tredici, M.R. Evaluation of *Nostoc* Strain ATCC 53789 as a Potential Source of Natural Pesticides. *Appl. Environ. Microbiol.* **2004**, *70*, 3313–3320. [CrossRef]
103. Abdel-Baky, H.H.; Shallan, M.A.; Baroty, G.E.; El-Baz, F.K. Volatile Compounds of the Microalga *Chlorella vulgaris* and Their Phytotoxic Effect. *Pak. J. Biol. Sci.* **2001**, *5*, 61–65. [CrossRef]
104. Berry, J.P.; Gantar, M.; Perez, M.H.; Berry, G.; Noriega, F.G. Cyanobacterial Toxins as Allelochemicals with Potential Applications as Algaecides, Herbicides and Insecticides. *Mar. Drugs* **2008**, *6*, 117–146. [CrossRef] [PubMed]
105. Marten, G.G. Larvicidal algae. *J. Am. Mosq. Control. Assoc.* **2007**, *23*, 177–183. [CrossRef]
106. Rankic, I.; Zelinka, R.; Ridoskova, A.; Gagic, M.; Pelcova, P.; Huska, D. Nano/microparticles in conjunction with microalgae extract as novel insecticides against Mealworm beetles, *Tenebrio molitor*. *Sci. Rep.* **2021**, *11*, 17125. [CrossRef] [PubMed]
107. Becher, P.G.; Jüttner, F. Insecticidal compounds of the biofilm-forming cyanobacterium *Fischerella* sp. (ATCC 43239). *Environ. Toxicol.* **2005**, *20*, 363–372. [CrossRef] [PubMed]
108. Becher, P.G.; Keller, S.; Jung, G.; Süssmuth, R.; Jüttner, F. Insecticidal activity of 12-epi-hapalindole J isonitrile. *Phytochemistry* **2007**, *68*, 2493–2497. [CrossRef] [PubMed]
109. Kiviranta, J.; Abdel-Hameed, A.; Sivonen, K.; Niemelä, S.I.; Carlberg, G. Toxicity of cyanobacteria to mosquito larvae—Screening of active compounds. *Environ. Toxicol. Water Qual.* **1993**, *8*, 63–71. [CrossRef]
110. Delaney, J.; Wilkins, R. Toxicity of microcystin-LR, isolated from *Microcystis aeruginosa*, against various insect species. *Toxicon* **1995**, *33*, 771–778. [CrossRef]
111. Saario, E.; Abdel-Hameed, A.; Kiviranta, J. Larvicidal microcystin toxins of cyanobacteria affect midgut epithelial cells of *Aedes aegypti* mosquitoes. *Med. Veter. Èntomol.* **1994**, *8*, 398–400. [CrossRef]
112. Cook, W.; Beasley, V.; Dahlem, A.; Dellinger, J.; Harlin, K.; Carmichael, W. Comparison of effects of anatoxin-a(s) and paraoxon, physostigmine and pyridostigmine on mouse brain cholinesterase activity. *Toxicon* **1988**, *26*, 750–753. [CrossRef]
113. dos Santos, D.S.; Rosa, M.E.; Zanatta, A.P.; Oliveira, R.S.; de Almeida, C.G.M.; Leal, A.P.; Sanz, M.; Fernandes, K.A.; de Souza, V.Q.; de Assis, D.R.; et al. Neurotoxic effects of sublethal concentrations of cyanobacterial extract containing anatoxin-a(s) on *Nauphoeta cinerea* cockroaches. *Ecotoxicol. Environ. Saf.* **2018**, *171*, 138–145. [CrossRef] [PubMed]
114. Hassan, M.E.; Mohafrash, S.M.M.; Fallatah, S.A.; El-Sayed, A.E.-K.B.; Mossa, A.-T.H. Eco-friendly larvicide of *Amphora coffeaeformis* and *Scenedesmus obliquus* microalgae extracts against *Culex pipiens*. *J. Appl. Phycol.* **2021**, *33*, 2683–2693. [CrossRef]
115. Dolma, S.K.; Singh, P.P.; Reddy, S.G.E. Insecticidal and Enzyme Inhibition Activities of Leaf/Bark Extracts, Fractions, Seed Oil and Isolated Compounds from *Triadica sebifera* (L.) Small against *Aphis craccivora* Koch. *Molecules* **2022**, *27*, 1967. [CrossRef] [PubMed]
116. Punia, A.; Chauhan, N.S.; Singh, D.; Kesavan, A.K.; Kaur, S.; Sohal, S.K. Effect of gallic acid on the larvae of *Spodoptera litura* and its parasitoid *Bracon hebetor*. *Sci. Rep.* **2021**, *11*, 531. [CrossRef]
117. Joshi, R.S.; Wagh, T.P.; Sharma, N.; Mulani, F.A.; Sonavane, U.; Thulasiram, H.V.; Joshi, R.; Gupta, V.S.; Giri, A.P. Way toward "Dietary Pesticides": Molecular Investigation of Insecticidal Action of Caffeic Acid against *Helicoverpa armigera*. *J. Agric. Food Chem.* **2014**, *62*, 10847–10854. [CrossRef]

118. Zhang, X.-Y.; Shen, J.; Zhou, Y.; Wei, Z.-P.; Gao, J.-M. Insecticidal Constituents from *Buddlej aalbiflora* Hemsl. *Nat. Prod. Res.* **2017**, *31*, 1446–1449. [CrossRef]
119. Saber, A.A.; Moussa, S.; Abdel-Rahim, E.F.M.; Cantonati, M. Insecticidal Prospects of Algal and Cyanobacterial Extracts against the Cotton Leaf Worm *Spodoptera littoralis*. *Vie Milieu Life Environ.* **2018**, *68*, 199–212.
120. Sigamani, S.; Chinnasamy, R.; Dharmaraj, R.K.; Ramamurthy, D.; Devarajan, N.; Narayanasamy, M.; Natarajan, H. Larvicidal potency of the extracts from *Chlorella* sp. against *Aedes aegypti*. *Biocatal. Agric. Biotechnol.* **2020**, *27*, 101663. [CrossRef]
121. Rahuman, A.A.; Gopalakrishnan, G.; Ghouse, B.S.; Arumugam, S.; Himalayan, B. Effect of *Feronia limonia* on mosquito larvae. *Fitoterapia* **2000**, *71*, 553–555. [CrossRef]
122. Aguilar-Marcelino, L.; Pineda-Alegría, J.A.; Salinas-Sánchez, D.O.; Hernández-Velázquez, V.M.; Silva-Aguayo, G.I.; Navarro-Tito, N.; Sotelo-Leyva, C. In Vitro Insecticidal Effect of Commercial Fatty Acids, β-Sitosterol, and Rutin against the Sugarcane Aphid, *Melanaphis sacchari* Zehntner (Hemiptera: Aphididae). *J. Food Prot.* **2022**, *85*, 671–675. [CrossRef] [PubMed]
123. Perumalsamy, H.; Jang, M.J.; Kim, J.-R.; Kadarkarai, M.; Ahn, Y.-J. Larvicidal activity and possible mode of action of four flavonoids and two fatty acids identified in *Millettia pinnata* seed toward three mosquito species. *Parasites Vectors* **2015**, *8*, 237. [CrossRef] [PubMed]
124. Ghatrehsamani, S.; Jha, G.; Dutta, W.; Molaei, F.; Nazrul, F.; Fortin, M.; Bansal, S.; Debangshi, U.; Neupane, J. Artificial Intelligence Tools and Techniques to Combat Herbicide Resistant Weeds—A Review. *Sustainability* **2023**, *15*, 1843. [CrossRef]
125. Rani, L.; Thapa, K.; Kanojia, N.; Sharma, N.; Singh, S.; Grewal, A.S.; Srivastav, A.L.; Kaushal, J. An extensive review on the consequences of chemical pesticides on human health and environment. *J. Clean. Prod.* **2020**, *283*, 124657. [CrossRef]
126. Zhang, A.; Luo, W.; Sun, J.; Xiao, H.; Liu, W. Distribution and uptake pathways of organochlorine pesticides in greenhouse and conventional vegetables. *Sci. Total. Environ.* **2015**, *505*, 1142–1147. [CrossRef]
127. Balmer, J.E.; Morris, A.D.; Hung, H.; Jantunen, L.; Vorkamp, K.; Rigét, F.; Evans, M.; Houde, M.; Muir, D.C. Levels and trends of current-use pesticides (CUPs) in the arctic: An updated review, 2010–2018. *Emerg. Contam.* **2019**, *5*, 70–88. [CrossRef]
128. Liu, L.; Pohnert, G.; Wei, D. Extracellular Metabolites from Industrial Microalgae and Their Biotechnological Potential. *Mar. Drugs* **2016**, *14*, 191. [CrossRef]
129. Hickman, D.T.; Rasmussen, A.; Ritz, K.; Birkett, M.A.; Neve, P. Review: Allelochemicals as multi-kingdom plant defence compounds: Towards an integrated approach. *Pest Manag. Sci.* **2020**, *77*, 1121–1131. [CrossRef]
130. Qureshi, H.; Anwar, T.; Ali, Q.; Haider, M.Z.; Habib, N.; Fatima, S.; Waseem, M.; Bibi, Y.; Arshad, M.; Adkins, S.W. Isolation of natural herbicidal compound from *Lantana camara*. *Int. J. Environ. Anal. Chem.* **2019**, *101*, 631–638. [CrossRef]
131. Cheng, F.; Cheng, Z. Research Progress on the use of Plant Allelopathy in Agriculture and the Physiological and Ecological Mechanisms of Allelopathy. *Front. Plant Sci.* **2015**, *6*, 1020. [CrossRef]
132. Soltys, D.; Krasuska, U.; Bogatek, R.; Gniazdowsk, A. Allelochemicals as Bioherbicides—Present and Perspectives. In *Herbicides—Current Research and Case Studies in Use*; Price, A., Ed.; InTech: London, UK, 2013; ISBN 978-953-51-1112-2.
133. Balaji-Prasath, B.; Wang, Y.; Su, Y.P.; Hamilton, D.P.; Lin, H.; Zheng, L.; Zhang, Y. Methods to control harmful algal blooms: A review. *Environ. Chem. Lett.* **2022**, *20*, 3133–3152. [CrossRef]
134. Yu, S.; Zhang, Y.; Ran, Y.; Lai, W.; Ran, Z.; Xu, J.; Zhou, C.; Yan, X. Characterization of Steryl Glycosides in Marine Microalgae by Gas Chromatography-Triple Quadrupole Mass Spectrometry (GC-QQQ-MS): Steryl Glycosides in Microalgae Analyzed by GC-QQQ-MS. *J. Sci. Food Agric.* **2018**, *98*, 1574–1583. [CrossRef] [PubMed]
135. Cichoński, J.; Chrzanowski, G. Microalgae as a Source of Valuable Phenolic Compounds and Carotenoids. *Molecules* **2022**, *27*, 8852. [CrossRef] [PubMed]
136. Latif, S.; Chiapusio, G.; Weston, L.A. Allelopathy and the Role of Allelochemicals in Plant Defence. In *Advances in Botanical Research*; Elsevier: Amsterdam, The Netherlands, 2017; Volume 82, pp. 19–54. ISBN 978-0-12-801431-8.
137. Fidor, A.; Konkel, R.; Mazur-Marzec, H. Bioactive Peptides Produced by Cyanobacteria of the Genus *Nostoc*: A Review. *Mar. Drugs* **2019**, *17*, 561. [CrossRef]
138. Mendes, L.B.B.; Viegas, C.V.; Joao, R.R.; da Silva, R.B. Microalgae Production: A Sustainable Alternative for a Low-carbon Economy Transition. *Open Microalgae Biotechnol.* **2021**, *1*, 1–7. [CrossRef]
139. Grand View Research GVR Report CoverAstaxanthin Market Size, Share & Trends Report Astaxanthin Market Size, Share & Trends Analysis Report by Product (Dried Algae Meal or Biomass, Oil, Softgel, Liquid), by Source (Natural, Synthetic), by Application, by Region, and Segment Forecasts, 2023–2030. Available online: https://www.grandviewresearch.com/industry-analysis/global-astaxanthin-market (accessed on 1 March 2023).
140. Villaró, S.; Ciardi, M.; Morillas-España, A.; Sánchez-Zurano, A.; Acién-Fernández, G.; Lafarga, T. Microalgae Derived Astaxanthin: Research and Consumer Trends and Industrial Use as Food. *Foods* **2021**, *10*, 2303. [CrossRef]
141. Li, X.; Wang, X.; Duan, C.; Yi, S.; Gao, Z.; Xiao, C.; Agathos, S.N.; Wang, G.; Li, J. Biotechnological production of astaxanthin from the microalga *Haematococcus pluvialis*. *Biotechnol. Adv.* **2020**, *43*, 107602. [CrossRef]
142. Kumar, D.; Singh, B. Algal biorefinery: An integrated approach for sustainable biodiesel production. *Biomass Bioenergy* **2019**, *131*, 105398. [CrossRef]
143. Zhu, L. Biorefinery as a promising approach to promote microalgae industry: An innovative framework. *Renew. Sustain. Energy Rev.* **2015**, *41*, 1376–1384. [CrossRef]
144. Branco-Vieira, M.; Martin, S.S.; Agurto, C.; Freitas, M.A.V.; Martins, A.A.; Mata, T.M.; Caetano, N.S. Biotechnological potential of *Phaeodactylum tricornutum* for biorefinery processes. *Fuel* **2020**, *268*, 117357. [CrossRef]

145. Sivaramakrishnan, R.; Suresh, S.; Kanwal, S.; Ramadoss, G.; Ramprakash, B.; Incharoensakdi, A. Microalgal Biorefinery Concepts' Developments for Biofuel and Bioproducts: Current Perspective and Bottlenecks. *Int. J. Mol. Sci.* **2022**, *23*, 2623. [CrossRef] [PubMed]
146. Reijnders, M.J.M.F.; van Heck, R.G.A.; Lam, C.M.C.; Scaife, M.A.; dos Santos, V.A.P.M.; Smith, A.G.; Schaap, P.J. Green genes: Bioinformatics and systems-biology innovations drive algal biotechnology. *Trends Biotechnol.* **2014**, *32*, 617–626. [CrossRef] [PubMed]

MDPI AG
Grosspeteranlage 5
4052 Basel
Switzerland
Tel.: +41 61 683 77 34

*Plants* Editorial Office
E-mail: plants@mdpi.com
www.mdpi.com/journal/plants

www.ingramcontent.com/pod-product-compliance
Lightning Source LLC
Chambersburg PA
CBHW041411210926
51850CB00013B/3244
*9783725834952*